MENTAL ILLNESS AND SOCIAL POLICY

THE AMERICAN EXPERIENCE

MENTAL ILLNESS AND SOCIAL POLICY

THE AMERICAN EXPERIENCE

THE KINGDOM OF EVILS

E[lmer] E. Southard
and
Mary C. Jarrett

ARNO PRESS
A NEW YORK TIMES COMPANY
New York • 1973

Reprint Edition 1973 by Arno Press Inc.

Reprinted from a copy in
  The University of Illinois Library

MENTAL ILLNESS AND SOCIAL POLICY:
  The American Experience
ISBN for complete set: 0-405-05190-5
See last pages of this volume for titles.

Manufactured in the United States of America

———————◆———————

Library of Congress Cataloging in Publication Data

Southard, Elmer Ernest, 1876-1920.
    The kingdom of evils.

    (Mental illness and social policy: the American
experience)
    Reprint of the ed. published by Macmillan,
New York.
    Bibliography: p.
    1. Mental illness—Cases, clinical reports,
statistics. 2. Psychiatric social work.
I. Jarrett, Mary Cromwell, joint author. II. Title.
III. Series. [DNLM: WM100 S726k 1922F]
RC465.S65 1973   362.2'0425   73-2417
ISBN 0-405-05227-8

THE KINGDOM OF EVILS

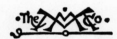

THE MACMILLAN COMPANY
NEW YORK · BOSTON · CHICAGO · DALLAS
ATLANTA · SAN FRANCISCO

MACMILLAN & CO., LIMITED
LONDON · BOMBAY · CALCUTTA
MELBOURNE

THE MACMILLAN CO. OF CANADA, LTD.
TORONTO

THE KINGDOM OF EVILS

Psychiatric Social Work Presented in One Hundred Case Histories Together with a Classification of Social Divisions of Evil

BY

E. E. SOUTHARD, M.D.

Late Bullard Professor of Neuropathology, Harvard Medical School; Pathologist, Massachusetts Commission on Mental Diseases; Director, Boston Psychopathic Hospital; President, American Medico-Psychological Association

AND

MARY C. JARRETT

Associate Director, Smith College Training School for Social Work; formerly Chief of Social Service, Boston Psychopathic Hospital

WITH AN INTRODUCTION BY

RICHARD C. CABOT, M.D.

Professor of Social Ethics, Harvard University

AND

A NOTE UPON LEGAL ENTANGLEMENT
AS A DIVISION OF EVIL BY

ROSCOE POUND

Dean of the Harvard Law School

New York

THE MACMILLAN COMPANY

1922

COPYRIGHT, 1922,
BY THE MACMILLAN COMPANY.

Set up and printed. Published October, 1922.

Press of
J. J. Little & Ives Company
New York, U. S. A.

To

THE MEMORY OF

JOSIAH ROYCE

WHOSE WORK ON
THE SOCIAL CONSCIOUSNESS
THE PROBLEM OF EVIL AND
THE PRINCIPLES OF ORDER
HELD OUR OWN WORK
IN SOLUTION.

PREFACE

The writing of this book had been completed, with the exception of a few passages, and the form of it had been planned before Dr. Southard's sudden death from pneumonia in February, 1920. He had said that he would do no more work upon it after February first, for one might continue indefinitely to elaborate a book such as this. We felt that its chief value would lie in the suggestiveness of the ideas presented and not in their completeness. It was not intended that the book should be either a treatise or a text-book, but a record of experience with comment. Such a work might serve several purposes,—to suggest ideas to social workers, to reveal to other professional persons the nature of social work, and to throw light upon the problems of mental hygiene for all persons interested in human life. Mr. Pound has said that "it is a book to quarry in."

Among the passages that Dr. Southard had not written were some on medical subjects, which his friend, Dr. Harry C. Solomon, was kind enough to write in accordance with views held by Dr. Southard.

The cases were not chosen as examples of successful social work, but were selected because they were believed to be instructive, whether by reason of success or failure.

The work of the social service of the Psychopathic Hospital during the period that this book records was the sum of much earnest and thoughtful effort on the part of many workers, assistants, students, and volunteers, to whom I wish that I might make personal acknowledgment at this time. Among the assistant social workers who had most to do with the development of the work were Mrs. Helen Anderson Young, Mrs. Maida H. Solomon, Miss Helen Wright, and Miss

Dorothy Q. Hale. Among the physicians who helped most to develop the social work of the hospital were Dr. Herman M. Adler, Dr. A. Warren Stearns, Dr. Abraham Myerson, Dr. Frankwood E. Williams, and Dr. Harry C. Solomon.

MARY C. JARRETT.

Boston,
    July 23, 1922.

INTRODUCTION

This book should appeal to a very wide public because it is a vivid transcript of poignant human experience—a record of human misfortunes and their healing. But this record should be especially illuminating because it is written by a man who was many men at once. He gathered these human documents as a student of mental disease and mental suffering; but he saw them also with the sympathies of a social worker and the insight of a philosopher. Philosophers do not often go to psychiatric hospitals. Psychiatrists are rarely of a philosophic turn of mind. Neither philosophers nor psychiatrists have until lately been concerned with concrete, moral, educational, or juristic problems, with which Dr. Southard grappled.

But Dr. Southard has in this book given us the mirror image of his many-sided mind, incurably interested in all human suffering, no matter where it led or whence it came, unwilling to confine his interest within any boundaries,—scientific, professional, or temperamental,—until he had understood a sufferer's troubles to the bottom. He has given us, therefore, a book full of cross-lights. He lights education from the side of medicine, law, and economics. He shows the doctor how he looks to the educator, to the lawyer, and to the social worker. He brings medical habits of thought into jurisprudence, economics, and education.

The book is full of technical terms not all of which are translated. But their meaning is soon clear from the context and their inclusion,—unexplained,—gives one a stimulating sense of looking straight into a busy workshop and gathering there the unexpurgated details of the situation. A heightened sense of reality and frankness results. Meantime, we get a satisfactory familiarity with the psychiatric jargon with which ere long pretty much all professions must be familiar. Army men will have to know it—since so many malingerers are psychopaths and so many mental tests (psychologic) are sure to be incorporated in the army routine of the future.

ix

Judges and lawyers have for some years past been getting inoculated with the terms, the mental habits, and concepts of the psychiatrist, since defective delinquents, epileptics, and the feeble-minded, as well as the insane, so often are before the courts.

Politicians and lawmakers must be familiar with the methods and concepts employed in this book. For our laws on sedition, our problems of free speech, the purposes and performances of our prison officials, almshouse superintendents, and asylum attendants can be judged only in the light of psychiatric tests and psychiatric results.

* * * *

The book is written in part to illustrate how doctor and social worker can co-operate in the care of the mentally deranged. It also illustrates, I think, how *fruitful* such co-operation can be, because the doctor, whose long suit is diagnosis, gets the aid of one much stronger than he on treatment, —namely, the social worker. After the diagnosis there is often little that the doctor, unaided, can do. The social worker comes to the front just there. Provided she can get a diagnosis and prognosis to start from, she mobilizes for the patient's good resources altogether out of the doctor's reach.

I think, myself, that if the psychiatrist were yet a little more broad-minded, he would call the clergyman as well as the social worker to his aid and would find his patients thanking him for a new sort of help now given by neither doctor nor social worker. But that is for the Utopian future when the clergy get their rights and come to earn almost the wages of hodcarriers.

* * * *

One fact certified to in this book is alone and of itself worth reading the whole for,—the fact that more than one man who was too crazy to get along at all in the community outside an asylum did perfectly well in the army! The army, apparently, is sometimes wiser than the doctors and social workers in its environmental guidance of certain poor chaps, who, as soon as demobilized, must again be clapped into an insane asylum. Surely this sheds light both on the army and on the asylum. Even though such cases are admittedly rare, even though many more are driven into asylums by army life, it is surely an arresting bit of information, that army life is good for the wits of *some*. Does this mean that the army provides more discipline or less than the non-military life, more work or less, more interest or less, more variety or less? All these possibilities are open. Indeed, I have seen them all fulfilled. But in any case a new remedy is added to the therapeutic accoutrement of the average psychiatrist when he learns (and if he believes) that army life did really suit some of the mentally diseased patients of Dr. Southard's clinic.

* * * *

Dr. Southard saw his profession as others see it. That is a rare and valuable power. He did not "claim everything" for psychiatry. Yet he claimed more, perhaps, than anyone else ever did, up to his time. For since he included "mental hygiene" in the domain of his art and believed that labor disputes, family rows, and international ambitions, as well as crime, alcoholism, and school-backwardness, belong in the field of mental hygiene,—it might at first sight appear that he set no limits to his profession or its scope. But in point of fact, *limits,* definitions, clear dividing-lines between adjacent fields of professional work, were almost a hobby of his,—as this book abundantly proves. He divides the *science* of psychology from the *art* of psychiatry, and the alienist from the psychiatrist. He refuses to confound (as psychiatrists and psychologists often do) the sphere of immorality with the sphere of disease. Not all sinners are sick—in his view, nor all criminals psychopaths.

This admirable clearness of definition is one of the outstanding merits of the book. He ranges everywhere through the emotions, struggles, diseases, weaknesses, delusions of humanity. We are beside him in the courtroom, in the laboratory, and in the homes of some very queer people. But he always keeps a clear head. He is never swept into a panic nor into a wide glittering generalization, never tempted into mergers that obliterate valuable differences. He has nothing of the fanatic or the doctrinaire except their energy, nothing of the imperialist except his sweep of vision.

I wish he could have lived to compress this book somewhat. It is perhaps too literal a transcript from his daily life and work. Yet there is an advantage in his very copiousness and reiteration. It is like life and teaches like experience. Its faithfulness to fact is in some ways more impressive than it would have been had he cut and selected his material more rigidly. Who reads this book will learn,—as the writer himself learned,—a body of balanced and cautious doctrine, docile under the "bludgeonings of chance." We can hardly forget teachings reiterated from so many points of view—just as real life reiterates them. In the end we are landed square in the middle of a moving train of thought, orderly and progressive, but by no means at the end of its run. We are abreast of the same difficulties, equipped with the same solutions that Dr. Southard was daily presenting to the current army of workers, —doctors, judges, social workers, parents,—who weave themselves in and out of these pages.

That is what he would have wished.

RICHARD C. CABOT.

CONTENTS

BOOK I—THE THREE MAJOR SPHERES OF SOCIAL WORK (Cases 1 to 7)

Public, Social, Individual

NOTE—The literal formulas (P, S, I; P, S; etc.) stand for *Public, Social, Individual*.

BOOK II—THE FIVE MAJOR FORMS OF EVIL IN THE *REGNUM MALORUM* (Cases 8 to 38)

Six Complex Cases (One Pentadic, Five Tetradic) Analyzed by Forms of Evil

NOTE—The literal formulas (M, E, V, L, P; M, E, V, L; etc.) stand for *Morbi, Errores, Vitia, Litigia, Penuriae*.

xiii

BOOK III—ELEVEN MAJOR GROUPS OF MENTAL DISEASES (Cases 39 to 100)

I. *Syphilopsychoses*

II. *Hypophrenoses*

IX. Clyclothymoses

X. Psychoneuroses

XI. Psychopathoses

THE KINGDOM OF EVILS

BOOK I

THE THREE MAJOR SPHERES
OF SOCIAL WORK

Public (Governmental)
Social (Voluntary)
Individual (Personal)

ANALYZED IN SEVEN SPECIMEN PSYCHIATRIC CASES

Then Job answered and said,

Be it indeed that I have erred,
Mine error remaineth with myself.

Behold, I cry out of wrong,
*   but I am not heard;*
I cry for help, but there is no justice.

All my familiar friends abhor me,
And they whom I loved are turned against me.

Have pity upon me, O ye my friends;
For the hand of God hath touched me.

Job, Chapter 19, Verses 1, 4, 7, 19, 21.

WOMAN ART STUDENT
IMMIGRATION SERVICE

In England	*In U. S.*
Bad Heredity	Convalescent Care
Quarreling	Unemployment (Voluntary)
Estrangement from Family	Insufficient Income
Threats Against Family	Charitable Aid
"Nervous Breakdown"	Suicidal Threats
Irregular Occupation	Public Nuisance
Sex Delinquency	Deportation

*Undesirable immigrant and pathetic nuisance: vicissitudes;
deportation.* Effects of a faulty diagnosis **and therefore
prognosis** *(neurasthenia in a woman not at all neurasthenic).*
To illustrate public, social, individual *problems.*

Case 1. Miss Agnes Jackson was sent to the Psychopathic
Hospital for observation from the Immigration Station at
Boston. She was a "mental" suspect and rather an appealing
figure. She herself said that in England she had had a "nervous breakdown." It seemed doubtful whether she could maintain herself on the small income she possessed, an allowance
from her family and a scholarship to cover art school tuition.
But finally she was admitted to the country in the joint care
of the director of the school she was to attend and the social
service of the hospital.

Correspondence with England shortly proved her the daughter of a professional man who had committed suicide a year
before. It appeared that her mother, brother, and sister were
living in England; but that she could not get on with them
and believed that they were persecuting her. Several years
earlier she had had a spell of bad temper and quarrelsomeness
after a love affair that did not come off. She won a scholarship
to study art in London, but had not fulfilled her contract.
About this time she had been observed in a London hospital,
where the (erroneous) diagnosis "neurasthenia" was made.
The parish rector wrote that she was "thought to be not right
in her head and her work as an artist was considered very
moderate." At the art school here, however, she was said to
have some unusual native ability.

After a week in the hospital she was sent to the country to
recuperate (through funds raised for the purpose) because
she complained of feeling weak and distraught as a result of
her detention at the Immigration Station under uncongenial
conditions. At the boarding house where she stayed she made
unreasonable demands and complaints, was untidy, and altogether made herself a great nuisance. She returned to begin

5

her studies at the art school, boarding at a working-woman's hotel. But in a few weeks she took to her bed and insisted on having her meals brought to her, saying that she would not return to her work, as she could not stand the atmosphere of the school. It was found that she had been very rude to her associates there.

Yet she went back after a time and gave no trouble for nearly six months. A piece of her work was exhibited at a well-known shop. As the pound-a-week allowance from England had stopped a friendly artist helped her out with small sums. Miss Jackson herself made no effort to sell her work and showed no industry. She talked a great deal about what would be done for her by this friend and another young woman, a fellow student, who had become interested in her. She continually talked about wanting to meet men, insisting that her friends should help her find a husband. She wrote voluminous rambling letters to them, and also to a physician at the Immigration Station, telling of her misfortunes and her unhappiness.

Meanwhile, she had turned against the social worker; but finally she came to the hospital, weeping and distraught, and was taken in as a voluntary patient. After a brief stay she was discharged, but pursued the same tactics. After two months the more serious step was taken of committing her to a state hospital for longer observation. In the course of time she was sent to England in care of a special attendant, to be returned to her family. This ends the American story of Agnes Jackson and the whole story so far as it has yet unfolded.

The American history of Miss Agnes Jackson thus lasted hardly over a year. The nucleus of these troubles was beyond a doubt psychopathic. Although a psychopath ought to engage one's sympathy and although Miss Jackson at the outset pulled every one's heartstrings, she remains in the minds of all more a pest than a patient.

From the immigration office standpoint she was an undesirable citizen, because a small art scholarship and the pound-a-week allowance plainly could not support her in America.

From the point of view of the social worker, the initial appeal of a young English art student of refinement, dropped from a Cunarder into the detention quarters of the United

States Immigration Office, was extreme. Yet whatever was done for her by officials or by new-found private friends, all ended in a pathetic tangle of minor troubles, amounting to a bit of a tragedy. Whether in England there had been anything really tragic may never be known, though our full accounts from London leave Love largely out of account and minimize the part that Money might have played in the unfolding of events. What tragedy may in future come to her in England we cannot say; but no doubt the same initial appeals and the same lapses into misunderstanding will continue to be her lot.

What after all is she from the medical point of view? Is the fact significant that an elder brother is badly affected with a disseminated sclerosis? On the whole, the hereditary taint in Miss Jackson strikes one as rather slight. Ample studies of her personality both here and abroad fail to place her case beyond cavil in any major group of mental diseases, though no doubt can attach to considering her in some wise psychopathic, and even possibly amongst that group of degenerative diseases so unfortunately termed *dementia praecox*.

As we study the case in detail we are not only able to bring out the governmental, social, and medical troubles, of which this "pathetic nuisance" was a paradigm, but we also find her more or less the vehicle of many, if not all, of the major sorts of evil that the world (according to our classification) has to face. As we hope to show in the sequel of this book, there are evils and evils. But amongst these, we may distinguish at least *five* great classes. There is, for example, the class of *Diseases* into which Miss Jackson readily falls by virtue of her psychopathy. Again, there are the evils of *Ignorance;* that is, of poor education, of misinformation, of the improper digestion of facts through lack of judgment, not necessarily in itself psychopathic, and of these, our paradigm case is not without good examples, of which her coming to America at all may serve as the greatest. There are also evils of which the sequel will supply far more striking examples in which various *Bad Habits* and *Vices,* non-psychopathic, form the chief constituents. Concerning these in the case of Miss Jackson, it may be difficult to disengage her laziness and tactlessness from the effects of psychopathy; but at first sight at least these ways of hers struck her friends and acquaintances as the effects not of disease, but of poor training. Sometimes again, the individual victims of trouble fall into the clutches of the *Law* or of public service in sundry ways. Miss Jackson was a good enough example of an "undesirable immigrant." Again there are evils of a purely economic nature, *Poverty* and other forms of resourcelessness —and it may be well supposed that under certain circumstances, if the Jackson family in England had been on a higher economic level, the life of Miss Agnes would not have been cast in its peculiar way, and in particular she might never have undertaken her American journey.

Hours spent by	Medical record, 65 pages
	Social record, 26 pages
Physician, 14½	Social work:
	Visits, 13
Psychologist, 1	Interviews at hospital, 14
	Telephone calls, 20
Social worker, 36	Letters, 20

Morbid altruist and boys' club organizer. Delinquency explained as due to mental disease (psychopathic personality). Recovery, in all **public** *and* **social** *senses.*

Case 2.   Richard Sully was a kind of morbid altruist. Like Agnes Jackson, Richard was beyond a doubt psychopathic, yet the psychopathic difficulty—a mild defect of the group of so-called constitutional inferiority—was not of such a sort as to perturb Richard's peace of mind or any other of his internal relations and self-adjustments. The trouble seemed almost wholly one of a social nature with occasional public contacts.

Richard first came under expert observation at fourteen. He became beset with the idea of starting boys' clubs. It distressed him, he said, to see boys idle on the street—they ought to get into clubs where they could read. He would hire a room, or perhaps a building, and give orders for suitable furniture. Sometimes he bought refreshments, hid them in his own house, and ended by eating them himself, as the proposed boys' clubs had as yet no members! Between these organizing efforts he worked hard, helping about the house and helping in neighbors' houses. He so helped his church janitor that he was even finally made janitor of the church at $3 a week. His earnings he gave to his mother.

His school work had been lapsing for about two years. A psychological examination at the age of fourteen showed him to be by the Binet Scale actually of a higher mental age level than his actual age; namely, fifteen. A test a year later showed a Binet rating of 12 2/5, but by the Point Scale he still rated at fifteen; in fact at the highest level which the Point Scale of Yerkes was at that time able to register. The psychological examiner reported that Richard was not feeble-minded and yielded no evidence of deterioration, that he was quick and accurate in learning. His analytic ability was especially good. So far as tests went, he was perhaps slightly limited in his power to interpret complexities (so-called "apperception" tests). As for the other mental faculties tested, they were of satisfactory quality, nor would one perhaps often find in a youthful psychopathic suspect like Richard so regular a test. In particular, he had grasped and retained his school knowledge well. On the basis that his imaginative and planning powers were not quite as strong and rapid as normal, the examiner risked the suggestion that Richard might possibly be a patient defective on the side of the will (and hence not defective within the range of many of the tests) and normal as to emotions and intelligence.

We here specify, concerning these psychometric tests, a little more detail than is strictly necessary; for we want to stress the great *negative* value of the mental tests. The patient's comparatively high intelligence is a factor to reckon with in explaining the peculiarity of his delinquencies, and a factor to be considered in building up a treatment procedure and a prognosis.

Now the outcome, at least in the six years during which Richard has been under observation, seems a comparatively good one. During the past four years there have been slight rufflings of the surface (occasional inquiries as to whether it was not now time to organize another boys' club), but these suggestions have been readily nipped in the bud by his advisers. Once even he went so far as to utter a small check, so that there is no doubt that the defect of will is still latent.

Along with Richard's rather minor individual difficulties,

chiefly a defect of will, it is plain that the bulk of his difficulties are in his relations with his family, with the church people, with the boys whom he tried to steer into his vaguely altruistic clubs, and with the tradesmen and others from whom he tried to obtain money. The public—that is, governmental—aspect of Richard's case was, with respect to the courts, rather more a matter of the "eternal not quite" (when brought to court the judge would tend to file the case, or not consider it, on the score of Richard's youth and the peculiarity of his offense); yet Richard was a pretty well-known figure to the local police, who would from time to time step in as good neighbors and help his mother straighten out his tangles. Another public, or governmental, feature of Richard's case was his commitment to a state hospital, which seemed advisable upon his attempt to float his fifth club enterprise. That he had a definite psychosis was perhaps never actually proved.

Richard entered the Psychopathic Hospital under the voluntary relation in a rather peculiar way in his fourteenth year. He arose from bed at home one night very late, took sixty cents from his mother's purse, climbed out of the window, hatless and coatless in a pouring rain, and reached the hospital drenched.

There was a kind of suggestion of the epileptic fugue in this and similar escapades, yet no convincing epileptic features were otherwise discernible. According to Richard, he read too much and got to day-dreaming. The physicians who committed Richard to the state hospital (under Massachusetts law physicians not connected with the state hospital staff must in the interest of the patient be called in) perhaps suspected that he was an early case of schizophrenia, (dementia praecox), as they called attention to a change in Richard's nature at the age of twelve, wherein he became less thoughtful and began to have things bother him. He told the committing officers that he did not sleep for six months at a time. He told them that he had formed about fifty boys' clubs of the same general nature. He was accordingly sent to a state hospital, and thence went home on a visit after a period of six months, for the greater part of which he was granted parole and helped about the laundry, a good and willing worker. He was there regarded as a "constitutional inferior." He was carried on the books of the hospital for six months and then discharged, with a request to report from time to time at the Psychopathic Hospital. There he took baths, as prescribed, somewhat regularly.

With the exception of the two small upsets mentioned above, he now became and still remains an industrious and faithful shoe worker in a factory. The clubable side of Richard's nature has now got its satisfaction in sundry church societies. Richard has always been on good terms with the Psychopathic Hospital and continually brings magazines for the patients, and at one time brought over his church club to entertain them.

We are not here attempting to expound the entire medical story of Richard Sully; yet it is clear that the diagnosis "constitutional inferior," accurate though it may be, might well give the wrong impression to laity and to physicians of the prognosis. At the age of twelve a boy undergoes a change of character and develops a sort of morbid altruism, endeavoring to organize boys' clubs and breaking rather obvious business rules in the process. He gets into medical and social hands, both under the voluntary relation and under the legal commitment relation in the state hospital system, and somehow works out of his psychopathic phase into a comparatively normal status. To be sure, in this normal status traces of his altruistic trend persist; he joins church clubs, sings in the church choir, is a member of the Massachusetts State Guard, of the Young Men's Christian Association and the like. Yet at present he cannot be regarded as much, if at all, outside the range of the normal.

Were there any features in Richard's earlier life which might have given a warning? It is said that he had been somewhat seclusive from early childhood, not caring to play with other children and preferring to read and study alone. He cared for no games or sports except skating. He rather early attempted to assume responsibility in his family and always wanted to escort his mother to the street cars and the like. He was for a long time troubled with tonsillitis, for which he was operated upon. Antitoxin administered for diphtheria at eight years of age partially paralyzed him for a time. The sex side was regarded as normal.

The boy's father deserted his mother, and during the father's numerous unexplained absences (before the final desertion and imprisonment) Richard grieved greatly and sat by the window to watch for his father. After the final desertion, the boy con-

ceived and stated that he now had a family to support, though
he was then but eight years of age. It is possible, or at least
conceivable, that a precocious ripening process in the boy's
mind was somehow started after his father's desertion of the
family. Both the father and the paternal grandfather were sex
delinquents, and the paternal grandfather was a suicide. The
paternal grandmother and two siblings were respectively unsocial, suicidal, and sex delinquent. A younger sister of the
patient is choreic. Upon the maternal side there seems to be
no taint, unless a certain tendency to vascular disease. So far
in Richard's history the other sex has not appeared, save in
his normal relations with his sisters. His interests have constantly attached themselves to persons of his own sex. A psychoanalyst who examined him was inclined to regard him as
showing a "conflict, somewhat homosexual." This diagnostic
suggestion was thought to be supported by the so-called "intelligence complex" shown in association tests, wherein twenty-
eight per cent proved to be "logical definitions." The thought
that after his father's desertion he must now be the head of
the family was also regarded by the psychoanalyst as supporting
the above mentioned "conflict." It seems that at the age of six
Richard had been excluded from some club of boys of his own
age, whereupon he had begun to dream of a club of his own,
which dreams may possibly have started the club forming habit
of his early teens.

The social worker at the state hospital where Richard spent
six months several years ago still supervises him. She wrote
us the following report recently:—

"Since I reported to you in March 1919, Richard has been
getting on exceedingly well. He has been working regularly
at Gordon's Shoe factory in East Boston and is now on piece
work and earns an average of four or five dollars a day, and
sometimes makes as much as seven dollars a day. He has not
attempted to take any responsibility in the Church, although he
has attended their young people's meetings faithfully and still
enjoys his associations there.

"During the summer he had a vegetable garden in one of the
lots given out by the City, in which he worked after returning
from the factory at night and during other spare hours. This
proved to be very beneficial, as it kept him outdoors and gave
him healthful exercise, as well as helping the family with the
food problem. His mother helped him in this.

"Although he had secured his discharge from the Local State Guard Company, in which he had been a Corporal,—upon our suggestion,—when the Police Strike occurred in September the men asked him to re-enlist and he felt it his duty to do so. He served with them during this trouble, but when the worst was over, he resigned again upon our urging him to do so, as it was keeping him from getting as much sleep as he needs. Because of his mental condition we did not approve of his doing a thing of that sort, although we did not know he was out on duty until he had been there a few weeks. As it was, nothing happened and he quite enjoyed the experience, and the factory made up his weekly pay to the average of what he was making at the plant.

"The local Red Cross Home Service has been visiting the family during the past year as Mrs. Sully discovered that her husband was in the Canadian Army and they helped her to get money from Canada. They have kept strictly off the problem of Richard individually, but I am glad to have them in closer touch with the family than I could be."

We have to deal, then, with a boy who apparently passes through a minor psychopathic phase for a period of three or four years about the time of adolescence, but before and after this phase shows but few signs of such a trend. Various diagnoses from the medical side, such as constitutional inferior, predementia praecox, early dementia praecox, even epilepsy and manic-depressive psychosis, were from time to time offered. The committing officers, bound to act on concrete data, were nevertheless in not the slightest doubt as to their duty to commit him to a state hospital. Before this latter decision was arrived at, all sorts of doubts had reigned concerning the diagnosis, some physicians proposing that he was not demonstrably psychopathic, but was, on the contrary, a rather pure example of a delinquent, deserving prison bars rather than the comforts of an asylum.

We analyzed the case of Agnes Jackson not only from the standpoint of the description of her troubles as public, social, and individual, but also (anticipating the considerations of Book II) from the standpoint of the kinds of social evil, of maladjustment, which she displayed. Following a similar plan with Richard Sully, we find him falling, of course, in the class of *Morbi* (*Diseases*) by virtue of his mild psychopathy. Whatever be the trend, or eventual outcome, of this psychopathy, (schizophrenic, epileptic, or otherwise), Richard Sully has at all events what physicians call a *forme fruste* of some sort of mental disease or defect.

How shall we classify Richard with respect to *Errores,* the evils of *Ignorance?* Unlike Agnes Jackson, who did show the effects to some extent of poor education, misinformation, and lack of judgment, Richard not only tested well by the set psychological tests, but seems, on the whole, to have been rather well educated and well informed. An adult insight and judgment should not be expected.

On the side of the *Vitia,* that is, the *Bad Habits and Vices,* Richard must be regarded as equally without pronounced defect, unless we regard with some authors any sort of exaggerated altruism as a form of vice! Shall we regard the forgeries and other delinquencies as at all the effects of moral perversion? Certainly, the tendency of the Psychopathic Hospital staff in its analysis of Richard was to regard these defects as rather more psychopathic (that is, falling within the group of mental diseases), than morally vicious. (We do not care to take up here the question of an eventual proof that some one may bring that moral perversion is in and of itself psychopathic. Such a proof may possibly arrive. For the present, however, we are employing the group of the *Vitia* to contain such *bad habits and vices as might conceivably be drilled out of the bearer by proper moral training, or even prevented by proper early management.* It is in this latter sense of the group of the *Vitia* that we do not regard Richard Sully as a morally dishonest or immoral person.)

Clearly Richard's case falls in the group of the *Litigia,* that is, of legal and similar entanglements; for as we have seen, he was frequently at least within the shadow of the courts.

It is true that the economic status of the family was at best "marginal," but no special effect upon the psychopathic status of the boy can be ascribed to the plight of domestic economy.

Hours spent by

Physician, 7

Psychologist, 1

Social worker, 12

Medical record, 47 pages
Social record, 10 pages
Social work:
Visits, 4
Interviews at hospital, 4
Telephone calls, 8
Letters, 13

PSYCHOPATHIC THIEF

WOMAN (ILLEG.) 27

1916
Arrest
Poor Health
Cut Off from Family

1917
Discharged from Probation
Care of Body (incl. Teeth)
Living with Friends

COMPLICATION : CHILDHOOD SEX TRAUMA

Thief. Infantile sex experience. Physical and psychical waves of disease. "Empathic index" question. "The patient's confidence." **Public** *and* **individual** *problems.*

Case 3. Jennie Walton's mother is said to have had some Indian blood. Jennie was an illegitimate child, and her paternity was never established. We present her as a paradigm of mental disorder leading to public (governmental) rather than family or other social complications. Medically, she should probably be placed amongst the psychopathies. She was arrested for stealing, and, although one might be tempted to make a diagnosis of kleptomania, on the whole the delinquency is probably a minor incident rather than the effect of a strongly marked special instinct, and the fact that simple and obvious social service measures served to straighten out the Walton case (without resort to elaborate and specially designed reëducation or moral reformation) permits us to think that her psychopathy was of a minor degree. Such merely social (non-governmental) complications as did exist were so slight as to be negligible.

Jennie Walton came under hospital observation at the age of twenty-seven, having been arrested for stealing patients' clothes, linen, a fur coat, and utensils from two hospitals, where she had been employed as a domestic for half a year previous. The girl had been of such exemplary character and had so many intelligent, good friends amongst previous employers that the arrest came as a shock to these friends, one of whom wrote that the arrest must be a "fearful mistake" due to a "conjunction of circumstances seeming to implicate her."

However, it appeared that her work at the hospitals from which she stole had not really been satisfactory and that for a period of some five years those who knew her well thought her disposition peculiar in that she was "almost morbidly sensitive, heedless, impulsive, and reckless with money." As for a previous history of stealing, there was none; but she was noted for collecting and hoarding buttons, ribbons, clippings, and

17

poems. She seemed to be rather ambitious and of the type known as a "born leader." She had a certain skill in making clothes out of cast-off things, but no motive of self-adornment could be traced in several of her pilferings. In thirteen years of work in various families she had saved no money whatever. One might naturally inquire whether such a patient as Jennie was more or less hypophrenic (feeble-minded). Mental tests led the psychologist to say that the patient was certainly *not* feeble-minded. She yielded a fairly even rating at the fourteen year level, losing some points on her association tests and on the tests for logical and practical judgment; that is, the seeing of analogies and absurdities and the like. Should she be regarded as, if not a moron, then perhaps a border-line or subnormal person, in the sense of being above the moron level but below the normal? The psychologist remained in doubt, but went so far as to say that the patient graded somewhat below expectation for her age and class. Now her "class" looked better to the psychologist and to any casual observer than it proved to be. She had a shell of special information, having taken special courses in domestic science and in first aid for the injured, but in the meantime had never completed her grammar grades.

When the girl was a baby, her mother was married to a man, not the girl's father, an alcoholic and abusive person who allowed the mother to support the family. Sex relations (age seven to fourteen) with this alcoholic stepfather formed a rather extraordinary episode in the girl's history, according to her own story. In the girl's conscious life this history played a considerable part. She complained bitterly of the robbery "of all that is dear to a woman." She would readily tell neither about the larceny nor about the sex history, nor was any one of several medical approaches successful in starting a stream of confidences. Finally a friend and confidante was found to whom enough of both stories was confessed that the main outlines of the situation were clear.

The medical side of the story was not without bearing on the patient's estimate of herself and upon the psychiatric diagnosis. She had had many and various children's diseases. At eighteen she described herself as having had a kind of general debility from overwork. Whether this was connected with her engagement to a man at nineteen, broken off when the man shortly afterwards entered a forced marriage with another woman, remains doubtful; but the old incest story and the breaking of this engagement "soured her," she said, "on all mankind," so that she was in a way "to become a man-hater." In this nineteenth year it appears that she had a sort of exhaustion attack for a fortnight. She was operated on at the age of twenty-four for appendicitis, and in her twenty-fifth year resorted to an osteopath for exhausted muscles. In her twenty-fifth year she was operated on for peritoneal adhesions; her ovaries were removed at this time. Concerning the oöphorectomy, she claimed that it was, in the opinion of her physicians, made necessary by the trauma of her childhood. She had then woven her incapacity to bear children into the general situation of disgust with the world.

Yet, despite all this checkered history and interweaving of embittered comment by the victim and although for the first part of after-care by the social service her behavior was in some respects queer and even psychopathic, at the end of a year she had so far restored herself to a normal attitude that her case was closed by the hospital social service and was placed on file by the court.

One's prediction about the future of such a case as that of Jennie Walton might well be influenced by preconceived notions. If we took her for an inborn psychopath of mild degree —the psychopathia being, as it were, stamped in by childhood sex experiences and at last emerging in the overt act of larceny—we might give her a rather unfavorable prognosis. At the time of hospital observation she was in rather poor health. Her teeth, especially, were bad. It transpired also that she had been for eighteen months at a state hospital for tuberculosis (pulmonary, no longer in evidence). We must remember the occasional spells of exhaustion, dating from the late teens, which though ill described, may possibly represent some sort of periodic or wave effect in her physique, reflected also in her mental life.

We have recorded that the psychometric rating left case Walton as certainly not a moron and as not clearly subnormal in a milder degree. Psychiatrically examined she proved not abnormal. She was, to be sure, somewhat sad at times, but a psychopathic depression could not be proved. The only question raised was that of delusions, as Jennie told a story of the conspiracy of fellow employees, suggestions to inaugurate a strike, refusal to admit sex advances by hospital employees, placement of articles in her room by fellow employees wishing to do her injury, and the like. These stories were interpreted by us as part of the defense-reaction of one charged with delinquency.

A systematic review of her case by physicians and social workers in staff meeting led to the diagnosis of "psychopathic personality," but without especial grounds therefor, except the patient's history and the general impression that somehow she was psychopathic rather than delinquent. Several physicians thought the outlook was medically bad. Some physicians thought she might be merely psychopathic in the mild sense of the so-called psychopathic personality, but that she might eventually turn out to be psychotic (in the sense of having a definite mental disease).

After the first six months of her period of social supervision, she seemed to bear out this idea of poor prognosis. In a variety of domestic places the girl did on the whole rather poorly, and from time to time rather suspicious things happened. A pin or two disappeared, which she might have stolen; a fire was set, possibly by her. One night she moaned in bed for hours and stayed in bed the next day. She sometimes resorted to osteopathy, and got a diagnosis at a general hospital outpatient department of "chronic arthritis (teeth)" whereupon she went regularly to a dental clinic. She came down with German measles and had a bad cold and the grippe. Meantime she kept endeavoring to get work and to do it as well as possible, and by the end of a year she seemed to have worked out of her susceptibility to illnesses and got upon a better level of physique (all this helped out by a pleasant summer with friendly people). There were no further suspected stealings or other bits of odd behavior. Accordingly, as above noted, her case was put upon file.

We note that the exceedingly few social complications in Jennie Walton's case rendered social service relatively easy, as throughout her adult life it still proved possible, after her misadventures, for her to find good and highly appreciative friends. It took some six months for her psychopathic phase (if it was such) to pass and for the social workers to establish themselves on a confidential basis. This was not so much a question of continued or increasingly clever efforts at gaining Jennie's confidence as it was a matter of the passing of what we finally concluded to be a pretty definite psychopathic phase. Whereas it would not be safe to think of Jennie Walton as clearly a periodical psychopath (in the sense, *e.g.*, of the so-called cyclothymic constitution), nevertheless a review of her entire history yields traces of such a phasic course.

Should she again appear in the courts or in the hospital and fall again within the medical and social service range, no doubt the procedure would be much clearer. In the meantime it would be medically impossible to say either that she is definitely periodic or that she is at all certain to have a further episode. Amongst the ill-defined psychopathias which fall short of the full-blown psychoses (which latter we find typically in institutions), there may be a kind of psychopath with a periodical trend, a sort of *forme fruste* of the out-and-out "manic-depressive" psychosis. Yet various other psychoses have periodical or phasic tendencies. After all, the psychologist did find a certain subnormality about the case, a certain lack of logical and practical judgment. Sundry misspellings and a certain simplicity characterize her letters. Thus (after receiving a Christmas present):

"I simply cannot find a thank you big enough to tell you how delighted I was with the dear little book you sent me. When I read it my delight was doubled threefold, for I think the good fairy whispered to you that it was a set of my favorite quotations which I have scattered around on scraps of paper and which never can be found when needed most to drive a cloud of the blues away."

Again we may try to resolve this case from the standpoint of the distribution of social evils. We have sufficiently discussed her disease and its rather doubtful end, yet there are plain somatic as well as psychic factors therein. As for poor education, there is a certain evidence of this, and a certain superficiality in the education which she had actually received; but it does not appear that her comparatively poor education really contributed much to her difficulty, nor is it easy to ascribe to her any altogether unfortunate moral attitude, despite the fact that her interpretation of her childhood misfortunes and of her later psychopathic complications were not always sound. Yet it is probable that the unsoundness of these interpretations is to be attributed rather to her psychopathy than to any actually poor moral training. Her legal difficulties are obvious and no doubt tended to obscure the physician's interpretation of her case on account of the defense-reactions so natural to men and women when entangled in court. Nor was the Walton case particularly a case of economic disability, though her state was "marginal" rather than on the so-called "comfortable" level. Nor was the will to earn her living ever lost. The difficulties facing the social workers in their general attitude to such a case are not easy to state. In the face of a rather poor medical prognosis (to say nothing of the prevailing general, though baseless, feeling of doubt as to the outcome in *all* psychopathic cases), the social workers had the duty of keeping up their supervision steadfastly until somehow the patient's mental state cleared up. This process of clarification of Jennie Walton's mind, running *pari passu* with a great improvement in her physique, took about a year to bring itself about.

Hours spent by	Medical record, 33 pages
Physician, 6	Social record, 26 pages
	Social work:
Psychologist, 1	Visits, 66
	Interviews at hospital, 4
Social worker, 112	Telephone calls, 17
	Letters, 40

Black sheep. Generalized **psychopathia sexualis.** *Neurasthenia elements removed. Moral improvement ("more of a man" suggestions).* **Social** *and* **individual** *problems.*

Case 4. Henry Loyal was a steamfitter. He had been for many years, at least since puberty, in constant social difficulties. Looking back over his life up to the age of forty-eight, one was tempted to relate these difficulties to drunkenness, gambling habits, sex escapades, and a sort of general irresponsibility in life. He was the acknowledged *black sheep* of a middle-class American family. An analysis of this so-called black sheep will prove conclusively that he was a psychopath, and that all his troubles, medical and social, could be, and have in fact been, greatly improved by the hard work of his official friends.

His friends, whether medical, social, or casual, could not

fail to be impressed with the profound irresponsibility of the steamfitter. What with the fitfulness of his trade and the numerous occasions in which his psychopathy would break out, the task of adjusting him to an environment was not easy. Nevertheless, in the end, what with advice to the man, advice to his wife, and an unusually close supervision, he has now become what, without straining the point, may be called an encouraging example of psychiatric social work.

The case was most unpromising, and, throughout our four years' supervision, it was never possible to avoid an occasional lapse into destitution on the part of the family, and recurrent dissipation on the part of its central figure. There was a slack, profane wife, who was alternately devoted and jealous, and there were four children, all variously affected by disease or defect (one choreic, another tuberculous).

The husband had long been so hopeless a figure that one's first impulse would naturally be to sever him from the family, try him a while, and perhaps finally set him adrift (as one says, "close the case"), and do one's best with the wife and children. The family, however, despite the centrifugal tendencies of the father and the profanity and extraordinary jealousy of the mother, was close knit with profound affection. The paternal affection was, in fact, the main social lever. The existence of this lever was all the more astonishing as the man had for years come home drunk and surly, or stayed away from home in irregular sex life, or loafed about for days, weeks, and months, gambling; every now and then subject to violent spells of rage and cruelty. When one learned from the history in his teens of all manner of unspeakable sex practices, and an early development of thoughtless and irregular tendencies, one was the more convinced that really nothing could be done. When one looked into the family history and discovered psychopathic taint in several near relatives, one could only feel the more certain that, after all, one's efforts might well be wasted.

What shall we term Henry Loyal medically? The strong heredity, though it strengthens our idea that there exists some unusual blot in this social defective, does not point to a particular group of mental diseases having a particular prognosis. When the man came before the Psychopathic Hospital staff, it showed diagnostic leanings in many directions. For example, he was suspicious of his hospital friends and rather apprehensive. If one stretched a point, one might think of him as subject to the so-called paranoid trend, and therefore almost think of dementia praecox. Yet on the whole, the suspiciousness and apprehensiveness of the man were hardly more than might be expected. Again, Loyal had been markedly depressed and his depression was in sundry details not inconsistent with the diagnosis of manic-depressive psychosis (in fact, he had feared that he was going to commit suicide about three weeks before he was observed in hospital). On the whole, however, there was no good reason for regarding the depression as psychic, and suicide might, with a certain type of mind, be regarded almost as a natural thought in the family abyss. Again, Loyal might be regarded as inclined toward the group of the psychoneuroses on account of his hypochondria and headaches. Headaches had been, in fact, for him the main medical feature in his life. Once, too, he had fallen and had an attack which, owing to his being drunk at the time, was called delirium tremens. Whether this attack was actually alcoholic, whether it was not in part hysterical, or whether it may have been at bottom epileptoid, was another group of questions. Amongst the ten or eleven great groups of mental disease recognized by most modern psychiatrists, one might therefore think of adequate reasons for putting him in more than half.[1]

When a case with numerous psychopathic features does not strike one as definitely epileptic, psychoneurotic, schizophrenic (dementia praecox), or cyclothymic (manic-depressive), one is likely to let it fall into a group for which the favorite psychic designation of the present day is "psychopathic personality." Though the psychiatrist might be put to it to define this term, it is enough to say here that the so-called psychopathic personalities are rather apt to bear traits that look in one or other of the directions just mentioned, and on the whole to strike even the lay observer as in some degree childish. This latter idea of the childishness of these patients is expressed by some authors by the phrase "infantilism," as if the "below par" level (*Minderwertigkeit* of the Germans) was somehow an expression of a slight lack of development. Some classifiers use the phrase "constitutional psychopathic inferiority" for these cases,

[1] See pages 436-491 for general discussion and charts dealing with the main groups of mental diseases.

and this phrase is even to be found in our American immigration laws.

But when we choose to term a man a psychopathic personality or a psychopathic inferior, we must constantly bear in mind the different directions which the mild infantilism may take. There was always a doubt in the Loyal case just what particular direction we could describe the psychopathy as taking, especially since there was, in addition to the suspiciousness, the depression, the hypochondria and headaches, and the possibly epileptoid attacks, also a tremendous hypersexuality, so that one might almost think of terming the man a sort of diffuse *psychopathia sexualis*. In most of these directions he was somewhat influenceable, and on the whole the psychoneurotic trend is perhaps to be preferred, if we must press Loyal into a single compartment. How profoundly important the choice of a diagnosis may be is to be seen from the fact that by pursuing the way of therapy (even in this very unpromising case), the year-long tendency to worry and the habit of headaches (fifteen years) were actually terminated by treatment.

At this point let us try to throw Henry Loyal into contrast with Agnes Jackson. Miss Jackson was for us a paradigm of medical, social, and governmental troubles, a victim perhaps of mild schizophrenia (dementia praecox), the primary solution of whose troubles lay in the proper adjustment of medical and social work to the Immigration Office rules and regulations. If we try to analyze the case of Henry Loyal from this standpoint, we find his troubles chiefly medical and social. To be sure, from time to time the Loyal family would fall into destitution and require public or semi-public aid mechanized by more elastic means than are ordinarily possible for strictly public agencies. In short, Henry Loyal was a public or governmental case only in an incidental or occasional way. He is a fairly pure compound of medical and social troubles, with the emphasis perhaps more upon the social than the personal side.

The case of Miss Jackson we found more or less the vehicle of all the major sorts of evil that we tried to classify under the five headings of disease (*Morbi*), ignorance (*Errores*), vices and bad habits (*Vitia*), legal entanglements (*Litigia*), and poverty or other forms of resourcelessness (*Penuriae*). Studying the case of Henry Loyal, we find that, as in the majority of instances in this book, he is the victim of disease;

at all events, of a degree of psychopathy that is sufficient to bring him into all sorts of personal and social difficulty. Shall we charge him also with being the victim of the evil we call ignorance? We found him on the verge of feeble-mindedness by tests, but the psychologists felt that on the whole he must be regarded as of normal mental level. He was neither a good nor a poor scholar. He was an adequate steamfitter. He proved amenable to persuasion if not to conviction, and no elaborate reëducation or implantation of totally new ideas had to be carried out in the process. His sex irregularities cannot on the whole be said to be due to ignorance or poor intellectual training. On the whole, there was a good deal to go upon in the practical handling of Henry Loyal, and we must count him as not falling to any extent into the evil-group termed ignorance.

Re the third group of evils, as in our paradigm case of Agnes Jackson, so in the present case, it is difficult to disengage the bad habits and vices shown from effects of disease. If our separation of the bad habits and vices, on the one hand, from the diseases and character defects on the other, is a logically sound separation, then there ought to be some cases in the world of persons who unfortunately have not been properly trained and given the proper moral set-up in life; and these persons ought, by hypothesis, *not* to be instances of mental disease or defect. Such persons ought to be trainable by suitable methods, either by way of telling them or showing them what to do, by precept, example, reward, or punishment. So far as mere precept and mere example and the common methods of reward and punishment were concerned, hardly anything could have been done with Loyal. Punishment would no doubt have failed. The kind of reward offered was the pleasing sense conveyed to him of increased responsibility for a family to which he was tremendously though interruptedly devoted. He was made to feel more of a man. That Loyal had sundry bad habits and vices aside from his psychopathia, we do not know for certain. But whether we are dealing merely with psychopathic instability or with the effects of poor moral training, no doubt the plan of reëducation is at first identical for a victim of either form of evil.

Of legal entanglements, our first paradigm, Jackson, was a prime example in that she was an "undesirable immigrant."

Loyal's succession of predicaments for the most part failed to lapse into the legal group, though he was in court four times for non-support and wife-beating. The wife never had to appear in court to make her point, and his official friends and supervisors made use of the point once only, when he was threatened with the prospect of a separation.

How far can the Loyal family difficulties be regarded as purely economic? That is, how far does the evil in question fall into the group of poverty and other forms of resourcelessness? We said that if the Jackson family had been on a higher economic level, the life of Miss Jackson would not have been cast in its peculiar way and that she might never have become an immigrant, desirable or otherwise. What can be said of this point in the Loyal case? The family as a whole is on a fairly high middle-class level, with a number of relatives regarded.as well-to-do. Some non-psychopathic relatives are successful in their professions. The courses in life of some of the psychopathic relatives indicate that their economic level, high or low, has little to do with the behavior adopted. Hence the social treatment of this case or of the Loyal family group as a *purely* economic problem would quite miss the point. In point of fact, Henry Loyal while at work could earn, both before and during war time, exceedingly good pay.

We shall now turn to a few further details of the case Loyal. Note should be taken of the slow and slight, but steady, and on the whole uniform, stabilizing which Loyal's character is undergoing. Doubtless he would have to live several lives tandem to get sufficiently stabilized so that he would no longer require supervision; but our general principle of *hope for stabilization even in the most difficult cases* remains a principle. Our records run to over a hundred pages, but for the purpose of this exposition we will limit ourselves to a few of the more striking episodes in the Loyal history.

Loyal first came to the Psychopathic Hospital on the advice of a social worker in a general hospital where his little daughter was under treatment for chorea. He was out of work at the time and for years had failed to support his family. The oldest girl was fifteen, the second one, who was choreic, was twelve, and the youngest child, also a girl, was five years old. A fourth girl was born four months later. At this time the family was living in a shack on the outskirts of a suburban town, and their economic condition was acute. On the ground that there might be a nervous cause for his headaches, which he claimed prevented him from •working steadily, Loyal was persuaded to come to the out-patient department for an examination and even consented to enter the hospital for a week's observation.

He got a job and moved to a good neighborhood. Some of the debts were paid off, and a much coveted piano was obtained on the installment plan. All went well for about eight months, when Loyal again became irregular in all his habits. He contracted gonorrhea and his wife became infected. Meanwhile, one of the children had developed a tuberculous hip, required long, patient treatment in a hospital, and was later boarded out in the care of a children's agency. Throughout her illness Mr. Loyal was in a state of anxiety and excitement which threatened to interfere with the child's proper care, but in the end the social worker prevailed and the little girl made a good recovery. The second child recovered from her attack of chorea under the exceptionally good nursing given her by her mother. The baby too was sick, but not seriously.

Work became slack and the landlady threatened prosecution for arrears of rent. From time to time it was necessary to give financial assistance, for which funds were given anonymously by a relative. Finally public aid had to be sought. In time, Mr. Loyal found new work on government buildings and had no more difficulty in getting employment, although he was likely to be idle for short periods between jobs. It was never possible to find out what he did with the high wages he received. Certainly the results were not evident. In one of these intervals of unemployment, nearly four years after the family became known to us, a crisis arose. Mrs. Loyal was sick and in need of hospital care (she had been having serious trouble with varicose veins), funds were exhausted, and the landlord had set a date for eviction. Loyal had a job in view, but could not get it until he was restored to good standing in the union. The way out was found by sending one of the girls to a relative, Mrs. Loyal to a hospital, and the two younger children to the public authorities for temporary boarding-out. The oldest girl by this time was married to a man considerably older than she, a distant relative with some means. She had developed a character much like her father's. Nevertheless with the family provided for and his financial condition revamped, Mr. Loyal started for his new job. In a few months he was able to take the children from public care to their mother, who went to live with her sister in a city near the scene of work. At last report, he and his wife were making efforts to get together a home again.

Hours spent by	Medical record, 42 pages
	Social record, 106 pages
Physician, 15	Social work:
	Visits, 120
Psychologist, 1	Interviews at hospital, 57
	Telephone calls, 105
Social worker, 245	Letters, 75

Adventuress, thief, liar—psychopathic personality. Mental level testing very high. A "public" problem in hands of the law, sent for observation by alienist.

Case 5. We possess numerous newspaper clippings about the possible deportation of the supposed wife of a famous British army officer. "Lady" Nora Campbell was brought to the Psychopathic Hospital by a social worker. Mrs. Campbell had been doing voluntary war work. Her husband, she said, had been a major in the army, killed on service in the war, leaving her a child, which about six months since had died at the age of eighteen months. Now, it chanced, she said, that she was the goddaughter of the King, a niece of a well-known general, had given from her ample estate a hospital for the use of English soldiers and had had some seventy per cent of her money taken over by the British Government. She said at one time that she was the illegitimate child of a person high in English society, who was paying her seven thousand pounds a year as sort of hush money.

From various physicians and Boston people with whom the patient had had dealings, a number of stories were collected concerning Mrs. Campbell. The biggest story hung upon the loss of a brooch by a fellow war worker, who had known her for two or three months and regarded her as a quiet, ladylike victim of the war who was only to be pitied for her wanderings, the loss of her husband and baby, and her present loneliness. To be sure, Mrs. Campbell it seems had flirted with a son of one of the war workers, and had on some pretext obtained twenty dollars from him. There also was a somewhat unlikely story about a man's coming to get two hundred dollars hush money and making away with eight hundred dollars more which was in her purse. Finally, a valuable brooch disappeared under very suspicious circumstances, and shortly thereafter Mrs. Campbell tried to sell a brooch on account of its "evil associations." Detectives were finally called in. Several inconsistent stories were told them. In the end the brooch was found, and after sundry vicissitudes, also the central stone, which at one time Mrs. Campbell tried to isolate by burying it.

The eventual diagnosis from the psychopathic point of view in the case of Mrs. Nora Campbell was that of psychopathic personality, a phrase intended to convey the idea that she was not a mere delinquent but that her tendencies were in large part psychopathic. Of course, there were numerous and sundry defense reactions of the true delinquent in Mrs. Campbell, who told many forms of tales and lied more or less expertly on all occasions (never, even in the end, confessing her theft of the brooch) about her life and status. Physically, there was no certain evidence of there having been a child born, and conditions were, on the whole, rather consistent with the idea that no such obstetric history could ever have occurred. The physical examination proved, in fact, to be practically normal in all respects.

Psychologically, she rated extremely high, achieving 95 points in a possible 100. She did many of the tests exceptionally well, was perhaps somewhat over-suggestible and fell off particularly in certain performance tests. Whether or not on account of her intentional and unintentional lying, she gave the impression of a slight memory defect.

The case of Nora Campbell is schematically simple. To be sure, from one point of view, if Mrs. Campbell was a psychopath, then it is clear that we must logically conceive that she possessed "individual difficulty." There is presumably no psychopath who is not a "damaged individual." In the first place, there remains judicial doubt and also doubt in the lay mind whether this adventuress, liar, and thief was really a psychopath at all. For example (the judge or the layman might say) an adventuress, thief, and liar might be such from faulty education, as the criminals taught by Fagin in *Oliver*

Twist were victims of faulty education rather than of disease or moral deficiency. So it might be that Mrs. Nora Campbell had been educated under conditions which made a life of adventure with the fleecing of society, subject to the accompaniment of picturesque lying, a natural career for a woman. Admittedly, this would be doubtful, but the hypothesis must necessarily be entertained, if only to be dismissed. A far more likely hypothesis concerning the intra-individual blemishes of Mrs. Campbell would be that she was a vicious person, a person of faulty mental and moral habits who had slipped into a life of crime of this "grafting" sort more than half intentionally. Such a hypothesis would, no doubt, fit a good deal of what we term crime (in the minds of the laity).

However all this may be, the point in *not* classifying Nora Campbell as a case in the "individual" group is that she did not fall under the sphere of authority which deals with the individual as such. She was and remained an almost purely legal case, despite the fact of her observation at the Psychopathic Hospital under much more lax conditions than most communities permit.

Should we not classify Mrs. Campbell as falling under the sphere of social influence or authority? To be sure, many interested society people and many social workers became interested in her and spent some time upon her devious ways. Nevertheless, throughout the whole situation, the hand of the law and the penetrative technique of the detective drew the red herring of public influence over all the social and individual interests which might otherwise have prevailed. The point for the general or psychiatric social worker to bear in mind is that, whatever may be the medical information concerning the profound and delicately balanced psychopathic interior of the case, nevertheless a case like Campbell is without the range of the physician to influence thoroughgoingly, simply because the iron of the situation remains in the hand of the law. Again, whatever the social worker may think as to the excellence of her own technique in managing a case like Campbell, she must always remember that the case remains one under public authority. She may supply a good deal of velvet for the outside of the glove, but the iron remains therein. Upon whatever logical or profoundly sentimental grounds the physician or the social worker may want to proceed, he or she is forthwith stopped, in all authoritative procedure, by the hand of the law. There are public interests here which are organized and crystallized from the habits of centuries on the part of the legal world. These old, crystallized judicial and institutional habits must prevail until they are bowled over or turned into dead letters by the new knowledge which may accrue in future systematic studies of delinquency and near-delinquency.

We concede that we have presumably no right to draw such heavy conclusions as the above from the case of the adventuress Campbell. Throughout the rest of the book, however, we shall find these public interests interwoven through the social and individual interests that we are tempted to think ought often to have the right of way. The interests of the state as a juristic person and the interest of the state as guardian of social interests (phrases of Dean Roscoe Pound) are interests often paramount to the individual interests in personality, domestic relations, and economic circumstances, and paramount over such general social interests as the security of social institutions, the maintenance of general morality, the conservation of social resources and general progress—all of these phrases borrowed from a legal statement of certain fundamental conceptions of the "legal order." "The legal order," writes Dean Pound, is "an adjustment of human actions and relations in order to conserve the goods of existence, prevent friction in human use and enjoyment of these goods, and eliminate waste of them." In the case of Campbell, it is a question of a brooch, borrowings of money, etc., an enormous waste of good people's time, and a question of prevention. Aside from imprisonment, it must be granted that the legal order does not seek the methods of prevention that social workers and physicians would be eager to establish. Punishment and redress are far more prominent in the legal order than prevention. But that is another story and one calculated to be extraordinarily developed by a systematic attack on the problems of general and psychiatric social work.

Hours spent by	Medical record, 61 pages
	Social record, 9 pages
Physician, 9	Social work:
	Visits, 4
Psychologist, 1	Interviews at hospital, 1
	Telephone calls, 3
Social worker, 9	Letters, 15

ALCOHOLIC PSYCHOSIS

IN A PACKER

November, 1915	*November, 1916*
Inebriety	Sobriety
Unemployment	Steady Work
Physically Disabled	Good Health
No Income	Good Wages

After-care of an alcoholic. Rationalization. Point of view of a hospital organization known as the **Men's Club.** *Non-psychiatric social worker likely to miss the point of such a case. Patient now better than he ever was. Problem* **social,** *rather than public or individual in the special senses of those terms.*

Case 6. Alfred Mack, an Irish elevator man, is now almost forty years old. We describe him, with some misgivings, as a paradigm of social troubles, occurring practically pure, that is, without any public (governmental) complications and without special medical difficulties. Mack was under our social supervision for some three years. A recent inquiry has shown him socially adequate, after a period of about five years since the medical incidents that brought him to the hospital.

Possibly the layman would not regard the episodes which brought him to the Psychopathic Hospital as mere "incidents," since he there got a definite diagnosis of mental disease, due to alcoholism, and since doubts were there raised as to whether he might not be a victim of very severe mental disease leading possibly to deterioration. No such deterioration has set in. The mental tests, in point of fact, yielded, five years ago, according to the Yerkes Point Scale, an age level of fifteen years plus. It is true that the Binet tests left him at an eleven year level at the time he was first examined; but the psychological examiners even then attributed his deficiency to the alcoholic traces which he still showed.

The alcoholic mental disease, severe as it was (he had definite delusions of persecution and even hallucinations of hearing, possibly of vision) ended in a relatively perfect recovery, so that he could be discharged recovered in nineteen days. According to the usual psychopathic hospital technique, Mack was discharged to the out-patient department of the hospital, where he has since been carried on the books.

Upon a further study of his situation, another bothersome, but rather banal medical condition was drawn into the foreground. He had, for a number of years, had ulcers of his feet which had been variously treated in general hospitals and which

35

have left him, up to date, quite unable to do certain kinds of work. At various times a packer and a shipper's assistant, he has finally settled into being an elevator man. (As to actual nature of the disorder of his feet there is doubt. The ulcers were apparently treated at one time as syphilitic, but our blood tests proved negative in this regard. On the whole, the disorder seems to be almost purely orthopedic.)

Far more serious than the severe, acute episode of mental disease through which he was carried, and of less consequence than the orthopedic disorder just noted seemed, at first blush, his twenty years' history of alcoholism.

Mack was a somewhat appealing little man, looking rather old for his years, with a pigeon breast, trouble with both arches of his feet, and poor teeth. A study of his heredity left one much concerned for his outcome. Both parents (the mother, a Roman Catholic, had married a Church of England father) were alcoholic, and the father died of cirrhosis of the liver, the mother of paralysis following five years "of being peculiar after her first stroke."

The father had been a sex delinquent and nothing was known of his brothers and sisters if, indeed, there were any. The mother's brothers and sisters were all alcoholic, two dying of paralysis (one of the aunts had a kind of mental disorder at menopause and died at a hospital for the insane after a paralytic stroke in the sixties). It is difficult to choose a general epithet for the family, whether "alcoholic," "paralytic," or "cardiac," though possibly these conditions are in this particular family closely interrelated. Nevertheless, Alfred Mack, himself alcoholic and given inordinately to tobacco, despite his somewhat melancholic self-depreciative and rather unsocial frame of mind, was always considered a man of normal intelligence and a fair worker. He held his first position for eighteen years and was not known by his employer to be the steady alcoholic that he really was. He may have been held in this position somewhat out of pity for himself and his mother, whom he helped to support for ten years. The rheumatism and ulcers of the toe were said to have followed a severe attack of scarlet fever in childhood. There is history of a supposed concussion of the brain from a fall at the age of seventeen. (The psychiatrist is apt to think of such concussion cases as subject to unusual intolerance for alcohol.)

There is a still more obscure history of a supposed love affair in the teens, but for the rest of the patient's life, at least, he showed no interest in girls, had a few male chums, but was never "hail fellow, well met."

In his thirty-fifth year, Mack had an attack which it would seem safe to describe as one of delirium tremens. The second attack, which came on at a general hospital to which he had reported for an operation on his foot, brought him to the Psychopathic Hospital.

Up to the time of development of the first attack called delirium tremens, there appears to have been no sign of mental or nervous disorder save that, apparently at about the age of thirty-two, he once had a sudden attack of blindness lasting a quarter of an hour. For the rest, in early life he may or may not have had certain fainting fits in the course of the "rheumatism" which followed his scarlet fever.

In this analysis we are intentionally overemphasizing and throwing into relief sundry minor points in Mack's medical history with the idea of showing that the main complications which social treatment had to face were either not medical or else were perfectly obvious matters to deal with. In short, if we are searching for a case of practically pure social difficulty and confine ourselves to drawing upon *hospital* cases, we shall rarely find a purer instance of social difficulty without public complications and with rather obvious medical indications.

Let us contrast the problems as they faced the medical man and the social worker respectively. The physician confronted a rather prematurely aged alcoholic of twenty years' standing who had had two rather serious attacks of an acute mental disease due to alcohol. The heredity was in several respects poor and the stock in general given to disease of the blood vessels. The situation was complicated by rheumatism, ulcers, and some obscure though slight nervous phenomena, apparently attributable to a severe scarlet fever in childhood. The general medical indications were merely those of proper hygiene (possibly with special reference to work that might spare the heart).

Confronting Mack's case in the same general way, the social worker found him on a basis of (*a*) inebriety, (*b*) a case of unemployment of about a year's duration, and hence (*c*) without income and even possibly (*d*) disabled industrially.

As for the industrial disability of orthopedic origin, the cure was relatively easy, and general hospital care soon helped his feet so that he could undertake a new job as elevator man. Meantime, until the disability for work could be removed, small sums of money were got for him (this the very well-intentioned man later repaid) and the next step was to get him another permanent job. As the man's general nature was such that he liked to work in one place (his "occupational orbit" was very small) and as, moreover, the foot trouble helped define the issue, it was fitting that he should go back to an elevator job. But the desirable permanent job did not come until he had tried several temporary ones. Yet to remove the foot trouble, tide him over his convalescence and to get him a job, was not to abolish his inebriety. For this purpose he was compliant with a plan of coming to the so-called "Men's Club" which ran at the Psychopathic Hospital for several years (up to war emergencies) and was a most effective agency for holding certain recovered alcoholics to a program of abstinence or temperance. Mack took no especially prominent part in club meetings, but drank his coffee and ate his cake with the other social convalescents every evening after the club business was discussed, namely—how to beat inebriety. The Psychopathic Hospital Men's Club would be worth a detailed elaboration as an interesting application of the class method in psychotherapy. Mack was simply "one of the boys" at these meetings, which were presided over by convalescents elected to their jobs and run in the presence of a social worker or two. From month to month the program of the meetings varied, but as a rule some physician would help lead the attack on alcohol. A deep analysis of the operations of such a club would have to take into account the frequent successes of a psychotherapy for alcoholism which did not utilize music, religion, or even ethics in the common manner of so-called "uplift." In fact, a plain rationalization of the alcoholic's plight was the mainstay of these meetings where each man's endeavor was to some extent bolstered by a certain sense of competition with his brother convalescents. As for spiritual appeal, the case of Alfred Mack might have been difficult. With a Roman Catholic mother and a Church of England but sexually delinquent father, a boy who had been embraced rather than guided into the Baptist church was no specially suitable vessel for spiritualization, unless indeed some complete conversion could have been undertaken.

The elements in getting hold of a case like Mack's were not complex. To adjust the simple medical care, to get him a little money in the meantime, and to get him temporary, and at last permanent jobs, to rationalize and support a proper attitude (through the Men's Club) to alcoholism, were measures to which but one other had to be added. It was necessary to secure and maintain a proper attitude on the part of Mack's family to his history and his outlook. This family consisted of a sister and her husband. The brother-in-law was not a drinking man and was friendly to Mack. It did not take long to patch everything properly up. It is worth noting that the patient's sister had herself, at one time, been a charity case on account of the drinking habits of her mother. But married, as she finally was to a non-alcoholic painter, she herself had made what might be called a social recovery. All of which leads one to ponder upon the entire family background of the Mack case which, absolutely black as it was from alcoholism and tendencies to blood-vessel disease, nevertheless gave room for successful social measures.

We must not say that the insight of the psychiatric social worker is extraordinarily more penetrative in a case like Mack's than that of the medical social worker approaching the problem from more general ground. Nevertheless we think it safe to say that many a case with as black a heredity and family background, a history of years of social failure, might well drop into the discard in the presence of ever so many more "promising" cases. Of course one does not know what, for example, the orthopedic division of a social service department would have accomplished for Mack. It is a little bizarre, yet profitable, to think that without an attack of outspoken alcoholic mental disease, Mack might thus have been handled by an orthopedic social worker after a successful course of foot treatment at a general hospital. It is a question whether his alcoholism would have been handled as intensively as the Men's Club allowed it to be handled at the Psychopathic Hospital. Perhaps we unduly malign the non-psychiatric social worker in the above reflection, but it seems safe to say that without a good bit of experience with the temperaments of alcoholics and of more pronounced psychopaths, the routine social worker of economic bent or with the everyday philanthropic point of view would scarcely be tempted out of the ordinary run of measures. The concrete thing which the psychiatric social worker here did was to utilize the Men's Club for rationalizing the patient's outlook on life, but more than that, to employ the entire fundamental plan of attack which underlies the Men's Club and all other social psychiatric measures—namely, the temperamental or characterological point of attack. To be sure, any human being with insight into human nature and considerable experience therein might have seen through the slight unsociableness of the patient, marked out his native timidity as an avenue of approach, and fed his waning self-respect in a variety of ways.

We cannot claim that the church has not accomplished as much or more with equally alcoholic patients. But the church would probably have been of lesser service in this man of mixed religious antecedents. Nor do we deny that the technique of conversion or regeneration by the process of the "twice born men" would have been applicable. The social psychiatric question is, as the child W. K. Clifford used to say, *"What is the particular go of it?"* At all events, whatever the technique, we can safely say that Mack is at this time medically a much sounder unit in the world than he was at the time of his alcoholic psychosis and for many years preceding. Whether on the account of the social treatment or by reason of unknown factors, there has been a decided up-gradient in Mack's life. For years, during his early employment, he was something of an object of pity and might have been thrown completely out of employment had his steady alcoholism been known. Now Mack is one of the most reliable and efficient minor employees in a big shop.

We need no extended analysis in the case of Mack to show how the major sorts of evil that we have classified in the previous cases fall out. Into the class of diseases readily fall the tendency to blood-vessel disorder, rheumatism, and other effects of scarlet fever, and more probably (although not demonstrable) a certain tendency of mind which naturally led him into alcoholism. With such a heredity as Mack's it would be impossible to deny that there was not at least more latent tendency to disease in him than in the majority of men.

Turning to the matter of ignorance or errors of education, we find Mack singularly free from these. To be sure, two parents not agreeing upon religion probably gave him little enough of true home education or moral training. Despite these lacks, the man is relatively free of their concrete effects. A long controversy might be waged as to whether Mack's alcoholism was a vice or a bad habit into which he was led by nature on one hand or by imitation on the other. The present tendency is to underscore the hereditary standpoint and to scout somewhat the factor of mere imitation of parental ideas and habits. As to the tentacles of the law, Mack failed to be caught thereby, save in the benign circumstances that the temporary care law (that mildest of all legal adventures for the psychopath) became available when he was out of his head at the general hospital. The existence of such a law as the temporary care law (see Appendix C) is, no doubt, of extraordinary importance in the potentialities of social service for psychopaths and psychopathic suspects in any community. But that is another story.

As for the fifth group of evils which we have discussed, the economic factor was drawn only temporarily into view. We are dealing then with an almost purely social case whose minor complications are, to be sure, medical, but whose central feature, the alcoholic tendency, must be regarded as a kind of psychopathic tendency, whose effects are distinctly curable. This, indeed, is a frequent lay point of view toward the alcoholic unfortunate. It does not do to throw the alcoholic out at the door, even if his history be a long and sad one and his hereditary taint even more terrible.

We must here leave the large question of temperament unanalyzed. Below we shall meet many instances of a more striking temperamental make-up which the disease itself will have brought out in exceeding sharp relief.

Hours spent by	Medical record, 36 pages
	Social record, 15 pages
Physician, 4	Social work:
	Visits, 12
Psychologist, 1	Interviews at hospital, 5
	Telephone calls, 6
Social worker, 23	Letters, 15

*Industrial injury (shell-shock analogue from civilian life).
Looked highly "organic." Problem chiefly* **individual**: *the
man's relation to himself. Resentful of sympathy.*

Case 7. James Bailey, a Jewish laundryman, twenty-four
years old when he was first seen, is presented as a case of almost
purely medical interest, whose social aspects (both from the
standpoint of diagnosis and from the standpoint of treatment)
were of an obvious nature and who presented no public service aspects whatever, (his coming voluntarily to an out-patient
clinic in the Massachusetts State Hospital system may be regarded as putting him in contact with governmental agencies:
and his damage case against the Elevated Railway was in the
hands of a lawyer).

Medically speaking, James Bailey was a rather intriguing
case, since his disorder not only followed a definite street railway accident, but also looked to the neurologist like an "organic" case. Yet, Bailey's nervous system was really reacting
(as was eventually determined) to a tuberculous pleurisy. This
pleurisy, we came to think, formed a perfectly genuine nucleus
of pain in the back, around which the peculiar, at first sight
"organic," disorder crystallized.

It was somewhat with Bailey's case as with sundry shell-
shock hysteria cases of the war group, in that there was a
genuine focus of pain of organic origin around which the
functional, and perfectly curable, disease grew. Many functional disorders of the back and legs in the war neurosis group
have apparently developed in precisely this way around strained
ligaments, small hemorrhages, or other lesions incidental in
the strains, falls, or "windage" of war service.

Here, then, we were dealing medically with a "shell-shock
analogue"; but the military factor in the situation is replaced
by a pleurisy which was perhaps, although not certainly,
lighted up by the railway accident. Curiously enough, Bailey
developed his peculiar gait and reactions (somewhat at first
sight resembling an ataxic paraplegia) in camp. For Bailey,
about a month after his railway accident, in which two ribs
were fractured in alighting from a car, was drafted into the
United States Army and sent to camp. Six weeks later he had
to be discharged on the ground of physical disability, as he

could not keep up with the drilling and dragged his foot. It is, of course, *post facto* obvious that Bailey should not have been accepted for military service. Yet even in the light of these subsequent developments, the draft board physician now assures us that there was certainly nothing demonstrable about the man which could possibly have led to his rejection as a draftee.

We present this case as an almost purely medical case. The social work of the case might be characterized as supportive, as a sort of splint to Bailey's will, to keep him in contact with medical officers who only could cure him.

Bailey is of rather a refined and meticulous nature. Although a laundry worker in this country, he had been a teacher in Russia (whence he had emigrated at the age of nineteen) and had nourished ambitions to become a physician. With characteristically racial intensity, he had tried to improve his status in the world, had studied hard and gone to evening school. It appears that his mother was a worrier, or as one might technically say, somewhat "psychasthenic." She also had the history of developing at one time a paralysis; whether this was of hysterical nature or not is unknown. The ambitions for medicine were interfered with by the accident, and Bailey lost some of his savings. The army service set him further back. He was now, as one might say, on the defensive and in the passive voice. He felt that, after all, he was not entitled to sympathy and resented any signs of it in others. Bailey looked with suspicion on jobs suggested for him because he did not want to take a "charitable" job.

Upon the examination table his lameness and peculiar posture of back and legs were no longer in evidence. The whole situation, with the exception of the hypothesis of something "periorganic" (the pleuritic pain above mentioned) seemed to the physicians hysterical.

Bailey is now somewhat better; his condition is theoretically curable. The function of the social service is to keep him in contact with the sources of proper psychotherapeutic suggestion. The black side of the problem is merely that, after all, he has a definite tuberculous condition of his pleura. This can, no doubt, be cured, whereupon the whole hysterical situation would have no longer any possible organic basis. But, if we are to give him the régime suitable to a case of tubercle, we must clearly somewhat alter his mental attitude, which, though unlike that of his worrying mother, is of a somewhat psychasthenic trend. After all, the *relation of the patient to himself* is the most important point here.

We thus conclude our exposition of seven cases chosen to illustrate the three major spheres of mental hygiene, public, social, and individual, into which psychiatric cases (as well, doubtless as all other cases falling within the purview of social work) in general fall. We do not intend to rehearse at this point the main features of these cases, reserving such general considerations to the main summary at the end of this book. Briefly taken, however, our considerations descended in complexity from (*a*) the immigration case of Agnes Jackson through (*b*) three somewhat less complicated cases of Richard Sully (the boys' club organizer), Jennie Walton (with her peculiar thievery) and Henry Loyal (the steamfitter of psychoneurotic trend), a series of three cases in which but two of the major mental hygienic spheres of interest are illustrated (Sully, public and social; Walton, public and individual; Loyal, social and individual) to (*c*) three cases of still simpler nature, namely,—Nora Campbell whose offense and nature was such as to make her dominantly a public service case with social and individual features overshadowed by her apparent criminality; Alfred Mack, an alcoholic, without special public-service complications, with comparatively simple diseases and characteristics to contend with and whose handling was a practical matter of straight social work; James Bailey, the subject of the present sketch.

How can we justify placing James Bailey amongst cases that are chiefly individual in their mental hygienic problem? The grounds of this claim are that Bailey's relation to the public service was of the most tenuous, consisting merely of his relations with the psychopathic hospital out-patient department, that the social work involved was relatively obvious, and that all the work involved led very directly back to the medical situation (injury, "functional" lameness and gait) and his character, somewhat resentful of sympathy.

The previous cases in this present group of seven have been analyzed also briefly according to the peculiarities and special aspects of the maladjustments or "evils" which they presented.

The analysis of numerous cases upon this schema of evils is to be pursued in the second part of this book and to be further synthesized in our summary at the end. In this first part of our analysis we have discussed cases from the standpoint of their falling into one or other or even into two or perhaps three of what may be called the major spheres of interest and of authority in mental hygiene. We have in this first part of our book discussed the practical status which the personality of a psychopath, with all its internal and environmental complications, possesses in the existent human world, subdivided as this world is into interests maintained by (*a*) organized government (courts, state hospital societies, etc.), (*b*) community interests of a less organized character (voluntary social agencies, and other efforts of citizens at large), (*c*) and the interests of the individual himself (as mainly controlled by physicians and by other personal guides endeavoring to effectuate such changes inside of the personality as may straighten out the entire tangle).

However, even in these cases, presented from the aspect of the three main spheres of authority or applied influence into which they fall, we have seen the main divisions of social maladjustment stand out. To take this last case, James Bailey, for example, we find him afflicted first with some obvious medical complaints requiring rather obvious attention. But he is much more importantly afflicted with a special attitude to life, a definite slight defect of character requiring very particular attention for its correction or compensation. *Re* educational defect, this young Russian Jew is rather well informed, despite his feeling that he is not as well educated as he should be. It would be a nice point to determine whether we shall regard Bailey's educational question as a matter of character defect or as a matter of a true deficiency in knowledge of how a young man in his plight ought to look upon his future. Of course, in a general way also, Bailey is (from the so-called middle-class standard in America) not too well informed, and this may be regarded as an effect of his origin in the Russia of recent years and his transplantation to the American soil of today.

From the moral point of view, Bailey is exemplary; from the standpoint of legal entanglements he has entangled himself somewhat in lawsuit preparations over his railway injury. As for Bailey's economic plight, he groups with the so-called "marginal" cases and would not prominently classify in the group of poverty and resourcelessness.

Hours spent by	Medical record, 7 pages
	Social record, 21 pages
Physician, 3	Social work:
	Visits, 14
Psychologist, 0	Interviews at hospital, 21
	Telephone calls, 21
Social worker, 42	Letters, 21

BOOK II

The land of the shadow of death,
without any order.

Job, Chapter 10, Verse 22.

THE FIVE MAJOR FORMS OF EVIL
IN THE *REGNUM MALORUM*

Arranged for the Purposes of
General and Psychiatric Social Work

Diseases and Defects of Body and Mind	**Morbi (M)**
Cure!	
Educational Deficiencies and Misinformation	**Errores (E)**
Teach!	
Vices and Bad Habits, Non-psychopathic	**Vitia (V)**
Train!	
Legal Entanglements In and Out of Court	**Litigia (L)**
Counsel!	
Poverty and Other Forms of Resourceless-	**Penuriae (P)**
ness Provide!	

ANALYZED IN
THIRTY-ONE SPECIMEN PSYCHIATRIC CASES

NOTE.—The order of evils here adopted is proposed for the purposes of orderly exclusion in psychiatric and other branches of social case diagnosis.

Intelligent sex delinquent. Difficulties in public, social, individual spheres. Medical, educational, moral, legal, economic factors: Morbi, Errores, Vitia, Litigia, Penuriae. Psychiatric point of view.

Case. 8. Rose Talbot is one of those rare examples amongst women of the very intelligent sex delinquent. She is an emotional and unstable girl with strong sex desire, now twenty-four years old, with a record of marriage at seventeen, the contraction of syphilis from her husband (dead two months after marriage), the birth of a syphilitic child (still living and apparently normal after elaborate and intensive salvarsan treatment), and a second marriage at twenty-two with a divorce a year later, said divorce being procured by her new husband, a respectable man, on account of her sex delinquency.

The immediate medical problem was the cure of the syphilis which went forward as well as usual (or perhaps better than usual in psychopathic cases, whom it may be difficult to make appear at due intervals) to a practical cure, but back of the problem of the acquired syphilis is the problem of the patient's own emotions and will, whose disorder expresses itself from the legal point of view as sex delinquency and comes to the clinic for diagnosis. It is worth eternally insisting that not every sex delinquent is by the same token necessarily a psychopath. If psychiatry is likely some day to prove that sexual and other delinquencies are somehow expressions of psychopathy, nevertheless psychiatry has not, up to date, proved that crime is always and necessarily a disease. It does help the task of the mental hygienists when overenthusiastic theorists make extravagant claims to the effect that crime is always disease, and criminology, accordingly, a part of medical science. Perhaps more than half of all sex delinquents that come publicly to the surface are in one way or other psychopathic (that is, either severely or mildly psychotic or more or less feeble-minded).

How does it stand with Rose Talbot? We have mentioned her considerable intelligence, which was eventually to be proved by her becoming an expert telegrapher. The psychological examination taught us at once that from the standpoint of available tests, she was of high intelligence. This mental level, thus scientifically indicated by the psychologist, was at first sight not at all borne out by her history when she came to the hospital. She then struck the ordinary eye as a hopelessly undependable, probably incorrigible instance of an oversexed woman with the added complication of acquired syphilis and a syphilitic child also to be cared for. As a social problem of fitting into some occupation, Rose Talbot was difficult. As soon as she was a woman grown she had married; she had learned no trade; she was of an intelligence rather superior to the level of the kind of work which she could readily procure; a lapse into sex life had been easy, and a continuation of it was to be expected. It is a matter of interest that social conferences held over this case left most of the conferees in a dubious frame of mind. Upon reference to medical experts, one could only point out the dangerous menace of the girl's syphilis to the community, whilst another physician, upon clinical data alone, felt inclined to think that the girl must be somehow "feeble-minded," and still another advised a reformatory. Rose was, in fact, for a time maintained in a home for wayward girls, but had such spells of violence here that she could not be managed.

The technique of the social treatment of Rose Talbot was briefly as follows: The girl left her husband one day in 1915 in a temper (due to the suggestion that she live with her mother-in-law) and tried, as a waitress, to support herself and child. She made application to the charity authorities for the support of her child several months later and the child was boarded out. She was thus under the eye of social workers, one of whom, under a misapprehension (as we now see the problem) had her arrested as above noted. She was then put on probation and placed in a home for wayward girls where came those spells of violence which now began to indicate that Rose Talbot was not to be a simple case of delinquency. At a special conference the majority of social workers agreed that her case was, for the present at least, a hopeless one and that although there were definite psychopathic elements, the only available policy was to wait for the "overt act" which would eventually allow her commitment and internment in some receptacle for delinquents. Meantime, the baby would, of course, become a public charge and minor ward of the state. It was already obvious to the social worker specializing in the management of psychopathic cases that this hopeless point of view was logically not well founded. Not only had there been previous experience of relative, and often absolute, social readjustment in cases of this general group of psychopathic sex delinquents, but also there were special features (considerable intelligence and well-developed self-respect and good general judgment in most matters outside the sex sphere) that made the social prognosis of Rose Talbot not absolutely dark.

Nevertheless, no psychiatric social policy was at once adopted. Rose was still carried on the books of the probation office. A job for her as waitress in the country was got, and she paid her child's board. She had promiscuous sex relations with boys about the place. (With unwarranted hope for sex hygiene and with a technique not advocated by social workers, an internist who had known the girl wrote a letter to the public health authorities of the town where she was; rather naturally nothing came of this letter.) Social workers, without psychiatric training or point of view, had previously made an endeavor to have the girl arrested as a prostitute.

However, it happened that Rose had already become friendly with a psychiatric social worker and had become well disposed to the Psychopathic Hospital on account of the unexpectedly gracious way in which she had been met by the physicians. In friendly, unofficial correspondence, Rose would write such sentiments as the following:—

July 24, 1916

"But perhaps I'd better tell you my honest, way-down-deep reason for writing. You did seem to understand me so well while I was there. Now please, Miss Carroll, I am trusting you so thoroughly. Please don't tell. Oh, I know I shouldn't write or tell anyone, but it does so prey on my mind. I'm trying so hard to be good. Course it's lots easier than at first, but I want so much to be bad. I actually get sick fighting temptation. Why it's almost like a curse or horrible misfortune. I'm afraid I didn't inherit a very good supply of will-power. One thing I am learning good is to control my tongue. And that's what puzzles me. Now, my tongue is learning to behave quite nicely, but my passions are the most unruly I ever encountered. And it is by the most tremendous effort that I keep good. But then I can be thankful that there's a little improvement. My first month at Trinity House was a veritable night-mare. A most hideous month. And I know if I give in now I shall have the fight to do all over again, or else continue to be bad, and with no helping hand near, it is impossible to be good, once I start bad. But then, I shan't, because I vowed to God that I never would. He will keep me good, won't He? Do answer soon cause I'm so tempted. And it's impossible to leave. I'm most stranded and Betty's board one month in arrears. Do think over the possibilities of my becoming a nurse and advise, your sorely tempted, trusting friend."

July 28, 1916

   . . . "But I will be good, for if I give in I might just as well throw up my hands. And besides, God would punish me if I broke my oath, wouldn't He? When I was in my cell at James Street, waiting for trial, I swore to God never to commit adultery or fornication again. I couldn't break that, could I? Yet if He wishes me to be good why, oh why, will he allow me to have such horrible unruly passions. And after all my prayers! I want so very much to be bad. At times I ache all over, I feel if I only could be bad just once, awfully bad, I'd be quite happy and satisfied. He's a student. Treats me with an almost brotherly affection. It is such a relief to be able to tell you everything. . . . And I'd give in so quickly only I do want to be good, and am scared too. I was so much happier before in my ignorance than I am now with my eyes open. I do feel so sick and miserable all the time."

August 3, 1916

   "Mrs. W. is going to send me a couple of pictures of Betty. I can hardly wait for them. I shall be so glad when I am home with her again. I'm just crazy about the little kiddo. I just love to work for her now. At one time I was feeling kind of provoked to think I could never spend much for clothes, but since I came so near losing her, and after being confined at Trinity House, it's just wonderful to be free and working for her. I'm being so awfully good, not even thinking bad. You see, it is just once in a while I have those spells, and they seem so terrible at the time they frighten me, but now, looking back, it was nothing and confiding in you has helped so very much. I am so glad I have you for a friend and true confidant. It is just like a headache (a thing I rarely have) but when I do I think I'm killed. But there, I've troubled you long enough with 'I.'"

August 28, 1916

"I've read Casqueline's (I think it is spelled) *Truth about Woman* and Havelock Ellis' *Psychology of Sex* which quite knocked all my good resolutions to smash. You see it was really the religious side of me that was keeping me good, and my fear of God. But Casqueline states that religion has nothing to do with a woman being bad.—So you see it is not wicked to have sexual intercourse with other men than your husband. It is merely not the fashion.

"Now with you saying to be good and this book to give free rein to any and all impulses and passion, what is one to do? Especially when there is so much bad in them, and if I was bad it would be to satisfy my own natural cravings. And I feel so much more fit, mentally and physically.

"But, my gracious, please don't tell Miss Ford, that I've been talking in this strain or they'll become alarmed, which is quite unnecessary since I've no intention of being bad yet.

"Grandma says she'll be very glad to see me and I'm going to live with her and Betty."

September 24, 1916

"Sometimes I'm almost tempted to marry him. Oh, dear, I do hope I keep a level head and not do any more foolish stunts. And besides I simply cannot marry. Anyhow, I merely like him and am by no means fond of him. Now, aren't you pleased to hear I'm not going to be bad, I mean, give in to sexual desire?"

November 6, 1916

"Now, Miss Carroll, this is an honest fact, that just as soon as I start my prayers at night and feel spiritually good, something always turns up to make me doubly bad. Last evening I felt awfully good and said my prayers with the baby and felt that I'd never be bad again, and behold, this morning, I awoke worse than ever."

January 5, 1917

"I really don't think I'll be bad, maybe once in a great, great while, but not in the promiscuous manner I have been. I just wish I could explain. I don't think I can, yet you're the only one to whom I could begin to explain. It is all on account of working in the rubber shop and wearing that peachy dress you gave me. Don't think that I'm all fussed up over myself, but just the same, I *am* nicer than any worker in my department, or in fact, that I've seen here.

"My thoughts run ahead of my pen. Of course I couldn't make it clear anyhow because it's not quite clear to me. I've a great conceited bump on myself. Just a wee bit too nice to be bad. I've thought of it a good deal and seems to me I've had symptoms a way back, but lately they are becoming no end developed!"

March 17, 1917

"We have broken partnership, it really was that you know. There we were, two perfectly mated, physically and mentally— human beings, each desiring one of the opposite sex without the binding and restraining tie of marriage. It really is too bad. He was awfully decent and I liked him thoroughly, in fact could almost say it was a good like. And again I say it is too con- founded mean that one can't have free love, or at least until the children come. But there, I shall have to see you to tell you all about it."

July 4, 1917

"Am going to dress Miss Betty up and take her for a visit. Oh, I do love her so much, so very much, that I have no room for any one else, which is rather good, considering I have been thru so many 'puppy loves'!"

October 14, 1917

"Yes I do (*i.e.* love her divorced husband) and suppose I always will. Time hasn't done much healing in my case, but I do think that God has given me a pretty poor hand, perhaps in the next deal it may be filled with brightness and I shall live and enjoy a happy old age, that is, if I do live. I strongly contem- plate suicide in every moody spell, and I feel quite justified for does not our Lord say 'Come ye who are weary and heavy-laden and I will give ye rest.' So why not accept such a wonderful invitation. Still I rather think I am too much of a coward."

There seems to be no reason why the sentiments of these letters should not be taken on their face value. When Rose was dropped from the books of the Probation Office, she felt that she still required counsel and voluntarily applied to the Psychopathic Hospital for supervision. During a period of two years that she has since been under the hospital's official care her life and aims have pursued a gradual up-gradient. She became aware that her intelligence was superior to that of her fellow mill workers (she had betaken herself to work in a rubber factory, somewhat against her wish for less confining work) and herself got the idea of going into telegraphy. She is now, at the end of these two years, getting seventy-five dollars per month, is paying for the maintenance of her child in the (paternal) great-grandmother's home, and is living a much more promising and orderly life than anyone could have predicted. A peculiarity of the situation is that she is now living with her divorced husband once more. The question of marriage has indeed been raised, but it is the girl, rather than her former husband, who remains in doubt of the wisdom of the procedure. To be sure, her syphilis is as well in hand as can be contrived; at all events, her blood serum test has now remained normal for some time.

Let us now analyze the Talbot case in two ways. First let us analyze it briefly, after the manner of the first part of this book, namely, as to the existence of public, social, and individual factors in the case, and their relative importance. We may then follow the analysis, according to spheres of community influence, with a further analysis according to the distribution of the various evils shown by the case, thus introducing the topic of Book II. It goes almost without saying that a case as complicated as that of Rose Talbot must have planes of contact of both a public and a private nature. We may count as of a public nature, for example, her arrest for adultery, socially ill advised as that arrest may have been. As of a social (non-public nature) we must count her promiscuity in sex relations and her quarrelsomeness with her spouse. The divorce complications touch both governmental authorities on the one hand and the more private social relations on the other. As the history of the case shows, very possibly the sex promiscuity and even the girl's quarrelsomeness, socially difficult problems though they are, may well be regarded as fundamentally of a medical nature. If hypersexuality and irritability are not regarded in the lay mind as necessarily examples either of mental disease or of mental defect, nevertheless, from the psychiatric standpoint and from the standpoint of the psychiatric social worker, these tendencies are coming more and more to be regarded as essentially psychopathic. Even if we, in the end, come to regard them as eccentricity rather than psychopathy, nevertheless cases of sex appetite and cases of anger instinct can best be understood in psychopathic terms. The public and private factors of this case, or (to use our preferred tri-partition of factors) the public, social, and individual factors of this case are not only all well represented but are commingled in such wise that it is extremely difficult to "factor" them out, as they say in books of arithmetic. The factors unite in a complex unit which is not the result of summation as much as of multiplication.

Without delaying upon the further analysis of the Talbot case from the standpoint of community influences (see, for examples of such analyses, cases of Book I, *e.g.*, case 4) let us consider her from the standpoint of the evils. This is not the place to descant either upon the completeness of our list of evils or upon its exactitude. The appraisal of this manner of analysis may be postponed, nor shall we be prepared to discuss it fully until the medical data of Book III are well in mind. As briefly in Book I, we proceed to a study of the medical, educational, moral, legal, and economic factors, under the guise of the evils of disease (Morbi), ignorance (Errores) vices and bad habits (Vitia), crime and delinquency and other forms of legal entanglements (Litigia), and poverty and other forms of resourcelessness (Penuriae). The medical side of Rose Talbot is evident; character defects and certain overemphases of instinct, to say nothing of syphilis. The educational deficiency in Rose Talbot is most obvious and stands out the more clearly because she was by no means feeble-minded and, in fact, responded notably well to the instructions given her, at first by the psychiatrist and later by the psychiatric social worker. It was clear, too, that in addition to an educational deficiency (both in the matter of school life and home instruction) there was a pronounced moral deficiency It is not incumbent on us to determine here (or perhaps anywhere in this book) whether there is a distinction between intellectual and moral education, and no doubt many of the moral deficiencies, so obvious in these cases, are not only grounded in lack of information or in misinformation, but can be abolished, almost at a blow, by suitable teaching of a very ex-cathedra type. But Rose's moral deficiencies were in spheres of emotion, which mere instruction out-of-hand could not relieve. In point of fact a good deal of her difficulty may be assigned to disease and not to mere inadequacy of moral training. It will be remembered that there was much to go upon. There was the girl's rather lively self-respect in all matters save those of sex, and even in the sex sphere there was finally developed the monogamous trend. The rather extraordinary improvement in what one might term the individual "morale" of Rose Talbot when a certain blue serge dress was given her (see letter in text) cannot readily be ascribed to education of the intellectual sort. That singularly successful step on the part of the psychiatric social worker was an ethical, rather than a psycho-logical, step.

It is clear that in trying to distinguish between the medical, intellectual, and moral deficiencies in a case like this we approach fundamentals in the definition of medicine, education, and ethics, definitions which are not always easy to get in textbooks of these disciplines. When we approach the fourth group, delinquencies, we naturally find the plot to thicken appreciably, as we have, indeed, the choice of regarding the delinquencies of Rose as, on one hand, purely medical in origin, and therefore not delinquencies, or on the other hand as due purely to faulty education (and therefore hardly matters for which she could be called to serious account), or even as matters of poor moral training (wherein again, the handling of the case as criminal or legal would not serve the turn). But in what consists the delinquency or legal entanglement in this broad sense? We are using the idea in a purely practical way. We shall find it desirable to analyze each case in succession from all of these standpoints. For practical purposes, no one can deny that it is important for the psychiatrist and for the psychiatric social worker to consider the legal entanglements and the methods of fighting them which are brought up by any case which demands social consideration and social management.

So again, when we consider the economic disabilities of Rose Talbot (with her lack of knowledge of a trade at the outset, her syphilis to be medically and perhaps expensively treated, and her child, also syphilitic) we need not deny that another lot in life would have entirely altered the complications of her particular fate, but the fact that good middle-class surroundings would have changed this particular fate does not necessarily mean that economics is the sole, or even the leading, feature in the whole circumstances. Accordingly, we find in Rose Talbot, good examples of what, upon common-sense grounds, we must

regard as deficiencies in all five fields of evil, as we have chosen
to name them.   The order in which these fields of evil have
been laid down is also, we surmise, not more ultimate than the
fields of evil themselves.   In fact, in social work at large, it
has always been thought that the economic factor must take
a leading place.   It is our impression that even in general social
work (and many social workers agree with us) the economic
factor is often, if not in a majority of cases, outweighed by one
or more other factors of evil that we here list.

Perhaps it is worth while to make one or two further comments upon Rose Talbot.   Her improvement under social-
psychiatric treatment was remarkable enough, particularly as
she had been *an unsolved problem with no less than three agencies before she was studied and treated from the psychiatric
point of view.*   It would be less easy to define exactly in what
the social-psychiatric treatment of Rose Talbot consisted, and
perhaps we had, at this point, best fall back on saying that the
fons et origo of the success lay just in the "point of view."   It
might also be inquired how genuinely successful the treatment
has been, and no doubt the Greek warning, that we can scarcely
assign happiness to a life until it is ended, is a warning that
we should particularly heed in social work.   At the risk of
repetition, let us insist again upon the extraordinary contrast
between the girl's genuine self-respect and her *amoralia,* or
what the old English psychiatrist Pritchard might have termed
"moral insanity."

It is of subordinate nature, perhaps, that during the years
of psychiatric social treatment, Rose has been under the personal charge of four social workers in succession and has,
nevertheless, responded properly to all four, despite their own
differences in personality.   This brings out strongly the point
we above made, namely, that *the success in treatment depends
more upon the point of view than upon the personality of
the worker.*   We know that such a statement as that in the
previous sentence may well be regarded as revolutionary by
some authorities who very particularly point out the great importance of the personal relation, the relation of being *en
rapport* in these subtle forms of psychotherapy.   (Of course
another way of controverting this revolutionary point of view
of ours would be to say that all four of our workers were, as
it were, of a superior quality!   This the psychiatrist might

be compelled to concede. Yet it is true that persons of a very special nature are just the persons that remain in psychiatric social work, at least in its responsible phases.) It is not so much the point of view of the worker as it is difficulties in effecting the new contacts entailed by the shifting. This at least is our general experience, into which we cannot here farther go. In point of fact, it would be singularly unlucky if the only personal relation which the psychiatric patient could successfully maintain with social work should be a relation with but one human soul, since, in the nature of things, in the course of years (and these cases are year-long in their symptoms and demand for treatment) there must be effected a number of such transfers of control.

Another subordinate point in the technique of social work in the case of Rose Talbot, is the singularly small part which, in appearance at least, the psychiatrist plays in the details of treatment, in fact, the general course of social treatment is not, in this case, one specially conducted by the psychiatrist; it was rather, the duty of the psychiatric social worker, on the basis of the medical diagnosis, to proceed to establish proper general lines of treatment. It is entirely doubtful in our minds whether a physician, either male or female, could have gotten into the right relations with Rose Talbot.

Hours spent by	Medical record, 23 pages
	Social record, 49 pages
Physician, 4	Social work:
	Visits, 37
Psychologist, 1	Interviews at hospital, 11
	Telephone calls, 14
Social worker, 102	Letters, 28

FEEBLE-MINDED YOUTH

24 YEARS

(BY MENTAL TESTS 9.3)

1915	*1916*
Unemployment	Employed
Homelessness	Good Home
No Income	Good Wages
Estrangement from Relatives	Reconciled to Relatives
Recidivism (Larceny)	
Arrest (Arson)	Stealing
Probation	Disappeared

1917
U. S. Marine

Feeble-minded recidivist who set a fire. On probation ran away. Later corporal of marines.

Case 9. Thomas Fuller's real name was Michael Kelly. Thomas was a reformatory boy and after he left the reformatory chose to avoid its stigma by assuming his mother's name. He was twenty-four when we first came into contact with him after his arrest for "maliciously burning a dwelling-house." We present him as a paradigm of evils, not quite so progressive as his predecessor in this series, Rose Talbot, for Thomas Fuller, despite the fact that he measured less than ten years by the psychometric tests, got on well enough in the economic sphere. He showed signs, however, of trouble in each of the other four fields, medical, educational, moral, and legal.

To be sure, there was no obvious sign of disease in Thomas. He looked younger than his years, but was of a stocky and well set-up build, as indeed, the United States government was eventually to find and to exult in. But from our chosen point of view, we must regard his low mental age as a medical disability.

Thomas Fuller's father had long since disappeared, leaving, at the time of our first observation of Thomas, three sisters in the late teens. The mother, who had cared for the children until Thomas was fifteen, had died in an almshouse; the younger children had been left in an orphan asylum by the father, who then vanished from the scene. Thomas got no schooling until his twelfth year, with a little further schooling at the age of fourteen, and with three years of reformatory life in the late teens. The boy's moral training had suffered throughout such a life. The marvel is that his moral adequacy could, in the long run, be maintained. His arrest for "willfully and maliciously burning a dwelling-house" was but a single episode, and unlike phenomena in some of our psychopaths, could not be regarded as in any case a perversion of instinct such as may be found in pure pyromania.

65

Fuller, one day, in a fit of despondency, set fire to his porter's uniform which lay on the bureau in his room. He had been discharged from his porter's job and apparently decided to let that whole part of his life go up in smoke. The understanding how this might be both the first and the last episode of this identical nature (as against the story of so many pyromaniacs who keep on kindling fire after fire, apparently for the gratification of a particular instinct) is made a bit easier by a study of sundry facts in Thomas's past life. Without going into these in detail, we may mention that he had at times stolen money and again clothing, and had even participated in a small "break" into a house with companions. He was, in short, a sort of youthful recidivist in a variety of not extremely serious crimes. It was as if a feeble-minded boy, not educated even up to his mental capacity, and with poor and fragmentary moral training, had become a delinquent despite himself.

In point of fact, the case, from the legal standpoint, was quickly resolved by the psychometric observations—Point Scale 9.3 years, Binet 9.2 years. His deficiency of mind was of what may be termed the truncated variety. The defect was an even and regular one, not affecting the years above the grade registered. Whatever intellectual and moral education could be given to Thomas Fuller must reckon with this fundamental mind lack. There could hardly be a stronger contrast than that between the cases of Rose Talbot and Thomas Fuller. The one was an intelligent woman, with much to build upon, both intellectually and morally, despite her hypersexuality and tantrums; the other was a moron boy, with no special sex proclivities. Both enjoyed, however, good physique, and both proved singularly accessible to social work.

Probably, in a large part because of his exemplary sex record, the judge who dealt with the charge of "burning a dwelling-house" did not even commit Fuller on the hospital determination of his feeble-mindedness, but on probabilities (or perhaps as a matter of speculation) he was put on probation and proved a ready subject of social work and remained a faithful supervisee for the six months that he was on probation. He was somewhat disheartened by the extension of his probationary period for a further six months, and a month after the extension was granted he disappeared from view after a charge (correct or false) that he had again stolen clothing. Letters from no address not infrequently appeared at the hospital assuring the workers of his continued success in life.

The dénouement was now to be altered by the World War. He enlisted in the marines and he wrote that he was now "some man"; that he was "satisfied and at peace with the world" and that he would "never forget his friends at the hospital."

We have a number of Thomas's letters, written in a large round hand. Almost always he begins "I write you a few lines 'hopping' to find you well as I am." Some extracts from letters with the war fervor are as follows:—

September 14, 1917

"MY DEAR FRIEND: I write you a very few lines. I hope to find you well, as I am. And that you will time to read the letter, or when you read it you may call it a book. I know that you like to read books so that all right. Well I like to write to friend's, So you are one that I could not forget, The old saying it a treasure to have friends. Well you would like to know all about me. Well hear gos. In the frist plase, I have maked good without no one help. It noting like trying to make good that me. I thought I like to be a marine, so I went in the U. S. Marine Corps, for luck. And I have luck all the way, so good. And I am going to tell you that I am now out off the past, and I don't mind tell you, that I am now "some man," And I feel like a man who has eaten a real dinner, very much satisfied and at peace with the world. What do you think off that. And let me tell you my friend, that I have not forgotten your kind advice yet. It is very indeed profitable to me. And started out to make good, I did you know. Well the last time that seen you, I have traveled over this world a bit, I rought it to france, Washington D. C. and I seen the best man that the big world of our love him, tell me the one that I mean see if you know the one man I mean. I love him with all my heard. And I don't mind tell you that I am now a man with some good experience. And I have live a pretty hard life. And I've been down pretty low, and now I am up, and that is what counts. And I have won out, I am going to forget the methods I used in the past life. I am going to make everybody else forget them. I want to enjoy the remainder of my earthly existence.

"Well Dear friend I will come to a close with this letter very. I am now in the U. S. Marine. And I am not Thomas Fuller, but I am the Private Michael Kelly. I would like very much to hear from a good friend like you Miss Carroll. And the 25th of Dec. 1917 you get sum thing from me, and if I go to war, you will have sum thing remmber by. Write and tell me how you are, and how very one. On my 27th birthday not one send me a brithday card. As I have no more to say this time I will come to a close.

"And to you My sincere appreciation to you and the good worker at the hospital.

"Wishing you all success."

September 21, 1917

"Well my Dear friend. I take the greates in writing to you these few lines to you dear friend. And was very glad to hear from you too. It was your postcard that you send to me, it is the boston state house, some place you know. And the State House looks very good to me, you bet. And I know that you wrote that card. I remember your good hand off writing, that you write. write again plase. Well dear friend I do not very well when I will be send to france but I may go any time to france to fight for freedom, and peace. And let me tell you that I will fight in earnest for our be love and dear presidend Wilson, the man off the hour. I like him with all my heart.

"And I will not forget my friends. I will think off them when I am over in france, and now I will not forget you as you are one off my friends. You said that they are knitting at the hospital for the soldiers. And you asked me if I could used and thing. Well I can used and thing that you send. I would be glad to get anything that you send to me. Will close hopping to hear from you."

March 29, 1918

"I write you a few lines hopping to find you well as I am. Well I have make good, as I am now an corporal in the U. S. Marine Corp, that mean that I am to get $6. more an month. So I am now getting $36. an month now. Well I am doing the best I know how, that whi I was make an corporal in corps. I hope that you will write me an letter and tell me how you like the way I am making good."

Hours spent by	Medical record, 25 pages
	Social record, 34 pages
Physician, 4	Social work:
	Visits, 18
Psychologist, 1	Interviews at hospital, 23
	Telephone calls, 40
Social worker, 50	Letters, 45

Hysterical sex delinquent, a persistent social problem.

Case 10. Bertha Greenwood is a case which we present as a paradigm of troubles in the medical, educational, moral, and economic fields. She is the second of a group of five cases in which the troubles are fourfold. Bertha Greenwood's case is less complex by one field of evil, according to our proposed classification, than was Rose Talbot (case 8) whose troubles were fivefold. Theoretically we should be able to subtract from the difficulties of Rose Talbot the legal entanglements and arrive at the case of Bertha Greenwood; so theoretically ought we to have been able to subtract the social difficulties of economic nature from the case of Rose Talbot and arrive at something like the degree of complication found in Thomas Fuller (case 9). Taken another way, the phenomena of Bertha Greenwood will have, in common with those of Thomas Fuller, three kinds of factor, and will differ in but one factor: both cases are fourfold with respect to their distribution of troubles; both have difficulties in the medical, educational, and moral fields, but whereas Fuller's difficulties were legal, Bertha Greenwood's difficulties were economic.

Bertha Greenwood, we must confess, for the present, after three years of social observation and attempted treatment, to be a good deal of a failure from the standpoint of psychiatric social work, but it is no province of this book to put necessarily the best foot foremost. Perhaps it is better to deal with the grounds of failure in sundry cases than to congratulate ourselves unduly over the most striking success.

The reasons for the failure of our social methods in Bertha Greenwood are obscure, but probably based upon our lack of grasp upon her attitude. That attitude is, no doubt, a psychopathic one. Her temperament is one of ups and downs that are apt to occur in waves of considerable length as well as amplitude. The term "psychopathic personality" which is, in general, a proper designation for this, as for many other cases, does not duly specify the peculiar difficulties, which are, perhaps, a compound of hysterical tendencies, with a cyclothymic (manic-depressive) tendency, expressing itself rather more in periods of depression, of weeks' or months' standing, than in any periods of pronounced elation.

In her periods of comparative normality, Bertha is extremely manageable, and amenable in some degree to suggestion, although there is not much doubt whether her promiscuity of sex life is continuously maintained; in fact, we are pretty confident that in her periods of what we term "normality" she shows neither any evidence of oversexedness, nor any continuation of sex irregularities as a matter of habit. Like Rose Talbot, with whose case, as above mentioned, that of Bertha Greenwood falls somewhat into line, Bertha shows a kind of monogamous trend; at all events she, for a long period, bore in mind and descanted upon a certain married man with \whom she proclaimed herself to have lived in sex relation. Our best evidence is that this ideal, or paramour, of Bertha's was fictitious. At one time she even showed a bruise of the face which she said was got at the hands of this paramour whom, however, the police failed to trace. We assume that her tales about him sufficiently indicate a degree of monogamous trend. In general she has been, and is, promiscuous in sex relations, and has even been pregnant twice (abortions). Except at times of economic stress, as after recovery from influenza, we believe that Bertha Greenwood, like Rose Talbot, has shown a large degree of self-respect, at least in the matter of not taking money for her irregularities. She is of good physique, and of considerable intelligence, at least of such a degree as to be able to support herself properly in her normal periods.

Medically speaking, we might wonder whether the diagnosis "psychopathic personality" was not, after all, far more vague than two other diagnoses which we might be entitled to make, namely—"hysteria" and "feeble-mindedness." To take the latter, and simpler, hypothesis first, we find that she grades psychometrically on the Binet Scale at 11.3 (actual age, at the time of examination, twenty-three), but on the other hand we find by the Yerkes Point Scale that she grades up to the adult level, or at least to fifteen years plus, which was the maximum to which any person could attain by the type of test then employed. The educational test of the Binet type probably yielded poorer record for Bertha Greenwood than her general efficiency would point to; moreover, we have in our possession a pathography or partial autobiography written by her which exhibits much more insight into men, women, and things than a moron is entitled to exhibit. The psychologists, it may be stated, despite the Binet grade of 11.3, gave it as their opinion from the psychological point of view that she was *not* feeble-minded. It may be parenthetically stated here that persons clearly feeble-minded (let us say in the moron division) may be sufficiently complex to show what is termed psychopathic personality. That issue we are not here raising; we are claiming for the concrete case of Bertha Greenwood that she is probably not at all feeble-minded and may perhaps be an uncomplicated case of psychopathic personality. Dismissing the idea of feeble-mindedness in the metric sense of that term, let us ask whether we could further define the case by stating that Bertha Greenwood is hysterical. It is recognized, on all hands, that the psychopathic personality may show hysterical trends; that (as French authorities call it) there may be a *forme fruste* of psychopathic personality which looks in the direction of hysteria. We mentioned above her appearance one day with a bruise on the face which she attributed to her ideal, but probably fictitious, paramour, a certain married man. That this affair was an hysterical one might be thought from the fact that she was picked up unconscious, or half unconscious. There are other, somewhat less well-defined episodes, such as fainting spells upon the street, and the resort in wild terror, to the house of a woman unknown to her. One night, in Boston, in fact the very first time that she devolved upon the medical scene, she was in a kind of stupor, out of which she emerged telling of her terror at a certain man. Could we see into the psychic interior and be sure of our observations, we might think of Bertha Greenwood as leading a sort of ideal double life, with an idealized monogamous companion of whom she stood in a sort of fear, that the light literature of the day is inclined to attribute to the so-called "cave-woman."

It will be remembered that in the case of Rose Talbot syphilis was early acquired. There might be more reason to suspect the arrival of syphilis upon the docket here than in the simpler sex life of Rose Talbot. Our serum reactions in Bertha Greenwood have constantly been negative. This is despite the fact that a medical consultant in private practice concluded from his examination that Bertha was suffering from local syphilitic disease of the pelvis of long standing. This physician went so far as to say that the nervous side of Bertha's life was secondary to the disease of her pelvis. He counseled operation and indeed thought such to be imperative. Another hypothesis concerning the nervous spells in Bertha Greenwood is that they are due to dysmenorrhea.

In point of fact, whatever be the pelvic complications in the Greenwood case, there is ample evidence from her early life that the psychopathic trend far antedates the immediate effects of her sex life. As a child she had hysterical spells of rolling upon the ground, and these began at about the tenth year and are thought by the patient herself to have followed a criminal sex assault. In the eleventh or twelfth year she is said to have become subject to certain sleeping spells about which we know little, although one of them is said to have lasted for some two weeks. Whether these indications proved hysteria as against some more vaguely defined psychopathic entity may be left undecided.

Let us now take up in order the items of Bertha Greenwood's case distributed amongst the four fields of difficulty. It has been a classical idea, somewhat shaken by the war data, that hysteria is essentially a hereditary disease, or, at all events, that amongst the relatives of hysterics will be found other psychopathic or neuropathic persons. We find in the Greenwood girl the second of five children of a rather alcoholic father, who worked irregularly and finally deserted the family, and of a rather slack mother, certainly ignorant, and possibly defective. The family was, accordingly, constantly known to a variety of agencies such as The Family Welfare Society, The Society for the Prevention of Cruelty to Children, the Children's Aid Society, and the like. In fact, we find that no less than thirteen agencies had to do, at one time or other, with the members of this family. With respect to heredity, we may conclude that neither the alcoholism, nor the wandering tendencies of the father, nor any actually known features of the mother, thoroughly prove psychopathic heredity, but at least there is a considerable ground for suspicion thereof. As for Bertha's own mentality, we must remain in doubt whether she is finally to be termed psychopathic, in some indefinite sense of the term, hysterical, or something else. Probably the psychiatric doubt which still exists as to Bertha is responsible, in a measure, for our inability to handle the case with as much success as the hours spent might seem to warrant.

Physically she might be regarded as an example of hyperthyroidism. The thyroid is palpably enlarged, the pulse is rapid, respiration is rapid, and there is a fine tremor of the fingers. Whether this thyroid situation is secondary to the sex-gland situation must remain doubtful, although modern work upon the effects of glandular secretions upon the temperament might be consistent with the idea.

If we turn to the educational field, we find Bertha's mother ignorant and Bertha at the age of eight with three other children placed out in various homes for some four years. Thereupon, at the age of twelve, she attended trade school for a time and then got a job which suited her. At the age of fourteen she began to work in factories in and about Boston and lived in lodgings, and at this time her sex delinquency began. Some quotations from her autobiography, which we give below, indicate her present educational status. She, in practical ways, has learned a good deal and has become able to earn twenty-five dollars a week in hat-making, and has held a variety of positions, ranging from six dollars a week up, for various periods of weeks or months, until such time as her alterations of temperament set in. As for her moral training and status, she has always been an affectionate, though not always truthful, girl. She has rather made it a point to keep her promises. There was, as is frequent with hysterics, a good deal of the histrionic about her attitude; for example, she would, half in earnest and half dramatically, instigate the appearance of social workers and a detective upon Boston Common to meet the alleged man who might be going to do her harm. Possibly this histrionic trend is more an intellectual matter than a matter of moral attitude; but the trend seems to be central in her moral life. Of course it would be possible to assert that her interest in the Ideal Man is a gigantic bit of camouflage; but if so, this interpretation would only be in line with our general suspicion that she is, if not hysterical, at least hysteroidal in her make-up. It is open to question how much proper moral training she got in her placings-out; or if she got proper training in these homes, she may also have got much improper training. Her knowledge of sex life she herself claimed to be practically *nil* at the time of her first intercourse, said to be at the age of sixteen (of course there was that other story of an assault at ten). If we classify the patient as falling importantly into the group of vices and bad habits, we ought, in all conscience, to be able to recommend some proper steps in moral training which might be taken, or at the least show why further moral training would be fruitless. As a matter of fact, we "closed" the case no less than three times on the basis of what might be termed its social incurability; but each time, at the patient's request, the case was reopened.

One of our most powerful lines of management was to find work and to secure good associates. These procedures were singularly successful for periods of a few weeks, whereupon the familiar lapse into depression and into the necessity or tendencies of sex life would emerge once more. The facile proposition for her disposal would be to place her in some sort of new-fangled and perhaps not-yet-invented institution, which could analyze her with absolute thoroughness and could secure some technique for overseeing the temperamental changes that are central in the social debacle. We can put the question whether the irregularities of sex life are matters of poor training, to be reasoned out by better education or smoothed out by improvements in tests, standards, companions who might be better models, and in general the entire morale. Whatever else be true, there can hardly be any doubt that the sex irregularity is grounded in something somatic, something temperamental. Whether this "something temperamental" is ingrained in the nervous tissues themselves, *i.e.,* in the modern medical language an endocrine matter, is doubtful.

The situation with Bertha is somewhat like that with Rose Talbot (case 8) ; but with Bertha there is far less of a nucleus of self-respect and far less will-power has been yet developed in her than in Rose who in the end was made to acquire the idea of "success in life."

Extracts from an autobiography that Bertha wrote for the benefit of one of the physicians are here inserted. Although falsifying was a leading tendency with her, she sticks reasonably well to the truth in this story of her life :—

"It seems that life has been one hard knock after another. If I had a few happy days there were double the days of sorrow afterward to make up for the happy ones. And yet we must live and endure till the end.

"My father was a good father in lots of ways, but like other people he had his faults. One awful fault which was responsible for all our unhappiness and the breaking up of our happy home was his liking for liquor. He drank terribly. I don't like to say it, but I feel it is the truth. My mother was to blame for my father's drinking, because she was so mean to him, always nagging and finding fault. He got discouraged and didn't care, then started to drink and went so far he couldn't stop it. I can remember when my father was good and never drank. He worked hard for us and was always kind to Mamma and us children. Then too later I can remember how he used to come home, at first only on Saturday nights so drunk he couldn't find the house and all his pay gone. Then he got so he was always drunk. Poor Dad, it was awful and I am so sorry for him. My mother hates him. Well, she may have reasons for it that I don't know anything about. I don't think my father is dead, and I have often wished I could meet him on the street sometime, somewhere when I am out. I would love to see him again. Poor father. That is another thing I don't understand in this life, is why people who love each other and should be happy together have to be separated. I will never forget the day my father went away for good. We were all in the house together (with the exception of my father). My mother was sick in bed, she had just given birth to my sister Jessie, who was only a week old then. My three brothers and I were in the kitchen sitting around the table, telling stories. It was early in the evening. We were right in the middle of a story when we heard a rap on the door. We all knew it was Dad, because he had a knock of his own, three little taps. We all ran to the door to let him in. We hadn't seen him for a week and we were awfully glad to see him then. My mother cried when she saw him, and she told him to go away and never come back, that she couldn't have him around any longer on account of his drinking. He didn't say a word, but we begged Mamma (as best we could) to give him another chance. But she wouldn't. She told him to go, so finally he started. I will never forget it. We all clung to him crying. I know he must have felt bad. He went away that night and none of us have ever heard from him or seen him since. That left Mamma with five of us children to take care of and none of us were old enough to work. So of course it was up to my mother to provide for us. She worked in restaurants or anywhere she could find employment. I being the oldest girl most of the house duties fell on me. I had to dress the others mornings and get them off to the nursery. We were awful children and I don't blame my mother for losing patience with us, as she often did. She would warn us to go to school in the morning before she went to work, and one of my brothers and I used to

go off by ourselves and play all day, and then go home to
Mamma dirty at night. We never even saw the school house
from one day to another. The truant officer was always after
us but Ma was never home to see him. Well, we were proud
kids and we did not have clothes like other children had, and
we felt bad about it, so thought we would stay away from
school. I remember one *uniform* I had, my mother's shoes size
six. Can you imagine a girl of eight wearing shoes of six, my
mother's skirt tied around the waist with a string and pulled up
over the top to make it short, and one of her old waists. I must
have been a picture, oh dear! When I think of how I used
to race the streets and all the things I used to do and the places
I went, I wonder that I am even half as decent as I am today.
Besides not having clothes, we very seldom had a square meal.
We were always hungry. In the morning I always got up
(because I was made to, not from choice). I had the job of
blowing the fire to keep it going to make a cup of tea for my
mother. There was never more than one piece of wood in the
house and often only one match.

"There was a crowd of us kids who always went together on
hikes. One day my brother and I got lost and Ma found us in
Cambridge police station. I was the only girl, and there were
eight boys with me, two of them were colored. When Ma came
to take me home I didn't want to go. One of the policemen had
made a bed on one of the benches for me and the matron had
given me a doll. I felt quite at home there. It was much more
bright and cheerful than my own home, even though it was a
police station. I was always getting into mischief. One day I
stole a red and white tablecloth belonging to one of our neighbors. They had their pulley line fastened to our window and
I took the cloth. I got arrested for it. The policeman scared
me and told me if I stole again he would put me away. We
didn't have a tablecloth and I thought it would be kind of nice
to have one. As long as we couldn't afford one, I thought the
next best thing was to steal it, but I decided afterwards that it
was better to do without one.

"After a while Frank and I were taken away from Ma and
put in a private family. We were very homesick. The people
were nice to us, but we missed the others at home. We were
sent to school in the morning and we went into the woods and
stayed till school was out, trying to plan how we would get back
to see Mamma. The people we lived with couldn't do anything
with us, so our guardian had to find us another place to live.
The second family we went to live with were not as nice to us
as the others were but we had to stay there. We were there

four years. We were on a farm. We were awful lonesome and homesick. Ma only came to see us twice in four years, and she had tickets sent to her to go every month if she wanted to. We went to school while with these people and helped with the work after school, I with the house work and my brother with the farm work. After four years we had to be separated. I had a chance to go to Hammond School, but Ma wanted me to go home and live with her. She cried and took on so, I felt bad for her and said I would. (That was one step I took that I have always regretted.) My guardian didn't want me to stay with her, but I thought if I could help Ma I would, she had to work so hard. I'll never forget the first day I came home, I was so glad to see her, I ran to her and threw my arms around her neck and was going to kiss her. She pushed me from her and said she never kissed me when I was a baby and she wouldn't kiss me then. I felt awful, I wanted her to love me; I was hungry for love. I would have done anything in order to win her love. But she didn't care for me. I couldn't stand it to stay with her. Everything seemed so upset and dirty to what it had been in the country. I went to my guardian and told her I couldn't stay. She made arrangements for me to go back and stay with the people I had been with for so long. But when the time came for me to go, Ma cried terribly and begged me to stay with her. I didn't want to stay because I wanted to make something of myself and I knew I never could do it there. But I didn't have the heart to leave her (another step in the wrong direction). There were James, Jessie and myself at home then. James and Jessie went to school and I worked. Ma treated my brother James so mean he didn't want to stay in the house in the evening. She was always nagging. He started to go out evenings and got in with a bad crowd of boys. They stole something one night and all got arrested. My brother was sent to a reform school. He stayed there for a while and ran away. They got him back and made him stay twice as long to pay for it, and the poor kid has been in reform schools and jails all of his life since then, up to a month or two ago, when he enlisted. He says now that as hard as it is, it is the happiest time he has known in his life.

"My sister Jessie started to stay out nights for the same reason my brother did. I couldn't bear to see her have the same thing happen to her that happened to James. I took her to Court and she was sent to a private family to live. The people have adopted her and as far as I know she has everything she wants and is happy. I am glad for her.

"When I was about sixteen years old I went out of town to

work in an institution for my board, room and clothes, just for the summer. It was on a town farm. There were all kinds of people there, sick, well and old. The people who ran the place had four hired men working for them. One of them liked me pretty well, or at least he thought he did. He tried his best to go with me, but I wouldn't let him. I did almost as bad though. He gave me five dollars not to say anything about it and I didn't say anything. I didn't fully realize then what it meant, but I realized soon afterward. I liked him and I let him do that right along all the time I was there. When I left there I was always lonesome for him, but wouldn't give in. I came to New York and tried to forget him. I tried to find someone to take his place. I was lonesome and unhappy all the time. I lived with my mother for a while, but she was mean to me and I left her. I met a girl that I grew very fond of. She liked me too. She was older than I. She was a bad girl, but I didn't care, I liked her. But she didn't love me as I wanted her to, so I had to make her love me. I didn't care how I did it. After a time I told her I had gotten in trouble with a fellow, so that she would sympathize with me. I knew she would. She did, but I had to pay the price. I had to go to bed and stay there for two weeks (until I was sick). I had all the blankets and hot water bottles in creation on me to make me sweat, and I had to take nasty medicine every half hour. I did this all for love and I would not give in and tell her I had lied. I bore it and kept quiet. She gave me the affection I longed for and that was all I wanted. She was awfully good to me from then on. I was quite happy while I had her to go to. She satisfied me in every way and we loved each other. I didn't want anybody else. Then she went away and I only hear from her now. She is so far away I can't see her. She is in Texas. Since then I have never found anyone to take her place, and I am lonesome and unhappy. I have lived an awful lie and I can't get away from it, one little lie has led to another till now it seems as big as a mountain. I have lied to so many people I don't know what I will ever do, and everybody thinks I am bad."

We have chosen to regard Bertha Greenwood as a fourfold rather than a fivefold case, and to think of her as minus the delinquency aspect; that is, the aspect of legal entanglements. To be sure, in one sense to be sexually aberrant is to be a delinquent (the terminology is still a little doubtful), but we are talking of important spheres of contact with the law. There were no practically important legal contacts in the case. There were one or two minor court appearances which have not influenced the main lines of her social treatment by the various agencies. It might be inquired whether the kind of authoritative supervision which courts could exert would be of value in such a case as Bertha's. We mentioned above that some sort of institution might be devised that would help, although in such institution we suspect cases like Bertha's would have to be the central figures. It is doubtless unlikely that the state will find itself able to build institutions around single figures of this sort. We are of opinion that, despite our relative unsuccess in handling the case, nevertheless no better results could have been obtained by judicial methods; that is, it would not have helped to have treated this patient as a prostitute and to have maintained her in prisons from time to time for punitive or correctional purposes. It must remain an open question whether, in so difficult a case, the "iron in the velvet glove" that might be afforded by a probation system would have helped. In some modern systems, the psychiatric viewpoint is, of course, maintained.

We turn to the economic sphere. Getting her work was, as above stated, one of our best lines of handling. Would Bertha Greenwood have been another person had she been supplied with a good-sized annuity; had she been, in short, somewhere in the third estate of the well-to-do? We do not see how either her histrionic tendencies or her depressive phases, to say nothing of the "man crazy" trends into which she would lapse from time to time, could have been ordered by a change of social level. Still it must be granted that financial worries may have had their subtle effects upon the body's functions, and in some indirect way have changed perhaps the thyroid gland, or even the sex life. Perhaps we should not reckon this case as very fundamentally an economic one. For example, it appears that no more than thirty-eight dollars were ever spent out of available funds directly upon the Greenwood girl; still her psychopathy, with its phases, was continually throwing her upon the brink of destitution.

We now turn from Bertha Greenwood to three other cases which will in succession demonstrate the fourfold distribution of the social evils according to our classification. From Thomas Fuller, in whom the economic factor did not come in question, and from Bertha Greenwood, in whom the legal contacts were minus or slight, we turn to case 11 (Lewis Goldstein) a complicated case of traumatic neurosis, in whom moral difficulties were practically nil, to case 12 (Elsa Albrecht), a case very possibly of dementia praecox, whom we may regard as educationally without particular social flaw, and to case 13 (Agnes O'Brien), a case in whom the medical difficulties were subordinate or exceedingly slight.

Hours spent by	Medical record, 13 pages
	Social record, 72 pages
Physician, 4	Social work:
	Visits, 133
Psychologist, 1	Interviews at hospital, 19
	Telephone calls, 80
Social worker, 293	Letters, 47

TRAUMATIC PSYCHOSIS
FOLLOWING INDUSTRIAL ACCIDENT

1915
Industrial Disability
Insufficient Income
Debts

1916
Compensation
Investment
Business Failure

1917
Irregular Employment
Minor Injuries
Charitable Aid

BEFORE 1915: ILLITERACY; IRREGULAR EMPLOYMENT;
BUSINESS FAILURE

Steady, illiterate workman disabled by industrial accident. Family case. Slow social recovery. Mental hygiene of industry.

Case II. We take up, in Lewis Goldstein, the third of our five cases, showing not the full display of evils in their fivefold distribution, but exhibiting situations in some respects less complex, namely a fourfold distribution. Whilst Fuller (case 9) showed no economic disability, and whilst Greenwood (case 10) was not, in any important way, legally entangled, the present case of Lewis Goldstein is one in which another element or factor of evil was lacking, namely the factor of moral disability. In fact this young Russian Jew of twenty-three years proved to be a man of high moral standards and ambition. (It would be almost true to say, curiously enough, that his high ambitions interfered a little with his social cure.) Goldstein was working as a roofer's helper one day when a twenty-five pound tar bucket fell from the fifth floor upon his head. He sustained a compound, depressed fracture of the skull. He lived for a time upon the weekly compensation granted him under the Industrial Accident Laws and did no work. The Industrial Accident Board, not being sure of the degree of disability or even of the existence of a permanent injury, sent him to a general hospital out-patient department, whose medical authorities assured him that he had not been seriously injured by the tar bucket and ought to go to work once more. In due course he was referred to the Psychopathic Hospital by the Industrial Accident Board, coming, as is usual with these cases, as a voluntary patient. Here the psychological examiners found that despite his twenty-three years of actual age, his mental age by the Binet tests was but eight and one-fifth years. To the psychological examiners he seemed to be a man of poor comprehension, diminished learning ability, practically no planning ability (so far as tests went), poor powers of observation and apperception, a memory of narrow span and retarded free associations. We mentioned these details of the

83

psychological results to show how general, or as we are accustomed to say, regular, was the mental loss; in fact, the exceedingly competent examiner thought that Goldstein's reactions throughout were those of a feeble-minded person of low moron grade.

Now such results obtained by the psychologists are, in these cases, of extreme value, particularly when we come to compare the results of one year with those of later years. Sometimes it is possible to trace the improvement of a patient recovering from brain injury most precisely by means of successive, properly spaced, psychological tests, but in the present instance, the psychiatric social worker examining the man's past would have been entitled to wonder how the diagnosis of low moron could have been made in a man who had been reasonably successful in a variety of positions and had even, at one time, managed a small business. He had been a steady and dependable fellow of good habits, cheerful, even-tempered, fond of his family. At a pinch it would appear, however, that everything he had actually undertaken to do could have been performed by a moron of a high grade. It would be a pretty inquiry, and one which should be carried out by scientific employment managers or the administrators of business schools, to classify types of occupation, particularly industrial occupation, with respect to the degree of mental capacity necessary for their carrying out. Possibly many of these industrial occupations range in their mental age capacity around ten years. Goldstein, however, made eight and one-fifth years.

Accordingly, although the mental level and the manner of its reduction both signify feeble-mindedness, the social inquiry inclines us to the belief that either the accident, or some other element in Goldstein's history, had reduced his mental level somewhat. The psychiatrist, reporting upon Goldstein to the Industrial Accident Board, putting together the psychological and sociological data, said that "accordingly it seems doubtful whether the patient could have been a low-grade moron before his accident and that it is probable that the accident is a large factor, if not the entire factor, in his present condition."

The medical examination showed some evidence of a skull depression in the upper occiput and there was a minor disorder of the reflexes upon the right side of the body, comporting with the probable site of the brain injury inflicted by the tar bucket. Upon investigation, it appeared that, after being struck down by the bucket, he had become unconscious, was cared for six days at the Relief Station, became blind a few days, later was cared for at a general hospital, and thereafter had been in bed for a period of five or six weeks, so that the total history of bed-fast debility was something like two months.

The prognosis given by the hospital was that "the patient cannot at present work, and for some time he will be unable to make anything like eighteen dollars a week" (his wages as a roofer's helper).

Although this is not a textbook of psychiatry, it may be of interest to the reader to learn how many symptoms such a patient as Goldstein may show between eight and nine months after injury. He came to the Psychopathic Hospital complaining of insomnia, of loss of appetite, of backache, of an almost constant headache; his vision was greatly impaired and he was most seriously troubled with attacks of blindness that would last a few minutes and be attended with dizziness. He would, under such circumstances, fall into the street and then take to weeping. He had become restless, irritable, readily angered by trifles, and thereafter lachrymose. His incapacity to earn money made him depressed and apprehensive. He described himself as having a tendency to chills and said that his memory was impaired. Several features of this catalogue of symptoms belong to the so-called vasomotor neuroses of certain authors, characteristically found after injury; the facile spells of anger perhaps belong to the so-called explosive diathesis of authors. Upon these data, the Industrial Accident Board, after a time, fixed a lump sum settlement, and the money awarded was put into a small store. The business, however, failed in a few months. Possibly its failure was due to the patient's becoming upset by complications following his wife's pregnancy and confinement in a hospital. He shortly became well enough again to work, but refused to take a job that paid less wages than he was used to.

We had Goldstein under supervision for some three years. By slow degrees he got back to habits of regular work in his old roofer's trade. About three years ago (1918) the case was closed, partly because other cases seemed to demand more from the social service than did Goldstein's. As a matter of the technique of social work, it is interesting to point out that no fewer than eleven agencies were called upon to deal with Goldstein. No single relief agency was available that could supply all the funds necessary for his family, which was ever on the poverty line. Steady relief for the rest of the family would have been the ideal background for the psychiatric social worker in the Goldstein case, but it is permissible to point out that there would have been no family problem of moment had there not been a central psychopathic figure on the scene, namely the traumatic neurosis or psychosis of the bread-winner. At one time we attempted to transfer the Goldstein family relief question to a general relief agency, but the psychiatric features of the whole situation failed to be grasped by that relief agency and the case had to be reopened by us.

Certain minor psychopathic complications are worth a word. Thus, the man's feeble-mindedness, or queer equivalent thereto, had something to do with the temporariness of his different jobs. Thus Goldstein might promise to apply for some vacancy and then do nothing further about it; then again he would, in working, run a nail into his foot, or strain his back, or fracture his wrist, in fact have so many kinds of accident that there can be little doubt that the complications were largely due to his low mental capacity. It is this kind of thing which, in industry, would go to make up a genuine problem that might be called the *mental hygiene problem in industry*, for it is clear that feeble-minded persons who have not had their mentalities diminished by the fall of tar buckets on their heads, may nevertheless very frequently be subject to accident. Of course, throughout all this talk about Goldstein's feeble-mindedness, it must be remembered that he is a fairly well built, well developed, well nourished man who presented so good a general appearance that, no doubt, any employer would be inclined, and properly inclined, to hire him on sight.

Our analysis of Goldstein from the standpoint of the distribution of troubles may be brief. The medical features dominate, whether on the one hand we point to Goldstein's original moronity or to his queer lack of mental capacity. The educational disability was not alone that of the feeble-minded person, but was also that of the Russian immigrant. With respect to vices and bad habits we can find no evidence thereof, except phenomena that might be explained more readily on the pathological, or poor education, basis. The legal entanglements with the Industrial Accident Board had a strong bearing upon the rate of social "cure" and medically there is at least a strong suspicion that the law's delay contributed not a little to the fixation of his neurosis. Economically he was forced to drop from eighteen or twenty dollars per week to nine dollars per week. When the lump sum melted, Goldstein was worse off than before. It is plain that all the phenomena in this case are so closely bound up with one another that the cure or removal of no single element in the complex will turn the trick completely.

Shall we regard him as a "successful" case of psychiatric social work? As hinted above, we should not have, under ideal conditions, closed Goldstein's case. At all events, we must say that he is decidedly upon the up-gradient once more. Whether we attribute this improvement to subtle mind changes due to the passing of the effects of his brain injury three years before, or whether we attribute the up-curve to environmental effects of assiduous social work may and ought to be left undecided. We say "ought" to be left undecided because scores more of such cases as Goldstein's ought to be on the social work record books of the world. Had not eleven agencies had to do with Goldstein, and had not the thread of psychiatric insight been shown in the social work, it is easy to picture the collapse in several fields of social trouble of the entire family.

Hours spent by

Physician, 11

Psychologist, 1

Social worker, 106½

Medical record, 37 pages
Social record, 41 pages
Social work:
Visits, 61
Interviews at hospital, 9
Telephone calls, 50
Letters, 10

Mother of two illegitimate children. Mental disease suspected. Referred as a "terrible case."

Case 12. The fourth of our five cases that are less complex by one element than Rose Talbot (case 8) is the case of Elsa Albrecht, who came under our observation first at the age of twenty-six. This case is one free from educational deficiency, and is, in fact, a girl of rather superior education. She

came to us as of the group sometimes referred to as "terrible."
During her three years in this country she had had two illegitimate children. She could hold no job; she was very shifty
and undependable in her accounts of her life; her responsibility was a grave matter of question. As for the illegitimacies,
she showed little or no concern over them, nor was the truth
ever learned concerning them. To make a long story short,
she was eventually dismissed from the Psychopathic Hospital
with the diagnosis of "paranoid dementia praecox," a diagnosis
which should probably be revised on the basis of further
observation.

We find in the hospital the following evidence which under-
lay the diagnosis that we now regard as erroneous: The little
concern which she showed over the illegitimacies, irritability,
resistiveness, overemotionality, hallucinations (history of three
years' standing), double thinking (heard her own thoughts).
Psychometrically she was regarded as of adult mental age,
tested by norms for non-English-speaking persons. Perhaps
the most striking feature in the psychiatric situation was the
alleged hallucinations. She claimed to hear distinctly the voice
of some unknown woman and sometimes other voices that
were talking about her in English, French, or German. When
the question of voices was brought up with her she would grow
somewhat disturbed. Toward the close of her stay she said
that she was not now hearing these voices so much since confessing about a false name that she had used. She talked more
or less about her conscience and its troubling her about this
assumption of a false name and of "voices" accusing her of
being false to herself and to God. Whether we are dealing
with definite hallucinations of hearing or whether we are dealing with pseudo-hallucinations is a fine psychiatric question,
but it would not do medically to ground a diagnosis of dementia praecox upon so slender a basis.

This diagnosis of dementia praecox must be accepted as a
serious thing in any social case, for once let the diagnosis
dementia praecox be grafted on any case and a sort of taint
seems to cling to the case for all time. This is no doubt largely
on account of the sweeping implications of the term "dementia."
Where the case should be put medically remains in doubt. We
are certain of many of the so-called psychogenic features, features that are found to some extent probably in all kinds of

mental disease, but which, when developed alone and intensively, place their victim somewhere in the group of the psychoneuroses or the psychopathic personalities with psychogenic features.

Rather unlike the victim of dementia praecox, and rather more like sundry of the psychoneurotics, Elsa made friends easily and even lay friends stuck by her through thick and thin, and especially through the complications of the two illegitimate births. Although she made lay friends so easily, Elsa was, in the eyes of social agencies, a good deal of a menace, perhaps the more so as she made friends so readily. At one time an attempt was made to deport Elsa as an undesirable alien. However, upon investigation, it appeared that she had, after all, taken fair care of her children for whom, indeed, she never failed to exhibit her love. Amongst other contrasts with which this case was so rife we should mention Elsa's own division of mind over herself, her future, and her children. She was, for the most part, self-confident in asserting her ability to care for herself and her children, worked as a governess to support them, and, for a long time, held the ideal of bringing them up as sisters should be brought up; namely, together. Again she showed a deep depression, in fact, such a degree of emotionality as was suited to her situation so that the psychiatrist would very naturally question her being a victim of dementia praecox. Another contrast in Elsa's case was that between her excellent general intelligence and her inability to keep a job. It might even be thought that a slight degree of wandering tendency was herein shown, although the obvious cause for each loss of a job seemed to be matters of her high temper and inability to stand critique. As intimated above, perhaps the strongest contrast lay between her general self-respect and her curious light-heartedness concerning the illegitimate births. She explained that she was, in each case, engaged to her lover and seemed to feel that these sins were comparatively minor.

The history of the social care of Elsa Albrecht is rather unusually exciting because of factors thrust in from without. Somehow Elsa veered from her attitude of keeping the children together for their growing up and decided to have them both adopted, if possible. The older girl, now four years old, was adopted by friends. The younger one, now two years old, went through the process of adoption, but there came about an annulment in the following manner: When these sudden developments forthwith came to the attention of the social workers, the warning was given to the intermediator for the younger child (who happened to be a physician) that the foster mother might properly know something of the situation. The physician agreed readily with this idea, and in fact, set about forthwith to have the adoption annulled. Whether Elsa had at this time contemplated the marriage with an Oriental that she now promptly executed is in doubt; at all events what happened was that she went to a distant city and got work. The social technique consisted in requiring her, on moral grounds, to come back and assume responsibility for the now unadopted baby. She came back, took the baby, and repaired once more to the distant city, where she married. The baby was then placed out, and provision made for her board to be paid for by the husband.

As a matter of the progress of psychiatric social work in the country, it is interesting to know that we were able to get coöperation with workers in the city where Elsa now is, so that due attention could permanently be paid to the upbringing of the child and to any complication which might ensue in the married life of a woman who seems to be undoubtedly some sort of psychopath. After an interval of two years the following report came from the social agency:—

"We have had a report on this case within the last month showing that the patient is fairly happy in her home which is comfortably furnished and well kept. You must have had a previous report on her marriage to Mr. R——, her subsequent worry over the fact that he did not make as much money as he did prior to their marriage, and also her upset over the death of her youngest child, Gretchen. In October, 1918, she had frequent fits of crying and was grieving over the death of this child and the adoption of Frieda the older one. In May, 1919, she gave birth to a little boy, Charles. The birth of this child has seemed to compensate her for the loss of the other two. Her husband is now in a better financial position than formerly; and when the patient's children were spoken of she showed no emotion whatever and seemed to have no regret for the death of the one nor the adoption of the other. She was very affectionate to her new baby and seemed very proud of it. About three weeks ago she wrote us that the baby was progressing satisfactorily, is now walking and talking and she herself is getting along nicely with her husband and is in good spirits."

To sum up from the standpoint of the distribution of evils, we have here a medical, moral, legal, and economic problem, without important educational complications.

Hours spent by

Physician, 3¾

Psychologist, 1

Social worker, 28

Medical record, 17 pages
Social record, 17 pages
Social work:
  Visits, 7
  Interviews at hospital, 15
  Telephone calls, 45
  Letters, 31

MORON, 29

HYSTERICAL, POOR HOUSEKEEPER

1915-1916

Forced Marriage
Jealousy: Separation
Another Child
Estrangement from Relatives
Unemployed

1916-1917

Child with Husband's
    Relatives
Under Public Care
Reconciled
Employed

Hysterical moron, divorced, with an illegitimate child. Such cases often known to social agencies.

Case 13. It is now our duty, for the sake of logical completeness, to describe a case without special medical complications, but one which shall show the four other types of complication with which we have become familiar. In a book on social psychiatry it is, of course, in the strict sense not proper that we should describe any non-psychiatric, or indeed non-medical, cases. Agnes O'Brien did show, as a perfectly proper ground for her appearance at the Psychopathic Hospital, an attack which it is probably safe to regard as hysterical; but thereafter her social care contained, although many difficult, no special medical complications.

Let us at first make her out as medical and psychiatric as possible. When she arrived, it was with a.history that her face had become twisted; that she was unable to chew or swallow and that she had been crying a good deal. These things had been going on for a day. She said she was going to commit suicide by taking poison; she said she was going to throw a pocketbook into the fire. Her sister-in-law thought that Agnes hardly knew what she was doing. She was a rather frail woman of twenty-nine who looked almost girlish. Her sister-in-law said that five years ago, when pregnant, Agnes had had somewhat the same symptoms. It seemed plain that they were hysterical in part. Examination showed that the girl was pregnant. Detailed medical examination showed the contracted or tubular vision characteristic of hysterics. Although Agnes claimed that she was unable to speak, and spoke of occasional paralysis of one side of her face, it was found that, when her attention was distracted, she could enunciate perfectly and showed no sign of facial paralysis whatever.

Thus, the first medical point to make is that the patient was clearly, though mildly, hysterical. The psychological examination showed that she was a subnormal person grading at 11.3. Her grading was fairly even; that is, she showed the

95

"truncate" deficiency of mind which is more characteristic, statistically speaking, of feeble-mindedness than it is of acquired mental disease. Perhaps, therefore, we should classify her as a more complicated case of social trouble; namely, as the fivefold case in which medical, as well as educational, moral, legal, and economic difficulties confront the social adapter. However, we are, convinced that many a social agency deals on non-medical grounds, and certainly upon non-psychiatric grounds, with case after case of this order   We believe that the records of social agencies the country over will be found to contain such cases as Agnes O'Brien's treated, and with considerable or perfect success, by the usual social technique. When perfect success is achieved in cases of this order, apparently from a non-psychiatric angle, we suspect that the technique implied is, at bottom, that of the psychiatric social worker. In the practice of social work, and especially in the practice of medical social work, the psychiatric viewpoint sometimes gets implanted subconsciously in the social worker's mind. It is a part of the program for progress in psychiatric social work to point out the tremendous percentage of situations demanding social work that encloses as a core some psychopath. Concerning Agnes O'Brien, we then insist that her case is not an unfair sample of cases handled sometimes successfully, perhaps more often unsuccessfully, by agencies that employ neither the medical point of view nor the psychiatric point of view.

The social technique had to take account, for Agnes O'Brien, of some place in which she could await her confinement. The attitude of the family, especially of the in-laws, was not too pleasant, as might be supposed when it is noted that the pregnancy was illegitimate. The priest's interest was enlisted. The first pregnancy, five years before, had led to a forced marriage, and now that the new child was on the way by another father, there was a threat of divorce by the husband. The legitimate child required care. This was managed by placing the child with the husband's relatives. Prenatal care was arranged for. Care during the confinement, care of the baby in its early days, and placing-out of the baby, were other steps. It was a little hard to convince the municipal authorities that this seemingly relatively normal mother could not well take care of the new child. However, the child was finally placed out. There was also the important question of proper counsel and encouragement for the woman herself. Aside even from the complication of her pregnancy, Agnes O'Brien was a rather frail, inert person, a little sullen and stubborn. At the end of a year the situation was somewhat as follows: The legitimate child was under the care of her husband's relatives; the illegitimate child was under public care; the girl had become reconciled with her own relatives, and to some extent with her husband's relatives. She could, from time to time, see her child with them. She can, of course, also see her child that is under public care. (Parenthetically we may remark that the monthly or bi-monthly "pass" system by which children under public care are allowed to come to the vision of their mothers by the public authorities of some of these institutions may be a necessary, but certainly seems a somewhat inhuman system: the better agencies so individualize their systems that the parents who would not be disturbing elements in the foster situations are allowed due access.) Agnes is, for the most part, sufficiently devoted to her children, at least to the first, or legitimate child, yet her temperament is such that a letter of the following description was sent to her husband:—

"DEAR WILLIAM: As long as you don't intend to do the straight thing by me, I don't by you. So come up and get your old kid or I will leave her some where on the street. I am half dead from everything and can't stand taking care of her any longer. Don't send that rotten old Jew up to me Saturday or I will insult him. I can't give him any money and try to pay back milk bills and back rent and everything. Come take your kid quick or you will see what I will do with her. I am smashing her, she is a regular pest. If I am going to live by myself I can't have a good time with her tagging after me.
"Your neglected
"WIFE."

But these sentiments of the neglected wife are entirely inconsistent with her actually idolizing the child.

Shall we regard the analysis of this case as essentially free from medical factors? It is facile enough to point out the moronity of this girl and say that feeble-mindedness leads to such complications as forced marriages and illegitimacies, yet it would be more accurate to say that feeble-mindedness is not infrequently followed by such complications. Certainly, however, no one can fail to be aware of sundry equally moving instances of forced marriage, illegitimacy, etc., that dot the lives of persons that are not feeble-minded, possibly not even psychopathic. Whatever be the truth of these contentions, we present the case as one in which four types of factor are predominantly in evidence, whereas the fifth, or medical, factor did not particularly influence, save in the most subtle way perhaps the social treatment.

Hours spent by	Medical record, 15 pages
	Social record, 32 pages
Physician, 4½	Social work:
	Visits, 43
Psychologist, 1	Interviews at hospital, 8
	Telephone calls, 34
Social worker, 86	Letters, 25

Deaf, syphilitic, unstable. Abusive and psychopathic husband.

Case 14. With case 14 we begin our group of threefold cases; namely, cases in which two of the five fields of social trouble are not predominantly in evidence, and we choose, for the first case, one with medical, educational, and moral difficulties, but without special legal or economic disabilities. The case is that of Margaret Hersey, whose social symptoms might be listed as follows: Marital discord, seclusiveness, deafness, suspiciousness. Margaret was an illegitimate child. Her husband was a sex delinquent and one of her stepsons was also a sex delinquent. It is of note (*re* general progress in the mental hygiene of the community) that Margaret Hersey came to the attention of the social service indirectly. First came to us the delinquent stepson who had gotten into some sex difficulties, not here to our point.

Abstracting, for the moment, from the difficulties of the rest of the family, let us consider the situation depicted in marital discord, seclusiveness, deafness, and suspiciousness. The psychiatric viewpoint would immediately try to connect up some of these phenomena. Psychiatrists believe that there is actually to be found in the world at times a so-called "psychosis of the deaf"; that is, a more or less well-defined mental disease directly depending upon sense-deprivation, viz., deafness. But psychosis of the deaf is not actually in question with Mrs. Hersey. The deafness was extreme enough and made communication very difficult with other members of the family. Mrs. Hersey may have been, to start with, a little paranoid; that is, given to ideas of being put upon, of being persecuted. If so, the at first indefinite ideas of persecution were, no doubt, driven further into her make-up by the deafness and her lack of power to verify or disprove sundry hypotheses about her husband and son.

Mrs. Hersey had been married at the age of twenty and was now thirty-eight. The very first night of her marriage, her husband was violent and abusive, and from him she promptly also contracted syphilis. Whether her deafness is syphilitic remains in question. It began about eight years after her marriage and grew worse some years later after her husband had struck her a bad blow upon the head. At one time (age thirty-three) the poor woman even attempted to commit suicide.

Medical examination showed that Mrs. Hersey had, besides sundry minor nervous symptoms, a positive Romberg sign and an ataxia of gait, both signs suggesting, with the rest of her history, a syphilitic involvement of her nervous system. In fact she had been treated at two general hospitals for this complication of syphilis, and at the time when she came under Psychopathic Hospital observation her spinal fluid had become negative—a finding which does not necessarily show that there is not still some active syphilis. There were also, in her history, two miscarriages, which might be thought consistent with the history of syphilis (though one of these miscarriages followed a trolley accident).

Deafness, incommunicability, suspiciousness, seclusiveness, formed a complex serious enough in itself; but it appears that from time to time she also had definite hallucinations of hearing, hallucinations, however, which she quite well understood to be perceptions of an imaginary character.

Our investigations showed that the family was economically upon a reasonably high level and that with proper family counsel that level could be well maintained. Perhaps we can indicate the kind of social treatment adopted in this case by the following notes:—

1917

9/28 Interview with husband to assist in persuasion for examination.

10/ 1 Interview with patient. Reassurance.

10/ 2 Interview with patient's mother. Encouragement and advice.

10/ 7 Interview with husband. Attempt to improve insight into patient's condition. Slight gain in coöperation.

" Interview with patient's son. Object: To appeal to his sense of chivalry.

" Interview with patient's daughter. Object: To suggest consideration for patient.

" Interview with husband. Object: Attempt to gain his coöperation by agreement to assist him in making a revision of his budget.

10/10 Interview with patient. Advice and encouragement.

" Interview with patient's mother. Reassurance.

10/17 Conference with entire family. Aims:

    1. To straighten out difficulties in misunderstanding over family finances,

    2. To give constructive advice along this line.

    3. To prompt a more friendly family relationship.

    4. To have all sides of the question presented impartially and thrashed out.

    5. To persuade that reconstructive measures should "let bygones be bygones."

    6. To encourage patient by suggestion of lip-reading.

" Dr. Basch interviewed to enlist coöperation and acquire possible evidence.

10/22 Conference at Horace Mann School to enlist interest of teachers and lay constructive plans for lip-reading.

11/ 4 Patient and husband interviewed. Aims:

    1. Financial advice given.

    2. A dietary manual given patient to stimulate her interest and enlist her coöperation in plan.

    3. General advice and encouragement.

11/10 Patient and mother interviewed. Advice and encouragement.

11/15 Patient and mother interviewed. Encouragement, advice, and reassurance.

11/22 Letter. Advice and encouragement.

11/25 Interview with patient and mother. Much reassurance.

11/30 Patient interviewed. Aims:

    1. To make plain continued friendliness.

    2. To encourage and advise.

    3. To give patient relief of fully expressing herself.

12/13 Letter. Encouragement.
12/14 Mother and stepmother seen in New York. Object: To secure coöperation.
12/23 Christmas gifts to the family.
12/28 Letter thanking patient for Christmas gifts. Encouragement.

1918
1/16 Letter. Education.
1/17 Talked with husband. Coöperation.
1/24 Lip-reading teacher talked with. Education.
1/25 Telephoned. Education.
1/26 Family seen at home. Advice, encouragement, coöperation, education for children, reassurance about treatment.
1/29 Letter urging treatment.
2/ 4 Same.
2/ 9 Same.
      Letter to husband urging treatment.
2/12 Telephoned (same as above).
2/13 Patient at hospital. Received treatment.
 "   Patient on wards. Encouragement.
 "   Telephoned husband. Education.
2/15 Husband seen. Coöperation.
2/16 Son, William, seen. Education of William in attitude toward patient.
2/18 Mother written to. Reassurance.
 "   Letter; arrangements for meeting.
 "   Mother written to. Arrangements for starting patient on trip to New York.
2/19 Letter to husband urging generosity toward patient.
2/20 Patient taken to South Station and put on train for New York. Reassurance.
3/11 Letter to patient. Object: To give her courage to tell husband that she had lost her money.
 "   Daughter taken to Dental Infirmary for dental treatment.
3/21 Telephoned to get patient to hospital for treatment.
4/ 3 Letter urging treatment.
4/10 Same.
4/24 Same.
4/29 Letter preparatory to visit.
5/ 2 Interview with patient and mother. Advice, encouragement, education.
5/ 8 Letter to husband urging that William report at out-patient department and that patient come for treatment.

5/14 Letter to patient urging treatment.
5/18 Patient and mother interviewed at hospital. Patient is
      finally persuaded to take treatment. Encouragement.
      Reassurance.

Let us call attention especially to the notes in the above
abstract under October 17; namely, those that deal with the
conference held with the entire family. That conference seemed
to straighten out a great many of the tangles. A very difficult
situation, the social care has now pretty well succeeded in all
respects, except in securing proper continuous treatment of Mrs.
Hersey's syphilis.

The reliance of patients upon the professional character of
the social worker irrespective of her maturity or personal experience was illustrated well in this case. The first worker
after several months of work with the Hersey family left the
department and the case fell to a young woman out of college
but a few years. The complications of marital discord with a
sex-delinquent husband might have caused the assignment of
the case to a more mature worker, if there had been a trained
and mature worker free to take it. The result, however, justified our faith in the ability of young women well trained to
deal with situations of even such deep-seated complexity as
Mrs. Hersey's. At one point Mrs. Hersey wrote the young
worker as follows:—

"You phoned Mr. Hersey last week—it had some effect, but
soon wore off, when he heard you had not been here. I do not
like to burden a young girl like you with my troubles but you
seem to know how to treat such affairs."

In analyzing this case for its distribution of difficulties, we
have tried to make it a paradigm in the threefold group. There
is no economic disability of importance. There is, in the patient
herself, no complication worthy of the term "legal entanglement." Of course, the characters of the husband and son
must be taken into account; these are doubtless also, in some
ways, psychopathic and may lead to important legal complications, even to separation or divorce. Yet all the complications,
aside from purely family ones, converge upon Mrs. Hersey's
sheaf of diseases: namely, syphilis, deafness, suspiciousness,
and hallucinations. In addition to these we found her somewhat deficient in general judgment and of a certain extrava-

gance in managing her household, but these deficiencies were such as to be rather corrigible by training. It would be rather difficult to draw the line in this counsel between a belated education, true moral training, and psychotherapy itself. So deaf a person should, long since, have been taught lip-reading, and her deficiency therein must be mentioned as one of Mrs. Hersey's educational disabilities. As will be noted from the above extract of the treatment records, steps were taken to teach her lip-reading. She was something of a moral problem for us, inasmuch as she seemed not to have the will to stand to her treatments persistently. Moreover she had been a nagging sort of wife.

On these scores we have made her a paradigm of medical, educational, and moral deficiency, but we regard her social problem as centering in her diseases.

Hours spent by	Medical record, 35 pages
	Social record, 35 pages
Physician, 10¼	Social work:
	Visits, 15
Psychologist, 0	Interviews at hospital, 24
	Telephone calls, 13
Social worker, 53½	Letters, 45

"Mystery girl" of the newspapers. Sleeping spells on the street. Feeble-minded, hysterical.

Case 15. Bessie Polski figured in the newspapers as a "mystery girl." The police officer found the nineteen-year-old Polish girl in a faint and brought her to the Associated Charities. Bessie said that she had been going to commit suicide. She had a letter which reads as follows:—

"I am awfly sorry, and am a Catholic girl, and know that I will lose my heart, but I cant help it because I am so hungry that I dont know what to do. I'm afraid to take poison but I cant help it because I cant live. I cant give another to my cousin because he said I am not his cousin [untrue]. I have not one cent and no money and I dont know how to live. I dont know where to go, and the next day I did not eat nothing for the whole day. I am a young girl, I dont eat nothing, only cry all the time. I have hurt my hand and didn't work for five weeks. Pleas who will help me. I am so poor that I sleep on the street, no one knows me, and I don't eat at all."

The statement about her cousin has been noted above as untrue and a variety of other statements failed to hold water. The day after the police found her she was brought to the Psychopathic Hospital and there was determined to be not insane (that is, in the medico-legal sense of not being committable to some receptacle for the insane) but to be hysterical. Bessie said that she was subject to long attacks of unconsciousness. Her "sleeping periods" lasted from a few hours to ten days, with convulsive attacks of laughing and crying and a localized anesthesia of the skin of the neck. Early in her stay at the hospital she apparently had another psychopathic sleeping spell which lasted about a day.

She now went from the hospital into the care of an agency, which agency tried to have her go to a state institution for treatment of syphilis, which she was supposed to have contracted (the blood serum reaction was positive according to the Wassermann test, and there was a slight, though distinct, evidence of inflammatory reaction, if we are to trust the cell count in the spinal fluid). Whether these findings indicate the acquisition of syphilis by this girl, or whether they possibly indicate that she was a victim of congenital syphilis (victims of congenital syphilis are not infrequently without any laboratory sign whatever of their syphilis) must be left in doubt. In any event, Bessie did not reach the state institution and further blood specimens proved negative to syphilis two months and a half later.

She went back home, and the case dropped out of social service contacts for about two months, when a rather extraordinary episode took place. While Bessie was going along the street, she was accosted by a man, to whom she said she was looking for work. The man said that she might go with him to a tenement house to meet his brother, the foreman of a candy factory who would get work for her. What happened in the tenement house was rape by three men. Bessie's outcries drew the police. The men escaped. The girl was held as witness.

Some convulsions shortly ensued and Bessie was brought once more to the Psychopathic Hospital, whence she was discharged, ten days later, with the same diagnosis as before, hysteria. She was observed in a so-called convulsion while in the hospital. The seizure lasted three minutes, during which she got red and gritted her teeth. She did not bite her tongue or froth at the mouth. Her attacks would in general begin with a feeling of pressure in the chest and a palpitation of the heart; then there would be a choking sensation in the throat, whereupon, apparently, unconsciousness would supervene, for the patient could not describe the rest of the attack during which she would laugh, cry, and toss her arms about. Curiously enough, the loss of sensation observed upon her first visit to the hospital was not now at all in evidence.

She went out to live at home, had an operation for appendicitis, and did not come under observation again until four months later. Then came the following newspaper clipping which may serve to show the attitude of newspaper men to the so-called "mystery girl."

"GIRL DEFIES DOCTORS' EFFORTS TO WAKEN HER

"Going to Sleep for Long Periods Has Become Habit with Bessie Polski.

"Bessie Polski, who goes to sleep for periods that vary from a few days to several weeks, is at the —— Hospital in sound slumber and puzzling the doctors. She lies in bed calmly, with her eyes wide open, and takes food when it is offered, but seems unconscious.

"About a year ago she had another long sleep at her home in ——, and was in a far more serious condition, as she was unable to take food, and had to be fed through the nose. Dr. —— of —— who attended her at that time, thought she was suffering from a form of hysteria. Her history, he says, shows a similar sleep of several weeks' duration when she was living in ——.

"She went to sleep on the sidewalk at Park and Madison Streets and was taken to a drug store, where attempts were made to revive her. Later she was taken to the hospital, where one of the nurses [sic] remembered that she was brought to the hospital several months ago in similar circumstances. At that time she was asleep for the greater part of five days.

"It is said that she has met with several accidents in places where she was employed, and that about two weeks ago she fell from a car at —— Street."

She was again observed at the Psychopathic Hospital, but had no longer any seizures and showed no further sleeping periods. There were no stigmata of hysteria. It was, however, decided that she might best be committed to a state hospital. The basis for such commitment was, not so much the hysteria, as the feeble-mindedness which she showed upon psychological examination. There were no marked irregularities in this examination, which gave her a Point Scale age of nine years, actual age nineteen years. Her attention was unstable and she was oversuggestible by the tests employed. In other respects she was rather generally deficient.

After a time she was released from the state hospital and placed out, but she could make very poor wages and was eventually allowed to go back to her family whom she aided by working in a restaurant. At last accounts she was earning a little money by working in a restaurant.

This case we present as a paradigm of triple disorder, medical, educational, and legal. The medical fraction of the count is clear: the two years' history of hysteria and the low mental capacity, not necessarily in alliance with one another in all cases, are no doubt combined in Bessie Polski to confuse results of social treatment and to complicate the economic situation. The educational deficiency was a marked one, centering chiefly upon a language difficulty, which was not merely the girl's own but was shared by all her relatives. A galaxy of Polish-speaking social workers might have been necessary to have made all the points desirable with Bessie's relatives. The legal complications with the police by reason of the rape attempts were dominant. It is perhaps well to say that not all the "mystery girls" who form so striking, if so small, a part of the psychopathic hospital clinic are feeble-minded. It might be inquired whether this girl, a probable victim of rape, a possible sex delinquent prior to her first period of observation at the Psychopathic Hospital, should not be considered as somewhat of a moral problem. Our evidence is, however, that she was, in general, not immoral in the popular sense of this term. We are not even sure that syphilis was ever acquired. In any event the problem of social care did not seem at any time to involve moral training. Bessie's "immorality," if such we may call it, was no doubt a matter of ignorance, and the total problem here was one of adjustment to the community, with due regard to the feeble-mindedness and hysteria on the one side, and the language difficulty and educational deficiency on the other.

There was no proper guardian for Bessie save the public institution from whose iron she might be saved by the velvet glove of social service. The only relative of this girl in this country was a well-meaning, friendly, but ignorant cousin, whose wife could, of course, not understand Bessie's feeble-mindedness, to say nothing of her hysteria, and assumed a rather hostile attitude to her. The proper answer to the Bessie Polski question was evident resort from time to time to a public institution. Obviously we cannot count this case as one of highly successful social practice, yet it is as well to demonstrate failures and negative results from time to time as always to put the very best foot forward. We above spoke of the desirability of public institutional care; but it is worth further specifying that the public institution in question should unconditionally be a medical institution and not of the prison system. The chief social service contribution in the case of Bessie Polski, then, may be summed up in the words "public care and supervision under medical auspices."

Hours spent by	Medical record, 34 pages
	Social record, 8 pages
Physician, 9	Social work:
	Visits, 6
Psychologist, 1	Interviews at hospital, 3
	Telephone calls, 3
Social worker, 11	Letters, 10

Grown-up "spoiled child." A motherly landlady found.

Case 16. Mark White is now nearing thirty-one years, but strikes one still as a rather overgrown boy. He is rather an inferior-looking shipping clerk, who came of his own initiative to the Psychopathic Hospital. He said he was afraid of crowds and that his memory was not as good as it had been. He dated his troubles from a time when his express wagon had run into a street car and stunned him. He had a damage suit brought after this accident. He told of hallucinations of several sorts, the absurdity of which he said he now realized.

Once he had thought a doctor had hypnotized him. He had very peculiar ideas about masturbation, which he said that he had done as a rebel against God and to displease God. The patient was a Roman Catholic. We found him to grade at 16.5 years on the Point Scale and to show few failures except in the memory tests; but in his memory he was more erratic than actually deficient. The question was raised whether he might be a psychoneurotic, or possibly a victim of dementia praecox.

A study of his family relations showed that he had been for many years rather extraordinarily dependent upon his doting mother's care; but she had died four months before he came to us. Up to this time he had been thrown only in the society of women of his mother's age and had made no friends amongst his own sex or amongst younger women. He was a sort of overgrown, spoiled child, a rather seclusive and very self-accusatory person. As for the hallucinations above mentioned, it is a question how gravely they are to be taken in the matter of the diagnosis of schizophrenia (dementia praecox). Certainly the notions about hypnotism and about masturbation are peculiar enough to suggest schizophrenia, and the so-called ideas of reference (people pursuing him on the street) might be used in building up that diagnosis.

He was discharged to the social service without a definitive diagnosis between schizophrenia and psychoneurosis. The ideal in such a case as that of Mark White might be to give him, in a popular phrase, some sort of "sublimation." The best social service could do appears to have been to give him compensation. A landlady of maternal type was secured through a room registry. Upon due explanation of Mark's plight, the landlady undertook his care. A position was found. The end crowned the landlady's work. Mark is now at least as well off as ever, perhaps better. Latterly he has even developed some fresh contiguities and interest in women of his own age. He became particularly interested in the nurse who took him through influenza. Formerly made fun of where he worked, he has now become well liked and sociable both with men and women of his own age. The socializing problem is going apace with the aid of church measures, the community chorus and the like. Aside from irritabilities at the doctors, Mark White seems to be approximating the normal.

Briefly analyzed, Mark White appears to be a threefold case

of social difficulty in which neither moral nor legal difficulties appear. His medical category must remain in doubt; but there can be no doubt that he is in some sense psychopathic. His curious up-bringing and maternal spoiling form an equally prominent part of the story; indeed some might claim that the medical difficulty traced absolutely and entirely back to his curious home environment. He was economically in the need of aid during the first months of observation, coming to us as an object of charity, with the history of being in debt and of having received aid from a relief society.

Hours spent by	Medical record, 42 pages
	Social record, 38 pages
Physician, 9½	Social work:
	Visits, 26
Psychologist, 1	Interviews at hospital, 13
	Telephone calls, 55
Social worker, 57½	Letters, 25

Alcoholic and syphilitic woman under the influence of divorced delinquent husband. Refused treatment. Aboulia (weak-willedness).

Case 17. Eva Collins, a sales clerk, thirty-one years old, is presented to illustrate the threefold combination of social difficulties: medical, moral, and legal—the educational and economic elements being absent or negligible. The prime medical reasons for her hospital observation were alcoholism and neurosyphilis. Indeed, her first diagnosis was that of locomotor ataxia (now universally recognized to be a syphilitic disease) and a "psychotic episode" due to alcohol. Mrs. Collins had acquired her syphilis from a sex delinquent and otherwise criminal (forger) husband, whom she had married twelve years before our observation of her, namely at the age of nineteen. It is probable that we must regard her as a rather indecisive and weak-willed person, and this native hypoboulia was at last to interfere gravely with her fate. She was for various medical reasons regarded as a most promising case for antisyphilitic treatment; but, owing to her indecisiveness of character and to a more or less ill-grounded desire to get away from the Psycho-

pathic Hospital atmosphere and sundry drawbacks of its publicity, she continued for but ten months under our social care
and medical treatment. Despite continual efforts our contacts
with her grew fewer and fewer during the last few months
before her case was closed on the score of her recalcitrance.

It is interesting to note that a poorer patient who could not
have begun to pay for antisyphilitic treatment would doubtless
have remained under our care despite objections on her part
to being hospitalized.

Doubtless under ideal conditions of social work, recalcitrant
cases of this sort would be pertinaciously pursued into the community so far as the rights of privacy of the individual would
permit. Relative to these selfsame rights of privacy, it is of
course a modern point of view that syphilitics of whatever sort
are hardly entitled to so much privacy as that which normal
persons enjoy. The house of a syphilitic is not his castle.
Moreover, we have to deal with a delinquent and vicious husband. It has for years been plain that only the very poor and
very rich get adequate medical treatment. Here Mrs. Collins
offers a peculiar instance of failure on the part of the moderately well-to-do person to get continued treatment from a mixture of pride motives, indecision of character, and husband's
influence.

Mrs. Collins felt that she was well-to-do enough to employ
a private physician, and this was no doubt the case, but in our
experience the proper tenacity of antisyphilitic treatment is
rarely shown in private practice partly for reasons grounded
in the old-time attitude of physicians to the syphilis problem
and partly because a patient without marked symptoms slackens
his interest in treatments that are on the whole rather annoying.

We have noted that the difficulties of moral adjustment
here were perhaps grounded in a degree of psychopathic indecision and perhaps also in part in the neurosyphilis itself.
There were also sundry divorce complications. When Mrs.
Collins first reached the hospital, she was endeavoring to secure
a divorce. Although she was prevailed upon to abstain from
her husband's company for a period of six months and although
the divorce proceedings were carried through, she reversed her
attitude shortly and began to get her alimony at the personal
hand of her former husband. How intimate her relations with

the former husband now became is a matter of doubt. Before we lost track of her, however, she had lost contact with her former husband and announced to us that she was now keeping company with another man, to whom she said she was to be married. Permanent loyalty to husband, relatives, physicians, or hospitals was apparently inconsistent with Mrs. Collins' character. These shifts in allegiance were regarded as probably part and parcel of the weak-willedness (aboulia) noted throughout, but it may be that there is a slight general tendency in Mrs. Collins of the sort sometimes termed paranoic, a tendency, that is to say, to the development of delusions of persecution. She was rather childlike in her attitude to ordinary affairs such as her money. After she was in straits about money, she fell into a sort of depression and thence into alcoholism. She drank with her husband. This lapse into drinking became ingrained and what might be called a conditioned reflex upon seeing her husband. Seeing him would precipitate a bout.

We have not up to this time mentioned the hereditary taint in Mrs. Collins; but when we put together the medical and moral features of her case, we are not unprepared to find that her mother and a sister had actually been committed cases to an institution for the chronic insane. The mother had suffered from involution melancholia and the sister from dementia praecox. Other brothers and sisters were normal enough. We have spoken of her as childlike in worldly reactions, yet she made an exceedingly high score upon her psychometric test, namely 18+, with a score of 93 points on the Point Scale. The only item of her psychometric record at all noteworthy was a certain degree of oversuggestibility. How far "oversuggestibility" of routine psychometric tests can be correlated with weak-willedness (aboulia) remains doubtful, and it is a stock and justified complaint that routine psychological tests have so far not quite measured up to our hopes of definite means of judgment concerning moral capacities and potentialities.

To justify our calling this case a combination not only of medical and moral troubles but of serious legal ones, we need refer only to the divorce complication. As a sample of record of social treatment we insert the following entries for three months :—

1917

8/30 Interview for purpose of enlisting patient's coöperation for future treatment by appealing to her intelligence and for purpose of bracing her up to point of decision of living away from husband. Friendliness of patient clinched by offer of visit to mother with view of arranging her treatment at home and incidentally gaining access in natural manner to patient's relatives.

8/31 Purpose of visit to patient's mother carried out. Family coöperation enlisted largely through offer of medical assistance to mother. Investigation made easy through this method.

9/ 5 Letter to patient to show continued friendly interest.

9/ 6 Encouragement of patient continued.

9/ 8 Patient's confidence strengthened by friendly advice which leads naturally to frank discussion on the subject of patient's use of alcoholics.

9/11 Lawyer interviewed for purpose of establishing good working coöperation with him and with idea of clearing his mind of any misapprehensions in regard to social service connection with case. Coöperation secured and constructive plan leading toward future change of work outlined.

9/12 Encouragement.

9/18 Evening call on patient for purpose of showing social friendliness as well as for purpose of sizing up patient's living conditions.

9/21 Visit to Mrs. Smith (an acquaintance of visitor) in hope of connecting her up with patient on friendly basis.

9/25 Letter to lawyer for purpose of keeping him informed in regard to social service interest.

9/29 Encouragement.

10/ 1 Encouragement and advice in regard to patient's family situation which is reacting upon patient.

10/15 Business course started according to plan of 9/11.

10/18 Encouragement.

10/20 Arrangement made for outside examination of patient by oculist in order to save working time and make examination as little of a nervous strain as possible to patient.

10/22 Encouragement and advice.

10/29 Call to show friendly interest.

11/ 3 Encouragement and reassurance in regard to situation in family of patient's sister.

11/12 Call for purpose of friendly advice and encouragement.

11/21 Conference with Visiting Nursing Association in order to gain their coöperation through explanation of mother's eccentricities.

11/23 Visit to patient's sister for purpose of getting over to her the fact that there is an intelligent and constructive treatment possible to use in the case of a boy of the make-up of her son. Patient reassured by this interview and coöperation of sister gained in making better plan for her nephew. Opportunity taken to straighten out situation existing between district nurse and mother.

11/27 Arrangements made with Dr. Jones in order to insure interest and reliable medical advice for patient's nephew on which to base future social action.

Hours spent by	Medical record, 30 pages
	Social record, 37 pages
Physician, 4	Social work:
	Visits, 27
Psychologist, 1	Interviews at hospital, 16
	Telephone calls, 30
Social worker, 46½	Letters, 25

Psychasthenic atmosphere about an eye trouble. Alcoholic, spoiled child.

Case 18. Hamilton Green, a rather under-sized, boyish-looking man of twenty-nine, came voluntarily to the Psychopathic Hospital at the suggestion of the social service of a general hospital. It was plain that he was in some important difficult way an "eye case," but the medical story would sound a good deal more complex if one took into account the indigestion, constipation, headache, dizziness, nervousness, fearfulness on the street, whisperings heard when going to sleep, temporary drinking to excess, "gas on the heart," and the like. Competent ophthalmological examination showed the man, who had recently been a porter and elevator boy, to have an actually severe astigmatism, such that exceedingly strong lenses were required. There was no small degree of hereditary taint; namely, a question of mental or nervous disease in the father, epilepsy in certain paternal cousins, and stammering in maternal relatives.

The second element in Green's case is the moral one. He was at times excessively alcoholic. But a more fundamental moral deficiency lay in his irresponsibility to his mother. Perhaps this is to be laid in part to his being a spoiled child. He was an only child. His mother helped him financially. Other relatives helped out also. Yet applications to the Associated Charities were from time to time made, but had to be refused because of these family resources. Finally, however, the mother ran through the small capital sunk in their house and mother and son became partial public charges. That there was a necessity, therefore, in Green's mental or medical condition is not likely. There was a question of moral attitude involved. This moral deficiency has now been in part made up through the counsels and insistence of the social workers. At this time it is fair to say that Green's own interior ambition has been aroused so that the social service splint may not for all time be necessary for him.

As for the economic deficiency, we have discussed it in general terms in the above paragraphs. After some two months of handling by the social service, no further grants of money were required for Green.

The situation now shows in the foreground the eye trouble, which is not only objectively somewhat serious, but has shown no signs of disappearing as an object of careful subjective concern. Green continually complains of the drawing of his glasses, of his not desiring to walk up a hill for fear of its rising to strike him, of his often misjudging distances, and so on. However, he has been prevailed upon to stick closely to a single eye clinic, and no doubt in the long run the subjective concerns, which now seem almost obsessive, will atrophy or gradually retire. Here we have an example of what is sometimes termed a "periorganic" situation. The term periorganic refers to the actual objective existence of a serious somatic trouble (in this instance astigmatism) around which develop by almost natural processes an obsessive or a psychasthenic atmosphere. Reference to the first paragraph of our discussion gives a catalogue of complaints forming this psychasthenic atmosphere.

Remarkable therein are the actual hallucinations, the hearing of whispers as he goes to sleep. These so-called hypnagogic hallucinations of hearing are interesting also in connection with the flashes of light which Green says he imagined after he had been dreaming about his landlady, whose rent was two months past due. Whether these phenomena are to be regarded as genuine hallucinations or as vivid fancies of a dreamlike world remains still in doubt. Some observers of Green have thought of him as possibly a victim of schizophrenia (dementia praecox) and would no doubt look upon these hallucinations or pseudohallucinations as consistent with that far more serious disease, schizophrenia, than the one we have elected to ascribe to this man. However this may be, practically all of the constellation of symptoms first set forth has now vanished, leaving astigmatism and its immediate sequelae in the center of the stage. We should make one exception. Green will still occasionally lose a job through getting drunk. Green claims that his drinking is somehow connected with his eye trouble, or at all events that the drinking habit is in general a matter of the last five years during which time the astigmatism came to the surface of his life.

Hours spent by	Medical record, 9 pages
	Social record, 17 pages
Physician, 5½	Social work:
	Visits, 16
Psychologist, 0	Interviews at hospital, 3
	Telephone calls, 9
Social worker, 28½	Letters, 12

Industrial traumatic neurosis in a competent steady family man. Family problem. Slow recovery with graded light work.

Case 19. John Flynn we present as combining medical, legal, and economic elements of trouble.

The legal elements in question are Industrial Accident Board complications. Although we have all along stressed the centrality of the individual in social psychiatric cases, we have not intended to give the impression that the family group is not equally in the practical eye of the social worker. John Flynn's problem would, no doubt, be very properly regarded as a family problem by the non-psychiatric social workers. The psychiatric social worker regards it also as a family problem (with even sundry psychiatric complications produced by the wife's ignorance or feeble-mindedness as indicated by her rating of 11.6 by the Point Scale) but finds the hub of the difficulty, after all, to lie in the psychopathic central figure.

The psychopathy in question was traumatic neurosis. By neurosis we mean a functional, that is, a theoretically curable disease, which, under proper treatment, ought to revert to the normality of the man before his accident. (It may be as well to say that traumatic *psychosis,* also at times suspected in John Flynn, means a disease of more serious character, often a condition of defect directly consequent upon brain injury, and hence, not to such a degree recoverable; and the rather poor prognosis early offered by the physicians for John Flynn himself was probably due to the suspicion that, *in addition to traumatic neurosis,* there might be some irrecoverable brain defect in him. The traumatic neuroses may be best classified under the psychoneuroses, though the traumatic forms of psychoneurosis offer rather special features.

A hundred pound weight struck a glancing blow on Flynn's head, causing a scalp wound. Flynn was not made unconscious by the blow. He has always stuck to the idea that the weight hit not only his head, but his back, and explains the persistence of pains in the head and back from that circumstance. Flynn was, at the time, in the midst of some rather complicated machinery. He saved himself by dropping some thirty or forty feet to another part of the machinery. He was able to work a day or two, but then had to give it up by reason of severe headaches and dizziness. The dizziness passed, and to some extent the headache, but he could not work, or felt that he could not work, on account of persistent backache. He did not arrive for treatment at the Psychopathic Hospital until seven months after the accident.

Meantime he had been in contact with the Industrial Accident Board, through which compensation was granted him at the rate of ten dollars a week, being six dollars less than his previous earnings. Some small savings he quickly used up.

There was no *mauvaise volonté* about Flynn. He wanted to be cured and made several unsuccessful attempts to work. The background was not bad. He had once been a hatter, earning as much as twenty-four dollars a week at one time.

Later he had become a machine oiler. He was interested in machinery, had been ambitious enough to attend evening classes for firemen, read and studied a good deal and had saved several hundred dollars. He was a good family man, amiable in disposition, energetic, and strong. Now, since the accident, he had become apathetic and seclusive. He read no more and was apt to be irritable when approached. His sleep was poor. He felt tremblings all over his body and felt sometimes as if his legs were going out from under him.

Meantime pressure was being brought upon the Industrial Accident Board to have his compensation stopped, as the medical examination by the company's insurer led to the view that there was no reason why he should not work. It appeared to his examiner that there was, or might be, a fixed idea of inability to work. Accordingly he was sent to the Psychopathic Hospital. There it was found that he showed some tubular vision, or so-called limitation of visual fields, a condition which seemed to us to indicate that he was either hysterical or inclined to hysteria.

The idea that he was suffering from a traumatic hysteria, that is, a traumatic neurosis of a rather particular nature, was also supported by finding evidence in him of sudden spells of sweating, sometimes confined sharply to one side of the body. This so-called "vasomotor neurosis" was another point looking in the direction of traumatic hysteria. There was also some evidence of diminution of sensory power, although no definite anesthesia. On the more psychic side of the man, his irritability, his fear of falling, and a newly acquired fear of walking in the open, to say nothing of a reluctance to working further with machinery, were other points fairly consistent with the idea of a traumatic neurosis. In short, John Flynn showed sundry features with which we have become so familiar in the so-called shell-shock group of war cases, cases in which, either with or without actual direct violence to a part of the body, symptoms of a general or special nature occur (the war neuroses, war hysteria, war-shock, shell-shock) and as in many of the war cases, the symptoms were somehow determined to a side of the body on which or near which the blow (windage) or sound occurred.

The medical diagnostician's impression of a case as psychogenic is, of course, tremendously heightened by the determination of symptoms to the side on or near which the exciting cause was delivered, since, by and large, a blow on one side (say the left) of the head, with injury to underlying tissues, should ordinarily lead to symptoms on the other side (say the right) of the body. This is not the place in which to go into the question of the so-called "mechanisms" of hysteria, yet it is of importance for the psychiatric social worker to know upon what a delicate knife-blade the diagnostic decision now and then depends. Another obvious point, here worth mentioning, is that amongst physicians themselves all such cases as John Flynn's deserve attention by special physicians.

As in all Industrial Accident cases, (particularly in view of their later possible improvement), the psychometric level was determined. He was not regarded as feeble-minded or as having shown intellectual deterioration, grading at 11.3 by the Binet Scale and 12.5 upon the Point Scale. (These differences are due to certain differences in the tests, which do not argue any fundamental divergence of opinion as to psychometric rating, but simply go to show that the methods of determining psychic levels are not yet absolutely *established*. The results are found trustworthy within certainly a year or so of the figure given. It is, of course, worth while eternally insisting that the determination of even a low level of intellectual capacity does not argue that the status is original; that is, that the patient is a feeble-minded person. The decision whether we are dealing with inborn lack or acquired loss of mind remains a delicate one, based upon psychiatric estimate of symptoms that pull down the patient's memory capacity below his normal level and of course must depend upon data as to the patient's social status. No doubt the previous record of John Flynn's life would absolutely prove that he was not feeble-minded in any ordinary sense of that term, in fact we felt that it was a certain psychopathic depression that pulled Flynn down even to the 12.5 level at the time he was examined.)

The prognosis was rendered that John Flynn would spontaneously clear to a large extent "within an unknown period," and it was added that our tests indicate that his feeling of inadequacy was rather an objective one, despite the fact that he had subjectively added a great deal of what the old books used to term "hypochondria." This suggestion of an actual objective feeling of inadequacy meant to show that the insurer's physician was, perhaps, not right in thinking that the patient was objectively able to work to full capacity. A diagnosis of plain traumatic neurosis would, on the contrary, have meant that Flynn would have been set down as a man objectively able to work though subjectively unable. There was, consequently, between the physicians, no issue as to adequacy for work at the moment *subjectively*.

The insurer would appropriately take the attitude that a man objectively able to work might soon become subjectively able (that is with the proper social or medical technique) and thus relieve the insurance company from its burden. There was, of course, no question throughout of simulation or a conscious "faking," as the man in the street has it. We are therefore dealing with a most delicate question of diagnosis, wherein the personal equation and acquired professional slant of the diagnostician must inevitably operate. But whether the patient is objectively unable to work, subjectively unable to work, or even (as in not a few Industrial Accident Board cases) actually simulating, at all events, the man is not at work. The Industrial Accident Board itself, having semi-judicial powers and impartiality of view (all sides of the compensation question being represented as a rule in its make-up) of course acts as a stabilized social service mechanism; that is, as a bit of public machinery that has rather recently grown out of the demands of modern social service. As is now familiarly known, the Industrial Accident Board representatives can be of direct community help and individual help in the advice they offer to the victim of injury as to whether he should or should not take a "lump sum" settlement or continued compensation. Which of these lines is technically better depends upon the case, and "dependence upon the case" means that adequate modern social investigation has to be before long undertaken.

A decision was made in John Flynn's case, whether for better or for worse, (and whether permanently for better or worse remains still in question), to grant continuing compensation decreasing with his wages. So judicial and authoritative is the Industrial Accident Board that an admixture of social work not of quite such public nature is often advisable in cases like John Flynn's. We at first sent him, whilst still in a state of almost complete inability to work, to a cement shop conducted on principles of occupational therapy at a near-by hospital.

Here he was able to work for only a quarter of an hour at a time. He was rather irritable when others were about and had to be given work by himself. The occupational therapy was so far successful that at the end of three months he had become ready for light employment. He became an elevator man in a college dormitory. He told his employer about his dizzy spells and gave the impression that he was likely to faint rather often. At first the prospective employer was fearful. The social workers explained the man's exaggeration of his own trend, and he got the job. With the help of one of the college boys he was kept under constant supervision, for he needed daily encouragement. The work was light and the boss favored him as much as possible. Days when he felt he could not go to work alternated with more hopeful days. He suffered from nausea, weakness of legs, dimness of vision. By almost imperceptible degrees he has improved, until now a year and seven months since he came under treatment, he is almost restored to a firm industrial footing.

He did not lose confidence when the college dormitory closed for the summer, but with guidance found another suitable job running an elevator in an apartment house. Recently his tenement was burned, and he lost many of his household goods; but he met the situation competently and with the help of relatives has gotten together another home. For over a year he has been in great anxiety about his baby, who is threatened with a serious illness. He still has spells of stomach trouble, which has improved under treatment.

In spite of all these difficulties he is practically well, except for minor pains and feelings of discomfort, and slight spells of irritability, symptoms which he has learned how to control.

That this case is a psychiatric one in the sense of a psychoneurosis there can be no doubt. It is worth the social worker's while to remember that all depends upon the point of view of the physician whether certain psychiatric cases are regarded as psychiatric. For instance, the nausea and indigestion of John Flynn secure treatment for him at a high-grade general hospital under the diagnostic terms "hyperacidity and gastroptosis." No doubt, good clinical proof was available for said hyperacidity and gastroptosis, but no doubt also, the bull's-eye was hardly punctured by the treatment.

The general lines of treatment in John Flynn's case may be

summed up as follows:—First in line comes encouragement. Work of graded difficulty to comport with the terraces in his improvement was indispensable; correlative arrangements with the Industrial Accident Board had always to be examined; Flynn's eyes had to be examined and payment arranged for by the Industrial Accident Board, to say nothing of the treatment just mentioned and payment therefor at reduced rates. No less than sixteen visits to the wife in her household were made in the period of thirty-two months. The wife we found to be a woman of even, pleasant disposition, well-meaning, but rather ignorant (her mental level stood, on examination, at about 11.6), a good and thrifty housekeeper. There were two children. A third came for whom some arrangements had to be made with the Milk and Baby Hygiene Association. Advice had to be given about the confinement, and a visiting housekeeper was called in.

It is unnecessary to rehearse the evidence for placing this case amongst cases of medical, legal, and economic difficulty. It might be questioned whether Flynn should not also be regarded as belonging in the group of educational difficulties. Certainly more or less advice had to be given to him and his family along lines of everyday information. Nevertheless, the educational defect in Flynn himself was no doubt directly medical; that is to say, traumatic in origin. Morally speaking, Flynn was throughout a good risk. Our latest advices about him are that he has now undertaken a more complex and difficult job, which he performs successfully.

Hours spent by	Medical record, 44 pages
	Social record, 63 pages
Physician, 14	Social work:
	Visits, 32
Psychologist, 1	Interviews at hospital, 34
	Telephone calls, 137
Social worker, 89	Letters, 15

Intelligent sex delinquent. High empathic index. Six months in a state hospital. Voluntary institution care.

Case 20. Dora Hadley, like Rose Talbot (case 8), belongs to that relatively small group of persons, the intelligent sex delinquents,—at least we may speak of them as relatively rare from their toll in clinic records.

We classified Rose Talbot as a psychopath. Presumably she would fit in the heterogeneous group known as psychopathic personalities. Perhaps we should classify Dora Hadley also here. It is clear that the term sex delinquent, like the term delinquent in general, makes no kind of psychiatric diagnosis. There are delinquents and delinquents, and it helps to solve no problem to call all delinquents *à priori* psychopathic. The plane which separates cases like Talbot from cases like Hadley is perhaps imaginary. Nevertheless around the circle of obvious psychopaths is another circle (or is it a matter of wider and wider circles?) containing persons who are merely in some sense eccentric and to a lesser degree off-center than the acknowledged psychopaths.

We are endeavoring in this section of cases to report all tertiary combinations of social symptoms. If we stretch a point in regarding Dora as unmedical, we shall not damage the main contention, which is that Dora Hadley presents no particular economic problem but is predominantly a moral problem with a train of legal entanglements (eventually leading to state hospital care for six months) and with the problem of moral and, perhaps more important still, intellectual instruction in the mid-center of the picture.

We shall give below the rather long summary of Dora's case as a sample of actual case records which the student may use for analytic purposes in preparation for the still more difficult analyses of original records on which such summaries are based (at the end of this book are examples of such complete records for analytical purposes), but before presenting the summaries we may give a still briefer résumé of Dora Hadley's case as follows:—

Dora Hadley was a girl of respectable family of fairly good New England stock. Dora's mother died in childbirth. Although very intelligent (her own psychometric tests gave her an adult age level) she got expelled from school for insubordination. She was an inmate of many homes which were scarcely "homes" to her. She lost jobs, ran bills, and resorted to prostitution. Under psychiatric social treatment there was at first little progress. She remained a slack worker and mischief-maker. She still lost jobs which were got for her. She remained promiscuous in sex relations. She even took to drinking. She rather naturally got blue at times over her plight.

The story would not be properly told if Dora's beauty of physique and vivacity of behavior should not figure therein. Everybody's empathic index (as someone has called it) for Dora was high—one somehow liked to see oneself in such a guise.

Here follows the summary of her history quoted from the social record :—

Social History:

Patient is a girl of nineteen, of American birth and parentage. Her father works in an eyelet factory. Her mother died when patient was one week old. From that age to two years, she was brought up by paternal grandmother, where she remained until fifteen. There were two half-sisters only a little younger than herself. From the age of fifteen to nineteen patient tried high school, but flirted with boys, whispered and did not do her work, so that she was asked to leave. She lived with several different relatives, and two families in which she worked. She spent six months at the Middlesex State Hospital. She tried factory work three times but was discharged for poor work and bad conduct, singing, talking, and disturbing others. In the spring of 1914 she became acquainted with Elsie Rich (also a patient here) of the State Reform School, who taught her prostitution. She and the other girl met men in a ravine and had intercourse for money. Went to hotels in Worcester for dinners. This period was of several weeks duration. During the summer, while working in a family she formed an acquaintance of a Harvard student of good reputation which lasted all summer. One time she was found in a dark hall dressed in a kimono sitting in his lap. In January she was sent to Trinity House by the Children's Society who had been trying to help patient's family to care for her in the past two years.

Physical History:

Patient was a seven months' baby but developed normally. She was six months in care of Middlesex State Hospital as a voluntary patient in 1912. Was in Psychopathic Hospital January 27 to February 15, 1915.

Her mother died of "peritonitis" ten days after her birth. She is reported to have had "queer spells" every few weeks, when she did not lose consciousness but was unable to speak. The attacks were preceded by a vision of her mother or hearing the voice of her mother. An aunt on the maternal side was demented before her death in old age. The paternal grand-mother was said to be a "gossip and trouble-maker."

The patient is lazy, but nervously active. She is strong and in good health, but is very susceptible to pain.

Mental History:

Patient went to school from six to fifteen years. When in the ninth grade she whispered and disturbed other students so much that she had to sit in the sixth-grade room because that teacher was better able to control her. She had one year of piano lessons. Reads some good classics.

She has been unsuccessful at work because she cannot apply herself continuously to one task. In housework she failed be-cause she was unsystematic and careless. She bothers others at work by talking or singing or direct conversation. The patient has no trade but wishes to be a nurse.

She takes very strong likes and dislikes but is fickle and turns against a person as soon as she finds he is no longer useful to her own ends. She is extremely vindictive and spends a great deal of thought on how she can "get it back" at anyone for a supposed injury. She says she must have excitement.

She is untidy in her personal appearance and takes no care of her clothes or room. She is nervous and fidgety, quick to anger and very fluent in expressing her anger. She is com-pletely wrapped up in herself and her own pleasures and ends, and considers no one else's feelings. The patient holds lewd telephone conversations with men, picks up men, deceives, and lies. She runs up bills. She spends her earnings on clothes.

From infancy she has had crying spells and when younger would hold her breath until she was blue in the face. She has always shown a brutal strain and a desire to torment someone or something—pinched a baby she cared for till he was black and blue. In the same way she makes up stories to injure people she knows. Insinuated to a woman for whom she worked that her husband made advances to her.

Patient thinks she has been ill treated and that her half-sisters have been given more privileges than she. Everyone has knocked her about she thinks. Has no fondness for parents, whom she considers hypocrites.

There seemed to be no change in her at time menses began, but a gradual development of this character from early child-hood.

In the light of most of the story above given the following letter, restrained and stable as it plainly is, is a bit astounding, the more so as Dora actually did make good her promises therein.

"MY DEAR MISS ADAMS:

"I'm very sorry I went away from you as I did Wednesday afternoon. I was feeling bad, and rather cross too, because of the way things had turned out in the last week. You'll forgive me, won't you?

"I have made up my mind at last, Miss Adams. I am tired of leading the life I have led for the last month. Now I have given up my freedom, my friends (?) and am going to put in six months here at Trinity House. I want to be good. I simply cannot trust myself as much as I hate everything immoral. I'm not immoral, Miss Adams,—I hate it. I've been unmoral, that's all. You understand me, don't you? And I think you believe in me. I want to be a real, true woman. I'm going to be one. I'm going to try so hard to please everyone. Miss Ellis is beautiful and good. I love her and Miss Mansfield and I want to be like them, just the kind of a girl they want me to be. I can do it.

"I shall miss heaps of things. I want to see someone but cannot. I shall be lonesome too—but I'll stick it out, if it will only help me to be what I want to be.

"I want you to come out and see me, and surely you will write to me?

"Sincerely,
"DORA."

She not only at our suggestion made voluntary resort to an institutional home, putting herself under its control for six months, but stayed with the home for six months longer than she promised. The Psychopathic Hospital social service was then emboldened to close her case. She is now doing well as a nurse in training. In a period of eighteen months or, if we count the state hospital term as sharing in her progress, two years, Dora climbed a considerable terrace educationally and morally. Lest we be regarded as over-optimistic, we may remind the reader that the White Slave Traffic Investigation in Massachusetts some years since—an investigation headed by Dr. Walter E. Fernald—gave a number of examples of prostitutes who if not highly intelligent were at all events not feeble-minded. In fact the obviously feeble-minded among the prostitutes of that investigation were but slightly over fifty per cent of those examined by strict mental tests. We are informed by Dr. Fernald that the woman of intelligence who resorts to prostitution and whose case is not otherwise complex is very often to be found in the course of a few years outside the temporary field. Many known prostitutes of this intelligent group have settled into stable married lives.

Hours spent by	Medical record, 39 pages
	Social record, 31 pages
Physician, 11	Social work:
	Visits, 21
Psychologist, 1	Interviews at hospital. 32
	Telephone calls, 43
Social worker, 54	Letters, 13

Unstable Jewish girl with obsessive ambition for education.

Case 21. Bessie Silverman, a nineteen-year-old Russian Jewess, came to the out-patient department of the Psychopathic Hospital of her own volition. She came by herself and said that she wanted to find out her mental ability. She gave her own history. Her family in Russia had been fairly well-to-do, the mother was dead, and her father had married again, and emigrated to America leaving Bessie in Russia. In her fourteenth year Bessie herself came over and interspersed factory work, which she shortly undertook, with periods of schooling. The dominant issue with Bessie was to get an education. It was rather a sharper issue with Bessie than with the typical Russian Jew of the recent American scene. Bessie must needs get an education and must go through college, and the issue was still sharper when her ambitions were compared with those of her father and stepmother, for the Silverman family had in a sense come down in the world since their immigration to America. Upon examination we found her to make a score of 17.5 years with 87 points. There were no special features in the examination to throw clearer light upon her character. Her answers were rather slow and she seemed to be rather less self-confident than most persons taking these tests. Physically we found her to be negative except for a spinal curvature. On the whole the best large category in which to place her seemed to be that of the psychoneuroses. One of our reports speaks of her showing a kind of fundamental disharmony in life, a disharmony based on the incompatibility of her ambitions with her immediate opportunities and perhaps with her own mental capacity.

The principal of a high school became interested in her upon our proffering him the case. He wrote that he thought he had succeeded in arranging a reasonable program for her and found her in a good frame of mind for work. Carrying this school work (in which she really needed a private tutor according to the school view), wearing a plaster cast for her lateral curvature, and earning money outside formed a triple weight which she was hardly able to carry. All the while she seemed to resent the social crutch, and her nervous make-up never failed to be in evidence.

The procedure was beset with difficulties. The central idea, that of going to college, we eventually decided to indulge. She must of course go through preparatory school first. A man of means who had taken an interest in the Silverman girl (she was rather adept at making friends) undertook to finance her going to a suitable and expensive preparatory school. This plan must needs fail on account of Bessie's determination not to accept charity. We seem to have reached an *impasse*. She says that if she only had money she could win in life, but as she has not enough money and will not take it she therefore denounces the American situation, particularly the school situation. In point of fact, the school work with the heavy collateral burden had proved too much for her. She has now reached a level of what we might from the general standpoint call compensation. She is doing housework for weeks or months at a time in different places.

We have not ticketed Bessie Silverman as distinctly a medical case, finding her problem to be one of moral training and of economic difficulty. Yet if pushed to explain her case we should be inclined to think that in a very tenuous way there are sundry medical difficulties at bottom. At all events there are temperamental faults which can best be understood by looking in the psychiatric direction. The social service and the school authorities, to say nothing of her general American experience, are teaching her, if not her level, then some potentialities in the present world. It might be easy to charge up her plight to something racial and it is indeed true that sundry Russian Jews do appear from time to time upon the social scene who have some features of Bessie Silverman. We are inclined, however, to think of her as rather specially affected by a psychoneurotic trend. Whether her general disabling through inconsistent ambition is so much an educative as a moral affair is also doubtful. The economic evidences are plain enough, but the attitude toward them which Bessie assumes is still more troublesome. It is easy to speculate upon the outcome.

Hours spent by	Medical record, 12 pages
Physician, 4	Social record, 77 pages
	Social work:
Psychologist, 1	Visits, 38
	Interviews at hospital, 64
Social worker, 139	Telephone calls, 123
	Letters, 40

"Little fiend," a neglected child, becomes "the pet" of a foster household.

Case 22. Elliot Calderwood was brought to us as a "little fiend." He came through the court. His aunt had found him unmanageable and was so incensed with this boy of eight years that she refused even to telephone to learn our findings and refused to have him in her house another night. His aunt told us that Elliot was wild in every way, could not eat like a decent boy, shuffled his feet, ate like a gourmand, and was a frequent and sometimes open masturbator who had attempted sex relations with his four-year-old girl cousin. One reason why the aunt felt so desperately concerning her nephew was a variety of facts which she knew concerning his father and mother, who both had somewhat checkered sex histories.

The small boy, observed in the hospital, was found to be a likable affectionate small boy, who admitted much, if not all that his aunt maintained. He was, however, so far as we could make out, in no sense a medical case. He measured up to normal psychologically. He had learned his sex practices from various adults and said that he had been taught also by them to steal.

The need of a careful education was represented to a children's agency which assumed responsibility for the boy's support and thus avoided his becoming a public charge. There was some likelihood that the father, who was now in the Canadian Army, might perhaps be reached to help in payments. (The father was located and actually did make an allotment.) At all events, the children's agency's decision was greatly justified by the outcome in the Calderwood case. The boy was circumcised and placed in a country town with a kind woman who became very fond of him. With her he gave no trouble, ceased masturbating and became the "pet" of the household.

We present this case as one of threefold disorder, minus the medical, and curiously enough, the moral complication. We say "curiously enough" because a case brought to us as a sort of fiend of immorality might, perhaps, be regarded as one of distinctly moral disorder. To be sure, the moral question had, forthwith, to be brought up for discussion, but the mental tests and the general hospital observation, to say nothing of his smooth history on placing out, will not allow his being classified in the moral group. The whole situation seemed to be one rather of education; and upon proper intellectual training, the moral pseudo-difficulty disappeared. We place him in the legal group because he came to the hospital through the court. He was a neglected child and an economic charge.

Hours spent by

Physician, 3

Psychologist, 1

Social worker, 5

Medical record, 12 pages
Social record, 3 pages
Social work:
  Visits, 2
  Interviews at hospital, 1
  Telephone calls, 7
Letters, 2

WOMAN, 43, LIVING AS MAN
12 YEARS

1916	*1916-18*
Man's Dress	Woman's Dress
Inebriate	Drinking Spells
Irregular Work	Steady Job
Bisexual Delinquency	Books and a Pipe!

Early History:

Married, Deserted
Abandoned Child
Put on Disguise

Woman who lived as a man. Psychopathic sexualis. Alcoholism. Became a steady worker, consoled by pipe and book.

Case 23. Julia Brown was a woman who lived as a man. She was probably in the late thirties when she first came to medical attention. Of old New England stock, she had lived with her family, father, mother, and two sisters in country towns to the age of eleven, whereupon Julia's mother died and her father married again. Julia went to live with her aunt. She left high school at the end of her second year to work in a mill. After a year in the mill she married a hard-drinking man who left her shortly after the birth of a baby boy. Putting the baby (whom she was never to see again) in her aunt's care, she went back to the mill and worked three years. In the late teens or early twenties, Julia Brown put on men's clothes and from that day forward never wore women's clothes again until she came under care. According to her story she was constantly teased for looking so much like a man. She thought she could get work more easily and get better pay as a man. Moreover she was very fond of girls. After donning men's attire she assumed the name of Alfred Mansfield. She began to drink and to smoke a pipe incessantly. She lost a series of jobs on account of her drinking habit. There were no other delinquencies except that she was once accused of stealing fifteen dollars. To all public observation she was well behaved and was seldom actually seen drunk. In general she led a happy life according to her own conceptions, and was accepted as a man, fitted into the social life on the chosen level, and sang in a quartet with three men, etc. For a year she kept house with a girl who for a time thought that Alfred Mansfield was a man, but in general, according to her story, she lived alone.

About a year before our observation she came to Boston with a clairvoyant for whom she had worked in another city. She helped the clairvoyant for some weeks. When he left the city she got work as painter and odd-job man, and then worked as a press-feeder.

133

Early in December, 1915, Alfred Mansfield was overcome by gas and next day found herself in a general hospital. She had been unconscious in the interval. She denied that she had turned on the gas with suicidal intent. The examination at the general hospital revealed that Alfred Mansfield was really a woman. She was shortly sent to the Psychopathic Hospital, no doubt in part because of the history of concealment of sex, but also because she had buzzings in the ear and complained of hearing children's voices. There was never, at the Psychopathic Hospital, any behavior which would suggest hallucinations and no further complaint of voices.

We found her a tallish, well-developed, and rather poorly nourished woman with somewhat heavy, masculine features, short coarse hair, some slight evidence of beard, and a low voice. She had a sizable scar on the left jaw. Her teeth were in very poor condition. She suffered from flat feet but otherwise showed little that was abnormal. There were striae of her pregnancy. Her gait was masculine.

The gynecological examination proved bacteriologically negative. She talked readily without reticence and gave a fairly consistent story whose dates we have not been able in all details to verify, but there was clearly no general tendency to concealment of her vital record.

Psychometrically she stood by the point scale at 12.5 years and by the Binet Scale at a slightly lower level; namely, 11 3/5 years. After the details of these tests, it seemed that her free associations were retarded and her interpretative powers (in the tests employed) rather poor. On the other hand, her memory span was fairly wide and she exhibited a fair degree of comprehension and powers of observation. Her learning ability and perception of form proved good and her attention fairly stable. She was noted as oversuggestible. The psychologist concluded from the psychological standpoint at least she could not be regarded as feeble-minded.

There was never any sign of a definite psychosis or of any progressive condition suggesting mental disease. It was clear that she belonged amongst the psychopathias or psychopathic personalities, or possibly she could be put in a group of eccentric persons that are not clearly psychopathic; that is to say, amongst a group of mild psychic anomalies. From her own standpoint, however, her life was fairly self-consistent. She on the whole felt that she had lived a happier life in her disguise and had more money. She was certain, and quite tranquil in her assertion, that she would forthwith go back to her life as Alfred Mansfield.

Psychiatrically we found her without active symptoms of any sort. She remained under observation at the Psychopathic Hospital for a month. She then had to be transferred to a general hospital owing to a throat culture positive for diphtheria. She remained technically under our care for a few more days, and was then discharged by court order to herself and to our social service. We determined that she was not insane and not feeble-minded, and expressed a question as to her being a victim of psychopathic personality.

The situation was on the whole rather more pathetic than ludicrous. The net result of the social work in her case is that Alfred Mansfield has gone back into Julia Brown who so far as we know (she was lost to notice for three months at one time) has constantly worked and has betrayed no masculine tendencies, unless persistence in smoking a pipe be so regarded. It is true that she has for the most part lived in somewhat questionable lodgings and that she has not been finically neat in her life there. She has had a number of drinking spells. One night she came home drunk. The next day a lodger missed fifteen dollars and charged her with the theft. At all events, the landlady turned her out. That morning she staggered away drunk with two suitcases. She sat down upon a doorstep to rest. Someone noted a pipe sticking out of her pocket. When the police arrived, Julia had vanished, leaving the suitcase wherein the police found men's underwear and quantities of strong tobacco. There was no proof of the alleged theft, the police on investigation found that she was giving satisfaction in her mill work (she had become a checker of stock and was well liked, even having been made secretary of an employees' war savings stamp club) and dropped the case.

With the social service, Julia Brown has been on the whole rather friendly and rather passive under treatment. When she gets into a fix she calls upon the department to help her. For example, her drinking at one time badly frightened her as to its possible outcome and upon her desire for aid, arrangements were made for sending her to a state hospital as an inebriate. There she stayed for some three months and emerged greatly improved. We feel that she has been restored to that level of normality, or subnormality, which could in all reasonableness be hoped for.

Apparently during her life as Alfred Mansfield this woman was rather sociable. Now she is a good deal more seclusive. She reads classical fiction, smokes strong tobacco, and cannot be broken of a desire for spirits which she drinks at home alone We have closed the case so far as all active steps are concerned, but naturally expect from time to time that she will resort to the department for aid. She has developed an ambition for learning some technical sort of work which can be performed at home, the textile products of which could be sold by the piece. The point seems to be that she wants to make a home of her own.

A number of rather human questions might be raised by this case. On the whole we feel that the present approximation of normality is a good deal superior to the previous plight despite the seclusiveness which has developed. A question might be raised as to whether she should be put in contact with her son, whom, as above stated, she has not seen since he was a few weeks old. For the sake of the individual happiness of her son, it has been for better or worse decided that no special efforts were imperative to bring mother and son together. In the course of a few years the mother's status may be so far improved and the boy's character sufficiently stabilized to warrant a set attempt at reëstablishing relations. The woman is herself turning her thoughts to the boy and the family relation. Recently one of the hospital social workers met Mrs. Brown on the street. She seemed pleased by the encounter and stopped for a chat. She was looking well in a new spring hat and she seemed quite satisfied with life. One of her favorite expressions is: "Life is sweet to me."

We have presented the case as one of non-medical and non-educational nature, although it would be easy to say that she is so far a victim of psychopathic personality that medicine has an important part in the plot, and it will also be easy to show that her life has been such that a part of her plight was due to ignorance. Nevertheless, we are not prepared to say that she is definitely a psychopath in the sense of sundry cases of overdeveloped instincts or of a definite psychopathia sexualis. She may belong as hinted in that wide and vague circle of eccentrics and cranks that lie in the limbo outside the circle of the psychopathias. Educationally, the woman is well informed and writes a good letter; there is no obvious gap in education to make up. On the other hand there was, of course, a large moral problem and the question of readjustment of the entire attitude of this woman to her life. We have purposely laid little stress upon the sex delinquencies, heterosexual and homosexual, which are suspected or implicit in some parts of Julia Brown's history. With a case of congenital psychopathia sexualis we question whether our social treatment would have been so relatively successful and so quickly productive of results as the above account indicates. In short, the readjustment problem was more a moral than a psychiatric one despite the fact that the psychiatric point of view was no doubt of the utmost service in picking the situation to pieces and parting out the moral from the distinctly psychopathic elements of Julia Brown. The element of delinquency needs no further analysis than what the history reveals and the economic problem, though never desperate, required a good deal of help and indeed from time to time actual money grants.

Hours spent by	Medical record, 27 pages
	Social record, 48 pages
Physician, 5	Social work:
	Visits, 49
Psychologist, 1	Interviews at hospital, 14
	Telephone calls, 53
Social worker, 95½	Letters, 21

Depressed cigar-maker; could not work; feared open spaces. Low standard of living; family problem.

Case 24. We now undertake a new group, the binary combinations of social trouble. We shall find ten binary combinations, the first four of which will be combinations of disease with some other form of social trouble.

David Stone was a Russian Jewish cigar-maker who came to this country at the age of five. We medically placed him in the psychoneurotic group.

By way of exemplifying the routine summaries of social, physical, and mental conditions with their results, we here insert the actual text (as usual with the names and certain other features changed) from the social record. The reader should bear in mind that the summary is of the *social* records and not of the medical records.

RESULTS: February 25–July 3, 1918
Social:

Work was found for patient in the stock room of a wholesale cigar plant at fifteen dollars a week. Patient worked there about three months and then he obtained work from the Standard Life Insurance Company, as an agent, on a commission basis, earning about twenty dollars a week. Patient's wife has not been working; two hundred and twenty-five dollars security for patient's new job had to be raised, patient's wife getting this through the Jewish Free Loan, and by pawning a few articles as well as by borrowing from relatives. Patient is paying back at the rate of five dollars a week on this.

After urging by social service family moved into better quarters.

Patient's son Arnold was ill for a short time at the county hospital. Made a good recovery, though he is still to report to the out-patient department here.

Patient's wife has complained of a uterine disturbance for which a private physician has treated her. Social service referred her to the county hospital for this.

Physical:

Nothing of note.

Mental:

Patient likes his new insurance work. Has grown less and less timid about going about alone, declaring himself cured the beginning of July, 1918, Dr. Myer saying he need not report to the out-patient department unless he wanted to. He took this new work as he saw in it more chance of advancement. Patient has reported to the out-patient department several times.

July 3–October 3, 1918
Social:

Family have moved to 47 Wall Street, Roxbury, a better section, where they have three large rooms; the rent being nine dollars.

Patient's niece is wife of a cosmetic specialist who uses the fourth room in front of the tenement as a store for his wares, and reduces the rent to nine dollars in return for occasional services of patient's wife in the store. Patient's wife is not doing any other work. Social service arranged for her and the children to have a vacation during the summer, which benefited them considerably.

Patient's wife puts off her own treatment at the county hospital or by her physician. She has not taken Arnold to the county hospital as she should.

Patient is still working for the Standard Insurance Company, earning twenty-one dollars a week. He works mornings, rests in the afternoon, and finishes work in the evening. Patient is still paying back at the rate of five dollars a week for the amount borrowed for security.

Physical:

Patient's condition is about the same. He was overcome by the heat in the summer but is able to do his work now.

Mental:

Patient's son or wife frequently accompanied patient at his work, the heat having made patient afraid to go out alone for fear of fainting. He has reported a few times to the out-patient department. His work is still that of agent at the Standard Life Insurance Company, which he enjoys very much.

October 3, 1918–January 3, 1919

Social:

Patient is still working for the Standard Life Insurance Company as agent, earning twenty-three dollars for the past quarter, which is almost up. He is still paying back his money borrowed at the rate of five dollars a week, and is paying one dollar a week on a fifty-dollar Liberty Bond recently taken out.

The family are still living at 47 Wall Street, Roxbury, which is proving a very satisfactory home considering the cheapness of the rent. They were very appreciative of the second-hand bed and mattress provided through the social service.

Patient's wife still has not had adequate medical attention for herself. She refused treatment in the county hospital because she does not approve of the medical students being present in clinic, and defers visiting the Norton Hospital on one ground or another. She and the three children have had influenza recently but did not have serious attacks.

Physical:

Patient probably had influenza in October, but did not have a serious attack. Since then he has been feeling stronger than he has for several months.

Mental:

Patient has been steadily improving in his ability to go out alone, his wife accompanying him less and less frequently. Now he goes to work alone practically all the time. For the past two months he has worked very hard to make up for the time he lost in the heat of summer. He works overtime when he takes a holiday, such as Thanksgiving and Christmas. He is very enthusiastic about his work and pleased with his increase in salary. Patient has been in out-patient department once. Seen by Dr. Jones, who prescribed medicine as a nerve tonic, which Dr. Jones felt sure would have immediate results.

January 3–May 3, 1919

Social:

Patient continues to work for the Standard Life Insurance Company from twenty-five dollars to forty dollars a week. His debts are almost paid off. He still lives at the same address. His wife has been examined by the physician who attended her in the first confinement. She thought she could afford this luxury. The doctor told her that she was in good condition, the only pathological finding being a nervous stomach which she could disregard. She is anxious to arrange a good vacation for the children in some way and thinks it would help patient if they could find a cheap summer home from which he could commute.

Physical:

Conditions are negative.

Mental:

Patient had one somewhat depressed spell in February, Dr. Jones, out-patient department, thinking it pointed possibly to manic depressive insanity as patient's real diagnosis. Patient's wife explained it as his usual reaction when seasons change, and as due also to the fact that his salary was not increased as much as he had been led to believe by a mistake on his employer's part. This did not keep him from work, however, and after a few days he was as well as ever. He says his own mental attitude has been his salvation since he came to the hospital.

He is concerned lest he be unable to give his children a good education. He came in willingly to be presented at a clinic for employment managers in April, and impressed the group as a fully recovered man. He says he likes to do anything he can for the hospital and for others ill as he has been, and he has inquired with interest for a patient to whom he gave vocational advice here six months ago.

We present this case as a combination of medical and educational difficulty. There is obviously very little actual character disorder save that which is involved in the psychoneurosis itself: On this account we do not classify Stone as a case in which moral measures need systematically to be explained. Nor were there any legal complications of note. The observer who found them living in their four dark rooms (five sleeping in one room whose window had to be kept closed on account of an odorous alley) might at first sight suspect moral difficulty. This, however, was not at all in evidence save for the facts noted above. The social symptoms summarized were as follows: spouse working, housing bad, employment irregular, failure in business, debts, and selfishness. If it be objected that "selfishness" is not in itself a social symptom in the strict sense, nevertheless selfishness has such a marked social effect that it may well stand for a whole sheaf of social symptoms.

David Stone's medical deficiency is plain. How can we define the deficiency we regard as educational? Here was a not infrequent family type, strongly anticapitalistic and socialistically well-read, yet their living and housing conditions were bad (perhaps one ought not to say bad deliberately but bad through a kind of lack of social sense, through a mind of social apathy or thoughtlessness). Such living and housing conditions obviously combined with David Stone's psychoneurosis to form in some sense a new compound sort of social defect. Neither psychotherapy alone however skillfully leveled at the psychoneurosis nor the cleverest neighborhood work directed at the cubical contents of the Stone tenement would, by itself, affect that social cure of the family plight. It is the obvious thing to say that David's fear of open spaces and the family habit of living in a sort of crevice in the world is somehow racial and a matter of the ghetto. How ingrained or how superficial the alleged ghetto loves of this race really are, we are not competent to discuss. Suffice it to say that not everybody in the ghetto is psychoneurotic and that many a Russian Jewish point of view gets in a rather brief time complete illumination on these and other matters in our American scene. Be all this as it may, the low educational level of a family like the Stone family was something social to be wrestled with.

Throughout these binary combinations of social trouble we shall find ourselves inquiring whether the two conditions each time in evidence are intimately or loosely combined. We shall ask whether they are combined so intimately as to form, as it were, a new compound such that the social treatment entailed is not merely a subtraction, one by one, of the two problems from the patient's life, but requires a novel form of handling. It is clear in Stone's case that a strict agoraphobia or fear of open spaces was primary in his psychoneurosis, was in some sense identical with the intentions or motives underlying a strictly unnecessary life in a tenement. We are tempted, therefore, to say that the Stone compound of disease and ignorance was a rather intimate product of the two factors working upon each other.

The Stone problem is now happily almost settled. Curiously enough the main problem that exercises the mind of the now stabilized paterfamilias is the education of his children.

Hours spent by	Medical record, 6 pages
	Social record, 21 pages
Physician, 14¾	Social work:
	Visits, 19
Psychologist, 0	Interviews at hospital, 10
	Telephone calls, 46
Social worker, 37½	Letters, 13

Steady employee of good character who pilfered. Epileptic wife: marital discord. Social treatment depends upon correctness of medical diagnosis.

Case 25. Alfred Stevens is, no doubt, a case of the so-called cyclothymia group. He has been three times voluntarily a patient at the Psychopathic Hospital and although the first time there was a question between manic-depressive psychosis and psychoneurosis the settled diagnosis was manic-depressive psychosis. We are not in this book discussing the medical aspects of psychiatry, yet it is important for the psychiatric social worker to remember that the cyclothymic (manic-depressive) group of disorders is on the whole theoretically quite separate from the group of psychoneuroses. The psychoneuroses (hysteria, neurasthenia, psychasthenia) are on the whole diseases both theoretically, and very often practically, influenceable by psychotherapeutic methods. It would be almost safe to generalize that the psychoneurotic group is the psychotherapeutic group *par excellence*. The cyclothymic (manic-depressive) group of disorders is theoretically noninfluencable by the psychotherapeutic technique, although cyclothymics, like all other persons normal or subnormal, are to some degree influenceable in subordinate features. On the whole the attacks of emotional disorder that characterize cyclothymia and are expressed in its Greek designation are self-limited in their course and not controllable in the degrees of their severity. The typical cyclothymia (manic-depressive psychosis) will show attacks of emotional disorder sometimes *depressive* and sometimes *maniacal* (the medical denotation of this term maniacal covers all degrees of excitement down to mere psychopathic illusion or hypomania), but not all cyclothymics show maniacal attacks and some of them never show any phenomena that are not clearly depressive. Alfred Stevens was in point of fact the victim of a sort of a *constitutional melancholia*. He was of a brooding and seclusive temperament without outside interests. He was, however, not of a complaining sort and had no tendency to feel persecuted.

For years he held a good job in a dry-goods firm, and, as transpired in the sequel, he was given to continual small pilferings, a habit of over ten years' duration. A moral complication of the Stevens case was that beyond question the wife knew of these pilferings but on some ground condoned them. A trunkful of ribbons, laces, collars, etc., was found in the house. The firm did not press the pilfering issue but discharged Stevens on another pretext. He was not without some sense of the real reason of the discharge.

Can we connect the pilfering with the man's cyclothymic temperament? Pilfering might on an oversimple schematic basis be regarded as a sort of overdevelopment of the acquisitive instinct. The acquisitive instinct might stand out in relief on the general background. This at least is the hypothesis for sundry of the special forms of psychopathia (kleptomania, wanderlust, etc.) with which we are familiar. In this instance, however, we are not so much inclined to attribute the pilfering to any trend toward kleptomania as to the effects of a certain *weak-willedness* or *hypobulia* more closely related with the man's general make-up.

He was a rather effeminate and timid man. Without suggestion of homosexuality, he has always been "a regular sissy," had been unduly finical about his clothing, had not smoked or drunk, had no sense of humor, had no interest in religion, had always preferred to be alone, made little sexual demands (sex interest absent for ten years), and did not want guests about the house. However, he did want to please his wife, and doted on his little girl. The wife was frankly an epileptic and had sundry seizures upon the street and elsewhere. Despite his kindliness with his wife, there was a good deal of irritability in the home, no doubt largely due to the wife's temperament. Indeed this epileptic wife has twice left Stevens and had in fact shortly before Stevens' appearance at the hospital definitely decided to leave him for good.

Psychometrically Stevens stood at 11.3, making a general intelligence score of 68 upon the Yerkes scale. At the time of examination his chronological age was forty-six, the irregularity in the tests stood at nineteen points, and the irregularities stood out especially upon the supplementary tests. He made at the time a very poor score on tests of immediate memory and upon the construction puzzles, despite the fact that his coöperation, interest, and attention were very good. The irregularity of his examination was interpreted as suggesting psychosis rather than inborn feeble-mindedness.

Manic-depressive psychoses and the cyclothymias in general are rather characteristically hereditary in the sense that there are frequently two or more relatives of a cyclothymic patient that also show psychopathy; often indeed the psychopathy of the relative is also cyclothymic. In point of fact, Stevens' father had died in an English hospital for the insane, and a sister's child has been fifteen or more years insane in an English hospital. However, two brothers are in the English Army and so far as known normal, and there is a second sister who is apparently without taint. The mother's cancer is, so far as we know, without significance for heredity.

With respect to social treatment, it will be remembered that the medical diagnosis upon his first appearance upon the hospital scene lay in doubt between cyclothymia and psychoneurosis. Indeed the man's general appearance was rather suggestive of psychoneurosis, and the constitutional melancholia shown in his history got rather easily an interpretation as psychoneurosis. Stevens' finicalness bore some resemblance to the psychasthenic obsessions of that form of psychoneurosis known as psychasthenia. He would sit in the out-patient department weeping, and strike the observer as greatly in need of comfort and counsel along lines that might be called psychotherapeutic or common-sense lines, according to the terminology preferred. Comfort and counsel would indeed cause him somewhat to brace up, though the underlying temperament obviously persisted.

The first idea of the social work was to rationalize the attitude of this supposed psychoneurotic pilferer to his stealing. Some progress was made in this rationalization process. Despite minor successes of our counsel, on the whole no progress was made in altering the man's entire attitude to his life, especially as to steadiness in employment and attitude to wife and child. Before he came to the hospital he had had no less than twelve jobs in eight months.

As soon as the medical diagnosis clearly pointed to cyclothymia instead of psychoneurosis, hospital care could rationally be advocated rather than out-patient counsel. He was sent, or rather voluntarily went, to a state hospital and the situation in the course of a few weeks was so altered that although he left against advice he had gotten upon another temperamental level and was prepared for steady work. In fact, he found such steady work for himself. Since this time no further special steps in social treatment have been necessary, his wife has come back, and a new home has been started. As to the pilfering history, Stevens' conscience does not now trouble him. He has rationalized the pilfering as due to his mental disease. Whether this is profoundly true or not, a solid readjustment toward his past has accrued.

It is plain that the treatment is not in any sense an "elaboration of the obvious." **The differential medical diagnosis betwixt cyclothymia and psychoneurosis proved a most important one for Stevens' quick restoration to self-sup-**

port. Medical practitioners as a group are not too well-informed with what they are rather apt to think a superfine distinction between mild degrees of mental disease. **Many a case of mild cyclothymia (manic depressive) and even of mild schizophrenia (dementia praecox) has been diagnosticated psychoneurosis over periods of months and years.** Close observation, psychological examination, and social history (including points got from the non-effect of some of the early steps in social treatment) here combined in a comparatively brief period to assure the correct diagnosis, and the correctness of this diagnosis meant shifting the whole front of treatment.

In summing up the analysis of Alfred Stevens, we need dwell no further upon the importance of the medical side. There was no important gap of ignorance to fill. Luckily the pilfering never reached a legal phase, the economic difficulties were implaced in the medical situation, and on the whole rather easily met. Whether Stevens is, narrowly speaking, an ethical case might stand in question; yet we do not regard his pilfering as either implaced in the manic-depressive psychosis or in any plain psychopathic trend. There was distinctively a moral attitude assumed by him and by his wife toward pilfering habits of ten years' duration. A new moral attitude toward stealing had to be instilled.

Hours spent by	Medical record, 53 pages
	Social record, 36 pages
Physician, 10	Social work:
	Visits, 21
Psychologist, 2	Interviews at hospital, 23
	Telephone calls, 28
Social worker, 52	Letters, 9

Arrested under "work or fight" law; a case of mental disease. Commitment. Provision for the family.

Case 26. Kevork Ardinian was suddenly arrested under the "work or fight" law, but was shortly thereafter sent to the Psychopathic Hospital, being committed from the court for observation. The situation was somewhat strange. Ardinian was an open-faced, smiling young Armenian who had, until very recently, been a hospital porter. He worked alongside his wife in a general hospital and he had saved a little money so that they could be classed as "independent" rather than marginal in our economic classification. Ardinian's wife was already advanced in pregnancy when he was discharged for refusing to do part of his assigned work. He said that he had headaches, and stood about complaining on the streets in an Armenian neighborhood. He occasionally smiled to himself. (This causeless, silly smiling is a characteristic symptom of the disease schizophrenia-dementia praecox—from which Ardinian was later thought to be suffering, but it does not do to draw definite conclusions from any single symptom in mental disease.) As for any adequate reason for his suddenly ceasing to work, Ardinian could give none, but simply replied gently that he did not need to work as he had enough money in the bank for a time. He said that more money would come to him, possibly from the government. In line with his silly smiling, he was observed to be rather detached in manner and a bit playful, although not saucy, with women. He had a somewhat oversweet manner with them. He fell into silence when reproved, kept to himself, and was inclined to tease his neighbors, for example, leaving laundry baskets in the aisle for the fun of making the people walk around them.

That a man could be both smiling and stubborn, as was Ardinian, seemed to argue an abnormal mixture or compound of emotions. Such queerly mixed emotions (sometimes termed by the psychiatrists "parathymia" or even "schizothymia" having reference to the dissociation or split in emotions found in schizophrenia) would rarely appear in any other disease group than the schizophrenia group.

Psychologically they found Ardinian to rate at 13.3. The non-English norms were used, and an interpreter was present. The psychologist reported that Ardinian would perhaps have done better if he had not refused altogether to do the form association test and the three-words-in-a-sentence test. His cooperation was rather poor. When non-English norms are used in determining the psychological level, the practice, of course, is to allow sundry points for the supposed inability to do some of the tests that require certain educational capacities. Accordingly it is always possible to allow too much or too little to patients who are tested by the non-English norms.   There was no question, in any case, of moronity or feeble-mindedness, which would argue a mental age from nine to eleven inclusive. Here was a man with some deficiency on test.   We are probably able to argue from his social history that he was not, at the outset, feeble-minded even in the slight degree that lies above moronity and below normality.

We are not, in this book, discussing psychological levels or their determination, but it is clear that the social worker, like the psychiatrist, must never view the psychological level as determined completely out of its social-psychiatric setting. Viewed in the social and psychiatric setting, these psychological level determinations are amongst the most powerful agents we possess in diagnosis.

Physically we found no special signs of disease or abnormality.   It would not do to regard overactive knee jerks and irregular pupillary margins as of great importance.   There was, however, a slight protusion of the eyeballs that his friends had latterly noted as unusual.   Whether this slight exophthalmos could be regarded as pointing to some slight degree of Graves' disease is doubtful.   The thyroid was not palpable, and the pulse was not increased.   There were, however, some tremors of hands and tongue.

Psychiatrically he proved, for the most part, normal.   There were of course the free, broad smiles upon insufficient occasion. There was a certain resistiveness at times, though whether Ardinian's refusal to have a bath on entrance should be regarded as suggestive of dementia praecox must be doubted. He said that he ought not to be compelled to do anything he did not want to do.   That there was a certain delusional trend seems possible if not probable.   The government had not treated him right. , He should not be made to work unless he wanted to.   On being asked several times over why he had refused to work, he replied "me too much work."

It seems that he had been born in Armenia twenty-five years before; that one brother was an elevator boy at the hospital where he himself had worked, and that another was in Russia. He had worked in mills as a laundry helper.   He had once gone back to Russia and come around the world in returning.   He had been making eleven dollars a week.   When he had first come to Boston he had been remarkably ambitious and went to night school a few months so that he might read and write English. Although he was better coaxed than driven, he had never shown stubbornness or lost his temper with his employer. On the other hand, it appears that he was not at all liked by his fellow employees as he was rude to them and swore at them. On the whole, he was inclined to keep by himself. After he brought his new wife back from Russia his employer noticed a change. He had become moody, had begun to tease and irritate other workers and refused to do anything beyond the bare routine of his job. He "did not feel good," had shaking attacks at night, and his eyes began to stare. The fact that his wife was still working, although far advanced in pregnancy, shamed him not at all.

At this time Armenians of the neighborhood arrested him under the "work or fight" law. Ardinian was rather carefully examined and his case was placed before two staff conferences at the Psychopathic Hospital. There seemed to be no doubt that he was a victim of schizophrenia (dementia praecox) yet the disease was of such slight degree that Ardinian was not at first regarded as committable. It was thought that some kind of close and effective social supervision might encourage him to work. Supervision was imperative, however.

The fact that he had in the late teens or early twenties been able to teach school, but had in recent years lost his capacity to do more than such work as dish-washing, seemed to warrant the assumption that there had been a slow-moving loss of mental capacity over a longer period than recent facts indicated. In short, the schizophrenia process may have been going on even before Ardinian's marriage.

Ardinian showed, under social treatment, a somewhat peculiar attitude to work. He took a great deal of interest in the occupational worker (a graduate of one of the courses in occupational therapy established for war work) and worked rather effectively at weaving for her. He said that he would work to please her, but that she was making him a great deal of trouble. The moment the pilot was dropped, so to speak, that moment he refused to work further. There was thus a sort of psychopathic altruism of small dimensions, but there was no ambition or effective egoism which could be worked on. If the worker said "please" to him he replied "do not say 'please.' If you say 'please' I have to make and I cannot make."

Ardinian became mildly but annoyingly flirtatious at the end of three months. He asked his wife to go out and work for him. He was making no progress in work for himself. He got excited at times and even struck his wife. In playing with the baby he swung it wildly about.

The money the Ardinians had saved was now practically exhausted and no progress was likely toward immediate cure or self-support. The psychopathic altruism which allowed Ardinian to work a little on the immediate suggestion of the worker was too tenuous to build upon in community life. That Ardinian might become a fair worker under hospital conditions was possible. The answer to the questions on this case seemed to be "commitment." Ardinian was committed fourteen weeks after he left the hospital. Looking back upon this case, one might wonder whether Ardinian should not have been committed to a state hospital forthwith upon his first period of observation. There was no change in the medical diagnosis during the fourteen weeks that elapsed between hospital observation and eventual commitment. No doubt much time now proves to have been wasted by the occupational worker, who, save for her own experience, secured nothing in exchange for her time, either for the world at large or for the Ardinian family in particular.

The problem facing the court in a case like Ardinian's would be exceedingly difficult if there were not adequate social supervision available, for the court would, on the one hand, not be able to find enough in Ardinian's record to warrant commitment. To be sure, he received from an acute medical observer the diagnosis "dementia praecox," but this would not in itself indicate commitment forthwith. On the other hand, the experienced court would bear in mind numerous cases in which mild dementia praecox had blossomed into exceedingly dangerous excitement, violence, or destructiveness. Such "waiting for an overt act" is unfortunately the rule in sundry communities. Here, with the proper social supervision, there was less likelihood that the advance of Ardinian's process would go unobserved and catastrophes would very probably largely be avoided.

Meantime, as a matter of social technique, the social care of the wife and arrangements for her pregnancy and confinement and for her offspring were carried out by a family agency. Upon his commitment the family was then turned over to the family agency on the ground that the psychiatric part of the problem had been removed or sufficiently disposed of.

We have put the case of Ardinian amongst the binary combinations and classify him as a combination of medical and legal difficulty. The medical difficulty we have sufficiently analyzed. Legally, Ardinian came to an arrest and was committed to the Psychopathic Hospital under a special law for observation. He was thus a court case of mild mental disorder whose problem got its solution in commitment to a permanent receptacle for the insane. There were no special legal complications attending this commitment. Had Ardinian committed some overt act of violence or destructiveness before his first appearance in court and his observation at the Psychopathic Hospital, no doubt he would have been forthwith committed. His mental disease was such a peculiar one and in one sense so mild at the outset, that this solution of commitment was delayed. In the long history of legal process, however, no doubt we may think of Ardinian as a relatively simple case of a man arrested under the "work or fight" law on the ground of behavior for which he was quite irresponsible.

Hours spent by	Medical record, 30 pages
	Social record, 21 pages
Physician, 5½	Social work:
	Visits, 22
Psychologist, 1	Interviews at hospital, 6
	Telephone calls, 27
Social worker, 35	Letters, 7

Intelligent clothes-presser disabled by occupational neurosis. Large family in Russia to support.

Case 27. Herman Simonson left his family in a little village of Russia ten years ago and came to America to advance his fortunes. He lived frugally and uprightly and was a man of high character and some education. The work he found to do, clothes-pressing, paid good wages, but yet not more than enough to keep him and support the family in Russia—his wife, six daughters, and the wife's aged parents. As the years passed, he began to fear that he could not earn enough to bring them over; they were growing restless and hard feeling began to creep into their letters.

In the end Simonson acquired a severe neurosis with pains in the legs that became unbearable when he worked at his trade, and deprived him of strength to operate his pressing-machine. When he came to our out-patient department he had been the rounds of a number of general hospital clinics without improvement. His legs were cold and blue in spite of the five pairs of stockings he wore. His mental state was one of utter despondency; if he could not get well he could never see his children again; he had lived for them and now they had not enough to eat in that little Russian village and he could earn nothing to send them; would it not be best for him to commit suicide while his life insurance was paid up? If he could not be cured, almshouse life, never to see his wife or children again, was a fate tragic enough. He was cured after three years of persistent work. He first and last resisted treatment, wanted to try another doctor, objected to every kind of light work suggested and found fault with everything the social workers did for him, but was restored to competency, one might say, in spite of himself.

It was decided that the best prospect of making the patient self-supporting lay in setting him up in business in a small store, and a sum of money was raised for this purpose. After many attempts to find a store that would be a safe investment, an opportunity for trading in coal was arranged. Meanwhile a number of temporary occupations were tried, which the patient would give up after a brief effort. He was under treatment as an out-patient continually, and for six weeks was in the hospital as a voluntary patient. He complained that the doctors did not help him; thought that the lodge members who were obtaining financial support for him were adding to their reputation as charitable individuals by helping him; claimed that the money raised for him belonged to him and should be given to him unconditionally; repeatedly said he suffered "every minute of the day" but had not the courage to kill himself though he would if it were not for his children.

As the pains in the legs decreased and he admitted feeling

better, we insisted that he take a position as porter in a small factory in order to prevent his becoming completely disused to work. This was a job that he considered beneath him, and it paid only ten dollars a week, but it was the only thing open that he could do. He still holds on to this job at higher wages, although he has since developed the coal business. In the factory he is regarded as a man who must be humored, for everybody near him must hold his opinion or none. The foreman sums him up, "Well, you know, he's Simonson!" He has been elected president of a benefit organization to which he belongs. He is said to be "as cranky as ever" but is alert and in good spirits.

We analyze Herman Simonson as a binary combination of medical and economic disorder. We regard him medically as belonging to the psychoneurotic group of disorders. His fleeting pains, his rounder's history in several hospitals without relief, and his constipation were features. Whilst in hospital he woke up five or six times in the night worrying about his family in Russia. He felt cold sensations in the legs and sometimes had prickling sensations in the calves of both legs. Sometimes his hands were overwarm and sweating. He complained of a bad headache. He was neurologically normal.

The impression which Simonson conveyed to the physicians was one of relatively hopeless psychoneurosis. Accordingly, when it proved possible to get several hundred dollars to set Simonson up in business there was considerable concern expressed by the physicians lest the money was being thrown into the sea. The results above described speak for themselves.

It is worthy of particular medical inquiry whether there is any adequate and obvious physical cause for such a psychoneurosis as Simonson's. Cases numerous enough in this collection yield no such physical cause, but the failure to find such on the surface does not mean that such may not really exist. Moreover, there may be a kind of psychoneurosis due to special physical causes working directly or indirectly upon the mind. Thus in Simonson's case it may be inquired whether the steady, hard work and confining work at clothes-pressing with its persistent cramped postures may not have worked after the manner of the so-called occupation neurosis. The best example of occupation neurosis is, of course, the familiar writer's cramp, but even in writer's cramp there is an admixture of physical with psychic conditions, a mixture not always easy to analyze.

Some authorities who have gone very deeply into the matter of occupational neurosis find physical causes in not a few. We give below a partial list of occupations which have given rise to occupation neurosis (Southard and Solomon in Kober and Hanson's *Diseases of Occupation and Vocational Hygiene,* 1916).

Auctioneer	Lathe-turner	Sewing-machinist
Bicyclist	Letter-sorter	Shaver
'Cellist	Lithographer	Shoemaker
Cigar-roller	Locksmith	Singer
Clarionetist	Mason	Smith
Compositor	Microscopist	Tailor
Cornetist	Milker	Tawer
Dancer	Miner's nystagmus	Telegrapher
Diamond-cutter	Money-counter	Tennis-player
Enameler	Nail-maker	Tinker
Engraver	Organist	Trap-drummer
Flower-maker	Painter	Treadler
Flutist	Pianist	Trumpeter
Gold-worker	Preacher	Turner
Hammerman	Sailor	Walker
Harpist	Sawyer	Watchmaker
Knitter	Scissors-sharpener	Zitherist
Laborer	Seamstress	

Hours spent by	Medical record, 18 pages
	Social record, 22 pages
Physician, 5½	Social work:
	Visits, 15
Psychologist, 0	Interviews at hospital, 14
	Telephone calls, 15
Social worker, 35	Letters, 12

Series of feigned suicides. Psychopathic girl who desired to be some sort of heroine.

Case 28. Aimée Prévost stands on the Psychopathic Hospital books as a psychopathic personality. Her history, with its series of feigned suicides, some of them most neatly staged, is possibly in some sense a history of instincts unchecked. Aimée constantly saw herself in other people's eyes and relentlessly tried a variety of expedients to succeed. The desire to be *some sort of heroine* was Aimée's desire. We confess to some hesitation in taking all such as psychopathic! In any event, we have classified her as virtually non-medical in her display of troubles and have regarded her as a combination of educational and moral difficulty.

When Aimée first appeared on the hospital scene, she seemed rather illiterate. In due time she was examined psychologically on four different occasions, at periods about a year apart. It was clear from the examinations that she was not feeble-minded and had good native ability, yet in all four examinations the variability of her attention and her lack of effort in carrying out the tests were striking. So far as the mental tests went, her difficulties looked in the general direction of a disorder of the will.

If we choose to disregard the vague aspects of psychopathy in the Prévost case, we shall see her problem as virtually the combined problem of reëducation intellectually and retraining morally. The legal contacts and even the economic problems remain minor.

Aimée Prévost was the oldest of four children in a French Canadian family living in a Massachusetts town. By the time she was eight years old both parents had gone to hospitals for the insane in Canada, and the children were scattered. Aimée went to live with an aunt. At sixteen she was working in a mill in another city and had begun her life of independence with little or no knowledge of her family. She came to Boston at seventeen and worked for periods from a few weeks to several months in hotels, restaurants, and hospitals.

She was twenty when we first knew her in 1913. A pretended attempt at suicide brought her to the Psychopathic Hospital. She had taken iodine and then gone to the police for safety, no doubt reassured by a similar experience six months before when she had sought the police after drinking chloroform liniment. Some months before she had swallowed a corrosive tablet in the presence of a medical student, who had carried her to an emergency hospital for treatment. She now said that she was despondent because this same student, who had lived with her as his wife, and whom she had expected to marry her, had left her. She said that she would "get revenge if it should take ten years." She had already written with vindictive intent to his father and a girl he knew at home.

When Aimée left the hospital the social service undertook supervision. She was a likable girl with a certain sweetness of disposition in her good moods, and with ability to reason intelligently. She had a rather touching desire for refined and attractive surroundings and surprising discrimination in recognizing educated tastes and manners. She prided herself upon holding a reputation for always having "classy fellows," and was never without one or more students to take her about. Her desire for "good times" was insatiable. Although the extent of her sex delinquencies could never be learned, by her own admission they were many. She had had two gynecological operations during the last three years, and was even now in need of treatment for gonorrhea. The blood test for syphilis was positive.

It was clear that the girl had had a poor chance in life, and she herself felt bitter about her lack of opportunity. She said she wanted "to take a fresh start" and to try with help provided by the social service "to make something of herself." A comprehensive program was planned, for work, recreation, a church connection through a sympathetic priest, treatment for gonorrhea, and a good boarding place. The social workers saw her frequently. Attempts to find recreation to compete with the "good times" of the past fell flat. Jobs were found and at once lost through the girl's incompetency. "We don't want her type of girl," the report would be. She ignored the church, found excuses for not living in the boarding places chosen, and neglected her treatments. She refused to go into an industrial school, to which there was no way of committing her against her will. Untrained for any work that might appeal to her intelligence and satisfy her ambition, she was despondent because she had "no future." So after a few months it was arranged for her to attend a trade school. Her board was paid by a friend of the social worker, who had had experience with girls in similar plights and undertook to help in the reëducation of Aimée. For a few weeks she was happy, but her work proved unsatisfactory, and in the second month she gave it up. A commercial school was tried (to learn typewriting and the use of the billing machine) and, when she was discharged for poor work and bad conduct, a second school was tried with the same result. "She made almost no progress, and was inattentive and troublesome, taking other students' attention and not following rules or instructions. Her personal appearance was much against her, as she was untidy as well as painted." The three school attempts covered a year. Meanwhile Aimée had improved a good deal in appearance and manners. She took better care of her clothes and person, although she was still rather inclined to be dirty. She had a series of admirers, and "good times" continued. She was asked to leave the girls' lodging house where she had been placed because she was "a bad influence on the girls."

Aimée had now to look again for an uncongenial job. She was discouraged and unhappy, and wanted to be with her own people. A sister had been located, well married and living in comfortable circumstances in a rural neighborhood in Canada. Aimée was sent to visit her. After a few days her brother-in-law in righteous indignation turned her out of his home and found her a refuge in the almshouse. We brought her back and found her a position at housework.

Soon she announced that she was to be married to a college senior, the son of wealthy parents from another state. The boy came at once in response to a letter asking him to call and said he did intend to be married to Aimée, and that, although he had believed that he was the first man to have sexual intercourse with her, he did not think the knowledge that he was not would make any difference. He said that he was willing to "break it off," but Aimée seemed so unhappy at the idea of his leaving her that he felt he ought to marry her, though he did not exactly love her. He was a fine-looking lad with nice manners. Learning that he was about to leave town, Aimée had him arrested for breach of promise, but agreed to drop the case under advice from the boy's lawyer. In compensation his father gave her five hundred dollars, and she fitted herself out at once with new clothes in remarkably good taste. The young man on release from jail went directly to her room and spent the night with her, again offering to marry her. He departed, however, and Aimée followed him to New York and threatened to bring another suit. But she came back and arranged the most dramatic of her suicidal episodes. She left by the river bank an old hat and coat with a note to the hospital saying that she would be drowned when it was received, and later returned to the spot to join the crowd watching the river dragged. Two days later the police, who had been notified, found her drawing the last of her five hundred dollars from the bank and brought her to the hospital. She was amused by the success of her "frame-up," and somewhat consoled for the loss of her lover by the newspaper notoriety she had gained, but she still swore vengeance upon him.

After this Aimée refused to keep in touch with us and we felt that our supervision would alter but little the course of her life. She was clever enough to find work and make friends and to keep out of court. The life of the professional prostitute disgusted her and she would probably continue to have promiscuous sex relations of a private nature and to work intermittently.

We heard of her six months later as nurse in training in a hospital for mental diseases in another state. A social worker there who had known her said that she was doing well in her work and seemed greatly changed. She appeared ambitious to lead a regular life and intelligently interested in her work. But soon she gave up the training and left claiming that she was afraid her history would be known, since she had been recognized.

Hours spent by	Medical record, 33 pages
	Social record, 51 pages
Physician, 9	Social work:
	Visits, 35
Psychologist, 4	Interviews at hospital, 61
	Telephone calls, 91
Social worker, 100	Letters, 75

Portuguese who got into a tangle over his draft papers and was arrested for "desertion." Epilepsy.

Case 29. We found it hard to get a good example of the binary combination of educational and legal troubles. It actually seems as if this particular dyad of evils is statistically very infrequent. At all events this is true for the Psychopathic Hospital group of cases. Yet if we think of the matter in the most general way, can the world be otherwise built than to show many instances of persons who through ignorance are unable to cope with legal difficulties? Naturally, plain combinations of educational and legal difficulty without psychopathic or moral twists would not in the first instance get to the Psychopathic Hospital clinic.

The Portuguese, John Manaos, whom we choose, was a man of about thirty years, who may have been somewhat feeble-minded, though there is no definite evidence of this. He could speak English, but spoke it very imperfectly. Though he had forgotten most of his Portuguese, he was fairly well Americanized. Yet he got into a tangle concerning draft papers in connection with his war service and apparently quite through ignorance was unable to straighten out the technicalities. He was arrested and put in a guardhouse for failure to fill out his draft paper. The fact was that he had really filled out a draft paper and returned it. A second blank was given him which he returned, saying that he had already filled out a blank. Thereafter came the arrest, technically for "desertion."

At the police station he began to show a psychosis. In the midst of normal talk with his relatives he would all of a sudden become mute and tense, staring fixedly at the wall. He was tense and staring on admission to the Psychopathic Hospital and was very resistive during the process of undressing. He said he had been in the hospital ten minutes and immediately afterwards said that he had been there all night. When asked the date he said "January 5, era first year, that is what they keep saying." He told of having fainting spells every week with loss of consciousness. Something dropped in his throat, he said. At other times he had been unable to talk. He said, "My mind is getting blank." He had had influenza about three weeks before admission. His eyes were somewhat prominent, hands tremulous, and his knee jerks hyperactive.

Under observation he was at times overactive and talkative, at times quiet and mute, at times hallucinated (women were talking about him and voices called his name). After about ten days he became pretty clear and began to take an interest in time, place, and persons. Asked about his phrase concerning the new era, he said: "They say the world is changing. They were talking amongst themselves. There was the first era, the Babylonian, Syrian, and Greek. I thought this was going to be the German or something like that, you know." About this time he seemed a case not only committable but deserving commitment forthwith. He was accordingly committed February 5 (about three weeks after admission), but was sufficiently well to be dismissed about seven weeks after admission in a condition "improved." The diagnosis was epileptic psychosis (clouded state).

Like so many psychopaths of various sorts, Manaos had the reputation of being a nervous and delicate fellow. His work record was studied rather intensively by a worker employed in industrial researches, and we therein find a history of many jobs dropped for a variety of reasons, no one of them particularly suspicious of psychopathy, yet taken on the whole suggestive of general inadequacy. In less than three years he had worked in ten different places as porter, car-cleaner, kitchen boy, milling-worker, machinist's helper, etc. Manaos had the idea of being a machinist. The bare record of condensed entries concerning the various jobs and the periods spent on them during the last three years fill five typewritten pages.

A record was found of his having been arrested as idle and disorderly for hanging about street corners at the age of twenty. The difficulty again seems to have been one of ignorance rather than of any moral defect. Of course, the hypothesis might be raised that he was already epileptic at that time, and if we felt that these episodes of arrest for idleness and for "desertion" were really arrests of a man who was in a clouded state of mind, then we should perforce have to regard Manaos not as a combination of ignorance and legal trouble but as a combination of disease and legal trouble. After giving due prominence to the hypothesis of epilepsy and its accompanying clouded states as a cause of Manaos's difficulties, we are still inclined to think that he is a man who could be and can be taught to do much better. For example, he was once employed as a night watchman. The owner found him sitting with his lantern on a curbstone outside. Upon being told that this was not proper watching, Manaos was thereafter (so long as employed) a perfectly good watchman. He had not been a stupid boy at school. He had started school late and left it at the age of fifteen in the eighth grade.

This is of course a case whose outcome cannot be stated. Many epileptics remain in this community doing perfectly good work throughout their lives. Indeed, there are no doubt many epileptics who accomplish unusual things and are actually eminent men. This Portuguese was actually committed (although released after a few days) as a victim of epileptic psychosis, and it may be thought that he will finally be committed once more. In the intervals, however, aside from the persistence for a few hours or days of a clouded state, Manaos is to our minds much more of an educational than a medical problem.

A community that should elaborate its mental hygiene to the last point would no doubt devise a means for light and non-disturbing contact with Manaos for a period of many years and no doubt the entire cost of such mental hygienic measures would be amply compensated for by the preserving of another industrial life from undue interference either by his lack of information or by the complications of epilepsy.

For a further account of epileptic phenomena, see Section III in Book III.

Hours spent by	Medical record, 11 pages
	Social record, 11 pages
Physician, 6¼	Social work:
	Visits, 11
Psychologist, 0	Interviews at hospital, 4
	Telephone calls, 9
Social worker, 23½	Letters, 7

Overworked young mother harassed by scolding husband.

Case 30. Emma Marburg came to the out-patient department by the advice of another patient because she felt she would not "be able to hold out much longer." She had married at seventeen John Marburg, a Pole, ten years older than herself, and had never been happy with him. She was now twenty-six and had five children. The family lived in three dark rooms at the back of a ground floor tenement. Mr. Marburg had earned only ten dollars a week as a mechanic until recently when he began to make fifteen to nineteen dollars a week. He had kept out of debt and his wife even suspected him of having some small savings; but as the weekly expenses for maintenance were between sixteen and seventeen dollars a week, their life was a struggle for existence. A legacy of several hundred dollars from Mrs. Marburg's father a few years earlier had helped out.

Mrs. Marburg was frail and lacked vitality. Her chief

symptoms according to the medical record were "fatigue, un-happiness, and worry." She felt hopeless about her ability to give the children proper care, and was terrified at the thought of having more children. She had lost all ambition to keep the house in order (it was unspeakably disorderly and filthy), for their tenement was unwholesome and even the necessary house-hold utensils were lacking. More fundamental than this ma-terial resourcelessness was the poverty of her relations with her husband, a man of good but peculiar disposition. He had always "nagged her" and quarreled with her, complaining of the disorder of the house and the poor quality of the food, and blaming her for having so many children, which he attributed to "her laziness." He suspected her of relations with other men (without justification) and a year before had openly accused her of sex relations with the godfather of one of the babies, who left the house and never returned. He seemed afraid of his wife: at night he would bolt the door of his bed-room, he would make the children taste the food before he ate, would move away if she came near, and look around if she passed behind him. At one time he complained to a children's agency that she neglected the children. No action was taken, but Mrs. Marburg was deeply mortified, as she said she had always tried to do her best by the children and stayed with her husband only on their account.

Mr. Marburg had come to our out-patient department three years before complaining of "nervousness and sleeplessness." The examination showed no evidence of mental defect or psy-chosis; and his symptoms were attributed to excessive use of coffee and tobacco.

The marital discord seemed to center around the question of thrift. Mr. Marburg came of a family of frugal, successful workmen and his mother had kept a clean, comfortable house in Austria. Both he and his brother were disappointed in the bad housekeeping of their American wives. Marburg wished to live well and also to save money. He wanted his wife to take lodgers, and to go out and work to earn still more money. He could not understand her refusal nor her inability to give him nourishing food and provide a clean home with the ten dollars a week he gave her. He was fond of the children and helped at times with their care; and he was fond of his wife to the extent of saying that he could care for no other woman, but he said that "the man must come first" and he was not so much worried by the fact that the children were thin and undernourished and the failure of his ambitions to have "a good home" as he was by his inability to save. He was the only well-fed member of the family. Yet he was a well-meaning man and sincerely troubled about the state of his family affairs. He had been many times to his physician with his tale of woe, until he had become "a pest." He offered to pay a fee for these social calls, which was not accepted, and finally the physician had to refuse to see him.

Mrs. Marburg had not had a happy life up to the time of her marriage at seventeen. Her mother died when she was a baby and her stepmother was unkind to her and her sister and fed them scantily, for the most part on bread and tea. She was kept out of school to help at home, so that when she was taken out of school at fourteen to be put to work she was in the seventh grade. She graded well in the psychological examination. After three years in a rubber factory she married to get rid of the "nagging" at home. Six years later her father committed suicide.

The social problem here was one of educational and financial deficiency, an untrained woman with an income insufficient for the needs of her family. If Mrs. Marburg could be taught good standards of living and educated in good housekeeping and sufficient funds could be provided to maintain the family suitably, it seemed probable that there would be no medical difficulty, and that the marital dissension would subside to a normal level. No question of conflict with public authorities ever arose in this case. Our efforts were directed then toward the better education of Emma Marburg and a more provident use of John's wages. In time he should be earning more. Although he sought to give the impression that he had saved a few hundred dollars, it was pretty sure that he had only about seventy-five dollars stored away.

The first steps toward this end were to secure John's sympathy and coöperation, which he yielded fairly readily, with occasional changes of mind; to keep Emma's courage up; and to rally around the family the friendly interest of relatives, physicians, teachers, and priest. A new tenement was found, whereupon Mr. Marburg committed the extravagance of furnishing a parlor in mission style, a hopeful sign we felt in a man with habits of excessive thrift. Some gifts of household goods and clothing were used to cheer Mrs. Marburg. There was not enough clothing in the house to dress all the children completely at the same time and Mrs. Marburg's apparel was depressingly shabby. The children were taken to a hospital for examination, and a tonsil operation was performed upon four of them. The baby's feeding was regulated also. After tremendous efforts to overcome Mr. Marburg's opposition to the novelty of the idea, Emma was sent to a convalescent home for a four weeks' vacation, while the children were boarded. Incidentally she acquired some housekeeping notions and brought back a sheaf of recipes. A visiting housekeeper was secured to undertake her instruction. Unfortunately one of the children brought home an infection of scabies which ran through the family and interrupted education; and Emma was laid up with a scalded foot. Then came the discovery that she was again pregnant. In spite of the terror she had shown when she first came to us a year before, she accepted the fact calmly. She had become somewhat happier and more reconciled to her husband, who showed a very much better disposition and took more responsibility for making the home comfortable. He had an occasional relapse into his scolding habits, but on the whole had become fairly considerate. The case was left in the care of a prenatal clinic. We felt that at least another year of intensive social treatment would be required to effect any lasting improvement in so deep-seated a case of ignorance and poverty, but we could not carry the case longer because (according to prevailing custom) our staff of social workers is not large enough to carry one-half of the current work of the hospital, and urgent and acute cases demand for the most part first attention.

Hours spent by

Physician, 4¼

Psychologist, 1

Social worker, 100

Medical record, 9 pages
Social record, 39 pages
Social work:
Visits, 62
Interviews at hospital, 6
Telephone calls, 18
Letters, 12

SYPHILITIC DELINQUENT—I

GIRL, 21

1915

Poor Stock (Alcohol, Sex Delinquency)
Placed Out, 3 (Troublesome)
Kidnapped Home, 12 (Incest)
Reform School, 13 (Good Work)
Parole, 18 (Lewdness, Temper, Blues)
Suicidal Attempts

(SYPHILIS CONGENITAL?)

SYPHILITIC DELINQUENT—II

GIRL, 21-24

1915-1918

Good Work at a Job but—
    Unmanageable
Suddenly Married a Black Sheep—
    Kept House Well
Baby Took a Prize
Illness—in Hospital
Discord
Another Baby Sick
Husband in Prison—Paroled
Third Pregnancy
Improvement Under In-Law's Care!

Wayward, syphilitic girl married to a black sheep. In the end a devoted mother.

Case 31. Alice Nardini, an American girl of twenty-one, married in haste to Joseph Nardini, an Italian youth about her own age (the "black sheep" of a good family) is presented as a case whose outstanding features were moral and legal. She had received a fair education, and although her early training was of the poorest, a term in an industrial school had taught her the essentials. Financially she could always "get along" although fairly near the margin of poverty. Strictly speaking, she was not without medical difficulties (presumably every case under care at the Psychopathic Hospital has some medical complication), but the positive Wassermann test probably due to congenital syphilis and the psychopathic aspect of her quick-tempered, moody disposition were less conspicuous in her case than her unreliable conduct. Legal complications appear from time to time. She seems to be one of those persons who are always on the verge of association with the court.

When Alice was three years old she was taken by the court from her parents, both of whom were alcoholic and sexually delinquent, and placed in the care of a children's agency. She was boarded in homes of the best sort, and given up by one after another because she was troublesome. When she was about thirteen her parents kidnapped her. They became drunk and quarreled, and the father after having the mother arrested took the child to a shack in the country where he practiced incest. She was rescued by the police and committed to an industrial school as "a wayward child, growing up in circumstances exposing her to lead an immoral, vicious, and criminal life." At the school she made a fairly good record and was a great help in the sewing room as long as she was allowed to be prominent. She would do almost anything to attract attention.

In childhood she had fits of temper when she would scream for an hour at a time. She showed such a tendency to vulgarity

167

that she could not be allowed to play with the neighbors' children in the respectable homes where she was boarded. If crossed she became sullen, refused to eat, threatened to kill herself, and finally got into a state of nervous excitement that alarmed her friends. A physician who saw her thought that she should be kept under restraint for the public safety.

When she was allowed to leave the industrial school to do housework in private families she used obscene language and was lewd in her manner with men upon the street.

Alice was sent to the Psychopathic Hospital because she threatened suicide when a girl whom she had known at the school spread stories about her in the town where she was working. Five months later she was returned after an attempt to take poison. On this occasion she had been allowed to visit her mother, now married a second time to a steady, respectable man, and no longer alcoholic. Her mother accused Alice of being in league with her stepfather to run the house and a quarrel arose that led to Alice's attempt to kill herself. The medical diagnosis the first time was "not psychotic." The girl was distinctly not feeble-minded, according to the psychological examiner. She appeared bright and quick. The second time she was in the hospital the final conclusion of the medical staff was that there was a question of early dementia praecox. The Wassermann reaction was positive and antisyphilitic treatment was given. As the mother had syphilis, the presumption was in favor of the opinion that Alice was a case of congenital syphilis.

The family chart of this girl is very black. Her mother is a high-grade moron; both parents were alcoholic and sex delinquents. On the father's side the grandfather was criminalistic, the grandmother hysterical, the great-grandfather a sex delinquent. On her mother's side, the grandfather and great-grandfather were alcoholic, the grandmother was feeble-minded, had tuberculosis and was alcoholic, and sex delinquency appeared among the great-aunts and uncles, a cousin was insane. Ten of the family were confined in institutions of one sort or another.

When Alice left the hospital the second time, she had become of age and could therefore no longer remain under the authority and care of the industrial school, so she was taken under supervision by our social service. In the position found for her she did satisfactory work but was unmanageable because of her pert and independent manner. It was impossible to tell what she did in her leisure time; but she could not live at home because she and her mother could not keep the peace when long together. Soon without warning she announced her marriage to Joseph Nardini, who had been given to drink and the use of morphine, but for a while had been sober and industrious, working as a grocer's clerk. The results of our supervision until a year and a half later, when the family moved to another state where Alice's stepfather had found promising work for Joseph, are summarized in the social record as follows:—

May 28, 1914–March 11, 1916

Social:

After leaving the hospital in June, 1914, a position at the Roxbury General Hospital was secured for her where she remained until October, 1914. She left without serving notice and was married without visitor's knowledge to Joseph Nardini, an Italian of good family. Just before this, she was going out with two different men, both of whom she alleges made improper suggestions to her. Boy was born July 24, 1915.

With the exception of a month in the fall of 1915, when the patient lived with her mother in Westbridge while husband was working in Eastboro, they have lived in the South End. Patient's husband has worked in a grocery store, for a roofing company, driving an automobile, cleaning streets, and as porter in a bank, earning from ten to sixteen dollars a week. The family has been in debt most of the time, and while they have made regular payments, one debt would no sooner be paid than another would be contracted. The parents of both patient and husband have regularly supplied them with money and with clothes. Of a bill of thirty dollars at the Maternity Hospital, five dollars was obtained through the efforts of Miss Fuller, a visitor to the Nardinis from the Charity Organization Society. When the family went to New York state, March, 1916, they were in debt over one hundred dollars.

Patient's husband has had periods of drinking, and for over a year before marriage used cocaine and morphine. He and patient quarrel. When husband is intoxicated, he is ugly and will strike patient. But since baby was born, July, 1915, he has treated patient better. He seems devoted to the baby.

For a time patient's mother and patient's husband were not on friendly terms, and patient did not dare let her husband know when she had seen her mother. Husband's parents have tried to hold up to both patient and husband a high standard of conduct. They have a strong sense of responsibility for patient since she has married into the family.

Physical:

Patient was given antisyphilitic treatment here the first summer and has been under observation of Dr. Scott since. When the baby was born in the Maternity Hospital patient was given ether. The delivery was normal. Patient had trichaniasis and was in the Roxbury General Hospital twice in fall of 1915. She is not living according to the diet prescribed. Patient is looking fairly well, but has lost weight since leaving the hospital. Is kept awake at night with the baby.

Mental:

She is fond of her husband and craves affection from him, and is devoted to the baby although she does not wish any more children. There has been a gradual change from the high-tempered, self-willed disposition to a more docile and obedient bending to husband's wishes, so that there is less quarreling at home. In February, 1916, threatened to leave husband, but after quarreling one half day and sending for visitor, went back to him. In December, 1915, had a noisy quarrel with mother at her home. Other less important squabbles occur.

Patient is a poor housekeeper, but mother says she is improving. She depends upon her mother to do a good deal for her.

When they returned to Boston after two or three months we reopened the case and results during a period of nine months follow :—

June 1, 1915–February 29, 1917

Social:

Family returned to former address in the South End because they found it impossible to live on husband's wages. Husband has worked more regularly since his return and makes from twelve to sixteen dollars a week. He has straightened out and no longer drinks or abuses patient. Debts are paid except fifteen dollars at the Maternity Hospital. Second boy born December 28, 1916.

Physical:

Patient no longer requires antisyphilitic treatment. Two weeks' rest in the country was urged before confinement, but she could not be persuaded to go.

Mental:

Patient shows marked improvement in housekeeping and personal appearance. She takes a real pride in her home and has shown marked ability in sewing for the children, even making some dresses for her husband's young sisters.

She is less impulsive and seldom quarrels. She allows herself to be ruled by her husband, and seems happy and content with her life. Her voice is subdued and she has poise and dignity of a grown woman.

She is now stated as not psychotic. She is considered a psychopathic individual who has been compensated socially.

Alice was much improved and the case was again closed as the supervision of the in-laws seemed adequate. But a friendly call three months later brought to light the fact that Joseph had been sentenced to the house of correction for a year and a half for drawing a revolver upon an officer who interfered in the advances of himself and his companions to some girls upon the street. Apparently Joseph had no malicious intentions, but the law had its way with him. Alice was being supported by public aid and her father-in-law. We joined Mr. Nardini in an effort to bring about the release of Joseph, who after serving six months of his sentence was paroled. By this time the original problem of the training of a somewhat psychopathic girl had been eclipsed by the "family problem" of the Nardinis, and we asked a family agency to take the case. When we heard of the Nardinis recently, Joseph had been drafted into the army. Before he went he had been drinking and taking morphine and had been abusive to his wife. He had gone about openly with a woman whom Alice styles "a regular bum." She is now endeavoring to discover an opportunity for the police to arrest the woman; and is thinking of going to court for separate maintenance when Joseph comes home.

The improvement in Alice herself (aside from the condition of the family) during the four years we have known her is a matter of some surprise. Considering her bad heredity, and unfortunate early experiences, and her unstable character, we did not expect as much stability as she has developed. In spite of many handicaps she has shown continued progress. Joseph, while he has had his good spells, has been a difficult husband to manage even with the help of able in-laws. Alice's mother, though kind and helpful for the most part, has an uncertain temper and once at least was intoxicated and "disgraced" her daughter in the eyes of the Nardini family. Alice herself has had a good deal of sickness and the first baby had ear abscesses and the second child was in a hospital at eleven months for feeding troubles. The third child was never well and died at three months. The uncertainty of their income has been another burden upon Alice, for although funds have always been forthcoming, Joseph's irregular habits of work and tendency to gamble as well as drink have kept the family most of the time in debt.

During the first pregnancy Alice was given antisyphilitic treatment regularly, and the baby was a fine child. Before the birth of the second child she was under medical observation, but treatment was not considered necessary. This baby also is well and sturdy. When we referred Alice to a general hospital for treatment for syphilis, the diagnosis upon our medical record "question of early dementia praecox" proved to be a snag, for the superintendent of the hospital to which we wished to refer her replied that in view of the diagnosis "the patient was directed to return" to our hospital, since if there was "any question of mental disease in her case" he felt she belonged in the care of our hospital. The matter was finally adjusted, with some difficulty, upon a statement from one of our physicians that Alice Nardini was "not a mental case."

Hours spent by	Medical record, 17 pages
	Social record, 31 pages
Physician, 5¼	Social work:
	Visits, 48
Psychologist, 1	Interviews at hospital, 11
	Telephone calls, 6
Social worker, 76¼	Letters, 16

Incompetent young wife quarrels with in-laws, then quarrels with husband, who deserts.

Case 32. Although Catherine O'Connor by psychological tests would be classed among high-grade morons (she graded at 11.6 years by the Point Scale and was twenty-three years old when tested), she was bright and teachable, fairly intelligent, and even capable when she exerted herself. She was not mentally different from many women coming to social agencies whose intelligence is never questioned to the extent of psychological tests. While her case might be regarded as presenting difficulties in the group of morbi, owing to her somewhat defective intelligence, yet the factor of intelligence defect played a relatively small part in her treatment, and the main difficulties to be dealt with lay in the moral and financial fields. After the desertion of her husband the question of support for herself and the children was the pressing consideration. Her moral difficulties were faults of "temper." Up to the time of her marriage she showed an easy-going disposition and had no particular trouble. As a child, however, she was somewhat peculiar, having sullen spells when she would go two and three weeks at a time without speaking to anyone in the house. After the birth of her first child, she quarreled continually with her husband and lost no opportunity to be rude to his family, whom she disliked. She would burn presents that they sent to the baby. At times she had thrown dishes at her husband and refused to cook his meals. She never did justice to her housekeeping, and was slack and untidy. The husband also was of an easy-going disposition and quick temper and bore up his end of the family quarrels. After one particularly violent scene, in which Catherine became very much excited and obsessed with the idea that her sister-in-law intended to take her baby away, a doctor was called, who advised sending her to the Psychopathic Hospital for observation. She said he told her "the hospital would be a good place to rest in" and she was willing to come.

The story of social treatment during two years and nine months is briefly told in a summary from our record prepared for the Associated Charities in another city to whom the case was referred after Mr. O'Connor had returned and the family had been transplanted to a new neighborhood. We asked that a friendly visitor keep in touch with them. Both Mr. and Mrs. O'Connor had shown marked improvement apart, but it remained to see whether they could attain stability in their common life. A copy of the summary follows :—

SUMMARY

Social History:

Patient is an American born woman, twenty-six years old, of Irish parentage. She is a pretty woman, short and slight, has pleasing manners and an attractive smile. Patient was married six years ago to Frank O'Connor. For a time they were happy together, but after the birth of the first child, 1913, there was constant friction. The husband earned fourteen dollars per week, and patient had great difficulty in making both ends meet. Patient also did not get along well with her husband's family. She felt that they were trying to take her child from her. Finally the husband had patient sent to this hospital, June, 1915. They were advised to separate, but decided not to and apparently were happier. Five months after birth of second child, January, 1916, patient's husband deserted her. Patient was sent to Peterboro for a vacation. She enjoyed the place so much that she decided to remain.

For fourteen months she and her baby Marion, now a year and a half old, lived in Peterboro, where the patient worked as stitcher in one of the Fox & Blake shoe factories. Patient earned between seven and ten dollars per week with which, together with the small amount given her by her sister Mary, she supported Marion and herself. Patient was well liked by her employers and made many friends in Peterboro. While there she lived in three different places in each of which there was someone to care for Marion during the time patient was working. Patient's older child, Winifred, four years old, is well cared for by Mrs. Edward O'Connor, 36 Troy Street, Foxbridge, mother-in-law of patient.

Early in the spring of 1917, patient heard that her husband had deserted from the army in which he had enlisted under an assumed name. In June he returned to Boston and went to see patient several times. He gave himself up and served a sentence of eight months at Blackport Island.

In October, 1917, patient was not able to work more than three or four days a week because of fatigue, due to pregnancy. November 13, she and Marion went to board at 12 Ford Street, where they had an attractive bedroom, a sitting room, opening on an enclosed porch, together with board for nine dollars a week.

Patient's board was paid by the Red Cross until February 9, 1918, at which time the sentence of patient's husband expired, and he returned to Boston. Previously patient's husband had been an unstable, irresponsible young man, lacking in ambition. Since his return, however, his entire attitude has changed. He at once sought work and secured a position as meat-cutter at fifteen dollars per week. The second week he was raised to sixteen dollars. He was desirous of leaving this city and making a new start. He chose Lawrence, went to the Y. M. C. A. there, secured employment at seventeen dollars per week in a factory and in addition worked as meat-cutter for Saturday afternoon and evenings. Eighteen dollars was lent him to pay patient's board for two weeks; of this he has already paid back sixteen dollars. Three dollars additional was given to patient, so husband now owes this hospital five dollars.

On February 28 patient was confined at the Maternity Hospital, where she gave birth to a boy weighing six pounds, four ounces, and where she remained eleven days. She then returned to 12 Ford Street for two weeks, her board being paid by Country Week. Patient and baby then spent a few days with patient's sister Mary, in Arlington. March 30 patient joined her husband in Lawrence.

During patient's confinement, baby Marion came down with scarlet fever and is now in the Contagious Hospital doing fairly well.

Physical History:

Patient had a normal birth and development. Her children's births were normal. While her husband was in, she became pregnant and was confined in February. During early part of last pregnancy patient was examined at Suffolk General Hospital and while at 12 Ford Street attended a prenatal clinic. There was nothing unusual during her confinement.

Mental History:

Patient went to the seventh grade in school. She is fond of reading and dancing, but had had little recreation since marriage. She is untidy and slack as a housekeeper, but when she tries she keeps herself and her baby neat and clean.

Patient's psychological examination at this hospital showed that she graded at 11.6 years. Diagnosis was: Not insane. Since leaving hospital in 1915, patient has been under the care of the social service. She has done her best to carry out suggestions made to her, especially recently, and is always appreciative of what is done for her.

Patient is optimistic about the future and greatly pleased

because of the change in her husband's attitude. She is eager to have a happy home and realizes that she must do her share to make it so. She also has become more interested in hygiene and in the health of her children. At present she is greatly worried about Marion, to whom she is devoted. She is amenable to social treatment.

A year after the family left Boston, one of the social workers who had dealt with them (three social workers had in turn charge of the case) happened to be near their new home and called. She found Mr. O'Connor doing well, and Mrs. O'Connor happy in a good, well-kept home. The whole family had been sick with the influenza during the epidemic and Mr. O'Connor had nursed them. The oldest child, a beautiful little girl, died. Even under the strain of this grief, Mrs. O'Connor has remained reliable. Mr. O'Connor is still going "up the ladder" as he expresses it, in a letter we quote below:

"MY DEAR MISS GOODE:
    "Received your letter last week sometime, but as I am not much of a hand at writing it took me until today to answer it. I hope that you have thoroughly recovered from your illness. I suppose that you will be mad at me for writing to Catherine and having her come up here. I found two nice rooms near my work and I also thought that it would be better for Catherine to be here because she was worrying over Marion. Being up here might take her mind off thinking of her. Now of course I know she will be all right at the hospital under the conditions. As I understand from Catherine I have got to pay for her board and treatment there, also the other expense of two visits of the doctors. I am doing all I can to make good. I have secured a position in a market for Saturday afternoons and evenings. So you can see that I am trying my best to get up the ladder as soon as I can and I hope to continue. I am in hopes that nothing more will come up to greaten the expense any more. I am very thankful for all of the good things you have done for both Catherine and myself. I will never forget them you have been my friend. Now as soon as I can I will try and straighten out all matters with you. I would like very much to see you but it is almost asking too much to call up to see me. I want to keep in touch with both you and the Y. M. C. A.
                            "Sincerely,
                                "FRANK O'CONNOR."

Hours spent by

Physician, 5

Psychologist, 1

Social worker, 100

Medical record, 39 pages
Social record, 53 pages
Social work:
Visits, 49
Interviews at hospital, 18
Telephone calls, 75
Letters, 45

Persistent forger and "ne'er-do-well."

Case 33. Ignatz Simanski forged a number of worthless checks totaling $176 all within a period of eight days. Simanski was an American-born Polish Jew who had gone back ɔ Berlin in his teens, worked with various firms, and was an interpreter seven years. Apparently he lived very well in Europe, but never sent money to his mother or sister. He kept mistresses in Europe. He did not want to enlist in the war, was ashamed not to, and finally left Europe to keep out of the war. An artist divorcee with whom he became infatuated used up his money. The forging then began. He got out of prison in eleven months, without money or clothes. A friend of Simanski's sister advised him to go to the Psychopathic Hospital suspecting that, with his record, he might be a victim of psychopathic personality. He came and was put under a sort of supervision. Assistance was given him—a week's board and shoes. A job was got for him in a munition factory. Three months after there had to be a tonsil operation which was arranged for. Upon emerging from the hospital he was again destitute. That Simanski was in any psychopathic (except under that extreme view of delinquents which regards them as all in some sense psychopathic) was very doubtful. He was referred to an agency for homeless men and the case was, from the Psychopathic Hospital point of view, closed. It appeared from recent advices that Simanski was married and is making good in a small way. Of course, he is not cutting the rather wide figure which apparently he cut in Europe and shortly after his return. Whether, in the long run, he will turn out again a more markedly delinquent, or whether he will become obviously psychopathic is a question. Of a psychopathic trend we found no sign.

We have described Ignatz Simanski as a case without pre-dominant or certain medical disorder. Perhaps we should re-gard him as a moral problem and lay stress upon his irrespon-sibility and selfishness, which we ascribe to educational defi-ciency. Superficially viewed, this man has developed sundry vices, but whether he is accessible to moral treatment in the ordinary sense of that treatment is to be doubted. Just as some authorities view crime as a sort of disease, so others view crime as a sort of vice. We do not wish to enter the lists to argue these views. In any event, the problem of Simanski is one of low moral standards combined with economics.

Hours spent by	Medical record, 4 pages
Physician, 3¼	Social record, 8 pages
	Social work:
	Visits, 3
Psychologist, 0	Interviews at hospital, 7
	Telephone calls, 21
Social worker, 15½	Letters, 20

Psychoneurotic plumber unable to work for six years. Afraid to go out alone.

Case 34. Daniel Griffin is a case we choose to analyze as one of almost purely medical difficulty. Educationally he was rather unusually without blemish, achieving the highest mental age level consistent with the scales in use and achieving a gen-eral intelligence score of 97. The psychologist noted that Griffin's performance was exceedingly good in the construction puzzles for example, but that he took much longer time on a second trial than on the first, since he became very nervous and feared that the second trial would fall off in excellence, al-though he coöperated well and showed great interest in both tests. He afterward complained of being greatly fatigued as he had not slept at all the night before.

Thus, although psychological tests are not as a rule extremely good sources of psychiatric data (as we cannot carry over a specific deficiency in given tests, such as one for oversuggesti-bility for instance, to argue a general psychiatric oversuggesti-bility), yet Griffin's behavior during the tests suggested the disease of which we think him the victim. Beyond question he belongs to the psychoneurotic group. He came voluntarily to the Psychopathic Hospital, complaining of feeling tired. He had had, he averred, a nervous dread for some five years. It was not a particular dread, but there was a feeling that something terrible was going to happen. He was worried because he could not get on his feet and could not make a man of himself. He himself called his disease "neurasthenia."

He had been a plumber and said that he had contracted lead poisoning, which was the cause of his disorder. However, at another time he explained the beginning of his disorder in a bout of rivalry over some bit of technique in the plumber's trade with a man who beat him in performance. All this he had taken much to heart. Whenever that particular thing was to be done in plumbing he kept having precisely the same creepy feeling that ran over him the day his fellow workman over-reached him.

For some six years Griffin had not worked. Mornings he felt shaky and trembly, was without ambition, and could not seem to "get started." He felt a dread that "something might happen" to him if he were alone. Evenings he would feel better and might then take a solitary walk. Day times, however, he could never prevail upon himself to go out. Day times he read or helped his mother about the house. He was interested in lectures, in studying, and in serious conversation. He spurned moving pictures. Whereas he had for a long time been very fond of athletics, he now had no stomach for anything except treatment for his nervous trouble. His brothers and sister, he said, had ostracized him. He was angry with one brother, though in point of fact at least a part of his feeling might be attributed to his vexation at not having his doctor's bills paid by the family. There appeared to be no religious or sex concern in Griffin.

Griffin presented a good general appearance, though his manner was a bit effeminate. He was not sad but anxious in expression and, though for the most part agreeable, became at other times petulant. He had been referred from the out-patient department into the wards of the Psychopathic Hospital. As soon as he entered the wards he wanted to know how soon he could go home. Nevertheless, he stayed, being fundamentally willing enough. His fault-finding would run after this fashion: "This has been a strenuous evening for me," he would say. "I just got through with the lady with the puzzles and it has affected me."

Nothing psychiatrically other than the above was found in Griffin's rather short stay (six days) in the wards, whence he was discharged (as the clinic slang has it) "to self and to the out-patient department."

He has been under observation for a good part of a year and is perhaps a bit better. He is now being got to take more interest in housework and repairs about the house, upon which he spends several hours a day. He thinks, or at least states, that his visits to the department are of little avail. He insists that physicians should tell him concretely what will make him well. He would rather like to have his excellent psychological rating on paper to present to friends as evidence that he is mentally normal. In all the visits that he has made to the out-patient department, he had never yet been able to go alone although he has from time to time made elaborate plans to get to the hospital alone. Evidently the brief trip seems to him a complicated tour. He protests that he must not come in the car with a social worker because he will "look awkward." The family's attitude to Griffin is altered again to one of affection.

This case we have picked as one of relatively uncomplicated medical interest. As above noted, he is psychologically on a rather superior level. Morally one might lay up to him as a kind of vice or bad habit the attitude towards work which he has assumed. It is somewhat a question of terminology, whether we shall regard this psychoneurotic attitude as distinctly a kind of vice or bad mental habit. To be sure, the effects of the psychoneurosis are found in the moral sphere and affect both emotions and the will. But probably that analyst would go quite wrong who should feel that, by those moral measures that aid the normal person who falls into moral difficulties, he could restore Daniel Griffin. Naturally the proof of the pudding in this case, as in many others, lies in the eating.

Nor would we deny that some cases *called* psychoneurosis have been cured by the usual moral measures at the command of the adult person of common sense who knows something about the world and has a modicum of personality. Of course, too, in some wide sense of the term, these common-sense moral measures might be regarded as a form of psychotherapy. On this extremely wide (and we think excessively wide) interpretation, even the processes of normal education as well as those of moral training would fall under the caption psychotherapy. But psychotherapy, strictly speaking, is a form of therapy, and the term therapy has come to be used as signifying treatment of disease or defect. No doubt, then, in a case like that of Daniel Griffin, ordinary measures must be used just as ordinary devices of education and instruction must be used. But the stock moral measures of the community will not serve and (as Daniel Griffin's five or six years of proper contacts with an excellent family prove) have not served to turn the trick.

To be sure, our own efforts have not been crowned with complete success—nor may they ever be, despite the uninterrupted up-curve which we have in the past months noted. What the real cause of psychoneurosis actually is remains to medical minds a question. We do not need here to mention the various psychogenic explanations which have been offered. Griffin was in charge of a competent physician fully cognizant of various modern suggestions as to the mental origin of sundry kinds of psychoneurosis. Whether psychogenic causes were absent or whether they simply were not discovered, at all events, no single or removable cause has ever been alleged for Griffin. All legal and virtually all economic difficulties fail to complicate the case. There was indeed nothing in Griffin's life or history, as so far brought out, which could combine with his psychoneurosis to form a picture like many of those before described.

Griffin is the first of five cases, in which we are attempting to display comparatively uncomplicated instances of medical (Daniel Griffin), educational (John Henry), moral (Clara Perkins), legal (Nathan Blumberg), and economic (Margaret Dolan) disability. Thus the cases of slightly greater complexity with which Griffin's case could readily be compared, are cases 24 to 27. Of these four cases of medical trouble combined with one or other type of non-medical trouble, two (case 24, David Stone, and case 27, Herman Simonson) are also cases of psychoneurosis. The case of David Stone we regarded as a binary combination of medical and educational deficiency, whereas Herman Simonson we regarded as a combination of medical and economic trouble.

In passing it may be noted that case 25, Alfred Stevens, was also at first thought to be a case of psychoneurosis. That case of Alfred Stevens was in fact, the striking case in which alteration of the physician's estimate from psychoneurosis to cyclothymic constitution (constitutional slight melancholia) made so profound a difference to the man's happiness and self-supporting power.

Hours spent by	Medical record, 19 pages
	Social record, 23 pages
Physician, 4½	Social work:
	Visits, 22
Psychologist, 1	Interviews at hospital, 4
	Telephone calls, 20
Social worker, 45½	Letters, 45

Boy kept a prisoner by insane mother. Enforced seclusion did not prevent intellectual development.

Case 35. John Henry was a nine days' wonder in the newspapers. He was a fifteen-year-old boy who was "rescued" from a dark cellar where his mother had kept him five months. The older medical textbooks used to tell of certain "wolf boys," of whom the celebrated Caspar Hanser was one of the first to bring up the problem whether an absolute lack of normal education would so dull or retard development as to produce in itself insanity or feeble-mindedness. The wolf-boy question hardly admits a general answer. No doubt many of the wild waifs picked up in the woods are actually feeble-minded or victims of dementia praecox. John Henry was not in that sense a wolf boy. He had been kept in his cellar on a strange hypothesis. His mother had kept him back in school; she persuaded the teachers to hold John back on the score of his feeble-mindedness.

Naturally, after John's somewhat picturesque rescue, he became the especial object of the psychologist's attention. *Mirabile dictu,* John graded virtually at normal. At a chronological age of fifteen and a half years, his Point Scale level stood at 16, and his level on the Stanford scale stood at 15.5.

This case so well illustrates the peculiar and critical advantages of mental tests in certain instances, that we here transcribe a large portion of a special report made by the psychologist at the Psychopathic Hospital, Dr. Josephine Foster.[1] This report includes some notes upon John's present situation and progress.

REPORT OF A CASE IN WHICH ENFORCED SECLUSION DID NOT PREVENT INTELLECTUAL DEVELOPMENT

The psychologist who gives "mental tests" is frequently met by the statement: "This low mental age means nothing because the child has been sick and has not been a regular attendant at school" or by: "You can't expect a child who has lived on a lonely farm and who has had no playmates to test at age." In vain may the psychologist answer: "I admit that inability to read may lower the mental age with a scale like the Binet or the Point Scale. In other respects, however, school training has little influence on the outcome of psychological examinations." Such a reply usually fails to carry conviction to one who is not an experienced examiner. Instead, an objector is likely to depart, thinking that the psychologist is grossly exaggerating the importance of the tests, resolving to take mental ages in the future with as large a grain of salt as ever, and continuing to consider the mental age only when it agrees with his personal opinion of the case.

In our work at this hospital we have come to use the answer: "Let me tell you about a fifteen-year old boy we examined some months ago." The illustration has been so successful that we offer it here to other psychologists for similar use.

John Henry (this, of course, is not the real name, but it is like it in having the same second name, which the boy spelled Henery) was born in a rather poor district of a New England city on August 13, 1902. Of his remote ancestors we know comparatively little. Presumably his paternal grandparents were natives of Ireland. His maternal grandparents are said by one of our informants to have come from England and Scotland, and by another to have been born in Nova Scotia and Maine. We have one history which says that a maternal uncle died in an insane asylum. Another maternal uncle, who came to the hospital upon request, is reported to have been insane, and appeared to be very unintelligent and was consid-

[1] Foster, Josephine Curtis. A Case in Which Enforced Seclusion Did Not Prevent Intellectual Development. In *Journal of Applied Psychology*, June, 1919.

ered as "probably untrustworthy in his statements." This uncle denied mental illnesses in the family, but at the same time showed such familiarity with hospitals for the insane as to suggest personal acquaintance. Of the boy's immediate family, the father was born in Ireland, and was probably a horse-trainer. He was heavily alcoholic, abused the children, and some five years ago deserted the family. John's mother was born in New England. She was at this hospital for a time, and is now an inmate of a state hospital for the insane with a diagnosis of dementia praecox, paranoid. Four of John's siblings are said to have died of starvation in the first year. An older half-sister is apparently normal.

The schooling of John and this half-sister Julia was decidedly meager. They were allowed to attend school occasionally, but although both of them learned to read, they acquired little else. If we could add together all the days John spent in school, they might come to three years. We know that the family moved so frequently (at least eleven times in five years) that he could seldom have spent a full term in any one school. John was last in the fourth grade. He attended school in this grade irregularly for some years. Apparently he was not held from advancement on account of dullness, but because the mother went to the teacher and said: "Don't waste any time over this boy of mine. He is feeble-minded and will never learn, no matter how much effort you expend on him." Apparently, also, the teacher believed the mother who was so candid about the failings of her son, accepted her advice, and spent her energies on the other children.

As might be expected under the guidance of such a mother, home life was not an aid to John's mental development. Julia says that her earliest remembrances are of squalid surroundings, a room or two with the poorest of furnishings, which were never anything but filthy. She had very little clothing, and at times such a small amount that she was forced to stay indoors. John says that his mother would buy him new clothes and then lock them up till he had outgrown them. Moreover, there was never enough food, and the children were continually hungry. The mother and stepfather beat Julia and obliged her to chop wood and do all the work. In her presence they also indulged in perverse sexual practices. John was not abused to the same extent, probably because he was the father's own child. However, the only attempt to teach him anything was his father's instruction in obscene verses and songs.

John and Julia had not even the opportunity to learn from contact with other children. Their mother often kept them in the house, and this happened still more frequently after the father deserted. Even when the mother was away scrubbing in the middle of the day, the children dared not venture out for fear there might be some truth in their mother's statements that "there was a God overhead who would do various things to them, that the policeman would get them and do terrible things, that people would kill them," and later, when Julia was living elsewhere, the mother told John that "they would catch him in the draft,"—a hazy, but horrible fate.

John's story of his life is of a succession of moves from house after house, with periods of confinement varying from a few days to one that lasted thirteen months. Most of the day time he slept or amused himself by reading the Bible, the few religious books, and the few Indian stories which they owned. When the mother returned from her work, he seems to have been occupied with endeavoring to escape her wrath. He says that she would ask him questions and then answer them herself. If he attempted a reply, she usually slapped his face. She talked continually of the references which the newspapers made to her, and of the pictures the moving-picture men were taking of her. They had no regular meals. The mother probably ate something at the restaurant where she did scrubbing, but all she brought home to John was bologna sausage, milk, crackers, and bread. When he came to this hospital, the boy had not had a hot meal in months. At night he was often kept awake by his mother's talking, by what he called "mother's lies."

Things went from bad to worse with John, but they improved for Julia in the spring of 1917. At that time the mother accepted a position as "an experienced cook" and took the children with her. On the third day she was discharged as dirty and hopelessly incompetent. Julia, however, was retained and since that time has had normal surroundings. John and his mother returned to their squalid living, and the boy was confined even more closely until early in 1918, when the police and one of the children's societies found them and brought them both to this hospital.

When John was examined here, he was a large, overgrown boy, sallow and anemic. His voice was husky and uncertain. He did not know how to meet strangers, and was shy and reserved. His face was a little sober, but almost expressionless. He smiled slightly and then only after many interviews. He answered all questions as briefly as possible. The most surprising thing about his attitude was that he took practically no interest in his surroundings or in what was to happen to him. John's ignorance of the world about him was astounding. He could name the president, the governor, and several recent mayors, but when asked for the capital of Massachusetts he did not understand what was meant. He knew nothing whatever of geography. With the exception of reading, arithmetic was the only school subject in which his performance was at all creditable. He had never seen a moving picture or a baseball game.

We have here, then, a boy of fifteen and a half, who has had practically no school training, practically no contact with other children, and no home education save what he may have picked up from the reading of a few religious books, and perhaps a stray copy of a newspaper.

In spite of this overwhelming lack of information and of training, when given a psychological examination, John received a mental age of 16.0 (I. Q., 1.04) on the Yerkes-Bridges Point Scale, and a mental age of 15 yr. 1 mo. (I. Q., .98) on the Stanford Revision of the Binet. There is nothing in the examinations that would be unusual in a normal boy of his age. On the Point Scale the errors he made were in: repetition of seven digits, repetition of the longest sentence, failure to give interpretation for two of the pictures, failure to give definitions in terms of classification, acceptance of the line suggestion, failure in one of the memory drawings, in one of the definitions of abstract terms, and in one analogy. On the Stanford Scale, he passed all the 9 year tests, failed in designs from memory in year 10, an interpretation of pictures in year 12, in the vocabulary in year 14 and the succeeding years, in giving differences between abstract words, in repeating backwards, and in the code in year 16, and in the repetition of digits forwards and backwards and in giving the thought of a passage in year 18. His arithmetical ability is particularly evident in the Stanford examination. He did the Healy Construction Puzzle A in seven moves in fifteen seconds and Construction Puzzle B in twelve moves in thirty seconds. His attitude during the psychological examination was somewhat listless and a bit childish, but he coöperated well and showed occasional interest and pleasure.

The conclusion must be that, in this case, at least, lack of school education, lack of home training, and lack of normal intercourse with other children have not prevented a normal rating on intelligence scales.

John's subsequent history, while not of consequence for our purpose, is, nevertheless, interesting. He was discharged from this hospital with the diagnosis "not insane, not feeble-minded." We hoped that it would be possible to give an examination at the expiration of his first year of living in normal surroundings. This proved inadvisable because the boy is doing good work on a farm, and a trip to the city might encourage his present ambition to work in a store, a job which doubtless would not fit him just now. The society, however, sent us a detailed report of a "visit" made, and we give the substance of that report here :—

John is living on a farm with a family who understand his case and are anxious to assist him in every way possible. He has gained in weight since last year and he looks physically well. However, he is very slow in his movements, and appears to take no interest in his surroundings. He seemed little affected by the fact that the visitor had come from Boston to see him, and the family say that this is his usual attitude. In the year that he has been with them, he has never spoken of his mother and sister, has never asked questions about places to which he has been taken in the automobile, or shown any interest in them. The only exception was one trip to the ocean when he asked, "Why can't you see the other side?" He has never spoken of the trip since. His typical day is as follows: Rises at six without being called, feeds the horses without being told, milks three cows, comes into the house for breakfast without being called, eats a hearty breakfast, then, without any comment, returns to work, waters the cows, and cleans up the barn. He comes back to the house about meal time, gets the mail from a box at the end of the lane without reading any addresses or ever asking if there is a letter for him. After the noon meal he takes care of the hens and does odd jobs. In the summer time he goes for the cows. After supper he reads the jokes in the daily paper and *Farm Journal,* sometimes smiling a little. He never grumbles while doing anything he is asked, never asks a question, very seldom speaks without being spoken to, goes to bed without being told to at six-thirty and is perfectly willing to do this day in and day out. In fact, far from disliking routine, he is somewhat disturbed when rain prevents the performance of some of his usual chores. He shows no interest in anything. He is good to the animals but never pets them and the dog and cat never ask him for food. He never notices anything unusual. If, for example, a cow were in great distress and he had not been told to notice whether or not the cow was sick, he would make no comment. Neither is he at all interested in the fact that the farmer is willing to give him fifty dollars if he remains with him a full year. Besides this total indifference, the farmer and his wife have reported several facts which are of importance in the prognosis of the case. He has recently been smiling more often, and occasionally laughs heartily when alone at his work. When asked what he was amused at, he insists that he did not laugh. He has never made any attempt to play with a boy who lives in the next house, a quarter of a mile away. It seems likely that the boy may end by having dementia praecox, like his mother.

From the above account as published by Dr. Foster, it will be seen that our initial idea in presenting John Henry; namely, that he might be regarded as an instance of purely educational deficiency minus all four other forms of social defect that we classified in this book, medical, moral, legal, and economic, is destined to prove unsound. Perhaps, in short, we did regard John Henry as a combination of psychopathic trend and educational defect. He brings out so purely and picturesquely, however, what lack of education *cannot* do that we have determined to keep him in his place in the series to portray a singularly simple instance of educational deficiency.

Hours spent by	Medical record, 25 pages
	Social record, o pages
Physician, 4½	Social work:
	Visits, o
Psychologist, 1	Interviews at hospital, o
	Telephone calls, o
Social worker, o	Letters, o

*Girl who fabricated and ran away from home. Mother of
two illegitimate children.*

Case 36. Clara Perkins' difficulties are all in the moral
sphere. She was an average scholar, graduating from the
grammar school at fourteen; and she qualified for entrance to
a nurses' training school, where she spent a few months in
training. She had had no difficulty in supporting herself; and
her family, although they find it hard to make both ends meet,
manage to keep out of debt. With public authorities Clara has
had no contact. When she was under observation in the Psychopathic Hospital at the age of eighteeen, the diagnosis made
was psychopathic personality; but after she had been under
supervision for a year and a half, the opinion of the physician
in charge of the out-patient department was that this diagnosis
was a mistake. He considered her normal and sufficiently
stable to undertake nurse's training. By psychological tests
she graded at adult age and did still better in the supplementary tests upon another examination a year after the first.

The cause of her examination at the Psychopathic Hospital
was a series of fabrications that began about a year earlier.
The following account is taken from the social record:—

Since January, 1915, patient has systematically and successfully deceived her mother and associates as to the work she has
been doing. To her employer and fellow employees she told
stories of being engaged, of the abuses of her parents who had
"sold her into virtual slavery" at fifteen to a man by whom
she had a child. She told of being an illegitimate child herself.
To her dentist she told elaborate tales of abuses by her parents
and the discovery of her real father. She maintained the
family were trying to force her to marry someone she did not
want to. To her family and neighborhood friends she gave
minute details of her nurse's training course and the visiting
nursing among the poor which she was doing. She stayed
away from home, ten days at Hotel Cambridge and three or
four days at Tremont Street lodging house, on a pretext of
being "on cases." She wrote two long letters to her dentist
and once sent for him to see her at Hotel Cambridge which he
did. To her family and to employers' children she introduced
some man by different names. She explains later this was a
chauffeur friend of a girl working in neighborhood. No other
suggestion or positive history of sex delinquency.

During this period of lying patient's habits were as regular as before. She left her place of employment to be married she said, and her mother's telephoning there to find out where she was disclosed the truth. Patient went constantly to moving pictures and could remember a film a year back as vividly as though she had just seen it. They affected her so much that she imagined herself as playing some of the parts.

Clara's father had been alcoholic for a time and her paternal grandfather and great-grandfather were insane. Her mother comes of good stock, but is a delicate "nervous" woman. The other children, three little brothers, are well. A half-sister and a half-brother, who live in the city, are married and successful, and take a good deal of interest in Clara. Except for the narrow limits of the family income (Mr. Perkins earned about fifteen dollars in a garage) Clara's home life should have been on the whole comfortable and happy. They had been in more comfortable circumstances in Nova Scotia, but Mr. Perkins lost his position through drink, and so nine years before they had come to Boston for a new start. Mrs. Perkins had always "kept a girl" and had not been used to the heavy work in the house that she now had to do. Mr. Perkins no longer drank to the point of intoxication, but enough to affect his disposition at home. Clara was very fond of her family but afraid of her father and jealous of his attention to the younger children. She was very affectionate and would sometimes cry if she did not receive the attention she desired. With her mother she often got into little quarrels, as both were quick-tempered, and Clara was apt to feel that her mother did not understand her. She never went out in the evening and had no girl friends except her half-sister and sister-in-law; and she had never "gone out" with young men. The home was neat and pleasant, but she was ashamed of it, because "the stair carpet had been taken up" and not replaced.

After leaving school Clara worked in eight different places within four years as bundle girl, laundry worker, and nurse-maid. She was never discharged but changed about from restlessness. She had no ambition except a vague desire to become a nurse.

When she left the hospital she was taken to a general hospital for the removal of tonsils and adenoids and after some weeks in a convalescent home was gotten a position in a laundry. Her eyes were examined for glasses and a fallen arch was strapped at a general dispensary. After a few months she left her position when a raise of wages was refused, and for several days went about the city looking for work and concealing her unemployment. After this she seemed physically tired and could give no clear account of how she had spent the time. This was the only recurrence of her deceptiveness until over three years later, when, a year after the case had been closed, her mother came to us in alarm because Clara had "begun her fabrications" again. She had been telling extravagant false stories about her half-sister with whom she was living, which stopped at once when she heard that her mother had consulted the hospital.

Work away from home was tried next and a position as maid in a small out-of-town hospital obtained for her. She gave satisfaction in her work and was advanced to greater responsibility. Her conduct was satisfactory also. Two young men whom she met in the town proposed to her and her attitude toward them seemed to be sensible and dignified. To one of them she was about to become engaged when he enlisted and was sent to France. Clara decided not to be formally engaged to him until his return. She wanted very much to enter a training school for nurses and was not opposed. After a few months she was doing so well that we felt we could close the case. We were influenced in this decision by the fact that the social worker who had dealt with Clara's case from the beginning was leaving. Although we felt that another year of supervision would be required before we could feel satisfied that Clara was in a stable condition, between the difficulty of introducing a new social worker to the case and the pressure of new work, we decided to close the case, unwisely as the event showed. We inquired of Mrs. Perkins in December, 1918, and were told that Clara was doing well; that she had given up the nurse's training which proved to be too hard for her, but was working in a mill and living with her half-sister, and that she heard from the young man in France who had asked her "to wait for him." When three months later the family were alarmed at signs of a returning tendency to fabricate and Mrs. Perkins came to us for advice, she told the real reason for Clara's leaving the training school—she had become pregnant. When she left the maternity home where she was confined, she boarded the baby with a friend of her mother and went to live with her half-sister, whose husband was willing to have the baby come, too, when it should be a little older and less care. Clara claimed that she had written the whole story to a soldier in France to whom she was "half engaged" and that he had replied in a fashion that led her to hope he still expected that they would be married. The case was reopened for supervision of the baby's health (the child was found to be in poor condition), of Clara's health (for she had been having more trouble with the arches of her feet), and to steady Clara during this period, while she was expecting the return of her fiancé.

When the soldier returned, however, he disclaimed an engagement to Clara and married another girl. In the meantime Clara had become pregnant again. The only account of the parenthood of this child that could be obtained was her story of an assault. The first baby she placed for adoption against our advice, and with the second baby she went to nurse during confinement the wife of the young soldier to whom she had claimed to be engaged. She filled this position with a good deal of ability, and when her services were no longer needed, she went with her baby to keep house for a small family at their summer home in the country. Here she is well liked and is highly commended for her ability in cooking and managing.

Hours spent by	Medical record, 38 pages
	Social record, 54 pages
Physician, 7	Social work:
	Visits, 38
Psychologist, 2	Interviews at hospital, 53
	Telephone calls, 15
Social worker, 69	Letters, 13

Overfrugal tailor in court for non-support. Attention of legal authorities to social and medical facts.

Case 37. Perhaps the Psychopathic Hospital should not have handled such a case as Nathan Blumberg, presented as a paradigm of relatively pure legal difficulty. Yet we can readily show a dark reflex of legal trouble upon several other sides of the man's life. In no sense of heroic proportions, just such gray or drab difficulties form the stock-in-life of a number of "normal enough" persons, whose best aid will probably turn out to be aid from social psychiatry. As in novels of Balzac the characteristic legal troubles not unreadily find a psychopathic figure in their midst or at least a figure which has a *soupçon* of mental disease about it, so in cases like Blumberg's. Blumberg was even at one time provisionally classified as falling in the group of psychoneurotics, but on the whole no satisfactory diagnosis of the sort can be offered, or perhaps any psychiatric diagnosis.

Amongst the social symptoms in case Blumberg we find such items as the following: arrest, separation from family, partial industrial disability, unemployment, family dissension. In point of fact, Blumberg was never seriously disabled, industrially speaking, save as the immediate result of his legal tangles.

Blumberg was a Russian Jew, one of twelve siblings. There were apparently no psychopathic or especially neurotic features in his family. He had not attended school in Russia and maintained that there were no schools where he was born. Nevertheless, he had in America learned to read English. He had learned tailoring from his father in Russia. He had been in the Russian Army before the Russo-Japanese War and came to America in 1904 to escape service in the army. He had already married at the age of twenty-six a quarrelsome wife, from (as he said) a quarrelsome family. He came to America without his wife. Finally, in the course of eighteen months, he sent for his wife. He had now become a bushelman tailor. Soon, however, the wife's complaints about money and her extravagance began to grate on Blumberg, who himself had an ambition to save every cent. He loaned money to a prosperous brother-in-law, but when he tried to get the money back a year later, he found that his wife was spending some of it. By the time the whole of the money was returned, Mrs. Blumberg had bought a fur coat with two hundred dollars of the sum.

Then came quarrels. Once the Blumbergs came to blows. According to Blumberg, his wife struck him first, as she "would not take him right." Blumberg was forthwith arrested and was triumphantly informed by his wife that "in this country a lady can do as she pleases." The case was filed, but he moved to another city whither his wife followed him some months later. With Blumberg's money Mrs. Blumberg started to run a shop with one of the boarders that she had been taking. Blumberg became suspicious that his wife was not true to him, but the suspicion was rather of her general loyalty than of any sex delinquency. Now shortly the wife began a suit for separate maintenance, and the newspaper publicity caused him again to remove, this time with two of his children, to a relative's farm. Then came the decree that he pay fifteen dollars a week for the support and care of his children and that meantime all the children should live with the wife, but visit Blumberg with reasonable frequency.

Blumberg had not of late been working steadily. He finally appeared at the Psychopathic Hospital out-patient department, coming alone and complaining that for the past year he had often been chilly all over, that he had had pains in all his bones and dizziness in his head which was worse on windy days, that he had slept poorly, that he had had bad dreams and was sweating profusely at night.

Upon investigation it appeared that the cause of the legal entanglements was chiefly financial, due to a conflict between Blumberg's ambition to save and Mrs. Blumberg's contrary ideal. Blumberg could not pay the maintenance allowance. It is somewhat edifying, though not amusing, to find that when Blumberg could not pay the allowance, he was adjudged (after some correspondence) to be under contempt of court and actually was committed to jail until he should pay one hundred dollars. He was bailed out two days later and fled to New York City. He wrote asking what he should do next, was advised to return and try to make it up with the court and did, in fact, come back to Boston; but before he could be seen by the physician with whom he was on friendly terms, he walked out and has not since been heard of.

It is a question in our minds whether what might be termed the "frightfulness" of the jail order has not tended to sever connections completely between Blumberg and his family. Sometimes inexperienced courts talk about *"these cases"* without, so far as we are aware, defining to what group *"these cases"* actually belong. We are not ourselves sure that we are dealing fundamentally with a "case," medically speaking. A case with such indefinite mental symptoms or features suggests that profound allowances should be made for errors in handling ; much hangs on whether Blumberg is psychoneurotic or is not psychoneurotic. It seems clear that his legal handling has not been based upon as thorough a knowledge of the everyday facts *as lay directly at the hand of the court.*

It is not that the wife's story was particularly appealing in contrast to Blumberg's, for no one has asserted that Mrs. Blumberg's moral attitude was of the most exquisite. Our present point simply reduces to the feeling that proper attention is not always paid by legal authorities to social and medical facts. Nor will it much longer serve for the legal authorities in these modern days to justify themselves by the vague generality that we lawyers understand these things whereas you laymen exist in the penumbra. We are bound to say that sometimes these matters are not attended to *in extenso* and in all their profundities by the judges themselves, but rather by the clerks of courts and probation officers, some of whom are not yet educated (even by prolonged "practical" experience) in psychiatric social work.

Hours spent by	Medical record, 6 pages
	Social record, 16 pages
Physician, 4½	Social work:
	Visits, 1
Psychologist, 0	Interviews at hospital, 6
	Telephone calls, 1
Social worker, 9	Letters, 24

Poor old woman, worried and overworked.

Case 38. Though Margaret Dolan came to us as a patient, her difficulties were almost entirely financial. The medical opinion after she had been observed for ten days in the hospital was "not psychotic." Her mental condition was the result of well-founded worry. For nine months she had been in considerable anxiety about debts, doctors' bills, and even the means of subsistence. She suffered from indigestion, which four doctors in turn had not been able to relieve, and was afraid to eat for fear of increasing her stomach trouble. She was afraid that she would go insane and spoke of feelings of unreality, saying "I feel I am way off in some other world."

Educationally Margaret was not lacking,—after graduating from high school, she had studied bookkeeping; and she was far removed from conflict with public authorities. But her financial difficulties loomed large.

She was fifty-two years old, and her sister Annie, with whom she lived, was fifty-nine. They were two gentle little old ladies, of frail physique and brave hearts. Annie was the more optimistic and had "always looked on the bright side of things" but Margaret always worried a bit. They took two lodgers in their tiny apartment and while Margaret did the housework Annie worked in a shoe factory, getting from seven to twelve dollars a week. In this way they were able to have a more comfortable home than if Margaret, too, had gone to the shoe factory. She had expected to be a bookkeeper, but soon after she took her first position she was called back home to nurse her mother through an illness of years, and again after working for a short time went home to nurse her father until his death. fifteen years ago. Then she and her sister came to the city to keep house for their brother. He drank heavily and finally eight years before had disappeared. The sisters continued to keep their home and got along comfortably, until Annie was laid off during a slack season, one of the lodgers left, and Margaret began to have indigestion. For doctors' bills for Margaret and living expenses they had gradually borrowed two hundred and fifty dollars and they could barely meet their living expenses. They could not afford to pay for the refitting of Margaret's artificial teeth, which did not fit properly and caused her difficulty in chewing.

After reassurance and three weeks' rest in the country, and a new plate for the teeth, Margaret had gained fourteen pounds and felt much better. It was several months before she would venture alone on the street. She held two hundred and fifty dollars life insurance for her brother, whom the sisters believed to be dead. This money was finally secured through a friendly lawyer to pay off the debt that was worrying them. Lighter work was to be found for Annie, as army shoes made heavy work for the frail little woman; but she developed cancer and soon had to be sent to a hospital where she died in a few months. Aid from a relief society was obtained for Margaret, who kept the home and visited her sister every day in the hospital. After Annie's death, she was well enough to take a position at housework. During her sister's illness many of her old friends renewed their interest in her. She no longer had a sense of unreality or feared to go about alone and seemed quite capable of taking care of herself.

Hours spent by

Physician, 8

Psychologist, 0

Social worker, 90½

Medical record, 17 pages
Social record, 27 pages
Social work:
  Visits, 47
  Interviews at hospital, 10
  Telephone calls, 64
  Letters, 25

BOOK III

Oh that my vexation were but weighed,
And all my calamity laid in the balances.

Job, Chapter 6, Verse 2.

ELEVEN MAJOR GROUPS OF MENTAL DISEASES

Illustrated in Sixty-two Specimen Cases of Psychiatric Social Work

I.	General paresis, juvenile paresis, etc.	**Syphilopsychoses**
II.	Feeble-mindedness of various forms.	**Hypophrenoses**
III.	Epilepsies.	**Epileptoses**
IV.	Alcoholic, drug, and poison cases.	**Pharmacopsychoses**
V.	Focal brain lesion cases (mental).	**Encephalopsychoses**
VI.	"Symptomatic" mental cases (bodily origin).	**Somatopsychoses**
VII.	Senile, senescent, presenile cases (old age group).	**Geriopsychoses**
VIII.	Dementia praecox; paraphrenia.	**Schizophrenoses**
IX.	Manic-depressive psychoses; cyclothymic.	**Cyclothymoses**
X.	Hysteria, neurasthenia, psychasthenia.	**Psychoneuroses**
XI.	Dubious and special psychopathias.	**Psychopathoses**

NOTE.—This book is intended to give the physician a general view of the social-psychiatric problems in the main mental disease groups.

SECTION I

SYPHILOPSYCHOSES (NEUROSYPHILIS)

Costly delay of diagnosis in a case of general paresis that looked like neurasthenia. Industrial disability for five years. Social work—free treatment and home care.

Case 39. We begin now to present social cases from the medical point of view. The psychiatric social worker (and eventually the layman too) must learn that insanity is not a unit. There can be no better way of grasping the fact that insanity, though legally a unit, is not medically a unit, than by considering cases of syphilis of the nervous system (briefly put, neurosyphilis) giving rise to mental symptoms.

We may begin with the case of Greeley Harrison, a case already presented from the medical point of view in the case history, *Neurosyphilis* by Southard and Solomon, 1917 (case 9 in that collection). These authorities put Greeley Harrison first in every account of the systematic diagnosis of the main forms of neurosyphilis because they desired to impress the medical profession with the costly delay of diagnosis in that form of neurosyphilis known as general paresis.

"Why was not I told that my disease was syphilis five years ago?" Harrison was wont to say after he had come under medical treatment at the Psychopathic Hospital at the age of forty-six. In point of fact, we found that for a number of years past there had been symptoms which should have attracted medical attention. Five years before he came to our observation, namely, at the age of forty-one, Harrison had been apparently overcome when working near a stove, and afterwards went upstairs, talking incoherently. However, he recovered shortly, and nothing was thought of the episode. Spells occurred almost every month for a time, and later still more frequently. Finally these spells became associated with unconsciousness and with loss of memory.

It is no part of the task of this book to give the details of medical diagnosis or treatment. From the standpoint of the lay observer, the fact was outstanding that Harrison had for five years been unable to do regular work. What misled the medical inquirer, and this is a lesson for physicians and laymen in all forms of mental disease as well as in the present form, was that Harrison's constant complaining would set him down as a kind of neurasthenic or psychasthenic. It would be stretching a point to say that his ideas were delusions, that is, demonstrably false beliefs, but he continually dwelt upon bodily symptoms, after the manner of the psychoneurotic (under the so-called psychoneuroses the psychiatrist is apt to include neurasthenia and hysteria). Harrison approached sundry physicians for aid, complaining of nervous indigestion of years' standing, of headache, of insomnia, of nervousness, of failing memory, and of deafness. After one knew that Harrison was a neuro-syphilitic it was, of course, easy to point out that headache and failing memory might well have suggested syphilis. However, a number of physicians told him that he was a neurasthenic, and when he arrived at the Psychopathic Hospital he announced that neurasthenia was the disease from which he was suffering and that he had been treated for this disease by hypophosphites. The so-called six tests (blood serum Wassermann, spinal fluid Wassermann, globulin and albumen reactions of spinal fluid, cell count and gold sol. on spinal fluid) proved positive. The medical diagnosis seemed, beyond much question, to be that of general paresis.

The medical lessons of this case are:—

1. Neurosyphilis, even in its paretic form (so-called general paresis or "softening of the brain") may look to the physicians like that purely functional disease, neurasthenia. (For an example of pure neurasthenia see below, case 87.)
2. Neurosyphilis, in its paretic form, is not necessarily completely intractable to treatment. (This is a most important conception, not yet well established in the medical mind.) And on account of the doubt which prevails concerning general paresis and its inevitable non-responsiveness to treatment, we shall need to look further into the medical history of case Harrison.

Harrison has had a great deal of antisyphilitic treatment including injections into the ventricles of the brain. He has continued in about the same state mentally; that is, there is a considerable degree of deterioration and he has occasional seizures. He is in a state hospital where he has charge of the patients' dining-room. Physically he is in rather good condition. His laboratory tests are now quite normal. He seems to have been held stationary for the past four years.

The social work consisted in getting Harrison free treatment, encouraging his mother, and seeing for how long he could receive suitable care at home. His mother and sister worked and supported him. He had used up considerable savings when he came to us and had nothing of value left except a fur coat.

Hours spent by	Medical record, 55 pages
	Social record, 1 page
Physician, 23½	Social work:
	Visits, 0
Psychologist. 1	Interviews at hospital, 6
	Telephone calls, 0
Social worker, 3	Letters, 0

Widow with syphilis contracted from an abusive husband. Well for fourteen years. Now marked depression. Treatment, rest, employment.

Case 40. Another case from Southard and Solomon's *Neurosyphilis*, Greta Meyer, (107 of that collection) is one of neurosyphilis, not of the type of so-called general paresis or "softening of the brain" but of a more diffuse type of disease, or, as commonly termed in medicine, "cerebrospinal syphilis."

This widow of fifty-one came of her own volition to the Psychopathic Hospital wanting aid from the physicians for a marked depression. It seems that she had lain down one day for a nap and on waking up found that she could move her right arm and leg only with great difficulty. She got much better in a few days.

Going back in her history, it appeared that two years before, at forty-nine, a small swelling had appeared on the right side of the forehead near the hair line, a swelling that was firm and not sore. Treatment, evidently antisyphilitic, reduced this swelling but left a hollow space in the bone.

Going still farther back in her history, it appeared that

some sixteen years before her coming to the Psychopathic Hospital, namely at the age of thirty-five, she had developed some red spots on her hand which she learned at a hospital were due to syphilis. She was treated rather faithfully for these spots for a year's time, whereupon she seemed perfectly well and, in fact, remained perfectly well for fourteen years. Going still farther back in Mrs. Meyer's history, it seems that she was married at sixteen and lived with her husband until twenty-nine, but at this time she left him on account of his being alcoholic and abusing her, and on account of her discovering, through his physician, that he was suffering from a venereal disease.

As is mentioned more *in extenso* in the *Neurosyphilis* case history book, the diagnosis of a diffuse neurosyphilis, possibly associated with a plugging of arteries, was then made.

After she had improved under salvarsan treatment, she then became also a problem for social workers in certain respects. She was referred to the social workers for employment and rest. She was accordingly given some three weeks of rest in a convalescent home. Some temporary jobs were then secured. The depression for which she had originally consulted the hospital was greatly diminished during this treatment by rest and employment. The case could then, for a period of about a year, be closed by the social workers and then referred to the follow-up division of our department to insure the proper continuance of medical treatment. An incident of her care was that about six months after her original treatment for syphilis she slipped on a wet floor and fell, fracturing the pelvis. (The bones of some syphilitics are well known to be rather more susceptible to fracture than those of normal persons.)

From the standpoint of social case analysis, the case of Greta Meyer seems then, comparatively simple; namely, a case of practically pure medical disorder. Not even the economic factor came specially into evidence.

Hours spent by	Medical record, 22 pages
	Social record, 6 pages
Physician, 14	Social work:
	Visits, 0
Psychologist, 0	Interviews at hospital, 5
	Telephone calls, 1
Social worker, 3½	Letters, 2

Familial syphilis. Routine examination of wife and children: positive blood test in all. No other indications of syphilis: source of infection unknown.

Case 41. We borrow the case of Walter Heinmas from the medical, legal, and social part of the Southard and Solomon book on *Neurosyphilis,* (in that collection case 97), not because either he or his family ever came to the point of social treatment, but because the problem of familial syphilis seems exquisitely exemplified in the children. The situation is one which rather astounds even medical men who are not always too well aware of the caprice with which syphilis shows itself.

Heinmas himself was a case of general paresis of a classical type, with marked feeling of well-being (the so-called euphoria) and characteristic grandiosity.

It is the routine procedure of the Psychopathic Hospital to look into the families of syphilitic patients. The Heinmas family consisted of the parents and two daughters aged nine and seven respectively. Both the patient himself and his wife denied all knowledge of syphilitic infection, nor was the wife able to support the idea that she had ever had any primary, secondary, or tertiary symptoms; especially there had been no abortions, miscarriages, or stillbirths. Both children had been born at term and had been absolutely healthy. Upon examination, the mother had no physical signs which could be referred to syphilis. Both daughters were well endowed in mind, were of very good physique and showed no stigmata of congenital syphilis, yet the blood tests of all three (the mother and two children) proved positive. These tests were repeated several times with the children (both with and without salvarsan injections) and their bloods remained consistently positive.

In the Southard and Solomon series it has been found that about 15 per cent of the marriages wherein one spouse develops paresis result in sterility, in 18 per cent there are abortions, miscarriages, or stillbirths, in 15 per cent there are positive Wassermann reactions in one or other members of the family. The rather obvious motto can be adopted: "The families of paretics are the families of syphilitics."

Hours spent by

Physician, 3½

Psychologist, 0

Social worker, 9

Medical record, 2 pages
Social record, 1 page
Social work:
  Visits, 5
  Interviews at hospital, 3
  Telephone calls, 13
  Letters, 19

GENERAL PARESIS

IN A MACHINIST

October, 1916	*January, 1917*
Disabled for Work	Employed
Inebriety	Sobriety
Marital Discord	Happiness
No Income	Adequate Wages
Debts	Debts Reduced
No Money for Therapy	Treatment

Paretic machinist, alcoholic, neglected treatment: on the verge of complete breakdown. Restored in three months to industrial efficiency through combined medical and social treatment. Promoted to foreman.

Case 42. David Collins we present as a good example of social problems in that common form of syphilitic mental disease known as general paresis.

General paresis is a kind of mental disease long known by psychiatrists and has always been thought to have a fatal prognosis in a period ranging say from three to five years from the onset of symptoms. Patients surviving that period for any considerable length of time would ordinarily be regarded as either not cases of general paresis at all or very non-typical ones. Accordingly the psychiatrist and the medical man in general would feel very skeptical as to the value of spending overmuch time or money upon social work designed to bring out earning abilities or develop valuable changes of character in victims of general paresis. No doubt this skepticism is statistically rather well founded. Yet modern work seems to show that neither mental and nervous symptoms nor laboratory signs (blood serum, spinal fluid, etc.) alone, nor any combination of these symptoms and signs, will invariably suffice to establish the diagnosis of general paresis in the early months or, let us say, in the first year of its symptoms.

If a mental disease looking like general paresis is not going to prove to be general paresis, what form of disease is likely to develop? There is another form of syphilis of the nervous system (for which the abbreviated term neurosyphilis has come into general use) called cerebral syphilis or cerebrospinal syphilis or diffuse neurosyphilis, which form has a much more favorable prognosis with respect to duration and a much more favorable prognosis with respect to the self-supporting capacity and manageability of the victim. It may accordingly make a crucial difference to the man and his family whether he is discovered eventually to have the paretic form of neurosyphilis (*i.e.,* general paresis) or the diffuse form of neurosyphilis (commonly called cerebrospinal syphilis). The medical man should not, and the medical social worker cannot, neglect the other members of the paretic's family. The children of a paretic, are, of course, the children of a syphilitic (examples of the value of this slogan are given elsewhere in Section I of this book) and accordingly various steps in mental and physical hygiene must be taken. These latter we do not discuss under the case of David Collins, but call attention rather to the value of psychiatric social work for the family.

Disabled for work in October, 1916, David Collins had, in three months, found work with the firm that had previously employed him. From a condition of inebriety he had, under the social service influence, become sober. A state of serious marital discord had been replaced with domestic happiness. The family which had had no income in October had, by January, the advantage of adequate wages. The debts previously incurred had been reduced, and treatment for the man's neurosyphilis had been arranged for. The case had been an appealing one to the social service, and it proved easy to raise money by newspaper advertising, (under "Divers Good Causes") on the ground that he was in dire need of medical treatment and would otherwise lose his mind. It must also be noted that within the first three months of social work the wife had also gone under treatment (blood test of a child proved negative)

Collins, at forty-five, had had to give up his machine shop work on account of becoming tremulous and sometimes confused about his work. He fell down unconscious a number of times. When he arrived at the Psychopathic Hospital outpatient department with his wife, they had nothing but return carfare upon them, and it was found that they had no means of income whatever.

Already two years of possible treatment had been lost, since the patient had two years before been brought to the hospital by the police who had found him in convulsions on the street. At that time he had refused to return for treatment. Such a refusal is, of course, a matter of great regret to the ardent believer in social work and intensive medical treatment for neurosyphilis. No doubt, in an ideal mental hygiene situation enough force and ingenuity could be brought to bear to bring all such cases, even when like Collins exceedingly recalcitrant, under medical and social care. He had always been a hard drinker and was still drinking.

It seems that he had had three jobs in two years which he had been forced to leave, finding each one too hard for him. By arrangement with the social service, the manufacturing firm that had previously employed him allowed him two mornings off a week to come for his treatment, on condition that he make up the time at night. On this basis he got his full pay, twelve dollars a week. He was influenced to stop drinking, the wife becoming immediately reconciled with him again and said it was the best day of her life when she brought him, two years after his first hospital appearance, to the out-patient department. Now, she said, they had become "like sweethearts again." Besides obtaining treatment for the wife, work was found for her by the social service. Ordinarily it would be considered rather poor social work to cause the wife to go out to work but in this particular situation it seemed advisable, so that the debts of the family might be paid off. Shortly Collins himself obtained a raise of pay. Later on he was promoted to the position of foreman.

In some ways this case of Collins might seem a schematically simple one. We find in our notes, however, that the investigation entailed inquiries of (1) Mrs. Collins, (2) the priest, (3) previous employers, (4) neighborhood storekeeper, (5) daughter's teacher, (6) the landlord, (7) previous landlady, (8) a neighbor, (9) the social service of a hospital where Collins had once been treated. Valuable data were obtained from practically all of these sources. It is plain that without a considerable social service staff this kind of work cannot be done and that it is entirely out of the question to suppose that the administrative officer, whether medical or social, who sits at his desk in however well appointed an institution, can obtain these data in such quantity as to permit valuable work.

Let us remark, too, in passing, upon the tremendous change in the attitude of public and private charitable institutions toward such problems as these. Time was when each institution "passed the buck" to some other institution and hardly any board of trustees would advocate "borrowing trouble" by seeking cases to treat in the community. Yet we believe we are safe in asserting that this modern attitude toward the hidden sources of disease in the community is the only attitude which, in the long run, turns the trick of eradicating either venereal disease or any other form of widespread social disease.

Yet with all the rather optimistic features present in the early progress of Collins' social care, under pressure of work the case was too early closed and not followed up as it might and should have been. It was again reopened through the vigilance of officers having in mind the tremendous value of this program of social work in neurosyphilis, and Collins went again under treatment. He was particularly difficult on account of his alcoholic tendencies and on account of the usual story on the part of these patients, namely their tendency, as soon as they feel rather well again, to drop treatment and refuse to report. This is the story not alone in the social care of neurosyphilis but in that of many other forms of chronic disease. All in all, Collins received regular treatment by salvarsan for a continuous period of nineteen months and subsequently for further periods. He is one of the cases under systematic therapeutic investigation by the Massachusetts Commission on Mental Diseases. What is to be the outcome of that investigation which began in 1914 and has under observation several hundred neurosyphilitics can doubtless not be said until the period of a decade has elapsed.

Here, then, is a sample of mental disease clearly syphilitic in origin, clearly chronic in its course, if not likely to pass rapidly into dementia and death; yet by combined efforts of the medical and social service, a reasonably good front to the disease on the one hand and the world on the other was provided. We now have a history of five years since his first appearance in the hospital after falling into convulsions on the street, and we have a history of three years since the initiation of a period of regular treatment. Whatever be the pathological fate of David Collins, whether it be early or late, at all events partial or temporary cure by social service must be scored for the Collins family, as well as for its central psychopathic figure. His case is by no means an isolated one in our experience. We feel ourselves entitled to crave most earnestly the concession by medical men that social service energy shall be duly expended even upon these cases of such (statistically founded) unfavorable prognosis. It is, perhaps, also worth while to insist that neither the intensive medical care nor the elaborate social care undertaken in the case of David Collins would have been warrantable by itself alone.

Hours spent by	Medical record, 11 pages
	Social record, 26 pages
Physician, 8	Social work:
	Visits, 27
Psychologist, 0	Interviews at hospital, 15
	Telephone calls, 5
Social worker, 51	Letters, 9

General paresis in a soldier; at first thought to be dementia praecox.

Case 43. Carl Spindler came from a public health hospital with the diagnosis of dementia praecox. His case was found to be one of general paresis requiring commitment. He was incoherent, and very talkative, to the effect that he was going to Washington to take the President's place, that the girls were all crazy about him, and that he had plenty of money. He was a well-built man of thirty-three of German descent. He had worked in packing houses until he enlisted in the army. He had seen service in France, where he had got a number of shrapnel wounds and had been gassed. He was transferred to a state hospital for prolonged care.

Hours spent by	Medical record, 7 pages
	Social record, 1 page
Physician, 3¼	Social work:
	Visits, 0
Psychologist, 0	Interviews at hospital, 2
	Telephone calls, 0
Social worker, 1½	Letters, 2

Steady young soldier who began to sing, dance, and fight. Taboparesis. Symptoms following his mother's death.

Case 44. Thomas Scannell was drafted at the age of twenty-one and had been in the army fifteen months (of which seven months' service in France) before he was sent to an A. E. F. hospital. He passed through three hospitals in this country where he was thought in turn to be suffering from (a) dementia praecox, (*b*) general paresis, and (*c*) manic-depressive psychosis. He was excited and talkative (threatening, *e.g.*, to write to the President for a better room), sang, danced, and fought. In the Psychopathic Hospital he proved definitely a paretic (taboparetic form). Accordingly commitment was recommended. But his sister and her husband, both plainly of low mentality, insisted upon taking him home, saying that they should never feel satisfied if he were not given a chance at home. He is now receiving treatment as an out-patient only. His mother died while he was in France, and he himself attributes his illness to nervousness resulting from worry over her death.

He is the illegitimate child of a hard-working respectable woman married to a worthy man who died when the boy was eight years old. Scannell was a steady young man with a pleasant disposition. He "was crazy about his sister's baby." He did not use alcohol and had held one job for five years.

Hours spent by	Medical record, 10 pages
	Social record, 2 pages
Physician, 3¼	Social work:
	Visits, 0
Psychologist, 0	Interviews at hospital, 3
	Telephone calls, 6
Social worker, 3½	Letters, 6

Boy with congenital syphilis (juvenile tabes). Dropped behind in school at eleven. Difficulty of getting parents to have treatment for him.

Case 45. The physician's point in presenting Archibald Sherry, the twelve-year-old victim of congenital locomotor ataxia (juvenile tabes) would be to show special pride in his therapeutic results in a rare disease. The case has been presented briefly from the medical point of view as case 38 in Southard and Solomon's case history collection *Neurosyphilis*. We may here omit the medical details. The layman would, of course, readily observe the unsteadiness of the boy's gait, and would come upon certain oddities in his teeth (typical Hutchinsonian teeth). The psychiatric social worker, like other lay observers, should bring notes concerning superficial oddities of teeth for the physician's consideration and now and again the worker will be able to throw considerable light upon obscure cases under direct medical observation by retrieving sundry dental facts concerning relatives of the patient, superficially examined in the course of taking histories in the patient's home.

The Sherry boy, after the diagnosis of his syphilis had been thoroughly proved in hospital, was treated and certain pains of his, certain attacks of confusion, and trouble with his speech disappeared upon salvarsan injections, and his gait became steadier.

From the standpoint of social psychiatry, Sherry's family history was of interest. On the father's side there was nervousness (as well as alcoholism and degeneracy). The number of things which "nervousness" may at bottom be is legion; of course no conclusion as to syphilis in the family could be drawn either from a history of nervousness or of degeneracy. The fact that the maternal grandmother had cancer is, no doubt, of no importance. A sister, four years older than Archibald, was also thought to be "nervous" and unstable. One task of social psychiatry was to have this girl examined for syphilis and especially to have her blood and spinal fluid examined. Both blood and spinal fluid failed to yield signs of syphilis.

Instructive also is the fact that Archibald, although always a weak and sickly child, did well in school to the end of his eleventh year, when his capacity to keep up with the other children dropped and he became no longer so amiable and sociable. An odd thing in the case was that the eye-lashes of the boy had turned white during the year.

It was, of course, also the duty of the social service to secure blood reactions of father and mother, who denied syphilis. The reactions of both father and mother proved, in fact, negative, and also, as above noted, that of the older sister. The medical observers remained in doubt as to whether the case was one of syphilitic disease handed down from father or mother, or whether the case was one of a rare or unique condition, namely—"acquired" juvenile tabes. (Concerning the true meanings of the terms hereditary, congenital, and acquired, the psychiatric social worker should make absolutely sure.)

Social work in this case proved difficult by reason of lack of coöperation on the part of Archibald's mother. Treatment could not, in fact, be consistently continued. However, social workers from time to time visited the boy in his home, and he has apparently shown no setback since his initial improvement following a few injections of salvarsan into the blood that were made some six years ago.

Hours spent by	Medical record, 9 pages
	Social record, 18 pages
Physician, 5½	Social work:
	Visits, 24
Psychologist, o	Interviews at hospital, 3
	Telephone calls, 18
Social worker, 42½	Letters, 14

Industrial disability caused by syphilis. Under treatment returned to work.

Case 46. The full text of Harold Gordon's social record is given in Appendix A.

SECTION II

HYPOPHRENOSES (FEEBLE-MINDEDNESS)

High-grade moron, daughter of a good family. Stealing, sex irregularity. "Football of environment." Institutional care. Need of psychiatrist, psychologist, and social worker.

Case 47. Florence Warner, nineteen, brought to the Psychopathic Hospital for observation at the family physician's suggestion, turned out to be a moron, measuring 11.5 years by the Point Scale and 10 1/5 years by the Binet Scale.

It is worth while to premise that these minor differences in the mental test levels, as is clear from the data of many previous cases in this book, allow no doubt whatever that the girl so tested was a moron,—provided always that the tests were carried on under favorable conditions without (*a*) fatigue on the part of the examiner, or (*b*) on the part of the patient, without (*c*) any clouding of consciousness, such as infectious disease, alcohol, drugs or other condition might produce and (*d*) without any trace of stupor or dullness of mental faculties incident to many forms of the frank psychoses. None of these latter phenomena were shown by Florence Warner. She was at the time of examination perfectly clear-headed and capable of a very fair amount of attention to the tests. In fact we find from the report recorded that her comprehension was good and that she had a very excellent power of reasoning in the examples set for her. Her memory, to be sure, was only fair and her analytical power limited. Her loss of points in the mental tests accordingly was a rather general one and the separate items were valued from rather poor to fairly good or even good—being for the most part only fair.

We may further take occasion at this point to say that the detailed procedures of the mental tests, whether by the various revisions of Binet or by the Point Scale, are entirely within the scope of a social worker to learn and even to use, as (in point of fact) these procedures are within the scope of any well educated person. But we do not need to exhibit the prejudices of an overspecializing psychologist when we insist that these tests are not to be trifled with, and are not to be valued highly save when performed by an examiner of considerable skill and experience who "has his hand in" and who for the most part is doing little else in life. This is not to say that what Professor James called the Ph.D. octopus need dominate the field of practical mental examination, although for our part we feel that every laboratory executing routine tests in important cases should be managed by an expert psychologist who shall stand sponsor for the results. Those not familiar with the situation in applied psychology may not bear in mind how rapidly the field is changing and how numerous the modifications and improvements in psychometric tests will be before at last we reach the ideal set of tests. On the other hand, the time is past when anyone can safely doubt the present-day value of the tests we have within ordinary limits of variation and under the special safe-guarding conditions enumerated above.

The problem in the Warner case was stealing and sex irregularity. While we are discussing the psychometric tests it may be worth while to insist that these tests throw little or no light upon the causes of such bad habits or vices. The mental tests, being almost exclusively *intelligence* tests, throw little light upon either the quality or the level of the emotional or volitional sides of the person examined. To be sure Florence Warner was somewhat "suggestible" to test; but this "suggestibility" is a very specific one which does not necessarily argue that the one who shows it steals or enters into irregular sex relations on account of it. The chances are that Florence was the "football of environment"; but it would require a far more elaborate analysis by psychiatrists (or by persons otherwise expert in the world's ways) to *prove* that her irregularities were phenomena of weak will or suggestibility. How, we may ask, shall such analysis of all sides of the mentality be made as will throw the needed light upon the causes of stealing, sex irregularity, and the like? There is no certain answer to this question, although various psychiatrists and psychologists have suggested schemata for analyzing personality under various headings.

It seems that Florence had been in the habit of stealing from members of her family and from friends ever since she was ι small child. She could now no longer live in her brother's family unless means were found by which she could support herself. But, as she was given to stealing, she could not be recommended to any employers. To add to the difficulty she had recently begun sex relations with various men. It seems she had gone to a distant state to work as a telephone operator and had there fallen into bad habits—drinking, smoking, and irregular sex living.

Upon the discovery of her level as a high-grade moron, institutional care was recommended, on the particular grounds that she was a high-grade moron of such a trend that she might benefit by institutional care and would otherwise be in considerable danger of becoming a source of venereal infection. In point of fact Florence was still negative to test as to venereal disease, but was already being strongly urged by a girl friend to join the prostitute group.

As is the situation in most of our states in the present phase of mental hygiene, the waiting lists at the schools for feeble-minded were extremely long. However, upon the Psychopathic Hospital's representation, Florence was listed amongst the urgent cases. She was in the meantime sent to a small private institution which agreed to make exception to its general rule not to receive mental cases. The institution must have regretted its step at the end of three months since Florence had plotted to escape with another girl and had a bad influence on the other girls.

The feeble-minded schools' waiting lists were still long and in the interval Florence was sent to the state infirmary, i.e., the big almshouse hospital of Massachusetts. She promptly took a violent dislike to the women she was there thrown with and was given night work so that she might avoid them. After three almshouse months she was eventually admitted to a state school for feeble-minded. She immediately began to mingle with the older girls and seemed to become perhaps more happy than could be reasonably expected.

It may be remarked that Florence's family was on rather a high level. It was naturally rather hard to persuade her relatives to let her go to a state institution. Of course the general level of mental hygiene in Massachusetts, as in a few other states, is such that we may hope that the general prejudices against all state institutions will at last melt away.

Could such a case be handled by the social worker in combination with a competent psychiatrist *without the aid of a psychologist?* The psychiatric examination determined her to be not insane. The *positive* evidence for the moronity in Florence is derived almost wholly from the mental tests. The physical examination was largely negative; still it may be of some importance to the girl that diseased tonsils and a functional heart murmur were found. The medical examination also was of value to her in showing that she was not as yet a "venereal" case. It is especially important to her that the psychiatrist could find no evidence of a definite acquired psychosis. We feel that it is of the greatest importance to exclude psychosis from these cases of feeble-mindedness. We are familiar with numerous cases in which moronity has been confused with acquired and progressive psychosis. In short, we hold that the psychiatric examination in these cases has extraordinary *negative* values.

While we are comparing the practical values of the psychologist whose data made the *positive* diagnosis "moronity" and of the psychiatrist whose examination was exclusive of any such disease as dementia praecox, let us inquire whether the psychiatrist and the psychologist combined could have handled this case effectively, *without a social worker.* It will be noted that the eventual success in getting Florence into the right institution was a matter of very time-consuming and ingenious persuasive work. The more competent the psychologist the more valuable his work in the laboratory and the less likely he or she would be inclined to "hug the telephone" and do the traveling necessary. The same holds. for the psychiatrists. Moreover, as those acquainted with social service technique are well aware, neither the psychologist nor the psychiatrist has a knowledge of the institutional equivalents, institutional and other personalities, community and neighborhood habits and peculiarities, and the technical facts which training and experience give to the social worker. Happily we are able to say that, as the years pass, the psychiatrists and psychologists are becoming less willing to say that, just because they *understand* every social service device employed, therefore they can *perform* the steps effectively in proper sequence and without loss of time.

With respect to the relations of the general medical social

worker to the general problem of medicine, there is no longer any doubt of the necessity of a medical social worker in any community with high health standards. But if this is true for general medicine and the medical social worker in general, it is one-hundred fold truer still for the complicated relations of the psychiatric social worker. In fact we do not need to argue upon this line for those who have had any practical experience in the field. But we take occasion in discussing this first of our group of feeble-minded cases to insist upon a point which stands out most clearly in a case like that of Florence Warner.

Of course we do not know what the eventual outcome in Florence Warner's case may be, granted that the psychometric diagnosis of feeble-mindedness is correct (and there seems to be no doubt of the accuracy of the diagnosis in this case). Possibly it will be in some respects easier to handle a moron who steals and has sex irregularity than to handle a person of perfectly normal mentality with precisely the same trends; but there is no general rule to this effect.

Hours spent by	Medical record, 18 pages
	Social record, 5 pages
Physician, 3¼	Social work:
	Visits, 2
Psychologist, 1	Interviews at hospital, 2
	Telephone calls, 4
Social worker, 7	Letters, 4

A psychopathic family. Each member (parents and eight children) an individual problem. Syphilitic, feeble-minded father. Distinction between **hereditary** *and* **congenital**.

Case 48. The family is today, in many social service quarters, the unit of interest in social work. We do not deny that the family ought to be the object of social work, yet we feel that the psychiatric viewpoint has gone far to prove that every family should be analyzed in the first instance, not so much from any supposed general family tendency, and not so much from the standpoint of the family income as from that of the social situation presented by each member of the family taken as an individual. We are aware that many social workers will feel that this plan is carrying individualization to an absurd degree. Particularly in the case of the Newman family, whose plight we hang upon the individual case of Bessie, but which contained ten members (parents and eight children), it would seem a little preposterous to consider technically every member. But let us consider the situation of each member.

Bessie, the third child, nineteen years of age as we now write, is a case of feeble-mindedness belonging in the moron group, measuring psychometrically 9 4/12 years by the Stanford-Binet method and 9.7 by the Point Scale. Bessie whom we first observed at the age of fifteen was at once determined to be suitable for a state school for the feeble-minded. The waiting lists were too long, however, and she could not be admitted. She remained at home, finally became pregnant, altered her character somewhat thereafter so that she became something of a runaway and was delivered of a child which became a public charge (because of Bessie's obvious inability to take care of it and because the family otherwise had already too much on its hands). Bessie remains at home a good deal of a problem. There was at one time a question whether Bessie might not be a victim of schizophrenia (dementia praecox) partly on account of the history of her going over to New York to visit a prostitute girl friend and an episode of throwing clothes out of the window. Technically, however, on the whole no convincing proof of schizophrenia could be found. In any event such a process would have been one grafted upon an original feeble-mindedness.

It was not Bessie, but a sister Rachel, seven years younger, who first came to the hospital's attention. She was sent by her teacher for falling out of her chair, one day as often as three times in an hour. Rachel was found to grade approximately at her age (eight) at the time of examination, although there was the hint of subnormality in her comprehension, emotional control, and power of concentration. No definite psychosis was determined for Rachel; but a certain hyperkinetic tendency on her part might look in the direction of some form of psychopathic personality.

She came under hospital observation two years later, a nail-biter and thumb-sucker, still suffering from the hyperkinetic tendency which was termed "nervousness" and "instability." Under hospital observation, as is so frequent, the girl showed no sign of the hyperkinesis noted outside but when she returned home she was as bad as ever.

The most important individual problem next in order amongst the children is that of Isaac, the oldest son, now twenty-three. He is definitely feeble-minded, grading 9.7 years by Point Scale when observed at the age of eighteen and a half. Isaac's record shows a general leveling down of his mental capacities although his power of attention and his emotional control are more prominently affected than the other faculties (recalling the situation with Rachel). Isaac was unable to read or write but made five dollars a week. He was a domestic nuisance because he, without provocation, administered heavy blows to the children. At the present time he is working with fair regularity for a relative and gives no trouble, though he "knows it all." He often sits for long periods without talking and cannot eat if the other children are about.

His next younger sister, Molly, two years older than the third child Bessie, seems to be absolutely normal in every respect, is physically something of an athlete, and was found upon the Psychopathic Hospital observation to be normal intellectually. Were it not for the abnormality of all the other members of this family of ten, we should regard Molly's having an illegitimate child as not especially suggestive of psychopathy. Perhaps it is safer not to guess psychopathy even against the heavy atmosphere of the Newman family. Molly has also a so-called "doubtful" Wassermann serum reaction of the blood which so often turns positive later on and is always suspicious. (The father of the family was syphilitic to test.) Molly, with the aid of one of the children's agencies, made some effort to take care of her child but eventually had it placed for adoption. She later made what seemed to be a promising marriage. When her husband returned from army service, he failed to support her and became sexually abusive. Now she is back with her own family seeking a divorce. She claims that one of the reasons for her quarrels with her husband is his failure to keep the agreement he made when they married that he would take steps to find and recover her first child.

Having considered, first Isaac, second Molly, third Bessie, we come now to the fourth, Louis, two years younger than Bessie and five years older than Rachel. He tested, when his actual age was thirteen, ten years by the Binet and 11.3

by the Point Scale. He was a boy with an uncontrollable temper and hyperkinetic in various ways, making grimaces and jerky movements of the limbs. He is now in a special class at a business school but is doing very unsatisfactory work and will no doubt shortly drop out.

Daniel two years younger than Louis, is bright in school, a nervous, irritable boy with a positive Wassermann serum test. He seemed to be always in a fight. His brother, two years older (Louis) and his father were especial irritants for him. He was quite uncontrollable by his mother. This boy Daniel graded a few points higher than his actual age, eleven and a half, by both the Point Scale (11.8) and the Binet (11 3/5). He may be regarded as in a general way somewhat precocious and to test was deficient only in his learning ability and in a certain oversuggestibility.

Of the two remaining children, Leo, now eleven, is a good deal of a problem. He is also, like his brother Daniel, not feeble-minded. He is a restless, quarrelsome, and excitable boy who cannot sit still and (resembling Rachel's falling from her chair at school) often falls down when playing or walking. He has recently developed hysteria and has already had two sufficiently pronounced attacks with paralysis of a leg. This paralysis combined with pain in the back of the knee has at times been cured for the moment through persuasion and command by the psychiatrist.

Sally, now seven years of age and the youngest, was at three years regarded as a bright little girl and passed most of the four-year-old tests. She even now grades approximately to her actual age. She cries continually, has a violent temper, is given to biting herself when angry, hits herself against the wall and, like Leo and Rachel, has the falling tendency noted for them.

What kind of parents did these eight children possess? The father Jacob, examined at forty-four, proved to have a mental age of some 9 years. His blood serum showed a suggestively positive reaction for syphilis (three years later a test proved definitely positive). At the earlier age it was thought that some organic mental disease, presumably a form of neuro-syphilis, was developing. Jacob makes many complaints at home, grows easily angry but has not in three years of observation yet developed any progressive mental disease. Whatever he may develop, it seems likely that he is feeble-minded. It might be inquired whether Jacob acquired his syphilis or was perhaps the victim of congenital syphilis. He has no marked stigmata to external observation. There is apparently some enlargement of the right lobe of the thyroid. A heart examination taken in connection with the positive serum test suggests aortic disease. There was some tendency to clubbing of the finger nails and there was a pronounced cyanosis of both hands. He sometimes complains of attacks, which taken into association with his syphilis, might seem to suggest organic disease of the nervous system. Yet it is possible that many of these phenomena in Jacob are hysterical.

His wife, Sadie Newman, although a woman of somewhat limited intelligence (not tested but almost certainly not defective; has efficient brothers known to the social service) has some psychoneurotic symptoms (heat flashes, nervous spells with chin quivering and inability to speak, feeling of general weakness). Almost all the other features in Sadie's life are extraordinarily to her advantage. She has naturally had a most difficult life but has brought the afflicted family through more difficulties than a normal mother would like to face. Mrs. Newman has had in all twelve pregnancies. The first was a miscarriage and the second child died young (thought to be feeble-minded). Then came Isaac, the definitely feeble-minded boy. These first three pregnancies form the clinical ascending scale of improvement found in the syphilitic family and the fourth child, athletic Molly, might be regarded as showing that the syphilitic taint had run itself out. However, next came a definitely feeble-minded child, Bessie, an ugly, pugnacious child. After Bessie came the second and last miscarriage. Then came the grimacing, high-tempered Louis, followed by nervous Daniel with his positive serum test; then came Rachel, Leo, and Sally with their overactivity and falling tendencies, but between Leo and Sally came a boy that died four days after birth.

We spoke of Molly as possibly terminating the syphilitic taint shown in the first three pregnancies but will remind the reader that this good child (the best in the family) herself had a doubtful Wassermann reaction of the serum. Three members of the family, Molly, Daniel, and the father Jacob, have suggestive or positive Wassermann serum tests.

Of course if we should construct a chart of the mental and nervous diseases and defects in this family we might make out a strong case for so-called "heredity" if we, for the moment, forgot the syphilis in the situation. It is worth while for the social worker to remember that, after all, we must regard many of the phenomena in this family as preventable in view of the fact that most of these phenomena accord very well with our idea of what syphilis can produce. To be sure we do not know why the father Jacob was feeble-minded and it may be that the expert eugenist could trace the separate threads of inherited feeble-minded and syphilitic infection in the Newman group. We do not at all know that the father Jacob was a congenital syphilitic. It may be that he was a feeble-minded person who acquired syphilis. Furthermore we must point out a number of psychoneurotic traits in Mrs. Newman, though it would be almost fair to inquire whether many of these traits were not a rather natural acquisition for a housewife in her plight. At all events, as we have repeatedly insisted elsewhere in this book, the social worker should not confuse the hereditary with the congenital. What the feeble-minded part of Jacob transmitted may perhaps be hereditary. What the syphilitic part of Jacob contributed was, no doubt, congenital. We would not bore the reader to understand the distinction between hereditary and congenital by this repeated insistence; however we have heard some relatively expert social workers on the platform using in their propaganda terms which signify that for them at least at the moment, *the distinction between hereditary and congenital* did not seem to be a worth-while distinction. It will be observed that this distinction is a very important one psychologically and even from the standpoint of the budget. The philanthropist who wants to stop hereditary mental disease and defect may perhaps best proceed by endowing eugenic researches and propagandas. The man who has in mind the prevention of certain preventable forms of mental disease and effect (by well-known public health methods, now being rounded into marked efficiency) would raise money on the venereal disease propaganda supported by research.

Let us briefly sum up the social treatment of the Newman group: I. Financial assistance was got so that household goods might be procured with which more decent standards could be maintained, with the result that while six years ago the family lived in dirty and dilapidated surroundings (there was not even a bed for one of the sisters) now they live in a fairly well appointed apartment.

2. Numerous and changing arrangements had to be made from time to time for different children. Three of the children have been boarded out for periods of some two years each. To be sure these children were neither "dependent" nor "neglected" children in the technical sense of those terms so that the fact that a public agency was got to give them better care must be scored as a triumph of prevention.

3. Arrangements had to be made for two confinements (illegitimacy in both), and for the care of the illegitimate children.

4. The father had to be instructed concerning work and his attitude to the family.

5. Advice and encouragement was given to the mother in regard to the father and in regard to each of her children in turn.

6. The relatives had to be advised with respect to the mental condition of the family so that their coöperation might be maintained. It was natural that from time to time they should lose patience.

It may be noted that twenty-six medical and social agencies have been found so far on the records as dealing with the ten surviving members of the Newman family.

Hours spent by	Medical record, 145 pages
	Social record, 99 pages
Physician, 49½	Social work:
	Visits, 95
Psychologist, 15	Interviews at hospital, 38
	Telephone calls, 105
Social worker, 180	Letters, 98

Imbecile boy kept at work by frequent changes. Trained in special class. Feeble-minded father gotten a job: sick mother treated.

Case 49. The Rosenthal family pales into insignificance beside the Newman family. Yet amongst five members three are definitely psychopathic up to date. The boy, Nathan, was the first to appear under hospital observation. He was sent by a school teacher with a question as to his mental defect and yielded a Binet rating of 6 with an actual age of twelve years. Once later he tested at a rather lower level but at the last examination definitely tested at 6 3/5 by the Binet and 5.9 the Point Scale. He is accordingly classified as an imbecile.

It was plain that he should be sent to a school for the feeble-minded. There was for the moment no vacancy to allow his admission. Concerning the possibility of *commitment* it may be noted that the family refused to allow commitment; even had the family entertained the idea of commitment, no doubt the committed child would have been released from the institution forthwith on the ground that there were other cases more suitable for schooling. Nathan had, therefore, to be supervised at home. He was hard to manage, irritable, quarrelsome, and if crossed, disagreeable. He threatened with a toy pistol persons who, he thought, had injured him. He would wait behind a door with this pistol to shoot a boy who had hit him. He attended a special class at school and his conduct improved a little after his teacher obtained for him a newsboy's license. Nathan is now working irregularly; his mother finds fresh jobs for him when he decides to leave one. He is very sensitive to children's taunts and comes home to his mother crying because somebody has teased him.

Nathan's two siblings, a boy two years younger and a girl three years younger, are regarded as very "smart" and are in the high school and grammar school respectively in proper grades (tested at the hospital their age levels are well up to normal).

The social service work in the case of Nathan shortly brought out the fact that his mother Sarah (forty-three) had bad headaches and so-called "rheumatism" with numbness of the arms. She was examined in the out-patient department, took hydrotherapeutic treatment and gradually improved.

Mrs. Rosenthal had to take care of the family finances because her husband Abram, also examined in the out-patient department, proved to be nine years of mental age (actual age forty-seven). Mr. Rosenthal, a painter, seems to have had a fall upon his head at about the age of twenty-four. He had come from Russia at the age of nineteen. He was still unable to read English. Rosenthal's friends thought that he had not been normal since his fall. He had been getting gradually worse and had begun to suffer from spells of dizziness. He accordingly had to give up his painting. At his first examination in the out-patient department there were some signs of lead poisoning. He was sent to a general hospital for treatment (the same general hospital where he had been treated twenty-three years before for "concussion with question of laceration of the brain," evidently the basis of his traumatic defect-condition). At this general hospital he was operated upon for appendicitis. Aid had to be given to the family in the meanwhile by two charitable agencies. Dental work was arranged for. Upon recovery he was helped to get a city position. His general health had by this time much improved.

At the present time, what with the father's improvement in general health and the mother's improvement as to headaches, the general situation is as good as might be expected. Once when out of a job Rosenthal came to the hospital for aid in getting another city job. Of course it is naturally not advisable for any agency, and above all a public agency, to cause patients to lean financially upon it; but a little aid applied at a critical time to help restore physical or mental health does not necessarily encourage a dependent attitude. Our assistance is often sought in finding work when there is no thought of money help.

Concerning heredity in this family complex, we know nothing concerning Rosenthal except that he was one of six children, one of whom died at twenty-five years but the others of whom lived to more advanced ages. The like holds true for the mother who was one of some nine children, all of whom are said to have lived to a considerable age. Both father and mother are the only ones of their siblings that survive. A niece of the mother has epilepsy. The data, as in the case of many immigrants, are of no particular value from the eugenic side. We do not know of any hereditary or syphilitic features in the family. If Rosenthal is a true case of traumatic defect-condition (that is with mental symptoms due to definite structural lesion of brain tissue caused by the accident) then we should have no reason for thinking that the boy could have inherited his feeble-mindedness from the father, but of course, we do not know whether Rosenthal graded to normal at the time of his accident.

Hours spent by	Medical record, 39 pages
	Social record, 45 pages
Physician, 16¼	Social work:
	Visits, 31
Psychologist, 5	Interviews at hospital, 23
	Telephone calls, 20
Social worker, 64	Letters, 10

Street car conductor, steady quiet fellow; moron. Enlisted in the navy. Sex obsessions and delusions.

Case 50. Bernard Bornstein, a moron, seventeen years old, wanted to enlist in the navy to see the world. His parents refused permission because the father was out of work and the family dependent on the boy's wages (he was earning between fifteen and twenty dollars a week as a street car conductor). So Bernard ran away and enlisted. His first day on shipboard he met another Jewish boy, who became his chum and in the course of time told him that the other sailors intended to make him commit sodomy. Bernard believed this. In the hospital he insisted that there had been about a hundred and fifty of his shipmates who had followed him around so that he could not do anything; write a letter, or take a bath, or get to sleep. He said he would wrap the blankets about him in his hammock and they would come and tear them off. He had in fact complained to the officers, who sent him to the hospital with a statement that there was no basis in fact for his ideas.

This boy had attended the public schools in New York until he was fourteen, made there (*though a moron*) a fair record, and had then worked regularly earning increasingly good wages. He lived with his parents and gave his weekly pay to his mother, to whom he was much attached. He was a quiet fellow who spent his evenings at home and went about very little with other boys. In this protected environment he was contented and useful, until a sudden impulse to see the world carried him into a life of responsibilities beyond his capacity.

Hours spent by	Medical record, 29 pages
	Social record, 0
Physician, 4¼	Social work, 0
	Visits, 0
Psychologist, 1	Interviews at hospital, 0
	Telephone calls, 0
Social worker, 0	Letters, 0

Feeble-minded recidivist.   Honorable discharge from the army.

Case 51.   Howard Driscoll by psychological tests showed a mental age a little over ten years (twenty-one at the time he was examined). He had enlisted in the artillery at sixteen and had been after three years in camp sent to England for guard duty, and later to France where he was wounded several times and gassed. His army record was sprinkled with A.W.O.L.'s but in the end he got his honorable discharge. He came home but after a short time vanished, turning up only at intervals for a few days. He was even arrested once for vagrancy and served a reformatory sentence. Again, he broke into the house of an aunt and stole jewelry for which he was given three months in jail.

He now enlisted in the navy and was soon discharged for mental incapacity. Some months later he joined the state guard and was assigned to a machine-gun company. A week later, whilst guarding ammunition, he offered to relieve another guard so that the latter could get his dinner. When the other man had been gone for several hours, Driscoll got angry, left his post, and went off for four days. He was then sent to the Psychopathic Hospital for examination, where he was pronounced feeble-minded as above.

The family gave an account of a change of character at the age of nine when the boy had a fractured skull. After this he lied and stole and fought. He had been twice in a reform school. He never kept at a job for more than a few days or a few weeks, with the exception of a position as moving-picture operator which he held off and on for two years, leaving five separate times because he did not like the "boss" who "called him down." Two months after discharge from hospital, he was again admitted, sent in by the court on a charge of larceny. His mother was distracted, fearing that the boy might do some terrible thing that would bring harm to him and disgrace to the family. During the two months' interval between his admissions to the hospital, he married a girl whom he met on the street after a week's acquaintance and in the full knowledge that she was pregnant by another man. This girl, as it chanced, had also been at one time a patient at the Psychopathic Hospital, a moron suffering from chorea sent in from a reformatory where she had made an attempt at suicide.

For lack of suitable hospital provision for such defectives as Driscoll, the chances are that the rest of his life will be spent in intermittent penal sentences. The girl he married is a similar problem.

Hours spent by	Medical record, 13 pages
	Social record, 1 page
Physician, 3¼	Social work:
	Visits, 0
Psychologist, 1	Interviews at hospital, 2
	Telephone calls, 0
Social worker, 1¼	Letters, 1

Subnormal psychopathic girl. Illegitimate child that died. Unhappy, quarreling. Family known to twenty-four social agencies.

Case 52. Beatrice Cellini has never been in the wards of the Psychopathic Hospital. She has been handled as an outpatient and under the social service. She came to us alone, crying and telling about her unhappiness. We found that she had been sent from another out-patient department with the idea that she might be a mental case such as could properly be treated at the Psychopathic Hospital. It proved that she came of a family that had been the subject of attention by no less than twenty-four social agencies in the City of Boston before she came to the Psychopathic Hospital as the twenty-fifth.

She said her home conditions were poor and that she cried a great deal. It was partly her own fault. A man had been attentive to her whom she wanted to marry, but "how could a girl who has had an illegitimate child marry." She said she had never gotten along with her mother, who had nagged her. Moreover she quarreled with her brother and disliked her stepfather. (There were five stepsiblings.) She had worked in candy factories not earning more than eight dollars a week. At sixteen she had run away to another state with a man who, according to her story, assaulted her. This man afterwards went to prison. At the age of twenty, according to her story, she was raped; at all events she became pregnant and the offspring, turned over to the state, shortly died. It was this past that she had so much upon her mind. A brother was dying of tuberculosis in a hospital.

Beatrice was given the psychometric tests (non-English) and

was found to grade at 13.4 years. The examination was a so-called regular one. She appeared to be overhasty and thoughtless in answers though she coöperated perfectly well in the tests. No doubt Beatrice is to be regarded as somewhat subnormal or perhaps amongst the upper third of the morons. Accordingly only a relative adaptability to the social milieu is to be expected. The expected success was scored. Beatrice was got to canvass for a magazine and this work appealed to her. She went out amongst friends and acquired a more cheerful attitude to the world. Through the counsels of the social service and otherwise she got upon much better terms with her mother. In some way, either through the passage of time or the friendly conversations with visitors, the history of her rapes and of the illegitimacy was either erased from her memory or, as the phrase goes, "rationalized." We are inclined to insist upon the value of what may be called the "psychiatric touch" or attitude. One of the general social workers who had come in contact with Beatrice had fired the following adjectives at her; "vain, idle, lazy, selfish, untruthful, immoral."

The innermost nature of the psychopathic personality remains to be worked out (see Book III, Section XI) and the relation of subnormality and moronity to psychopathic personality is a little unclear (see, for example, comments under the case of Marian Spring, Case 63, and elsewhere). Beatrice varied much in her attitude to the worker. Upon one visit she would be perfectly amiable and compliant, upon another, sullen and disagreeable; even within the space of a single visit her mood might well vary from sullen to amiable. On the whole the variation was almost always polarized towards the more pleasing mood; that is, she responded well to friendly contact. It was noted above that she disliked her home atmosphere; nevertheless she could not be persuaded of the value of going away from this disagreeable home. Whether these moods correspond with a slight tendency on the part of Beatrice to the so-called cyclothymic constitution (see Book III, Section IX) we may suspect but leave doubtful.

Hours spent by	Medical record, 11 pages
	Social record, 17 pages
Physician, 3½	Social work:
	Visits, 6
Psychologist, 1	Interviews at hospital, 3
	Telephone calls, 13
Social worker, 15	Letters, 7

SECTION III

A reliable workman for two years past disabled by epileptic seizures. Drinking debauch after mother's death: attack of violence. Doing well at work on relative's farm.

Case 53. Luigi Silva was brought to the Psychopathic Hospital by the police. He had had a fit and become violent and destructive during a heavy drinking debauch. He was still noisy and excited upon his entrance, unclear as to mental processes, and quite inaccessible to the examiner. When seen he was trying to break windows; looked as though he saw animals and seemed to be trying to pick up some things and avoid others. He would cry out: "Why don't you take that thing off of my shoulder?" or again "It is a lie!"

Two days later he was perfectly clear. He remembered having hallucinations of hearing and had a proper insight concerning them. He was quite vague as to his time in the hospital. He seemed on the whole rather dull. Psychometrically he graded at 9.2 years; the grading was rather irregular, suggestive, that is to say, of an acquired deterioration. He was rather effective with the construction puzzles and fair upon the memory tests. Physically the only positive points of note were moderate impairment in hearing of both ears, slight nystagmus, and slightly excessive reflexes on the left side of the body.

Silva had been born in Boston of Italian parents, left school at the age of fourteen to go to work, and had sometimes earned (doing heavy nickel and brass work) as much as ten dollars a week. Later he earned as much as twelve to fifteen dollars a week. He had been a reliable workman, not especially alcoholic. At about the age of thirty-one he had had his first attacks of an epileptic nature, coming every three or four weeks. For the past two years he had been unable to work on account of the seizures. Of late he had begun to drink a good deal of whisky. Two weeks before his arrival at the hospital, his mother died, and after her death he had a very heavy drinking debauch whereupon ensued the violent and destructive attack above mentioned.

Upon his discharge from the hospital he went to live with a relative on a farm. The plan was to keep Silva away from the temptation of liquor. Now and then he was to come to town to go to the hospital clinic. This plan was carried out. The patient helped about the farm, doing light carpentry, feeding animals, and cutting ice. The cousin brought him to the hospital from time to time. Immediately after his discharge the attacks grew for a period more frequent and severe. He is still having attacks which for the time are of milder nature. He is said to be improved mentally, which improvement presumably means that there are fewer after-effects of the now somewhat mitigated attacks.

There are a number of medical problems in the Silva case still unsolved. Like all but a small minority of epileptics he exhibits a number of signs of structural disease of the nervous system. We do not know why the epilepsy began, as it is said to have begun, after the age of thirty. We have so far found no evidence of epilepsy in other members of the family.

Perhaps we might use our ignorance of certain features in the epileptic Silva to insist upon the importance of the whole problem of the epilepsies. Perhaps nothing is more harmful to the victims than to lump them all under one term "epilepsy." It is just as true that there are numerous forms of epilepsy as that there are various forms of mental disease. The relations of alcohol to epilepsy are particularly intriguing. It seems to have proved that alcohol tends to produce more frequent and possibly more severe attacks of epilepsy in confirmed epileptics. There are also cases to prove that alcohol can *de novo* produce epilepsy in a person without hereditary soil or acquired taint, and that this epilepsy may then persist even without the stimuli of further alcoholism. But these relations between alcohol and epilepsy cannot be said to be thoroughly established in such a way as to offer clear principles of prognosis. Alcohol is only one cause or complication of the epilepsies. Following, on page 467, is a grouping of the major kinds of epilepsy; without going into their special natures, it can be readily seen that in the field of epileptology, the social worker, to say nothing of the psychiatrist himself, must step gingerly.

Hours spent by	Medical record, 19 pages
	Social record, 6 pages
Physician, 5½	Social work:
	Visits, 10
Psychologist, 1	Interviews at hospital, 0
	Telephone calls, 6
Social worker, 17¼	Letters, 3

Epileptic who killed his mother. Convulsions after head injury.

Case 54. Patrick Donovan, thirty-six, killed his mother and an indictment was found against him for murder in the first degree. Patrick had given himself up to the police, saying that the beer he had drunk the night before had been drugged and he did not know what he was doing. His sister thought he had had convulsions the night before the murder. These convulsions were not necessarily "epilepsy." It is important for the social worker not to confuse every fit of convulsions with the disease, epilepsy. But these particular fits turned out to be very definitely epilepsy, due to an injury ten years before.

Patrick had never had any serious illness before the age of twenty-six, although he was said to have been always very quiet, sullen, and quick-tempered—more quick-tempered with members of his family than with strangers. In short even before the fracture of his skull at the age of twenty-six he might be thought to have shown somewhat of an epileptic temperament, at all events a psychopathic temperament. Patrick's brothers were all alcoholic; his paternal great-grandfather had had a mental disease; his father had become insane at the age of forty.

The patient was struck on the head by a ledge weighing sixty pounds and was in the hospital for some thirteen weeks. On the day of the accident there were nineteen convulsions. From that time forward convulsions occurred frequently throughout his life, as a rule at night. Patrick drank heavily of water and had a large appetite. He grew very jealous and was unsociable in his family.

There could be hardly any doubt that Patrick's action was epileptic. His mother's body was badly mutilated. Some time before, it now transpired, Patrick had assaulted also his sister, breaking her jawbone. He had at that time also been drinking.

The psychiatrists found Patrick well oriented as to time, place, and person, nor could much impairment of memory be determined. He told of times when his heart stopped beating for long periods whilst he was lying in bed. He told how he had a queer, shivery sensation in his body. Often he felt he was falling when he was not falling.

The psychologists found Patrick of the mental level of thirteen years. There were no irregularities in his mental tests (that is to say, no marked examples of his passing tests of high year levels while failing to pass the tests of earlier years). His associative processes proved to be slow, as well as all of his responses, although he coöperated well. His vision had been somewhat diminished since the accident and the psychologists felt that his rating was thereby somewhat lowered. It seemed accordingly that Patrick was not to be regarded as feeble-minded by the mental tests.

Physically there were signs of the old head injury. There was no marked evidence of heart disease. Neurologically he showed sundry effects of his old fracture in the shape of elimination of the fields of vision of the right side and some visual impairment. The X-ray confirmed the history of the fracture.

Here is a case in which the sphere of authority was in the sense of our Book I almost purely public—indicted for crime he could almost at once be determined to be irresponsible for an act done at the time of epileptic seizures. He could therefore promptly be sent to an institution for the criminal insane, where no doubt he will lead a tranquil enough life punctuated by occasional epileptic seizures. In certain epileptic cases there is a possibility of surgical aid. But in this instance the medical details of the examination were such that surgery was not recommended.

What is the province of the social worker in a case like that of Patrick Donovan? The social worker's task is practically confined to the collection of data of value in the medical and psychiatric judgment of the case. In this case various points concerning heredity were obtained. Thirteen agencies, relatives, friends, and employers were consulted by letter, telephone, or interview.

There is no special tendency to epilepsy in the offspring of the *injured* patient. It is often of value to reassure the relatives of traumatic epileptics upon just this point. The theory is that the injury to the brain which brings on cerebral convulsions does not injure the germ plasm and accordingly has no effect upon heredity. In this instance there were no epileptics in the family tree, but there was mental disease on the father's side and there the patient's brothers were alcoholic. Besides this his somewhat psychopathic temperament must be considered.

Hours spent by	Medical record, 15 pages
	Social record, 4 pages
Physician, 5	Social work:
	Visits, 2
Psychologist, 1	Interviews at hospital, 0
	Telephone calls, 6
Social worker, 5	Letters, 6

Drafted but discharged because of epilepsy. Beginning of symptoms after industrial accident.

Case 55. Charles Lovell was sent from the National Guard camp with the statement that he was depressed, apprehensive, and excited. He seemed to be trying to give an impression of more mental trouble than existed. He said he "was crazy a year ago," that his "mind gives way under strain." He was twenty-seven years old and had lived with his mother in a small town, where he worked for a florist. In school he went to the sixth grade, leaving at the age of sixteen. By psychological tests he graded irregularly at 11.8.

Five years before, it was learned, while at work in a foundry he had been hit on the head, had lain unconscious two hours, and next day became "raving crazy" and attempted suicide. He was in bed several months and according to his mother did not get "right in his head" for a year. Thereafter had had occasional dazed spells and lapses of memory, such as forgetting how he came by money that his mother had lent him.

The diagnosis was epilepsy (no doubt traumatic). The patient was discharged from the army and returned to his old job. Two months later his mother wrote a frantic letter to the social service to ask advice as Charlie had received another draft paper to fill out. A statement of the examination here was sent her, and a local physician was obtained to take oversight of the case.

Hours spent by	Medical record, 17 pages
	Social record, 1 page
Physician, 3¼	Social work:
	Visits, 0
Psychologist, 1	Interviews at hospital, 1
	Telephone calls, 0
Social worker, 1¼	Letters, 4

Soldier in whom seizures followed vaccine inoculation. Always subnormal, but a steady lad.

Case 56. Frank Wayne was helping his father on the farm in a southern state when he enlisted at the age of nineteen, in the coast artillery, in the spring of 1917. Ten months later, following several vaccine inoculations, he began to have "fits." These attacks came on at night, while he was asleep. He would run about, without regard to the danger of hurting himself and would sometimes bellow and froth at the mouth. He was discharged from the service after a period in an army hospital and sent home. His seizures now became so frequent (he had as many as eight in ten hours) that his father could not control him, and he was returned to the government hospital and then sent here for a period of observation.

Before enlistment Wayne seems to have been a simple-minded lad of good habits and few interests. He went to school irregularly because of work on the farm and left at seventeen. He was considered by his father to have "good health" and to be "sound mentally." A year and nine months after his first seizure his mental rating was 8 by the Point Scale. There had evidently been some mental deterioration, though he was probably always subnormal in intelligence. He had a speech impediment and seemed dull, but otherwise showed no peculiarities while in the hospital. After a few weeks in the public health hospital he demanded his discharge and was again sent back home. The diagnosis in both hospitals was epilepsy with deterioration.

Hours spent by		Medical record, 12 pages
		Social record, 1 page
Physician, 3¼		Social work:
		Visits, 0
Psychologist, 1		Interviews at hospital, 2
		Telephone calls, 0
Social worker, 2¾		Letters, 1

Policeman who enlisted and had night attacks after first typhoid inoculation. Epilepsy or hysteria?

Case 57. John Bristol had been on the Boston police force before he enlisted, and was taken on again after his discharge from service, but lost his position during the police strike of 1919. While in the army he was boxing instructor in a training camp.

After his first typhoid injection he had a queer attack in the night. These attacks continued to occur nearly every night, always coming during the night, always alike, and numbering from six to fifteen in a night. He would suddenly turn over in bed, bury his face and head in the pillow until he lost his breath, then lift his head to get air and awake partly conscious. During the attack he knew what was going on about him, but could not control himself. He would jerk about and sometimes hit himself in the face.

He came into the hospital as a voluntary patient because these nocturnal episodes kept him from feeling up to regular work. He was single and made his home with his family. The father had died in an alcoholic psychosis. His case was left undiagnosed, for although it was felt that the trouble was probably epilepsy, the possibility of hysteria could not be positively excluded. An X-ray showed a slight clouding in the pituitary area, but there was no positive evidence of glandular trouble as the cause of the attacks.

After four months' treatment in the out-patient department, the attacks fell in number to five or six a night, and Bristol felt encouraged and ready for regular work. He said if he could ever get the attacks down to four a night he should feel that he was completely cured.

Hours spent by

Physician, 3¼

Psychologist, 0

Social worker, 5¾

Medical record, 9 pages
Social record, 8 pages
Social work:
Visits, 0
Interviews at hospital, 7
Telephone calls, 4
Letters, 10

SECTION IV

PHARMACOPSYCHOSES (MENTAL DISEASES CAUSED BY ALCOHOL AND DRUGS)

Expert physicist: invaluable employee. Drinking spells when violent and abusive. Evidence of character anomaly. His fault mental or moral?

Case 58. John Logan, thirty-nine, is a very competent advertising man in a business wherein a certain technical knowledge of physics is of importance. Logan was born in Ireland and had an excellent technical education there. He had come to America in his thirty-seventh year, having at that time been married four years and having two children. Within a year of his marriage he began to drink, and he drank continuously for seven months, during which time he was under the care of male attendants. From time to time he had spells of drinking in which he would become abusive and even violent. His wife even left him at one time, but went back with him to his father's house in Ireland, where he recovered. Several more spells of drinking followed. After one very bad attack, his wife again left him, carrying with her the two children, and consulted a lawyer. Upon this, Logan sold his house, came to America, got a good position where his technical ability counted, and eventually persuaded his wife to join him once more.

Work piled up and, in the course of some six months, Logan again began to drink on the ground that he was helped in his work thereby. He again became abusive with his wife, and the landlord gave him notice to quit. He turned upon the landlord, finally said he was going to hire a man to shoot the landlord, and was brought by the police to the Psychopathic Hospital.

According to Logan's wife, her husband was, as a rule, considerate enough yet objected to her making friends or having any other associations save with himself and the children

244

He would not take her out of an evening, being content to stay at home, reading or talking. He had never allowed a door to be unlocked at night, or a window to stand open even in the hottest weather. He was apt to become irritable at any trifling noise or disturbance. If his wife complained, he would threaten to go away and drink. In point of fact, had it not been for the children, Mrs. Logan said she would not live a moment with her husband.

After two weeks' observation in the hospital, Logan was discharged and went back to his position. He was regarded as "not insane"; he was thought to have been a victim of acute alcoholism and not of any alcoholic *psychosis*. The question of his being a delinquent was left unresolved.

Is it worth while to try to clear up a point or two concerning the respective place in diagnosis of "delinquency," "alcoholism," and "alcoholic psychosis"? As we have repeatedly hinted in other parts of this book, it may well be that the psychiatrists and the criminologists of the future will show that all delinquents are *in some sense* psychopathic; but so far as we are aware, this proof has not been brought. Even in those instances in which the character anomaly of a delinquent is so outspoken that the term *psychopathic* fits pretty well, nevertheless from the legal and even from the moral points of view, this anomalous character may remain perfectly "responsible." Naturally, it is not here our duty to inquire the meaning of the term "responsible." We leave the issue at this, namely, that *delinquency is not a psychiatric diagnosis*. The question of psychopathy remains to be determined whenever delinquency of whatever type is asserted.

Somewhat the same situation holds with respect to "alcoholism." Alcoholism is obviously a social diagnosis. It is very possibly a medical diagnosis. Sir Patrick Manson has spoken of alcoholism as a disease due to the toxin developed from yeast! But assuredly *alcoholism is not a psychiatric diagnosis*. It is especially important for the psychiatric social worker to bear in mind that acute and chronic alcoholism are two forms of social condition which are not at all necessarily mental diseases.

Logan was dismissed the first time from the Psychopathic Hospital without a psychiatric diagnosis. That he was a victim of acute alcoholism was obvious. That he might possibly be a delinquent (from his abusiveness, violence, and threats of homicide) was obvious. That his character was a bit eccentric might also be alleged. But then the "benefit of the doubt" had also to be extended to Logan.

Logan's employer had supposed that the man would have to be discharged. The situation was explained to the employer, who remarked that Logan's work was of so much value to the firm that an occasional leave of absence might be granted to him if necessary. The patient readily agreed to do no more overtime work, to give up alcohol, and to take more interest in his wife's happiness and amusement. Logan began to take a great interest in the Men's Club. (For a brief description of this club, see case 6, Alfred Mack.) Logan in fact even undertook to act as its president. However, within four months he began to neglect the club, grew resentful of the hospital's continuing to take an interest in him, even threatened to leave the state, said he could not be dictated to, and began to think that everybody in his office was jealous of him and working against him. He began again to drink heavily and to abuse his wife, and even once threatened to choke her. Upon this his wife notified the social service and Logan was brought back to the Psychopathic Hospital by the police. The next day he said he was rather glad he had come. He said he could not believe that he had been dangerous, and it was with some difficulty that he could be convinced of his change of character.

He was discharged once more after a period of ten days, again with the diagnosis of acute alcoholism (not a psychiatric diagnosis), yet the notes show that this man's character anomaly stood out somewhat in relief, so that a suggestion of the diagnosis of paraphrenia was offered by some observers. This condition termed *paraphrenia* is a disease rather closely similar to the so-called paranoia, a condition with which even the laity has become more or less familiar. It is a disease in which to all external appearances the patient acts quite normally. Neither his will nor his emotions are at all out of keeping with his ideas. It is these ideas which are at fault. Characteristically, the disease runs a course through (1) a somewhat indefinite early phase to (2) a phase of feeling persecuted. In typical cases, the phase of persecutory delusions passes insensibly over into (3) a phase of grandiose delu-

sions in which the patient feels himself superior to or dominant in his family and surroundings. There was in point of
fact in Logan's case no very striking sign of any grandiose
trend, but his complainings, jealousies, and ideas of persecution by his working associates and his wife seem consistent
enough with this diagnosis. On the whole, however, there
was no sufficient argument for paraphrenia. Upon discharge,
Logan seemed "amiable though rather peculiar." He came a
number of times to the Men's Club; then he begged to be
excused, disliking, as he said, the hospital associations and
feeling that his fellow employees would see him on the way
to the hospital. In point of fact, so skillfully had his hospital
stays been guarded from knowledge that only four or five
persons amongst his working associates knew at all of his
having been treated in hospital for alcoholism.

Four years followed in which Logan's family life was reasonably successful. To be sure, he remained capricious and
unreasonable, haggling over every slight expenditure and giving his wife money for food only. However, he drank not
at all, enjoyed his work, sent his family on good vacation;
when his wife was away himself did some work about the
house, and all went well. A third child had been born. The
family had moved to pleasant suburbs, where garden work
was the center of interest.

It is to be noted, however, that the prognosis by the medical
staff upon his second discharge remained a bit dubious. That
he might return some day to the hospital was an opinion that
stood for four years in the records without confirmation.
Even when the old situation recurred and he was again a fit
subject for the Psychopathic Hospital, there was a good deal
of doubt whether a man who had never received a psychiatric
diagnosis was suitable for reception. Could the Psychopathic
Hospital dogmatically advise the family or the police to bring
a man like John Logan back under care? Here lodges a large
and important question in the mental hygiene of the community. We make no doubt that in the end such advice properly supported by medical, psychological, and social data will
be proffered in cases far less dangerous than John Logan's.
However, we are aware that in vast communities of the United
States no such interference with personal liberty and an
alcoholic's privilege of the pursuit of happiness would be

tolerated. No doubt sundry representatives of the judiciary, even in our own community, might raise their eyebrows at this kind of reaching out from government to the citizenry. Looked at from another point of view, however, we are sure that progress will be in the line of such "interference." If it be "interference" to preserve a man from his own anomalies (to say nothing of his wife and children), then one might say, Make the most of it! The ideal day when psychopathic hospitals throughout civilized communities shall be as open to the mental sick as general hospitals are open to the somatically sick, will see far milder cases than John Logan's brought to the examining table. No matter what the cake of custom fixates in the minds of uncivilized communities, the Psychopathic Hospital movement must and will irresistibly go forward, and perchance engulf those very superconservatives that everywhere block progress.

We wrote the above words before the critical first of July, 1919, upon which day national prohibition in our country began. As a matter of history, Logan, it appears, was influenced to start drinking again by the suggestion that July 1 was upon us and that a few last drinks might well be in order. He took these drinks, and during the next fortnight at home drank more and more until he became again in the familiar way excited, noisy, threatening, and abusive. Aside from trembling of his hands and tongue, he was quite normal physically. As always, he was psychometrically on a high level, getting the maximum year level that our tests permitted. Again he received the medical or social diagnosis "alcoholism," was regarded as non-psychotic, and was discharged. What is Logan's prognosis? National prohibition may settle his fate. If, however, his spells of excitement and abusiveness are really not socially alcoholic in their origin but represent some profound wave of emotional change in Logan, then perhaps a new picture will unroll itself.

What has the social work accomplished in the case of John Logan? Such cases have not been at all frequent. Physicians might well be entitled to doubt whether such cases belonged to the medical, and particularly to the psychiatric, field at all. The question has been raised several times whether John Logan was really a proper subject for the Psychopathic Hospital. Would he not perhaps have been straightened out as effectively by treatment in some other form of hospital, or even as a delinquent? We are personally, however, strongly of the opinion that the psychiatric point of view is the best available for the elucidation even of such mild character disorder as we find in Logan. Logan himself, especially after he had been drinking for some time, no doubt felt that the Psychopathic Hospital cast somewhat of a stigma upon him. He was always polite enough to the particular worker set over him; but his behavior was unmistakably that of a somewhat complaining, resentful man. His wife, on the other hand, felt that John Logan's fault was far more mental than moral. Perhaps she was taught by our social workers so to think. In any event, without the ægis of some hospital, and perhaps without the particular ægis of our own in this community, Mrs. Logan would have felt quite at a loss. No one would have picked up the loose ends of the family plight; and we feel that an enormous *débâcle* might well have ensued in this family without the support afforded by social work.

The only alternative that we can think of to the sort of support afforded by the Psychopathic Hospital social service would be a similar type of support that one might ideally think of as possible under a greatly reformed criminological system. Should it ever be possible for the present system so to develop a fine system of extramural threads running to all parts of the community of delinquents and near-delinquents, then we can ideally conceive that an extension of the probational system along preventive lines might turn the same trick that was turned by the Psychopathic social service in the Logan case. But we may be permitted to point out that, if it remains doubtful whether the Psychopathic Hospital has any right to spread its wings over John Logan, then it is perhaps more doubtful whether a benevolent and reformed prison system could quite so readily spread its wings. Moreover, we think that the wings of the Psychopathic Hospital will always be of whiter hue than the wings of any prison system.

For the administrator of such a beneficent system, whether it stretches its wings from a commission on mental diseases or from a bureau of prisons, the problem presented by such a man as John Logan is always a bit difficult. Shall he or shall he not be admitted as virtually a psychopath when much doubt rules whether he is demonstrably a psychopath? Whatever the system, all depends, as is ever the case, upon the operator of the system. Imagine a stickler upon fine technical obstacles and you will imagine an operator who will fail whatever the general virtues of the system. Wherever possible the community should be given the benefit of the doubt, and in our experience, giving the community that benefit incidentally inures to the good of the central figure in the tragedy.

Hours spent by		Medical record, 11 pages
		Social record, 22 pages
Physician, 4		Social work:
		Visits, 12
Psychologist, 1		Interviews at hospital, 8
		Telephone calls, 16
Social worker, 29		Letters, 16

First attack of delirium tremens. Drank to excess while wife was in hospital.

Case 59. Patrick Nolan, forty, is presented as a case of delirium tremens, that most frequent of the alcoholic psychoses. (In the discussion of the next case, John Sullivan, we make some note of the differences between delirium tremens and alcoholic hallucinosis so far as these are of importance to the social worker.) This man was, according to the mental tests made by the psychological examiners, of a very high rating, namely 15.5 years of mental age (close to the limit of age that can be tested by present-day psychometric tests) and scored in other ways his intelligence was high. This test was made November 19 and the patient coöperated well though he was at that time impatient to get to his family waiting upstairs. He had been admitted to the hospital four days before, namely on November 15.

Nolan was an Irishman, alcoholic from the age of twenty-two years. He had been drinking to great excess for some days and had become very nervous and tremulous. Two nights before admission, that is on the night of November 12, Patrick waked up a family that lived near him and asked the head of the house to come to the Nolan home and stay with him as he was nervous and afraid he would die. His wife was in hospital for a slight operation and he had resorted to whisky for companionship. He himself said that while he and whisky had always been good friends before that, after his wife had gone to the hospital he and whisky had become inseparable. His friend, Mr. Doherty, stayed with Patrick all night. Patrick slept not at all but wandered from room to room. He seemed a little better next day but in the afternoon talked about seeing his dead brother. Accordingly a physician was called who found all the lights in the house lighted and the doors locked. Patrick refused to see the doctor; the police came; Patrick then opened the door and went with them talking about devils who were getting him. So far as his friends knew or at least would say, Patrick had never had a similar state before.

For two nights in the hospital he continued to see devils under his bed. He was "somewhat depressed" but the line between depression and a proper sadness is naturally hard to draw. When he told his story he had become humorous. All are familiar with the humor of the Irish but it would appear from medical observations in alcoholic psychoses that the so-called "humorism" is not merely an Irish trend but is found as a somewhat differential effect of alcoholism in a variety of races.

Patrick Nolan failed to see the "animals" which one is supposed to see if a victim of delirium tremens. Perhaps "devils" will serve in their place. It is just as well, however, that the case we here choose to illustrate delirium tremens is a case without the so-called zoopsia or hallucinations of animals.

Physically Patrick was a muscular, gray-haired, ruddy-faced man having the somewhat characteristic weather-beaten alcoholic facies. Aside from a flushed face and widely dilated pupils, there was nothing of note in the physical examination save very active knee jerks. The victim of delirium tremens is rather apt to look more "sick," that is, physically sick, than the victim of alcoholic hallucinosis (to be considered in the next case, John Sullivan). The facial flush, the tremulousness, the dilated pupils, the look of a certain confusion and perhaps fear combine to give this impression of a delirium tremens victim as looking "sick." "Nervousness" is a term the layman is apt to use about this state; but the term is used for so many other states that it is of little or no value from a standpoint of diagnosis. He was discharged recovered on the seventh day and his frank psychosis had thus lasted apparently some nine or ten days in all.

252   THE KINGDOM OF EVILS

Patrick was now referred to the social service. He was a married man without children who lived on the top floor of a three family house. He was an unskilled laborer earning fifteen dollars a week. Both he and his wife were church members. In Ireland he had had schooling until his thirteenth year and had worked on a farm until he was twenty-four. A brother had died at forty of cirrhosis of the liver, a condition which many books describe as of alcoholic origin, and which, no doubt, is often alcoholic in origin though other factors must probably enter. Another brother had died at the same age, forty, of heart disease. Still another had died of tuberculosis at thirty-six, and the fifth of the five brothers had been a victim of delirium tremens at one time at the Psychopathic Hospital.

An arrangement was made for the patient to come to the Men's Club but this proved not feasible. However, without this aid, through the very light supervision necessary, the patient ceased to drink and it was possible to close the case two months and a half after he first came under observation. It may be queried whether this case was not closed too early and this must be admitted, though no doubt with the experience in hand any renewed resort to alcohol on Patrick's part would have been quickly called to the hospital's attention on account of the relations established with the wife.

Hours spent by	Medical record, 13 pages
	Social record, 2 pages
Physician, 3½	Social work:
	Visits, 2
Psychologist, 1	Interviews at hospital, 1
	Telephone calls, 0
Social worker, 5	Letters, 1

Alcoholic hallucinosis in discharged real estate agent. Other forms of alcoholic psychoses. Temporary care law.

Case 60. John Sullivan, forty-seven, was a victim of a so-called alcoholic hallucinosis, a condition which somewhat resembles the condition well known to the laity under the name delirium tremens and not always easily told from delirium tremens on the one hand and from various other forms of alcoholic mental disease on the other hand. Before the era of national prohibition both *alcoholic hallucinosis* and *delirium tremens* formed so important a group of diseases that no social worker could fail to take an intimate interest in their nature, especially touching their prognosis.

It is worth while stressing the fact that *the alcoholic mental diseases do not vary in severity in proportion with the alcoholism* which is indispensable to their production. Whether there are not some other more essential factors that lie at the basis of alcoholic mental disease in its various forms is, at present, unknown. *By the administration of alcohol one could not promise the production of an alcoholic psychosis.* To be sure there are some pseudonormal forms of alcoholic mental disease that seem somewhat closely allied to *drunkenness,* a condition which is not ordinarily, or perhaps properly, termed a mental disease. The periodic form of uncontrolled drinking called *dipsomania* and the rare disease known as *pathological intoxication* are two conditions which require the most thorough observation and expert judgment to diagnosticate. The victim of genuine dipsomania is, no doubt, as a rule, a psychopath on some broader and deeper basis than the mere alcoholic habit. The basis of the strange disease, pathologic intoxication, is perfectly obscure, though the condition may suggest, in its suddenness and relation with perfectly insignificant intakes of alcohol, some peculiar condition of sensitization that may finally be explained when all such matters as shellfish poisoning, strawberry skin eruptions and the like are explained. We insist rather upon these points because there is an almost irresistible tendency for the lay worker and for the inexperienced physician to regard the alcoholic psychoses as, after all, probably somehow based on the intake of greater and greater amounts of alcohol. While upon the general topic we may add that despite sundry assumptions to the contrary, it is doubtful whether particular kinds of alcoholic beverages have very especial outcomes in relation to mental disease. (The experimental absinthe convulsions form an important exception.)

But the great bulk of the alcoholic mental diseases with which the social worker or the court officer comes in contact is, no doubt, composed of the disease delirium tremens, an example of which is the case of Patrick Nolan given above. Some authors even deny that a differentiation can be made between the two conditions, delirium tremens and alcoholic hallucinosis, and they can point out numerous transitional and intergrading forms of alcoholic mental disease. Some cases looking like delirium tremens may run along for several weeks after the manner of alcoholic hallucinosis. Some cases of delirium tremens, instead of presenting the hallucinations of vision that are typical thereof, present hallucinations of hearing such as we may ordinarily find in alcoholic hallucinosis. On the other hand, alcoholic hallucinosis, though it is less likely to run the brief course of less than a fortnight which delirium tremens runs, may not seldom show hallucinations of sight like those of delirium tremens. It is easy to see that the lay mind would here run too readily upon diagnostic rocks. To illustrate this fact we may point out that owing to certain details in the Massachusetts law, the Psychopathic Hospital was not expected to take cases of delirium tremens any more than it was expected to care for cases of real drunkenness. Nevertheless, every year scores of cases of delirium tremens were admitted to the hospital under the false assumption that they were cases of alcoholic hallucinosis. To be sure humanity entered here to cloud the issue. No other institution in Boston was so well equipped materially or diagnostically to handle the alcoholic psychoses as was the Psychopathic Hospital. (It is to this day a sad commentary on the progress of the so-called general hospitals that they have not equipped themselves with baths, isolation rooms, corps of skilled attendants, and proper diagnostic specialists to meet the complications of alcoholism, with the result that the jails have had to serve as hospitals in states not properly equipped with psychopathic units.) Accordingly we were in the habit of receiving, on the ground of humanity, sundry cases that seemed to be *in extremis* but which turned out to be cases of delirium tremens. When all is said and done, the differential diagnosis, even in this group of mental diseases which the layman is apt to think he understands fairly well, is not easy.

The prognosis of these cases is particularly hard, not to say often impossible to lay down, and some cases of a disease, ordinarily fairly acute, turn inexplicably into chronic cases requiring institutional care or its equivalent, and persisting with a batch of hallucinations and delusions like those with which the disease began, or else subsiding into a deterioration or dementia in the midst of which any very definite alcoholic features are hard to descry.

Before dismissing this topic of the alcoholic psychoses in general, we may mention the existence of a third group of alcoholic psychoses of an insidious onset and a chronic course, cases that do not necessarily begin with any acute form of mental disease (though they may do so) but do not characteristically "hallucinate" (a slang phrase of the clinic having reference to the process of having hallucinations; that is, false perceptions in some field of sense, notably in the alcoholic psychoses in the spheres of vision and hearing). We offer a case of this third group in that of Michael Piso, a case of *jealousy psychosis*.

John Sullivan was a real estate sales agent. He said his business had been going wrong for some time, that he had gone up to Canada one day and returned on the next train, having the idea that a detective was following him; in fact he said he saw someone following him and that he heard some men on the train talking about him. Even after entering the hospital he said he heard people remarking about how he was using other people's money.

Technically the fact that Sullivan had an idea that a detective was following him would be regarded as a delusion or false belief. If, however, he actually saw real men and, noting their whispers, conceived that they were talking about him, then his status would be technically regarded as one of the so-called delusions or ideas "of reference."

Whether Sullivan actually had hallucinations is a matter of some doubt, though he admitted hearing voices of no visible source, but he heard them rather vaguely. The victim of a typical alcoholic hallucinosis should, perhaps, have heard voices much more definitely than did Sullivan. The theoretical line of separation between ideas "of reference" and hallucinations is sharp enough, seeing that the latter must be definite false perceptions, whereas the former are a kind of erroneous idea; yet the practical claim of separation between these two symptoms wavers tremendously.

He had had a history of several weeks of such delusions, believing that the police were after him because he had held back his rent, that people had scoffed at him, that he was ruined (he had actually lost money in recent sales). He said that his mind had become rather confused of late and that he could not think. In fact, he "must have been insane." He had once even gone so far as to threaten suicide.

With all this it may seem strange that Sullivan had actually come to the hospital as a voluntary patient. When it came to signing the application for his admission he, however, became suspicious and refused to sign. He was accordingly admitted under the Temporary Care Law (see Appendix C for discussion of the Massachusetts Temporary Care Law, one of the measures without which extensive state work with noncommittable psychopaths is impossible). As he admitted having hallucinations or other symptoms of a frankly psychopathic nature, it was perfectly proper to have a medical officer (not upon the staff of the hospital) make application for his admission. Upon these preliminaries, Sullivan went to the ward without protest. This was on May 23 and by June 29 it was possible for him to be discharged, as recovered, to the outpatient department. He had had seven days of so-called "temporary care," that is, of care under the law which did not carry him to the probate court, but upon the seventh day, that is, May 29, he was actually "committed," that is, his case was carried to the probate court upon the evidence of two expert physicians not connected with the Psychopathic Hospital.

He was then carried upon the books until December 29. Already by May 29 he had improved a great deal so that the commitment to the hospital was really a measure on the patient's behalf, to the end that he could have hospital care until his disease was over. He was under hospital care, therefore, for a period of about five weeks. At some time in the third week he got good insight into his past condition. At this point the social service took control, although the term "control" might seem a rather heavy one for this particular case. Sullivan was a very amiable sort of man with what may be termed a rather high empathic index.[1] The technique of this social care consisted in utilizing the Men's Club for hospital and human contacts and in counsel and encouragement.

John's mother had been for two months at a hospital for the insane some years before, also the victim of alcoholic mental disease. One of three brothers was also a very heavy

---

[1] Southard, E. E., M.D.: "The Empathic Index in the Diagnosis of Mental Diseases," *Journal of Abnormal Psychology*, October, 1918.

drinker though all three brothers and four sisters were physically well. John's father had died of accident. John had had little schooling but had educated himself. Though he had been a gardener in England he had become a real estate agent in America. His business had been good until it had gone downhill during the last year, obviously the result of his alcoholism. So far as the history was frank, it would seem that before that time he had been drinking more moderately though all through the twenties and early thirties he had been a very heavy drinker, apparently without any mental effects of a nature to interfere with self-support.

Physically he proved entirely normal save his thinness, and psychiatrically there were no abnormalities save those mentioned. He explained that he had taken the trip to Canada with a vague idea that he was going to start anew there.

We find medical notes of reports in July, August, September, November, February, March, May. These notes show that there was no return of symptoms and that Sullivan was making a good deal of headway with his debts and with his business. *Pari passu* with these medical notes we find social service notes in February, March, April, and May of the year following his attack and, in fact, in May the case was closed by the social service. The social-service notes had told of visits at Sullivan's home and of advice concerning his coming to the Men's Club. The economic problem was not in the foreground, as the wife kept a lodging house.

Hours spent by	Medical record, 10 pages
	Social record, 1 page
Physician, 7¼	Social work:
	Visits, 3
Psychologist, 0	Interviews at hospital, 2
	Telephone calls, 1
Social worker, 5½	Letters, 4

Root of family dissension may be disease of one member. Acute alcoholic hallucinosis; chronic inebriety; morbid temperament.

Case 61. If we examine a social case card-catalogue, we shall find case after case of so-called family dissension. We say "so-called" not because the term is meaningless, but because cases left with the designation family dissension are, we believe, cases not properly analyzed as to the form of evil at work. That form of evil may as readily be disease in one or other member of the family as any other of our major groups of evil. Thus Margaret Murray, a Scotch woman of thirty-nine, was living in New Hampshire with her six-year-old daughter Pearl, apart from her very reputable husband, an iron-worker earning some thirty dollars a week. The "symptom" catalogue stood as follows:

Social symptoms:
    Inebriety (chronic)
    (?) Insane commitment
    (?) Neglect of child
    (?) Immoral influence on child
    Marital discord
    Arrest
Social diagnosis:
    Family dissension
Medical diagnosis:
    Acute alcoholic hallucinosis

We hold that the medical diagnosis *in this case* is the social diagnosis and that family dissension, though a perfectly correct term for the social conditions found, is not the caption most helpful in determining social treatment. Chronic inebriety is set down as one of the social factors: *a fortiori,* acute alcoholic hallucinosis is another and even more commanding factor, since (*a*) this disease brought Mrs. Murray to the Psychopathic Hospital and (*b*) its prognosis and treatment (whether by costing confinement in a state hospital or not) will influence every social step taken. In short we would prefer to place this case among the *Morbi* rather than among the *Vitia* where family dissension would tend to leave it. Let the morbid factor be removed, and the moral factor can remain— *i.e.,* Mrs. Murray would then have her chronic inebriety to face (provided that in her case the habit is not itself a disease). Let the inebriety be removed, and there might still be a basis in morbid temperament or bad habits for family discord.

Let us examine enough of the facts to demonstrate the issue. Mrs. Murray had drunk to excess and had been twice arrested for drunkenness (*chronic inebriety*). She came to Boston and, whilst working in an institution, developed the symptoms that brought her to the Psychopathic Hospital.

There she had hallucinations of hearing and told (delusional) stories of her husband's abuse of her. There was even raised the question of commitment. The husband was by now disheartened and antagonized and had begun to regard his wife as irresponsible. There was discord over the question whether she should live with husband and daughter, should take the daughter with her, or leave the daughter with her father. Mr. Murray felt that daughter Pearl might suffer immoral influences from her drunken mother. Upon study of the case it appeared to the social workers that the child could hardly be unaware of her mother's drunkenness. It was on this account that the list of social symptoms contained the two questions "neglect of child?" and "immoral influence on child?"

The efforts of the social service were summed up as follows:—

1. In arranging for temporary care for patient and child upon the former's discharge from the hospital until the husband could be located and until employment was found for her.

2. In making an investigation of the family situation to understand the facts.

3. To give advice and coöperation to both the patient and her husband as they are working out their readjustment.

If we take the phrase "working out their readjustment" upon the simple basis of family dissension, we should hardly avoid being influenced by the phrase itself. Family dissension clearly points to moral difficulties within the sphere of what we have in this book termed *Vitia*. Family dissension does not at all necessarily point to disease (*Morbi*). The man in the street and the social worker can hardly help feeling that family dissension is a matter of ingrained temperament difficult to train by moral methods, difficult or impossible to reëducate by the intellectual route alone and, even if psychopathic, by the same token harder than ever to meet. In short, the social worker, should she content herself with the social diagnosis family dissension, might believe that she was doing the charitable thing by her patient. Family dissension as a moral matter sounds less heinous than family dissension as a matter of disease.

But let us look into the facts. As a matter of the actual situation and its outcome, the social condition family dissension proved to be almost entirely, if not quite, fear of a rather acute mental disease or the so-called hallucinosis. That there was any deep underlying psychopathic trend of temperament is extremely doubtful. Even if Mrs. Murray became alcoholic through some deep trend of her nature, there is no proof, theoretical or practical, that this temperamental trend would, in and by itself, lead to family dissension. Accordingly, we hold that our proof is positive, that the social diagnosis in the case of Mrs. Margaret Murray should be alcoholic mental disease, in particular acute alcoholic hallucinosis. We hold that the social prognosis depends upon the medical diagnosis and prognosis. We hold that family dissension is an effect rather than a cause and is probably removable. We hold that the questions raised concerning neglect of child and immoral influence upon the child by her mother are questions which would be removed by a solution of the mother's alcoholic problem. Likewise we hold that the arrest and the question of commitment of Mrs. Murray to a chronic institution (a question raised during her temporary care whilst she was recovering from the acute effects of her alcoholic psychosis) are likewise purely secondary products of the situation.

We should also like to call attention to the fact that the phrase "chronic inebriety" which stands at the head of the list of social symptoms in this case is likewise somewhat misleading. To be sure the acute mental disease known as alcoholic hallucinosis was, in this case, incidental to a chronic inebriety. It is also true, no doubt, that alcoholic hallucinosis is, as a rule, incidental to a chronic inebriety, but it is not at all clear that chronic inebriety must necessarily or in any large proportion of cases lead to alcoholic hallucinosis. As one author rather paradoxically said, "The causes of delirium tremens are still obscure." The same holds for the allied disease, alcoholic hallucinosis, the causes of which are perhaps still more obscure than those of delirium tremens itself. Neither of these diseases is at all proportional to the amount of alcohol consumed by the victims nor to the duration of the habits of inebriety. Nor can we say that the prognosis of cases of delirium tremens or of alcoholic hallucinosis at all varies with the duration or severity of the alcoholic bad habit. We may be permitted to add that chronic inebriety shares with family dissension the pretty distinct intimation that we are dealing with bad habits and vices rather than with deficiencies in the patient's education or psychopathic temperamental tendencies.

The general social worker must bear in mind these intimations of the social phrase. The psychiatric social worker quickly learns the more obvious pitfalls of phraseology, but each type of social worker and the physician himself must guard against throwing *all* cases of family dissension and *all* cases of chronic inebriety over into the disease group. It must be plain from the general drift of our contentions in this book that disease must be considered as a primary hypothesis and not necessarily as a statistical probability. Deficiencies in education leading to family dissension or to chronic inebriety are even less statistically probable as a matter of actual fact—still, we must consider the hypothesis of faulty education. Nevertheless, if we are entitled to give over the psychopathic hypothesis and the maleducational hypothesis, then we shall be reduced to the hypothesis of moral deficiency or perversion. If we are reduced to this hypothesis, we shall find far more trouble in the process of readjustment for everybody,—as some might say nine parts of internal readjustment to one part of external and merely social readaptation. Family dissension might conceivably be an almost purely legal difficulty owing to perfectly logical disagreements on the part of different members of the family concerning (let us say) financial arrangements; but of that rare possibility there was no question in the Murray case. Nor was there any question of a purely economic basis for the dissension in this family.

The social analysis of the Murray case leads us, in the end, to placing an acute and curable alcoholic mental disease sharply in the foreground. The social prognosis becomes extraordinarily brighter than it would be if we took family dissension *prima facie* as the root difficulty. We are dealing with another sample of the well-known, though somewhat paradoxical, plight, the situation that **it is rather better to be sick than to be vicious.**

Hours spent by	Medical record, 6 pages
	Social record, 7 pages
Physician, 3½	Social work:
	Visits, 0
Psychologist, 0	Interviews at hospital, 2
	Telephone calls, 22
Social worker, 7	Letters, 15

Feeble-minded teamster ten years married to a good wife, suffers from alcoholic "jealousy-psychosis." Violent, abusive. Improvement. Family difficulties: poverty, sickness.

Case 62. There are hardly more intriguing cases than those of jealousy in alcoholics. Psychiatrists recognize a peculiar alcoholic "jealousy psychosis," sometimes conceiving that the onset of sexual impotence on the part of the alcoholic leads up by somewhat natural steps to the belief that the spouse is in love with a rival. Now there is, perhaps, especially in alcoholic families, always a possibility that there is some actual fire under the delusional smoke. The psychiatrist, and even the social worker who comes in close contact with family conditions, may be for a long time in doubt as to the actual facts. In alcoholic communities the psychiatrist often feels himself entitled to suspect alcohol in any case of delusions of jealousy. Yet the psychiatrist has constantly in the back of his mind sundry exceptional instances in which jealousy delusions appear in *non*-alcoholic persons, for example in victims of schizophrenia (dementia praecox). The social worker's data become of prime importance in making exactly this decision between alcoholic jealousy-psychosis and dementia praecox with sex ideas.

Michael Piso had been jealous of his wife, according to his history, ever since their marriage. As a jealous husband he questioned her about everything—at one time accusing her of immorality with a lad of nineteen years. They had been married for ten years, and his wife was in point of fact an exceptionally good woman. There were three living children. Michael had been alcoholic for some fifteen years. He always made excessive sex demands upon his wife and twice tried to choke her when these demands were not met. He was a teamster and worked in one place throughout his married life. At one time he developed an abscess in the right ear and complained of severe headaches. The psychiatrist brought up a question, upon his arrival at the hospital, of organic brain disease but was even then convinced (by such portion of the story as was available) that he was probably a case of alcoholic psychosis and was at the same time feeble-minded. This combination of diagnoses proved in fact the final one, and he was discharged as a high-grade moron with alcoholic psychosis.

Just before entering the hospital he threatened to buy a pistol and attacked his wife. He had left work about a week before entering the hospital and had grown increasingly jealous of his wife and imperious as to sex. A year before he had had a severe headache which had thrown him out of work for ten days, and at that time he vomited and had blurring of the eyes. As to heredity, one of his children had had convulsions and a cousin died insane in a state hospital.

The psychologist could find no marked irregularity in Michael's reactions; and, finding his mental age according to the Point Scale to stand at 11.6 (Binet 10 3/5) years, made the diagnosis of feeble-mindedness. It might be inquired whether this feeble-mindedness was more apparent than real. Seeing that Michael had been heavily alcoholic for fifteen years, we might regard him as a victim of alcoholic deterioration. Some victims of alcoholic deterioration do give a low test of this sort, even without marked irregularities; on the whole, however, a victim of acquired psychosis is very likely to show some traces of inability to pass tests of the earlier years of the scale (*e.g.,* seven-year-old tests) at the same time that he passes the tests of the higher scale years (*e.g.,* eleven-year-old tests). Michael was a teamster, and his work no doubt did not as a rule require behavior more complicated than that of the mental age level of 11.6.

The psychiatrists could upon physical examination find no sign of brain tumor, nor, with the exception of pyorrhea, was there any marked condition of disease in the body.

There was considerable doubt whether he had ever had hallucinations, although there was a possibility of auditory ones. The delusion of infidelity on the part of his wife he now very well concealed. After some three weeks in the hospital he grew quieter, remarked that he had one night heard a voice about his wife, saying, "Do not trust her"—a voice which he knew to be imaginary,—and now claimed he had never suspected his wife of anything and that he trusted her absolutely. Upon his discharge he seemed to be quite normal except for slight sidewise movements of both eyes (nystagmus), which were however held very quietly when looking at some definite point. He was now discharged to the social service, which had to face family conditions of some complication. The picture of the results obtained may be got from

the following transcript (names, as always, changed). See
below for general comment on these results.

July 8–October 8, 1916

Social:

Patient has been steadily at work earning thirteen dollars a
week. Expected to go to Men's Club, but did not come to
September or October meetings.

Physical:

Patient has only once had headache of late. Has worn
glasses for four years and will have eyes reëxamined.

Mental:

Patient has not been drinking except once. Wife still complains of sexual demands but commends him in every other
way.

October 8, 1916–January 8, 1917

Social:

Family visited five times. Mrs. Piso pregnant and without
clothes to get outdoors in. Children's shoes worn out and no
warm clothes. Clothes taken and arrangements made to send
wife to Boston Lying-in Hospital as free patient with permission
of own doctor, Dr. McDonald. Patient could not be persuaded to let wife go, so visitor arranged to have district nurse
give prenatal care. Patient is working steadily and brings
home wages every week, and comes in every night at six
o'clock. Patient has walked to Boston two evenings with wife
and about Charlestown once or twice. Wife is anxious to have
everything in good order around the house before confinement.
There is nothing abnormal in wife's condition and she feels
well. Children are well now and have had no colds since they
have been able to go outdoors. Dr. McDonald to take confinement case.

Physical:
Patient is well.

Mental:

Patient is not drinking now, at least wife sees no signs of it.
He was very firm about not letting wife go to hospital.

January 8–April 8, 1917

Social:

A baby girl was born January 23 and baby and mother did well in care of Dr. McDonald and the district nurse. Patient has worked steadily and brought money home. Patient has had no recreation except to visit his father who is ill. He spends his leisure at home with the children of whom he is very fond. Wife took cold in her breast and had to stop nursing the baby for a few days, but recovered satisfactorily. Is having teeth treated. The baby has some stomach trouble and has not gained very fast, but dispensary doctor says she is all right.

Physical:

Patient has been well except for trouble with hemorrhoids which lasted about two weeks in March.

Mental:

Patient drank about a week after birth of baby but stopped because it was so hard on family. He is very agreeable and helpful at home. He came once to Men's Club meeting and would have come two other months but his wife was ill and the distance great.

April 8, 1917–July 8, 1917

Social:

Patient worked steadily and was kind and devoted to the family during April and the early part of May. Patient's father died May 12, and he drank steadily for a month. For the last four weeks he has drunk nothing. Wife and children are rather tired and run down and have been registered at the Country Week for a two weeks' vacation. The baby has been under dispensary care and is doing well.

Physical:

Patient's work has tired him and he has suffered from headache occasionally but has not been induced to have his eyes examined. He has not worn his first glasses faithfully.

Mental:

While patient was drinking he became exceedingly jealous and irritable. His sexual demands were excessive. When not drinking he has been agreeable and helpful at home. Attended the Men's Club.

July 8, 1917–October 8, 1917

Social:

Patient has been working steadily in spite of heavy work and long hours. His pay has been raised to seventeen dollars per week. He has not been drinking for four months. After Mary recovered from diphtheria, patient's wife and children had a Country Week vacation for two weeks, which was very beneficial to them all. Mrs. Martin kept house for patient while they were gone. Patient and his wife go to Boston together Saturday nights to do their shopping now, instead of patient's going alone and getting drunk. Patient and all the family are in need of warm clothes.

Physical:

Nothing of note.

Mental:

Patient has been very kind to and considerate of his wife. He missed the family greatly while they were away on their vacation, and met them at the station with his express team when they returned. He is very fond of the children, and says that he prefers to spend all he earns for his wife and them, "instead of wasting it for drink."

Thus, medically the health of the wife and children was supervised and a vacation procured for them. It proved possible also to improve the housekeeping by concrete advice as to procedure. The wife was told "to be nice" to her husband, to "dress up" Saturdays for the purpose of taking her husband shopping. She let him buy a derby hat, saying, "You have to let them have something when they work so hard."

On the economic side she was discouraged from working to supplement the family income, so that Michael should not be dissuaded from trying to get a better paying job. Economically also the family was helped out by means of clothing, because after all Michael's wages were too small for the family needs. This case showed all the forms of evil discussed in this book except the legal. No doubt the mental issue was the dominant one and the economic probably stood next; but in the family adjustment the social worker employed means quite beyond the merely psychiatric and economic range, to teach the housewife much of value to the family specifically and to improve the moral situation between the spouses.

Hours spent by

Physician, 6½

Psychologist, 1

Social worker, 78

Medical record, 36 pages
Social record, 33 pages
Social work:
Visits, 46
Interviews at hospital, 8
Telephone calls, 17
Letters, 27

Morphinism and alcoholism in a woman of psychopathic personality. Fantastic story of a murder. A social service failure.

Case 63. Marian Spring we present to illustrate *morphinism,* though there is hardly any doubt that she is an example of a so-called psychopathic personality (see Book III, Section XI for other examples).

Marian had been brought up in her middle-class family and upon leaving school at fourteen had spent two years in a convent. Then after living some years at home, at nineteen she began to work in mills. While she was a mill operative, she began, in her twenty-first or twenty-second year, to drink with another girl, and apparently this drinking began after the death of her mother. Finally she got to drinking hard enough to interfere with her work, and at last began to make her rather checkered round of institutions, spending two years in an insane hospital from the beginning of her twenty-fifth year, and then being confined in three reformatories up to a period of four months before her admission to the Psychopathic Hospital. In the brief intervals between these institutional detentions she worked at housework which she did very capably and nicely. Marian, however, had few friends and apparently had chosen her associates from amongst the most undesirable of the mill workers. These associates were so undesirable that they were not allowed at home and the family had become quite discouraged with Marian.

She was a well-developed and nourished woman with rather prominent eyes and a certain asymmetry of face. She was physically energetic and sturdy, but said she was somewhat unusually susceptible to pain. She had always been healthy, she said, with the exception of having every year a sore throat.

According to her story and various inquiries she was capable enough in all places that she undertook to fill but lost them through alcoholism and the morphine habit which she had acquired very shortly after beginning to drink. She was a rather winning sort of person and very successful in getting help for herself by various subterfuges. Thus she had the usual skill in getting morphine by surreptitious routes and she could, on occasion, obtain help in getting out of hospitals or institutions. At one of these institutions, she had been destructive and quite unmanageable. She told at the hospital a very striking story about seeing a girl friend murdered by a certain doctor who, as she said, had great influence over her own life and with whom she had had sex relations. This story remains quite unverified and is, no doubt, an example of the fantastic lying which not only morphine patients are apt to indulge in but which is likely to be shown by sundry psychopathic personalities without the influence of morphine.

She came to the hospital technically "left by herself" but was, as a matter of fact, brought in in a disheveled state by a man and a woman. The man had found her somewhere drunk and had brought her in an automobile to the hospital, where she had told the man she wished to come. She was quite incoordinated, excited, and restive and apparently was hallucinating. (She said: "Oh, how it stares me in the face. If he had only killed me instead of her.") It remains, we suppose, a question whether she was actually a victim of false perceptions or whether she was embroidering after the manner of the morphinist or psychopathic liar.

The diagnostic question at once arises whether Marian was not feeble-minded. The term feeble-mindedness can, as has been constantly shown above, be used in various ways and some authors speak of a pure defect of will and emotions (the so-called amoralia of authors in which intelligence is entirely preserved or at a normal level) as feeble-mindedness. This use of the term feeble-mindedness would, then, have reference to social rather than demonstrable psychical defect. The impression of certain psychiatrists who saw her when she first went to the hospital for the insane was that she was a feeble-minded person but at that time no special tests were made. When these tests were performed she was found to be somewhat deteriorated, but the detail of the tests seemed to indicate that she was really not fundamentally feeble-minded. As we insist elsewhere, the things Marian did that brought her to social attention would not be explained by a low intelligence rating even had she shown such demonstrable defect outside the zone of will and emotion. Put briefly, the psychopathic personality may be feeble-minded to test or may test out not at all feeble-minded; the psychotic trends remain somewhat independent of the intellectual level, though no doubt the patient's degree of responsibility must hang somewhat upon her intellectual powers of judgment.

This case might be counted as a social-service failure. No doubt the social worker will, until the end of time, have certain failures to score. Supervision has failed to reform Marian despite her capabilities in the line of work and despite a high "empathic index" or attractiveness which means that she will, no doubt, always have friends. Unfortunately she makes friends amongst other psychopaths. The well-known gregariousness of morphinists may play a part here and this gregariousness of drug addicts has always to be borne in the social worker's mind. How much this gregariousness is a matter of morphinism or heroinism and how much it is a matter of a certain mild integrating psychopathic trend must be left to the future to decide.

Marian Spring will be what the English call an "in and out" for many years. Such forces as national prohibition and an effective Harrison law and other devices for the successful removal of alcohol and drugs from her habitat will, perhaps, in the end, leave her a not very socially dangerous character.

Hours spent by	Medical record, 32 pages
	Social record, 16 pages
Physician, 6½	Social work:
	Visits, 9
Psychologist, 0	Interviews at hospital, 3
	Telephone calls, 7
Social worker, 20½	Letters, 18

SECTION V

ENCEPHALOPSYCHOSES (BRAIN DISEASE)

Psychoses of old age. Prognosis in arteriosclerosis. Salesman with moments when he "lost himself." State hospital care or private measures?

Case 64. A psychiatric social worker always has to contend with the feeling on the part of many physicians, many fellow social workers, and the majority of laymen that mental disease is incurable. Even if something by experience has been done to diminish this feeling for sundry types of mental disease, the feeling of poor prognosis and of probable incurability still hangs about most patients developing mental symptoms in the fifties, sixties, or seventies. We give two instances later in this book, those of Catherine Cudahy (case 69 and Jeanette Burroughs, case 68), in which psychoses developing in old age were still not inconsistent with remarkable amelioration and easy accessibility to social-service measures.

A very firmly fixed medical prejudice is that "one is as old as his arteries." Accordingly a victim of the hardening of the arteries (arteriosclerosis) is assumed to be by the same token a victim of old age or its equivalent. Since old age has universally so poor a prognosis, then hardening of the arteries is dropped into the same basket of poor prognoses. Now, in point of fact, there are various kinds of arteriosclerosis, only some of which characterize old age, and many forms of arteriosclerosis are not in any respect characteristically senile. One of the greatest surprises of the youthful physician is to see cases of severe arteriosclerosis, looking to be at the point of death, come around in the course of weeks or months to a phase of comparative normality and even capacity of self-support.

Thomas Warren, sixty-four, received the diagnosis of arteriosclerotic dementia at the Psychopathic Hospital, whence

270

he could be discharged somewhat improved after about three weeks' observation, for the most part as a voluntary patient. The term "dementia" has almost invariably, to a physician as well as to a layman, the suggestion of permanence and incurability, although there is nothing about the prefix *de* in this word *dementia* which necessarily signifies that the deterioration is either permanent or temporary (in fact some of the older psychiatric textbooks talk of certain *acute* dementias which often led to complete recovery). Sometimes the term "deterioration" is used for milder degrees of "dementia." Perhaps it would have been safer to call the case of Thomas Warren (with some of the physicians) a case of arteriosclerotic "psychosis," thereby dodging the suggestion of permanence that now sticks to the term "dementia." At all events, as above stated, Thomas Warren was discharged somewhat improved.

Little is known of Warren's early history. His father had died of a shock. Warren himself had worked as a salesman and buyer from youth up and had never had any symptoms of nervous disease until some six or seven months before admission, when a hemorrhage of the eye had occurred and he had found some difficulty in working. He kept at work, but began to lose his memory. At times during this period of six months he completely lost himself for a few minutes at a time. He made mistakes in his work and knew that he had to be watched on this account.

These spells of losing oneself are amongst the most suggestive features of arteriosclerosis in men of his age, especially so when associated with gradual loss of memory and other signs of deterioration. (The layman should not, however, feel too great assurance as to the nature of such spells, since epileptic and epileptoid conditions might likewise bring them about.) It is worth while to insist that these "seizures" are *not signs of senile dementia,* but are signs of either arteriosclerosis or some other form of disease not necessarily senile. The important point we here try to make is that they do not necessarily argue an invariably down-grade process on the part of the patient. They may very well correspond with exceedingly slight destructive processes, due to blood-vessel disease, in the brain and may very well go alongside an almost complete normality of the whole brain mechanism. Moreover, the progress of these cases is not seldom highly irregular.

Persons with very definite and severe apoplectic seizures, involving the paralysis of an entire side, may not only recover to a large extent the functions lost at the time of the so-called "stroke," but may live to perform important functions in life and even to carry on complex business affairs. In short, let us insist that no very definite prognosis, either of regular or irregular down grade or of improvement should be offered. Nevertheless, it will be in the interest of the patient from the social standpoint to give him the benefit of the doubt with respect to his outcome. Not rarely will the worker be rewarded by a very fair compensation in the patient's life as a result of the execution of right social measures.

Warren was still a rather well-developed and nourished man, with a slightly increased blood pressure. His gait was unsteady and rather stiff. There was a certain incoördination also in the movements of his arms, and with eyes closed he would fall to the ground. Both fingers and toes were tremulous at the time of his hospital observation. He had been rather depressed before coming to the hospital. It would, of course, seem natural to the normal observer for a man thus affected to be depressed, and it might seem that the depression was a perfectly normal sadness; yet depression and emotionality with a tendency to rather disproportionate weeping have been observed to be symptoms in arteriosclerotic brain disease. The depression is often much more a symptom due to sundry stimuli working directly in the tissues or from the juices of the body than a rational effect of deliberate thinking about one's desperate situation.

It became a question whether Warren should not be sent to a state hospital for permanent care, partly on account of his dementia, which might be better cared for at a hospital than at home, and partly on account of the low state of his savings. It becomes a delicate question of some practical difficulty whether to advise that such rather gradually deteriorating persons shall remain in the community or be committed to a state hospital. On the whole, in most communities of a proper degree of civilization, the state hospital will prove to offer better facilities at a less total cost to all concerned than private measures can readily equal. It is of course possible with these cases, as with almost all others, to construct an "institutional equivalent" by turning some home into a hospital. Some years ago public authorities upon the insane used to bring up the question whether the state might not soon be asked to take care of many persons who could as readily exist outside the institutions. If we look at the subject from the standpoint of the total cost to the community, regardless of its exact and temporary source, we shall probably be compelled to agree that on the whole the modern trend toward state hospital care of persons hard to manage outside is the right trend and one to encourage. On the whole, there is an invisible, but none the less actual, insurance in the community, through the processes of state care, over against all manner of friction, wasted time, energy, and money spent by inexpert relatives of mentally sick persons. As the almshouse stigma disappears from state hospitals, as the insanity stigma diminishes to a hardly visible point, the trend toward state care of unfortunates of this group will no doubt become stronger still. Sentiment will turn into sentiment for, instead of sentiment against, state care.

Hours spent by	Medical record, 19 pages
	Social record, 11 pages
Physician, 8¼	Social work:
	Visits, 10
Psychologist, 0	Interviews at hospital, 8
	Telephone calls, 14
Social worker, 23	Letters, 4

Choreic girl with illegitimate child. Outbursts of temper; lying. Improvement in maternity home. Persistent social problem.

Case 65. Though from the psychiatric side Helen Fitzpatrick gave somewhat the effect of a psychopathic personality, she was a victim of chorea. Her mental symptoms accordingly gave rise to the question whether she was not what psychiatrists call a "symptomatic" psychosis. These "symptomatic" mental diseases appear incidentally in the midst of other well-recognized diseases of a somatic nature, for example, typhoid fever or pneumonia. Chorea, in the form in which Helen Fitzpatrick showed it, is itself probably an infectious disease.

Looking at the Fitzpatrick girl from the side of social factors, we find the following list:—

Stealing
Lying
Sex delinquency
Outbursts of temper
Industrial disability
Family discord
Separation from family
Lack of early training
Insufficient income

The major social diagnosis was set down as delinquency.

Upon her admission to the Psychopathic Hospital Helen remarked, "We are all a high-strung bunch, the whole of us at home, and that is all the trouble. We get on each other's nerves." It seems that, a fortnight before, a probation officer was called in by Helen's father, because she had cut up her sister's hair ribbon and thrown flatirons about. Her choreic movements were very marked while she was in the receiving ward. She explained she was untidy in dress because she had been taken from her house at five o'clock in the morning. In point of fact she had refused to dress at all.

Physically she was found to have, besides choreic movements, slight heart trouble (often found in choreics). All the reflexes were very active. Mentally she was quite inaccessible to the examiner, although she was plainly oriented in every way and very emotional. Later she grew more accessible and rated by psychological tests pretty evenly at fifteen (she rated at good or very good in the supplementary tests, except in those for motor coördination wherein she was fair and in those for voluntary attention where she was poor). While in the hospital she grew quieter and the chorea was even somewhat lessened.

The court, on representation that supervision for Helen should be undertaken, readily accepted the offer of supervision for Helen by our social service. After a few weeks in a convalescent home, where it was determined that she had become pregnant, she was sent to a maternity home and remained until after the birth of her baby three months later. She improved in health and recovered from the chorea. Her mental attitude improved and she took a mature and sensible view of her situation. She was brighter than most girls in the home. She showed no conduct irregularities or signs of bad temper while there.

Her marriage with the child's father, a boy, Thomas Lynch, was seriously considered. In the beginning her father insisted that they should be married, but, as the shiftlessness of Lynch and the rather low standard of his family came to light, Helen's parents became persuaded that the marriage would be an additional misfortune. Lynch was willing to marry, but left the decision to his mother. Mrs. Lynch objected to having her son "tied for life to a girl like Helen." As the boy was under age, his mother's consent was necessary, and in the end she flatly refused to give it, although she did agree that Thomas should support the baby. The final conclusion of all concerned was that a marriage between the two would lead only to further unhappiness. The priest coöperated by advising against the marriage.

When Helen was ready to leave the maternity home, she was referred to a children's agency with the understanding that she and her baby should be boarded in a family where Helen might be trained in the care of the child. She was fond of the baby and proud of her. Her attitude in general was so much improved that she was allowed instead to go home, but, though she took good care of her baby, she shirked all other responsibilities and got on so poorly at home that she was sent to board with the baby in a country home. The baby after being weaned was boarded separately, and Helen was placed in another family to do housework. This she did not at all like, and she proved unsatisfactory to her employer because she was untruthful and untidy. After three months she was allowed to go to a relative, who conducted a small sanatorium and who undertook to be responsible for her. Mrs. Fitzpatrick took the baby home.

Here then is a case which promises to be a persistent and year-long problem.

Hours spent by

Physician, 3½

Psychologist, 1

Social worker, 34

Medical record, 21 pages
Social record, 20 pages
Social work:
Visits, 22
Interviews at hospital, 6
Telephone calls, 10
Letters, 18

SECTION VI

SOMATOPSYCHOSES (BODILY DISEASE)

Mother of illegitimate child, with dubious mild psychosis.

Case 66. Ethel Murphy, twenty-seven, had been somewhat depressed, or at all events sad, since having an illegitimate child two months before admission. Her eyes were somewhat prominent, her thyroid gland was enlarged, her pulse was rapid. She thus presented many of the features of a Graves' disease which was, however, of mild degree. She had never expressed any suicidal ideas. It was suspected that at one time she had had auditory hallucinations.

The social worker at the hospital where she was confined brought her to the Psychopathic Hospital on the ground that as the baby was to be adopted it was important to have the mother examined for her mentality, so as to reassure the foster mother.

The psychologists found that Ethel graded very irregularly at 11.3 years. She coöperated very well but she made several illogical errors in the picture puzzle test. The irregularity (see discussion under case 19) presumably signifies an acquired psychosis rather than an original subnormality, but there is really no evidence of a definite psychosis unless we are to think of her as a victim of *a slight or minor psychosis due to hyperthyroidism.* Various diagnoses suggested were subnormality of mind, hyperthyroidism, epilepsy, and exhaustion, but the psychological examination appears to dispose of the subnormality of mind, at least as a fundamental and original state. There was no good evidence of epilepsy. The remaining suggestions of hyperthyroidism and exhaustion place her in an undefined group of mental diseases due to bodily disease. (See remarks under the case of Helen Fitzpatrick, case 65.) The child was, at the suggestion of the physician, placed under state care and separated from the mother.

The case was followed by the social service and Ethel is now at work in a contented frame of mind. That the social service had positively something to do with this result cannot be contended; although only the usual technique of counsel and assurance was followed. The earlier difficulties of technique had centered about getting this girl, who was (in her own judgment) only slightly ill to take the step of going into the wards of the Psychopathic Hospital from the out-patient department from which she had been first referred. No doubt the advance of psychiatry in the far future will bring more and more of these exceedingly dubious and (from the ordinary medical viewpoint) extremely mild cases under early suitable observation.

Hours spent by	Medical record, 25 pages
Physician, 5	Social record, 9 pages
	Social work:
Psychologist, 1	Visits, 20
	Interviews at hospital, 4
	Telephone calls, 9
Social worker, 34½	Letters, 16

Attack of mental disease following influenza.

Case 67. Joseph O'Brien is an example of *influenza psychosis* incidental to the influenza epidemic in Boston in 1918. He was a case of *toxic delirium*. His mental symptoms developed in the period of defervescence, in fact seven days after the temperature fell. It seems that his mind became affected immediately thereafter. He wanted to wander about, thought he was on board ship, did not recognize his family and had to be restrained by his relatives, would fall down, once set fire to a bureau. He himself said that he had been taking a good deal of alcohol but this was denied by his relatives.

Upon admission he seemed to be confused and was probably hallucinated as he reached out his hands to grasp imaginary objects, apparently looked at the object, and then began picking at the mattress. His hands were tremulous. He remained in the hospital four days short of two months and was discharged in greatly improved physical condition. His periods of confusion kept recurring for three weeks after admission and he developed from time to time a temperature which reached 103 degrees on the fourth and fifth days after admission. For the rest, the physical examination proved negative.

The task of the social service is here simple. It is a question of *follow-up*. The return of symptoms in influenza psychosis is naturally a matter of research at the present time. Letters are from time to time received from O'Brien showing that he is getting on well and, in fact, "could not be any better."

Hours spent by	Medical record, 11 pages
	Social record, 0
Physician, 5¾	Social work:
	Visits, 0
Psychologist, 0	Interviews at hospital, 1
	Telephone calls, 0
Social worker, 1	Letters, 4

SECTION VII

Senile psychosis. Widow saw her son who had been dead forty years. Improvement: proper care arranged.

Case 68. Jeanette Burroughs, a widow of seventy-two, was found getting her meals on a gas heater and doing needle-work for an art society, with her son paying the board bill. She went to church and to the movies and called upon her friends from time to time. She entered the wards of the Psychopathic Hospital from the out-patient department. She had had dizzy spells for two or three years, though she had never fallen down. Sometimes she had a peculiar feeling in her head like rushing water. She was in many respects very well preserved, looking younger than her age. She had at one time been treated for diabetes. Just before coming to the out-patient department, she had imagined that a son, now forty years dead, had sat beside her and talked to her. A man in black had walked up and down in front of her house. She felt, she said, prostrated with grief, and her sleep had become disturbed and fitful. She was a voluntary patient at the hospital, but there could be no doubt that she was legally committable on the score of the clear hallucinations and delusions.

Physically she was well developed and nourished. There were no obvious lesions of the heart and lungs, and there was no special disturbance of blood pressure. There were no evidences in the neuromuscular examination that there had ever been any degree of destructive brain disease. A certain emotionality and a feeling of loss of memory were the most outstanding mental symptoms, except the ideas revolving about the resurrection of her dead son.

Admitted April 16, 1917, it was not until June 1 that she gave up her delusions, admitting at that time that, though the ideas still did "come up at times," she was now "able after struggling always to put them down." She said she was less

279

collected in the evening than in the morning and night, perhaps better be spoken to earlier rather than later in the day.

The only point concerning the discharge of Mrs. Burroughs now lay in the question whether she would have proper care on leaving the hospital. This became the province of the social service to accomplish. During the period of a year the social service was able to keep her properly boarded out (with some aid from charitable organizations) and saw to it that she was visited by friends from time to time. She resumed her habit of attending church and the movies. She fell and injured her hip one winter's day—an accident which in an old person is ordinarily very dangerous. The hip trouble proved to be merely a contusion, and Mrs. Burroughs recovered. At the end of this time the case could be closed so far as the Psychopathic Hospital social service was concerned. She was left under the care of a non-psychiatric social agency. She has throughout continued to make a little money by needlework but so far as can be seen must remain for the rest of her life somewhat of a charge.

Is Mrs. Burroughs mentally normal? She is at all events now not a victim of any acute delusional psychosis, whether senile in causation or of any other origin. Nevertheless from time to time it appears that she still sees her dead son, and it is probable that she still bears inside some traces of the former psychosis. However, if she had never shown more psychopathy than she now shows, no doubt, she would never have appeared on the records of an institution for mental diseases.

Hours spent by	Medical record, 28 pages
	Social record, 10 pages
Physician, 8	Social work:
	Visits, 16
Psychologist, 0	Interviews at hospital, 0
	Telephone calls, 12
Social worker, 21½	Letters, 2

PRESENILE PSYCHOSIS

WOMAN, 55

February	*June*
Unoccupied	Occupied.
No Pleasures	Friends Call
Outbursts of Temper	Husband Told Why

Presenile psychosis. Scolded by the clock. Home life altered: improvement.

Case 69. Catherine Cudahy, fifty-five, kept hearing the big clock on the mantelpiece ticking at her vindictively. She had become violently enraged by this ticking at least twice in a period of two months. At last her husband had to send her to the Psychopathic Hospital. She thought a Holy Father was on the roof.

Her case was put by the psychiatrists in the presenile group and was called *involutional psychosis.* They found her a victim of hallucinations of hearing, but found that her delusion about the Holy Father was not very definite or fixed. She finally admitted that the ticking of the clock at her was only imaginary. She had not heard the clock ticking after the arrival at the hospital. Her memory seemed to be poor for details both of recent and remote events, but she could remember excellently the main events in her life. She was physically rather obese and, since an operation two years before, had not been able to go to church. She had begun to feel tired all the time and had been hearing the clock talking for about five months. Mrs. Cudahy did not use alcohol (an important negative fact for the psychiatrists).

The problem for the social worker came upon her discharge "improved." She was somehow to alter her home life; she was not to be left alone so much or spend so much time unemployed. These suggestions were carried out and she was made to take daily exercise outdoors. The relatives were persuaded to coöperate. They visited her and kept her busy. She reported regularly at the out-patient department every fortnight, and the clock went definitively out of her life.

Hours spent by	Medical record, 11 pages
	Social record, 3 pages
Physician, 7	Social work:
	Visits, 3
Psychologist, 0	Interviews at hospital, 6
	Telephone calls, 1
Social worker, 7½	Letters, 5

SECTION VIII

SCHIZOPHRENOSES (DEMENTIA PRAECOX)

Case of dementia simplex self-supporting in the community. May look like feeble-mindedness. Training. Simple environment provided.

Case 70. There is a form of schizophrenia (dementia praecox) to which the adjective *simplex* is added. In this form of the disease there is a certain deterioration and dulling of the emotional life which fails to be accompanied by the various so-called catatonic (formerly termed cataleptic) symptoms or by the delusions which are so frequent in most cases of schizophrenia. Moreover, in these so-called simplex cases the emotional deterioration may itself be slight, and it is commonly thought by psychiatrists that a great number of these cases of dementia simplex are found in the community at large, perhaps self-supporting or nearly self-supporting, with a history of having sustained a slight regression in their mental capacity insufficient to warrant or to suggest their internment in any hospital for the insane. It is, perhaps, a little difficult for the layman and even for some of the old-time physicians to think of cases of schizophrenia (dementia praecox) as "not insane." Until the concept of *mental disease that is not* (medico-legal) *insanity* becomes deeply imbedded in the lay mind, as well as in the minds of medical men and social workers, we shall not come through with a proper program of community mental hygiene.

Dana Scott, an unmarried man of thirty-seven, was brought to the Psychopathic Hospital for observation. The woman with whom he boarded told of violent fits of temper on Scott's part, during which clothing was torn and furniture knocked to pieces. As a matter of fact, the landlady greatly overdrew the story about Scott, as investigation failed to substantiate any destructive tendencies, nor was the landlady herself a good sort of person to live with. Nevertheless, with all the smoke there was some fire. It was generally agreed that Scott lacked ambition and initiative and might perhaps be the victim of some sort of mental defect. Had it not been for the landlady's character (an angel from heaven, it was said, could not live peaceably with her), Scott might have remained in the community even to this day without being noted by any expert to be psychopathic. He had been a rather queer child. It was told of him that he took books to the attic and stayed all day with them, omitting meals. The country neighbors who saw him daily did not consider him at all harmful. A nurse who brought him to the hospital said that he was one of the most willing and obedient patients she had ever had.

Here then was a man who was plainly in some sense a psychopath. Perhaps by straining a point he could have been committed to an institution. He was in charge of a guardian and had some little property, so that board could be paid for him. A place in the country was found in the family of a widow and her daughter. Here Scott could help with chores and might perhaps obtain some work in the neighborhood. Shortly letters were received from Scott telling how much he liked his new home. The family were well satisfied with him and pleased at having a permanent boarder who was so helpful.

It may be permissible to point out that with the old system, under which the public or private charitable institution "borrowed no trouble," the hospital work might have ceased with the diagnosis. In point of fact the social service was at first merely requested to secure a history. Yet, when such history was secured, perfectly obvious and valuable social-service measures stood revealed as the proper procedure. In institutions where psychiatric social work is carried out effectually this is no infrequent event, namely, that the social worker, sent out to secure a few facts, comes back with a series of rational measures.

Victims of the so-called simplex form of schizophrenia are often looked upon, even by physicians, as feeble-minded, nor is it at all possible in routine examinations always to determine medically with which condition one is dealing. The psychometric tests, executed by a properly grounded mental examiner, are sometimes of service: for instance, in the case of Scott, the Binet record stood at 12 1/5 years, and he was set down as beyond question not feeble-minded. His deterioration was not intellectual. The mental impairment was, as it characteristically is in all cases of schizophrenia, in the field of the emotions. There was a marked dulling of them. He was, from some points of view, not at all unintellectual; was. for example, a great reader of books on science and art, and conversed very fairly on current topics. Although psychopathic in this particular way, he had no savor of feeble-mindedness and would have been quite above the level of the majority of the teachings, which are so skillfully carried out for the feeble-minded in the schools appropriate for that group of defectives. There can be no doubt that his life with the widow and her daughter upon a farm was exactly the right fate for him. As with the psychological examination, so the physical and mental examination by psychiatrists at the hospital failed to show any striking deviations from normal, and the psychiatric impression of the case, based upon the medical and social history, was accordingly left at the diagnosis schizophrenia (dementia praecox) of the simplex form.

Of course many cases of schizophrenia, particularly of the catatonic group above mentioned, are not unlikely to become suddenly excited or violent; nor can it be absolutely excluded from the range of possibility that Scott may turn catatonic through some sudden access of the structural or functional disease which underlies his symptoms.

The layman, as well as the physician, must have forced upon his attention a certain sexuality in the symptoms of the majority of cases of schizophrenia (dementia praecox) ; but it would be an injustice to many examples of the disease to think of the sexuality as socially dangerous. Whatever bad habits in the sexual field and whatever bad table manners and other impolitenesses Scott might have been guilty of, probably all of these matters may never fall within the social danger zone. No doubt many of these psychopathically bad manners and customs can be, to a great degree, trained out of patients of this order by proper methods. Just as it is possible to train or tame certain animals without the employment of the methods open to a Socrates or a Plato, so it is possible to get sundry effects sometimes termed *reëducative* in cases of the schizophrenic group. Whether the training is in all cases a genuine rationalization with the Socratic or Platonic echo may be doubted. However this may be, the well-managed hospital for the chronic insane, harboring as it does so many victims of this disease, shortly becomes a very effective *school for schizophrenics*. In some governmental units, colonies for such schizophrenics have been developed, whose star patients are not those who, like Scott, are very easy to deal with from the outset, but patients who have passed through most violent and dangerous phases or phases of extreme apathy and utter economic worthlessness, only in the end to be schooled into a very fair efficiency. With respect to Dana Scott, then, we may perhaps regard the non-angelic landlady as really something of an angel in disguise.

Hours spent by	Medical record, 38 pages
	Social record, 4 pages
Physician, 4½	Social work:
	Visits, 2
Psychologist, 1	Interviews at hospital, 1
	Telephone calls, 9
Social worker, 5	Letters, 2

DEMENTIA PRAECOX

IN A MACHINIST

January, 1916	*January, 1917*
Industrial Disability	Good Health
Unemployment	Regular Work
Debts	Out of Debt
Suicidal Attempts	Cheerful

Vagrant: irregular worker: alcoholic: attempted suicide.
Men's Club. Peculiarities indulged at home. Steady, reliable
workman: a compensated schizophrenic. Economy of social
care.

Case 71. Ralph Johnson left home at thirty-one and was
not heard of for the next seven years. In point of fact he was
roaming over the country on foot, jumping freights and working off and on in railroad gangs. Wanderlust over, Ralph got
back to Boston and worked as an automobile repairer for the
next nine years in six different places. He then ceased to work
altogether for a number of months. It seems that he had had
an infection in his hand for some three months. He felt "run
down and weak," one night grew suddenly talkative, said he
saw dead people, friends of his, and cut an artery in his wrist
with a razor. He had been drinking, and a diagnosis of alcoholic mental disease was made. There were no sexual contents
or ideas of jealousy in Johnson, but he did show delusions of
persecution (people were going to kill him) and ideas of reference (the people that he saw outside of his house seemed to
him to be "laying for him"). There were no genuine hallucinations (false perceptions) in any sensory field.

Johnson was now referred to the out-patient department and
when jogged by letter reported from time to time. He ceased
to take any alcohol and for the most part felt "fine, though
somewhat unsettled in my mind with thoughts constantly
changing." After a few months he came in one day agitated
and weeping, maintaining that "his left side was dead" and
that he had "done terrible wrongs to several people"—could
he not be chloroformed or have his head cut off? Nobody
would hire such a man as he was and consequently he would
not ask for a job.

However in the course of a few weeks he came in again much
more clear-headed and alert, laughing about the death of his
left side, etc. Again he complained of "lack of concentration
of his thoughts" and talked somewhat ramblingly. He was
fading away, having lost he said, fifty pounds. From time to

time he reported rather regularly for the Men's Club and after a time became one of the most regular attendants at this Club which he found his only recreation. However, finally he stopped coming and, upon being visited, assumed a hostile attitude and feigned indifference to the hospital, its staff and its attendants. He said he had other things to do than to attend a men's club.

The entire history, since his first appearance at the hospital, has occupied five years. There was, however, a second appearance in the wards of the Psychopathic Hospital some eleven months after the first admission. Some days before entrance to the hospital he had begun to cry out aloud at night. He said his mother was calling him. For several days he cried out, talking rather desperately at times yet laughing at other times, and told of a feeling of electric currents over him. He was a readily committable case, telling the committing physician that he had heard God's voice and could hear it in the hospital as well as at home.

The diagnosis upon his discharge from this second admission stood at a question of dementia praecox, where the diagnosis should, perhaps, still stand. There is no longer any question of alcoholic mental disease, despite the rather certain view of the psychiatrist at his first admission that he was a case of alcoholic paranoia. Concerning the very existence of any such disease as alcoholic paranoia psychiatrists have registered doubts, and it can readily be seen that a commixture of schizophrenic symptoms and alcoholic traits can easily confuse the issue; many psychiatrists hold that the only true form of mental disease of delusional nature produced by alcohol is the so-called jealousy-psychosis, an example of which, from the social point of view, is given in this book under the case of Michael Piso (case 62).

Johnson remained in the hospital four months after this second admission. On his discharge he went to work once again in an automobile repair shop. They said he was a good, handy man at this work, although he worked somewhat slowly and if at all hurried got nervous and tired. He had to be laid off once when work was slack. He readily got another position at eighteen dollars. They said he was a very steady and reliable workman. Once he had a petty argument with his foreman and lost his job. Immediately he secured another job, this time at twenty-five dollars a week. Johnson's home was on a fairly high economic level. He lived with his sister. She had to be instructed concerning the indulgence of eccentricities on Johnson's part. She learned not to irritate him overmuch and was got to manage him with exceeding intelligence.

Is this a case of schizophrenia (dementia praecox)? It is, at all events, a case with definite psychopathic phases and probably belongs somewhere in the general group of the schizophrenics. Yet we may think of Johnson as in some sense a compensated schizophrenic. Perhaps no one would regard him as entirely normal, though it would certainly stump the ordinary observer to pick anything psychopathic out of his behavior for days and weeks at a time. There seems to be no question whatever that the social service here aided and abetted the process of character compensation. Again, we may not unduly insist that the ordinary method of letting such cases go adrift in the community without supervision and follow-up is, in the long run, a much more expensive process to the community than the cost of proper medical and social care and supervision (to say nothing of the effects of a non-compensated schizophrenic in the matter of possible violence, and disturbance of the peace). There was also to consider the alcoholism, to which this wanderer had fallen victim when he first came to observation at the age of forty-eight. How many of the wanderers on the countryside and persons found jumping freights may really be schizophrenic is a statistical question whose answer might vary in different communities and countries. Whether the tally reaches fifty per cent may be questioned. A good many epileptics, manic-depressive psychotics, and psychoneurotics may also be found amongst the hoboes to say nothing of queer characters whose abnormalities are of a milder and not easily classified form. (There is even a group of so-called victims of *poriomania* that seem to represent a specially developed instinct of wandering.)

Hours spent by	Medical record, 11 pages
	Social record, 18 pages
Physician, 7½	Social work:
	Visits, 7
Psychologist, 0	Interviews at hospital, 12
	Telephone calls, 7
Social worker, 27	Letters, 5

Litigious vagrant: counterfeiter.   Case of paraphrenia systematica.

Case 72.   Manual Rizzo is, no doubt, a victim of so-called paraphrenia systematica, a new name now rather frequently used for the so-called *délire chronique à évolution systématique* of the French psychiatrist Magnan.   Although the task of the social service here was more contributory to diagnosis than to treatment or care, the Rizzo case is presented because the social worker ought to have in mind some general picture of this condition.

Born in the Azores, Rizzo had come to this country at seventeen and was now sixty years of age.   For some seven years he had been a vagrant.   He was of a rather villainous appearance on account of a turning out of his reddened eyelids.   He was in general docile and affable but would now and then flare up.   In the admission office he said he thought the officer who arrested him had it in for him.   In fact that same officer had arrested him seven years before.   He was very circumstantial in his talk and gave the impression that he felt he was a rather important personage.   He said he was quite able to support himself.   He told circumstantially about his trip from the Azores and the various jobs which he had held.   According to his own story his trouble had begun in his forty-eighth year over some trade dollars which he exchanged for legal dollars. He said that ever since he had had a lawsuit over these dollars with the United States Government.   He had studied law and was now able to handle his cases perfectly well.   He said he was a strong temperance man and gave a long harangue on temperance.   He explained his not working for seven years on the ground that he had been too busy looking after his affairs in court.   He said he did a little work now and then and lived on it.   However, he did not live very well for he was alive with vermin.   Upon inquiry at the courthouse it was found that there were actually docket entries of nine cases.   He had lost all of these cases except one.   It appeared that he came to court daily when not in jail and went to file a suit against someone every time he had the necessary three hundred dollars. As for the jail, it was found that *he had been sent to jail at least twelve times for vagrancy.*   Apparently he had once had a small tailor shop and a man was found who had known him for some twenty-five years and knew him as "queer but harmless." It appears that in those early days he had been very religious. He had gone to church daily, sometimes had gone up to the altar and followed the priest about imitating everything he did toward the celebration of the mass. He bored holes in silver coins and plugged the holes with other material. Of recent years he had been seen getting food from garbage pails. He was also much of a collector, keeping pieces of paper and other objects that he happened to find in ash cans. He had served *three prison sentences for counterfeiting*.

The emotions and the will in the paraphrenic are theoretically supposed to be normal or to suit the nature of the ideas entertained. Rizzo would grow irritable at times, particularly when telling of his troubles, but this irritability was a very superficial one and soon disappeared. He assumed rather an oratorical attitude when speech-making but here again the action suited the idea and there could be no question of a primary disorder of the will. The imitation of the priest at mass may very possibly be so regarded; yet on the whole, we are better entitled to regard this old habit as a sign of his belief, even at that time, in his being a good deal of a personage.

Hours spent by	Medical record, 14 pages
	Social record, 3 pages
Physician, 5½	Social work:
	Visits, 3
Psychologist, 0	Interviews at hospital, 0
	Telephone calls, 1
Social worker, 4	Letters, 0

Diagnosis between schizophrenia and cyclothymia. Skilled salesman who lost his position through peculiar behavior. Recovered: remained steady: works regularly.

Case 73. It is an open secret that it is not an easy psychiatric distinction to draw in every case between schizophrenia (dementia praecox) and cyclothymia (manic-depressive psychosis). The two diseases are paired in the psychiatrist's mind as sister diseases, the former rather more frequent than the latter, both in the number of first cases developing and in the number remaining in state hospitals under observation. When the diagnosis lies between schizophrenia and cyclothymia, apparently the psychiatrist is statistically somewhat more likely to be right if he decides upon schizophrenia. It should be insisted that psychiatrists chiefly familiar with chronic institutional material are somewhat more likely to take a pessimistic view of the prognosis of mental disease in general than are the consulting neurologists of out-patient departments or of special practice or the specialists in charge of sanatoriums. In the ten-day period of observation which the law tends to procure for the majority of cases at the Psychopathic Hospital in Boston, there will, perhaps, be an error in diagnosis between these two diseases of something like fifteen or twenty per cent; sometimes the error will be upon one side, sometimes upon the other.

The present case of Paul Ernst is not the first in this book in which doubt has reigned concerning the diagnosis schizophrenia as against some other form of mental disease. At least three diagnoses, psychiatrically speaking, have been offered for Paul Ernst; namely, alcoholic hallucinosis, dementia praecox, and manic-depressive psychosis.

Ernst has been a patient twice at the Psychopathic Hospital, once in 1913 and again in 1914-15. At the first admission there seemed no doubt at all of the diagnosis of dementia praecox. He had run about his house nude, broken up furniture, and attacked members of the household. He refused to talk and became very sullen and obstinate. Just before this he had begun to worry over business matters and had grown morbidly depressed when an advance in salary was refused. One Saturday night he had been quite broken up and discouraged and unable to sleep. Sunday he had been normal, but Monday grew wildly excited. His excitement had lasted twenty-four hours.

In the hospital he became very violent, at times requiring seven or eight attendants to put him in the wet pack. He shouted, screamed, swore, and cried out, talking either sarcastically or very angrily about his treatment. During inactive periods he assumed a disagreeably sullen manner. He remained for the most part quiet, inaccessible to the examiners, but evincing some flight of ideas in his talk.

He was committed to the Boston State Hospital where he remained a month but was discharged with the diagnosis manic-depressive psychosis. He became entirely clear in his mind

before discharge. He now went back to his work as a salesman of a special kind of goods. He had never been alcoholic,
so that the initial suggestion of alcoholic hallucinosis was
unfounded.

After a time he began again to worry about finances. One
day at the department store where he worked, he began to act
peculiarly and left for home. There he smashed windows and
brought down a chandelier. He was again brought to the
Psychopathic Hospital and was there acutely maniacal for
some three days, but after this interval a physical examination
became possible, and he was found to be practically negative
in all respects. Mentally he was suspicious, rather facetious,
and non-coöperative upon admission but obviously perfectly
oriented for time and place. He tore blankets and night shirt,
was profane, obscene, and noisy and was treated by the prolonged baths and by packs. He either was not, or assumed not
to be, interested in his surroundings, kept his eyes staring
wide open, and winked constantly. He lay in bed in a rather
strained position. For a while on the first day he stood in
front of a window, talking, but there was a large question
whether the behavior was in response to hallucinations. The
psychiatric reader will note how difficult a diagnosis must be
with such phenomena between schizophrenia and cyclothymia.

On about the seventh day there was a change of phase: he
now appeared confused, was quiet but restive, and threw himself from the bed a number of times. He would burst into
noises now and then, but was at other times apparently quite
rational. Things going on about him he took in quickly and
was rather mischievous in his remarks and actions. He began
to speak of his wife and family and talked about wanting to
go home. At the end of three weeks from his admission, it
was possible to send him home in a clear state of mind. He
thought that he really had heard false voices just after admission, but conceived that they might possibly be the talking of
the attendants misinterpreted by him. He had however once
thought that his brother was there talking. He tried to read
The Three Guardsmen, but could not keep his mind on the
book. He was discharged with the diagnosis dementia praecox,
unimproved, despite the fact that his general status was for
the moment markedly improved.

The social service now took charge of him, and for a period

of some two years there is a running record which gives no sign of deterioration whatever. To be sure his former employers refused to take him back, though he had been formerly six years employed by the firm in a rather difficult job. He now had to take temporary jobs as salesman, acting from time to time as an extra. Amongst the measures of the social service were help to the family in the matter of clothes, more or less continuous reassurance of the wife as to the nature of her husband's situation and prognosis, advice concerning work on his part and the securing of vacations for the children.

Then came the death of the wife, upon learning which it was thought best to reopen the case from the social service point of view. However, despite the strain of the situation the family succeeded in adjusting itself, with the oldest daughter, a capable girl of seventeen, keeping the house. Meantime Ernst had remained steady, was working regularly, did not drink and showed no sign of deterioration. The success of the family adjustment is the more remarkable when it is considered that there are nine children (one of whom is choreic).

Is or is not this a case of schizophrenia? Perhaps the shrewd psychiatrist might say that time only would tell. Others might say that it was a case of dementia praecox that had gotten well or had made a compensation practically equivalent to recovery. Others might insist that the case was one of cyclothymia. For our part we may content ourselves with insisting that, whichever of these diagnoses is rendered, there is a certain statistical likelihood of error in diagnosis with our present knowledge (especially perhaps in the war group of cases). There may be noticed many instances of cases looking even more like schizophrenia than the present case of Ernst and yet turning out to be curable or capable of decided remission. Also it is worth while stressing the fact that the term "dementia" in the phrase dementia praecox should not be allowed to dominate anybody's conception of the disease schizophrenia. The so-called "dementia" is from the standpoint of all clear-cut cases a matter of deterioration of the emotions and not at all necessarily or characteristically of the intellect. The layman, social worker, or psychiatrist makes a grave error who carries over any ideas that he may possess concerning dementia and dements of the old age group into the so-called dementia of dementia praecox. Perhaps no more unfortunate term than dementia praecox has yet been devised for an important group of psychopathic patients.

Hours spent by	Medical record, 9 pages
	Social record, 4 pages
Physician, 7½	Social work:
	Visits, 2
Psychologist, 0	Interviews at hospital, 3
	Telephone calls, 0
Social worker, 2	Letters, 1

Spoiled child. Suicidal attempts: state hospital: dementia praecox? Marriage to soldier after birth of child: deserted.

Case 74. Nora McCarthy was rather a spoiled child coming from a not too intelligent, quarrelsome, and alcoholic family. She could not finish high school because she got "tired out" and "nervous." It seems that she got depressed rather often and several times tried suicide, once being taken to a state hospital for a month after a suicidal attempt and therein receiving the diagnosis of psychopathic personality from which, perhaps, there should be no dissent.

For some two years she had been at home doing nothing whatever. Then she became engaged to a very excellent young man whom she had known a year and who was about to enlist. They wanted to marry. Nora's mother refused, whereat Nora cried continually for a month, refused to eat with the family, was sent to the Psychopathic Hospital for observation and was there thought to have schizophrenia (dementia praecox).

It was now discovered that she was pregnant. The fiancé was unable to get a furlough for marriage. There were even preparations for an eleventh-hour marriage as he was en route for overseas. In point of fact the detachment had been hurried from train to ship and there was not even time to wire. An attempt at a proxy marriage was made but there was some doubt of its legality. Her fiancé wrote regularly and sent her money.

At the hospital she was given mental tests and was found to grade at 14½ years on the Stanford-Binet Scale. Her failure lay not so much in intellectuality but in impulsive and hasty answers. She was physically quite normal,

psychiatrically some of her talk about her family might give
ground to the suspicion of her being paranoidal, but on the
whole her statements seemed to be accurate or merely exaggerated. Emotionally she was somewhat depressed and at
times gave the appearance of apathy. It was, no doubt, upon
this latter ground that the idea of dementia praecox obtained.
In retrospect it would seem that a good deal of this abnormal
emotional appearance was really due to her feelings about her
pregnancy.

She remained for a time as a voluntary patient under observation and then went home, where she at first did nothing.
Gradually she became interested (in part under the visitor's
stimulation) in making baby clothes. The baby was born before its father returned from overseas. She worried about the
supposed nervousness of "the poor little thing." She gradually
became interested in housework and grew interested in taking
care of the baby even to the point of absorption. A proper
marriage had been celebrated.

At this point the social service closed the case. It appears
from the record that this decision was influenced by Mrs. Mc-
Carthy's statement that Nora was "very happy and well and
not at all depressed, taking an interest in her baby and in the
household." The closing note reads: "Case closed since patient is doing well and further visits would simply antagonize
her and her mother. Her mother is keen enough to recognize
new mental symptoms quickly and to insist upon patient's reporting to the doctor." Perhaps the fact that the McCarthys
lived at some distance from the hospital and on top of a steep
hill may have influenced the decision to close the case. Possibly the fact that several times the visitor climbed the hill only
to be told that Nora was out had also played its part. At any
rate, it was judged that her husband could not take care of
Nora; and it was left to Mrs. McCarthy to explain her condition to him. The young couple were to live with the
McCarthys.

Five months later the social worker received a letter from
Nora saying that her mother would not allow her to talk with
the social worker in the past but that she must see someone
now as she was in great trouble. Her husband had gone to
make a visit to his father several months before and had not

returned. He had communicated with her several times, but without letting her know his address. The explanation of this unexpected conduct in a man of excellent reputation has not yet been found. She was advised to take legal action to trace him. Meanwhile she is working as cashier in a department store, and living at home. She still complains of her family but manages to get on with them.

Hours spent by	Medical record, 36 pages
	Social record, 28 pages
Physician, 5¼	Social work:
	Visits, 53
Psychologist, 1	Interviews at hospital, 3
	Telephone calls, 10
Social worker, 81	Letters, 18

Girl committed after three years' observation. Intensive social treatment. Diagnosis altered from psychoneurosis to schizophrenia.

Case 75. We cannot regret the kind or the degree of social work carried out in the case of Clara Goldberg; yet in the sequel it might be thought that a good deal of someone's time was, for Clara Goldberg at least, wasted.

We choose the Goldberg case as one of dementia praecox. In the end, over three years after our original observation, the girl was duly committed to a state hospital, with the usual prognosis of cases of dementia praecox, that is, with the great likelihood of a persistent deterioration.

We noted above in the case of Alfred Stevens (case 25) an instance wherein the change of medical diagnosis proved of the utmost importance. The alteration of the diagnosis from psychasthenia to cyclothymia (manic-depressive psychosis) in the case of Stevens worked out tremendously to his benefit; for his stay in the state institution led to the smoothing out of his depression and his rehabilitation. Clara Goldberg is an instance of alteration of diagnosis from the psychoneurotic group to the schizophrenic (dementia praecox) group. The commitment of Clara Goldberg to an institution for chronic cases no doubt makes it somewhat easier for the girl herself and straightens out many family problems. In the present phase of medical science this will no doubt be the issue in the majority of cases of schizophrenia (dementia praecox).

Let us first consider her appearance and behavior at the time of her final commitment as a case of dementia praecox. She was then twenty-two years of age and had just entered the hospital with a record of not having eaten anything for several days. She volunteered the statement that she was a bad girl and a flirt and did not deserve to eat. Direct questions she answered correctly, but often wore a silly expression, hiding her face. For the most part she refused to talk. When asked a question she sometimes appeared as if about to say something but her words failed to come; she was "blocked." She was constantly seen sitting in a chair with her head inclined forward and the saliva running from her mouth. Now and then her hands and arms would shake violently. Her pupils were dilated. For the rest the physical examination was not remarkable.

A psychological examination would have been at this time impossible. Clara had, however, been under out-patient department observation for three years and had twice had a psychological examination. The second time, about a year before her appearance in the above described characteristically schizophrenic state, she made by the Point Scale a level of 13.5 years, grading, in fact, somewhat higher than she had graded on the previous examination a year before. She did, however, show on the second examination much poorer planning ability than she had at first shown.

Looking back upon her history, it is now easy to see schizophrenic traits. She is described as having had many mannerisms from the early teens, such as touching her face and teeth constantly and continually moving the muscles of her face. Efforts to curb these mannerisms—she felt that her expression was silly and even made definite efforts to change her expression—resulted in movements worse than ever.

In the later teens it appears that she became untidy in her person. It was wasteful, she thought, to have money spent on clothes. She would eat dry bread between meals so that the bread might not be wasted. A habit of masturbation had begun at thirteen. It is not even impossible that her deterioration had begun at school days (for instance, she spent three years in the seventh grade).

Clara's mother had had two attacks of manic-depressive psychosis, and Clara had a sister known to be excitable.

A year before the conditions described above, Clara Goldberg was the object of considerable attention. The social workers described themselves as at the end of their particular rope. They wanted to know what to do. The impression of this earlier phase was different. Notes, for example, ran at a staff meeting: The patient came in shrinking, with eyes reddened from weeping. She sat herself down and kept twisting in her chair with her head downcast. She was apparently laboring under great emotion. She answered haltingly and in a low voice. In response to questions she said that her conscience did not work, that she was not the right sort of person, that she had caused a certain social worker to leave the hospital, and finally she burst out weeping loudly.

After the interview and a presentation of all available facts, there was a remarkable split in the opinions of the staff, some of the more mature and experienced physicians lining themselves on both sides of the question, psychoneurosis *versus* schizophrenia. The purposefulness and emotionality of her reactions suggested psychoneurosis to several competent workers. Still it was noteworthy that when the "pragmatic rule" was applied and the question was asked *whether the patient was committable or not,* eight persons out of eleven felt that she was at that time committable and but three felt that she was not committable. Now, inasmuch as on the whole psychoneuroses are probably best treated outside of state institutions, whereas on the whole schizophrenics are best treated in state institutions, this opinion on the part of the staff is noteworthy. Observers who saw a large psychoneurotic element in Clara Goldberg were nevertheless inclined to think she would do best in a state institution.

It sometimes appears that the application of this "pragmatic rule," *What would you do for the case?* is technically superior to asking the question, *What particular disease is this patient suffering from?* To be sure, great authorities agree that one cannot make the generic diagnosis of mental disease safely without specifying the particular kind of mental disease that the patient is assumed to have. No general statement that a patient is "insane," "unbalanced," "deranged," is quite safe to accept. When the particular type of mental disease cannot be agreed upon by a large and active medical staff, it appears to be good technique to ask the pragmatic question as indicated above.

With respect to social treatment, some recommendations early made were as follows:

1. Mother's attitude should be changed to one of encouragement instead of fussy concern over Clara.

2. Occupation should be secured for the patient, an occupation interesting to her; if possible, with small remuneration.

3. The girl should be educated by being placed, if possible, in a domestic-science class.

4. She was to be influenced to mix more with girls of her own age.

5. She was to report regularly to the out-patient department for medical observation and treatment, and she was to attend a gymnasium for her physical development.

The results of treatment cannot be very briefly stated. While (a) living at home she failed to show improvement. She went from one relative's home to (b) another, thence to (c) a convalescent home and thence to (d) a working girls' home. Finally money was raised to send her to (e) a small summer camp for girls, whence she went back to (f) the home. Arrangements were made for (g) medical treatment through payments by her sister. She was engaged (h) to tell stories to children at a settlement playground and she was even somewhat successful in this. She was got to go to (i) a cooking class and then to (j) a pottery class. She was taught (k) to knit and kept persistently at the task of knitting a muffler, though the winter was over before the muffler was finished. She learned (l) to do simple office work in a fortnight at a public stenographer's office and then did (m) voluntary work for some weeks in the office of a civic organization. Then she served (n) as an errand girl in a dressmaking shop. All these employers reported that she was useful and willing. She received no pay for this work which was regarded as educational. At the summer camp she entered into all sports and games such as basketball, archery, and swimming. Physically she was greatly improved by her stay at the camp. (o) Her teeth were filled.

Whereas at home she had made no physical improvement, she improved steadily after her first stay at the convalescent home. The mannerisms that she had had since the early teens became less noticeable. She became able to meet and talk with other persons without much embarrassment. She looked rather pretty and appealing and dressed attractively. She spontaneously bought Christmas presents for social workers.

About ten months before she fell into the utter dilapidation described at the outset of this description, Clara began to fall off in her working capacity. She obtained work in a biscuit company but had no confidence in her ability to do the work and shortly gave it up. She became slower in all her processes. She began to accuse herself and said she was not earning her board. Her employers in the biscuit factory liked her well enough but found her in the end "impossible." Her statements and phrases became peculiar. She said, "I have burned my sister inside of me." She told the forewoman to discharge her, saying that she (Clara) was silly-looking and no good and that she had turned the hair of two of the doctors gray. She was reticent, seclusive, and very forgetful at the mill. At lunch time she would disappear with her package very mysteriously and return in time for work. If addressed by the forewoman she would tremble and shake and be unable to work.

Here then was a fairly promising case, as cases go, of dementia praecox. Here was a case with a good deal of emotionality and apparent insight with considerable ambition. It was always possible up to the last to exert the kind of influence upon her which occupational therapeutists desire to use. Her mannerisms had developed very early and appeared to have but a superficial relation to the main currents of her emotions and will. Was or was not the progress of the schizophrenic process in Clara Goldberg postponed or slowed down by the social work, rest, treatment, and occupational therapy?

Aside from the obvious physical improvements above noted, can we safely allege that her psychosis was slowed up? The only concrete point we can make is based upon the two special psychological examinations at a year's interval, the second about a year before her commitment (at which time a psychometric estimate would have been impossible). These two psychological examinations, so far as they go, give the impression that, up until about a year before the final slump, Clara Goldberg's deterioration was not actively in process. This conclusion is in accord with the maintenance of her general social status and working capacity up to and beyond the time of the second psychometric examination. Clara, it is worth noting, found her own jobs for the most part during the years of our treatment. The last one in which she failed was no doubt too hard for her.

Can it be that with superior light and power over what we have at command, a simpler job without the disturbing elements of exact and monotonous mill work and without the presence of great numbers of fellow workmen would have saved her from immediate deterioration? The question, some might say, is of little importance, since in the long run a patient like Clara Goldberg is bound to decline. This, some would say, is the almost universal history in true cases of schizophrenia (dementia praecox). Even concede this unhappy trend to be the rule, it is nevertheless of the utmost importance to pursue more intensive studies of just this sort, punctuated by occasional psychometric examinations, so that we may get some further light upon the interior of the schizophrenia problem.

No doubt, under the conditions favoring occupational therapy of modern state institutions, the Goldberg girl will become a sufficiently effective hospital worker, though of no great industrial value. Accordingly, although we probably should not have carried out quite such extensive therapeutic measures in Clara Goldberg unless she had shown many psychoneurotic features over and above schizophrenic traits in the early period of her medical observation, we cannot be sorry that so much work was done.

Hours spent by	Medical record, 44 pages
Physician, 20¼	Social record, 42 pages
	Social work:
Psychologist, 2	Visits, 45
	Interviews at hospital, 33
Social worker, 90	Telephone calls, 32
	Letters, 116

Negro soldier cited for bravery. Dangerous paranoid condition after discharge.

Case 76. George Stone, a negro soldier, who enlisted early in 1918, made an honorable record overseas. His discharge papers stated that he was in several battles, received a citation for bravery in escorting an officer through shell-fire, and was cited for the *croix de guerre*. He was gassed and in consequence was declared eligible for compensation on the ground of "pain in the region of the heart and lung defects." He was first sent in as a voluntary patient by the Red Cross, four months after his discharge from the army.

He had married immediately upon his discharge a widow about his own age (he was thirty-seven), who had shortly after joined a religious sect that absorbed a good deal of her time. Stone began coming to the Red Cross office nearly every day complaining that his wife stayed out all night and read the Bible all day in bed, would not cook for him, and did not care for him "since she got that religion." He talked incessantly and laughed a good deal in a silly manner. As he thought the pains around his heart were being made worse by his troubles, it was easy to get him to go to the hospital. He was very jealous of his wife and thought she was trying to injure him. He told her if she bowed to a man on the street he would kill him.

The case was diagnosed as a "paranoid condition" and commitment was advised. But as Stone was not considered dangerous he was allowed to go home. Within a month he was brought back by the police, to whom his wife had turned for protection. Meanwhile he had gone to Washington for a physical examination, in order, he said, to prove to his wife that he was not well, as she said he was. Now he accused his wife of infidelity and believed she was trying to get rid of him in order to obtain his pension money. He wrote letters to prominent officials complaining and asking protection from his wife. He believed that he had two hundred thousand dollars invested. He said he felt wonderfully healthy and was happy because God was in his soul. This time he was committed but escaped from the hospital and started to his old home in the South. Through Red Cross channels he was steered into a hospital in Washington and returned here.

Hours spent by	Medical record, 37 pages
	Social record, 2 pages
Physician, 7½	Social work:
	Visits, 0
Psychologist, 1	Interviews at hospital, 2
	Telephone calls, 0
Social worker, 2½	Letters, 6

Left a state hospital and enlisted.

Case 77. George Mullen was a single man of twenty-five, who was born in Canada but had spent most of his life in a New England state where his family live. In 1915 he was in this hospital suffering from dementia praecox. He was committed to a state hospital for mental diseases and discharged after five months. He immediately sailed for England and enlisted in the British Army. He fought in France, was wounded, and returned home. He seemed indifferent to his family, was excitable, talked continually about money. After a week at home he attempted to cash a check that he had signed with the name of a prominent financier, whose partner he claimed to be. After observation at this hospital he was again committed to a state insane hospital with the diagnosis of dementia praecox confirmed.

Hours spent by	Medical record, 13 pages
Physician, 3¼	Social record, 1 page
	Social work:
Psychologist, 0	Visits, 0
	Interviews at hospital, 1
Social worker, 1	Telephone calls, 0
	Letters, 2

Discharged from the National Guard as a case of dementia praecox. Drafted: again discharged. Claimed to be faking mental disease.

Case 78. Paul Dawson was first admitted to the Psychopathic Hospital two years ago. At that time he was twenty-three and had recently married a girl of seventeen. He had always been a great liar, had never worked long at a time, and had loafed a good deal between jobs. A year before he had joined the National Guard and been sent to the border. He claimed that he had "faked mental disorder" while there with his regiment and that he knew the symptoms since he had worked at times as attendant in state hospitals. He was discharged from the service with the diagnosis dementia praecox (the diagnosis of the Psychopathic Hospital physicians also).

He was sent home from the border to his father under guard. He and his wife then went to live with her family, but Dawson got into a quarrel with the in-laws and they were put out. They were taken in by his family, but when Dawson made no attempt to get work, his father refused to keep his wife, now pregnant. She returned alone to her own home, where she received a somewhat cold welcome. Dawson continued to loaf and drink, insisting that his wife return to him, but making no attempt to support her. Although several positions were suggested to him, he failed to go to work. His wife insisted that she would not "give him up," but finally she settled down to the necessity of making her home indefinitely with her family. When later her husband was drafted, she received an allotment. After the birth of a fine boy, her attitude was that she would return to him if he would "make a man of himself."

When war was declared Dawson at first decided to enlist, saying it would be better to do that than be drafted, but then he came to the conclusion that he would wait for the draft. He was taken into the army in the spring of 1918 and four months later was sent to the Psychopathic Hospital from camp with the following statement on the admission blank:

"Insomnia, weakness, pains, and poor appetite. Feared return of old mental trouble. Hears voices and sees people about his bed; has delusions that he has put electric wires about his bed to keep enemies away; believes wife trying to poison him and wants to do his own cooking. Will not speak to any patient or be spoken to."

He claimed again that his mental disorder was "faked." He had written his family from camp that he meant "to put up a game," because he did not want "to go across" and that he would "give the doctors a run for their money." The physicians believed that he had delusions, which he denied and tried to conceal, and made the diagnosis of unclassified paranoid psychosis. He worked for four months at a state institution and then joined the merchant marine where he became chief petty officer on a ship sailing for China.

Hours spent by	Medical record, 23 pages
Physician, 6½	Social record, 17 pages
	Social work:
Psychologist, 1	Visits, 22
	Interviews at hospital, 5
Social worker, 41¼	Telephone calls, 35
	Letters, 4

Corporal who developed dementia praecox in camp.

Case 79.   Howard Lancaster when drafted was doing exceptionally well in a bonding house.   He worked hard and efficiently and spent his leisure time studying law.   He had always been inclined to be seclusive and a little suspicious, and he had times of being depressed, when he thought he was not doing his work well and that his associates were talking about his falling-off.   He tried to enlist and was rejected because of a defective eye; but later he was drafted.   After two or three weeks in camp, he was promoted to corporal.   After two months he became ill, acting and talking in a silly manner, saying that he heard voices forbidding him to perform his duties. The diagnosis was dementia praecox.   He was committed to a hospital, but in a month had improved enough to be discharged "on visit" to his family.

Hours spent by

Physician, 4½

Psychologist, 1

Social worker, 2

Medical record, 34 pages
Social record, 2 pages
Social work:
    Visits, 1
    Interviews at hospital, 1
    Telephone calls 0
    Letters, 2

Army captain with dual personality.   Arrest for forgery.

Case 80.   Major Dobson (who proved to be Captain James Hill) was sent for examination by federal authorities after arrest on the charge of having forged a check for one thousand dollars under the name of Major Mark S. Dobson. He claimed a dual personality but could not explain it.   He said that he used two names, because he had two fathers, one of whom was dead, the name of the living one being Hill.   He believed that he had the rank of major and that the check he tried to cash was his pay check.   He thought that Captain Hill had been discharged but that Major Dobson was still in the service.   Although he had lived all his life in Florida, he claimed that part of him had been educated in Europe.   His conduct had been peculiar for several months,—in France he had wandered about for a month (he said he knew what he was doing but could not control it).   He had been hearing people say such things as, "Kill him." He was worried about himself and anxious for help in solving his problem. The newspapers had his story under the headline, "Afflicted by Shell-Shock."

Captain Hill had seen several terms of army life. He enlisted in 1912 and purchased release in 1913; reënlisted in 1914 and again purchased release in 1915. In 1916 he went to an officers' training camp and was commissioned. He served eighteen months in France and was once wounded. While overseas he cabled a proposal of marriage to a girl he had known for two years, a dancer in a comic opera company. They were married on his return and the week that Hill was taken into custody, his wife went on tour. The court charge of forgery was dropped when the hospital physicians submitted the diagnosis dementia praecox and the captain was sent to his family for hospital care.

Hours spent by	Medical record, 19 pages
	Social record, 8 pages
Physician, 4¼	Social work:
	Visits, 1
Psychologist, 0	Interviews at hospital, 2
	Telephone calls. 11
Social worker, 5½	Letters, 4

SECTION IX

CYCLOTHYMOSES (MANIC-DEPRESSIVE PSYCHOSES)

Young woman with spells of wandering and eroticism. Three diagnoses rendered—psychoneurosis, dementia praecox, manic-depressive psychosis. Importance of diagnosis in treatment.

Case 81. We find stretched on the records in the case of Winifred Reed three different psychiatric diagnoses; namely, psychoneurosis, dementia praecox, and manic-depressive psychosis.

Of all the diagnoses in the whole of psychiatry no doubt these three offer the maximum of difficulty. To be sure, we place in an eleventh or miscellaneous group of psychoses sundry conditions of still greater obscurity, both as to their nature and frequently as to their diagnosis. Yet these eleventh group cases of psychopathia are indeed so obscure that they practically defy analysis, but the three diagnoses that come in question with Winifred Reed fall into groups which in our Psychopathic Hospital experience we place just ahead of the eleventh group. The schizophrenic group (dementia praecox) we have placed eighth in our list; the cyclothymic (manic-depressive) stands ninth; and the psychoneurotic group stands tenth. In short, after we have swept aside the major diagnostic groups of a more definite character, we find ourselves confronting groups of cases of great diagnostic difficulty and very doubtful genesis. It will be the task of the psychiatry of the future to unravel the cause or causes of the schizophrenic, cyclothymic, and psychoneurotic disorders. Nor can we undertake in this book to expound at any length the psychiatric nature of these or any other conditions. Let us insist that whatever doubt may at bottom prevail concerning the nature and causes of these types of disease, nevertheless their treatment, once a particular diagnosis is rendered, is almost always specifically indicated. Let us insist with all emphasis that *it makes every dif-*

312

ference to the medical and social treatment of a case of mental disease whether it receives the diagnosis schizophrenia (dementia praecox), cyclothymia (manic-depressive psychosis), or psychoneurosis. Moreover, let us insist that it makes a difference to the patient even when the diagnosis is incorrect. We have above considered the interesting case of Alfred Stevens (case 25) to whose fate the matter of a psychiatric diagnosis was of extreme importance. It will be remembered that Alfred Stevens was erroneously classified as a psychoneurotic, was amply treated therefor, failed to make progress, and was promptly put on the right road again when the correct diagnosis (manic-depressive) was rendered. It will be recalled that as soon as Stevens was called a manic-depressive he was forthwith prevailed upon to enter a state hospital, wherein all his troubles quite smoothed out.

Winifred Reed was not very long seriously considered a psychoneurotic; nor was psychotherapy of the sort indicated in psychoneurosis used upon her. (In this instance, as everywhere when we speak of psychotherapy and its applicability or non-applicability to a case, we are obviously not talking about such advice and counsel as are properly given to every normal person; we are talking about psychotherapy deliberately chosen and planned to affect the particular rationalization of a particular difficulty.) The vital issue lay between the diagnoses of dementia praecox and manic-depressive psychosis. In the end, Winifred Reed proved, we believe, to be a victim of manic-depressive psychosis, but still she was for a long time regarded as a victim of dementia praecox. Omitting consideration of the medical data for and against these diagnoses, what are the prognostic features that bear upon social treatment? The psychiatric social worker must, of course, rely upon the medical diagnosis (erroneous though it may be in fifteen or twenty per cent of cases amongst these dubious groups) and must proceed on the hypotheses that underly these respective diagnoses.

We ordinarily think of dementia praecox as a progressive mental disease without characteristic tendency to recovery. *Per contra* we ordinarily think of manic-depressive psychosis as a disease with a strong tendency to recovery and to recurrence. If these ideas are taken boldly at their face value, then the logician might conclude that this victim of dementia praecox tending to an incurable dementia might as well forthwith proceed to his finish in some receptacle for the chronic insane. *Per contra* the logician might conceive that this victim of manic-depressive psychosis being likely to get well at least of this particular attack, might well be tided over his attack at home. But these conclusions of the logician taking the classical prognoses on their face value would land us in many a quagmire. The fact is that the schizophrenic, flattened out and leveled down as he may to a greater or less extent become, can often find a suitable nidus in his own home or somewhere in the community outside hospital walls. Contrariwise, the manic-depressive can be tided over his attack at a home only with extremes of difficulty which are quite unwarranted. You may perhaps at any time set up an institutional equivalent in a private home, with day nurses and night nurses and constant medical care, but ten to one you have not helped the patient's own attitude to his disorder in the slightest and there has been a very trifling gain in the avoidance of whatever stigma now remains for the mental case in the modern community. Far better is it that the tiding over shall be more effective and safely accomplished within the walls of a hospital. Moreover, if we attach to the benefits of the hospital stay the value of precise records for comparison with the data of future attacks and the potential virtues of social work in family adjustment, then we feel that there can be no doubt medically or socially of the propriety of sending these particular curables to hospitals. We again arrive at *an apparent absurdity; namely, that curables should be forthwith hospitalized and that incurables shall be kept in the community.* Obvious though this conclusion is, it nevertheless proves difficult to make the world understand it.

Winifred Reed was first admitted to the Psychopathic Hospital when twenty-four years of age. The physician who suggested that she ought to be observed said that she had been much depressed and thought she was "crazy." There was a history of her having wandered for two days and a night in the late autumn, hoping to die from starvation and exposure. Again, in the dead of winter, she had walked off knee-deep in snow, to the point of freezing her feet, again with the idea of dying from exposure. Upon examination there was little psychiatrically to find; she had a considerable insight into her situation. Aside from depression and over-active reflexes, she seemed mentally and physically normal enough. After elaborate discussion at staff meeting, the staff felt inclined to make the diagnosis dementia praecox, though psychoneurosis was also considered.

She was then dismissed to the social service, who fell into sundry difficulties with her. Her father was alcoholic. Her mother was a Christian Scientist. It seems that the father had become intemperate when Winifred was about ten years old, and had steadily become more and more of a drunkard (appearing at one time in a state hospital). The girl had been a stenographer without special responsibilities. It is not quite certain what the first mental symptoms were and when they occurred. It appears that she lost her job through an odd bit of behavior which has never been explained (she charged a fellow employee with stealing another's hat). She then lost another job after some three weeks and then tried to act as a salesman for her father. It appears that Winifred talked rather boldly about being "sporty." Some employers thought that she was "man crazy." It was difficult to decipher the course of her conduct because of the unreasonable character of the father. At one time the girl was kept in the back part of her father's shop, and customers were assured that the girl was kept there because she was going crazy. Just before coming to the hospital, Winifred had become careless and indifferent, though previously energetic and bright. In fact, Winifred had obtained unusually good grades at the high school from which she had graduated.

It is difficult or impossible to unravel some of the features of her history. There is no doubt that she was, in the stock phrase of the employers, "man crazy" from time to time. She herself dated her excess of erotic passion from the age of twenty-one, when, according to her story, she had sex intercourse for the first time. According to the girl, she had tried to fight against her intensity of passion but was not able to control it. In the same (twenty-first) year, there was also a period of depression which lasted about three months. Nothing connects this depression directly with the initial sex intercourse. These periods of depression have come on from time to time every year since, and in fact have increased in frequency as well as in duration.

If one read the history as we have just reviewed it there might seem to be little doubt of the patient's being a victim of manic-depressive psychosis. Her general excitability of temper, her attacks of depression, and her erotic episodes and trend would be entirely consistent with the diagnosis. If we look back, however, at the picture which she presented upon her first admission to the hospital after her fugue-like wanderings into the woods and snow, and if we bear in mind her change of character and indifference, to say nothing of the oddities of her behavior, then we shall readily see how the diagnosis of a mild dementia praecox could have been set up.

At all events, such is the general opinion of Winifred Reed. The best line appeared to be to manage her in the community with such moral support of the girl herself and of the family as might keep her on a fair level of social efficiency. Despite the fact that the prognosis of dementia praecox would run to a certain impairment of personal and social efficiency, yet from our social endeavors with the girl and with her associates much might be hoped. An endeavor was made to separate her from her alcoholic father and socially inadequate mother and to put her at suitable employment. The first step consisted in sending her to a convalescent home. From this house she forthwith escaped and repaired to her own home. Twice afterward she was also placed in convalescent homes, but whether from a convalescent home or from good conditions in some job that was got for her, Winifred Reed never failed to leave; she would repair to her home and there keep in hiding for a time, eventually telephoning to the hospital for help. Her eroticism and her odd behavior did not abolish the fidelity of a patient admirer who stood by her throughout, and though practically engaged to the girl, never married her.

Eventually, after some seventeen months, *the overt act* which so often supervenes with psychopaths occurred. Apparently she had a fresh outburst of eroticism (which is medically to be regarded as a form of attack in her disease). She was arrested for cohabitation and again brought to the hospital. The diagnosis seemed now to be much plainer than in the beginning. Instead of community care, with the securing of jobs for which she was not ready, and difficult supervision, she was accorded hospital treatment. In two months she could be discharged to probation. Her attack of slight mania had subsided. The further steps in this case, in which similar attacks are only to be expected, are part of a rather clear program. With this diagnosis in hand, it seems as if Winifred Reed could in future be managed with considerable if not with absolute success.

Hours spent by	Medical record, 64 pages
	Social record, 50 pages
Physician, 13	Social work:
	Visits, 23
Psychologist, 2	Interviews at hospital, 13
	Telephone calls, 122
Social worker, 81	Letters, 16

Cyclothymic waiter came to the out-patient department because he lacked initiative.

Case 82. William Donahue, thirty-six, came of his own volition to the Psychopathic Hospital, out-patient department, saying he had had depressed spells from a boy up. He said he was confident enough of his ability to work, but "lacked initiative." He said too that he had considerable trouble in getting on with other people, being regarded as a "grouch." It appeared upon conversation that he had had short periods of exhilaration. The diagnosis of manic-depressive psychosis was soon made by the psychiatrist, and Donahue was referred to the social service for employment. This was procured at a department store. He worked there for a number of months, but reported from time to time that he had not quite got back to his best form.

Donahue was never referred to the wards of the hospital, but was handled from the out-patient department and the social service. It seems he had worked always rather irregularly, usually as a waiter. His head had been split open when he was knocked down by a runaway horse at the age of eight. Donahue had never been very strong, had never taken much part in games with other boys, and had been out of school a great deal owing to sickness. His father was a heavy drinker. No special mental tests were made upon Donahue. He often left his jobs, which rarely lasted over a few months, for no reason whatever. He always wanted to work on his own responsibility. He wanted to be let alone and, if he was not let alone, he did not want to stay. He was self-supporting except between jobs, when he was dependent upon relatives. He was now in debt to relatives and to the dentist.

Amongst the measures of treatment given the patient, it was suggested that he attend the Men's Club. He became a most regular attendant thereat. One important measure was the explanation to his employers of his exact condition and reports to them of his improvement as it grew. Social treatment included such items as follows:—

> Interview to discuss possibility of advancement at his department store;
> To persuade patient of the necessity of more aggressiveness on his part for the purpose of getting promoted;
> To increase his self-confidence and to widen his interests and increase his acquaintance.
> A letter would occasionally be sent to express the visitors' regret at not seeing him at the Men's Club.
> The situation was explained to the secretary of a voluntary association in which he took out membership.

As a result Donahue did greatly improve although he remained supersensitive and somewhat lacking in confidence and aggressiveness. He became more interested in reading and current events. His aggressiveness wore off. He felt he was now doing a man's work and was filled with the idea of getting ahead in the world.

This is an example of the handling of what may be termed a cyclothymic constitution (mild manic-depressive psychosis). The more we look the more examples of such mild or severe cyclothymic constitutions are found in all corners of the world. Precisely these patients make rather good workmen, indeed sometimes extraordinarily good workmen if their psychopathic sides are understood and proper adjustments made. Of course neither the psychiatrist nor the social worker should attach too much significance to improvement in cyclothymic cases, at least from the point of view of claiming such improvement as the result of treatment.

As demonstrated elsewhere in this book, there have been numerous cases where such patients have improved over periods of months and years under influences beyond our knowledge. Still there can be no doubt that direct effects are obtained upon the under and over activities of some of these cyclothymic patients by counsel, encouragement, and direction of interests.

Hours spent by	Medical record, 1 page
	Social record, 19 pages
Physician, 1½	Social work:
	Visits, 6
Psychologist, 0	Interviews at hospital, 14
	Telephone calls, 18
Social worker, 32	Letters, 19

Governess with attacks of excitement and depression, requiring hospital care.

Case 83. Marie Dubois, forty, was a bookkeeper, very competent and well educated, of French-Canadian origin. She had a spell of depression at about thirty years of age, whereupon she came across the line and worked variously as a governess and a bookkeeper, holding her positions for long periods except during the year preceding her arrival at the hospital. We surmise that her succession of jobs during her fortieth year was due to the gradual appearance of the second depressive phase. Yet there was a more striking occasion for the eventual necessity of hospital care,—her mother died and two days later her cousin. This cousin she had been living with as his wife but without legal sanction, since her religion frowned upon a cousin marriage. She then fell into a depression. She was profoundly in love with this cousin. She wrote in her diary of how he died of a Sunday and how every Sunday following she grew sad.

It was some six months after the paramour's death that she got into a rather small difficulty which brought her to the hospital. She appeared at a place where she had formerly worked and was well liked and wanted to sell some tickets for a charity. She was allowed to set up her booth. She set this booth up rather inconveniently to the shop but claimed that God told her just how to do so and that the Cardinal had blessed her sales. She got very angry when requested to move the booth. During her depression she had been rather religious. She tells in her diary of having gone eighteen times to see, understand, and enjoy Billy Sunday's pantomime remarking that "it was a splendid derivatif from my recent sorrow" and that she "admired his perfect subtlety and his complete understanding of the masses of people."

While in hospital she narrates in her diary how "in my soul then I did see at first a beautiful grave of white marble, the top stone covering herself slowly with a small quantity of tulle (material for both dresses and veils). It was a young lady in the grave. I was helping the lover. It was growing and growing in my very presence until it was a beauty. Then appeared under this soft mass some wonderful stems of white lilies. I have never seen anything so beautiful in a funeral marble yet. This stayed with me all night, but in the meantime something was going on to prepare a wonderful Caliban that the committee has never heard of. (Too bad it is only in my imagination.)"

The first attack, as noted, had been one of depression and her mood after the death of her mother and her lover had been chiefly a depressive one. The episode of the ticket-selling was a sample, however, of excitement and the diagnosis rendered at the hospital was that of manic-depressive psychosis-manic phase. Miss Dubois was very restless and irritated at the time she was examined. She could not concentrate her attention. She grew restless and required packs and baths. She would sing and play about the room dramatically. She remained nude a part of the time but seemed not so much erotic as to have lost for the time being her delicacy. (In point of fact her diary records a considerable delicacy with respect to her early handling by the nurses.) Now and again she would seem to react to hallucinations of vision and hearing and above has been given an example of the sort of visual hallucination, if it be one, which she had. The imagery was more of that fixed and solid sort which psychologists have recently discussed, than of the fleeting, cinema-like sort which we are accustomed to find in the psychoses. She assumed no fixed attitudes at any time, took her nourishment willingly, and apparently had a rather good insight into her abnormality of mind. Physically she was almost normal, though her eyes were a bit prominent.

Upon discharge she reported from time to time to the out-patient department and the notes indicate that she remained exhilarated for some six months further. After a year it seemed to the out-patient medical staff that she need report no longer as a patient. To be sure she was a little overemphatic in her speech but perhaps not more so than a French-Canadian woman should be

Hours spent by	Medical record, 22 pages
	Social record, 15 pages
Physician, 9½	Social work:
	Visits, 20
Psychologist, 0	Interviews at hospital, 2
	Telephone calls, 8
Social worker, 35	Letters, 6

Hypomanic boy on probation: ran away. A "bad actor" in school.

Case 84. Joe Marino, fifteen years old when he was first referred to the hospital from a juvenile court, is a kind of adolescent delinquent that psychiatrists feel belongs pretty certainly in one of the more definite groups of mental diseases, namely the so-called manic-depressive or cyclothymic group. He yielded the impression of the so-called "hypomanic" manner of mild overexcitement when he first came to the hospital and his entire history seems consistent with his being fundamentally a cyclothymic.

He was a short, stocky Italian boy with rather an old-looking face. He was very talkative and noisy, easy enough to control but apt to get into mischief when not under immediate supervision. It seems that he had had an idea, perhaps an obsession, about going to California. He was opposed in this idea at home and became abusive and rather violent there. He boarded a train and got as far as Providence, when he was picked up by the police. He was brought back to the juvenile court where he had twice before been and from which he was even at that time on probation. Employers had always found him wayward and impertinent, and he had never stuck to a job longer than five weeks, for the most part leaving a job after only a few days. He had been arrested for breaking and entering, had ripped off plastering in unoccupied houses, and was regarded as a "bad actor" in school, where he had shouted and broken windows.

He was one of seven American-born children in an Italian family that lived in cramped and rather squalid quarters. His father got rather irregular employment but was somewhat intelligent and well disposed. The mother was an ignorant and excitable woman suspicious of interference and unreliable. The other six children were lively, jolly children and not especially troublesome. The family regarded Joe's visits to the hospital as rather a joke. They regarded his activity and pugnaciousness as due to his being "a kid and full of fun." Joe was under hospital observation in all for about seven weeks at two different times. His associations and his replies to questions were very rapid. He showed very well the symptom called distractability, picking up all the features of his immediate environment and weaving them into the conversation. Upon staff rounds, for example, he talked as if he were in a courtroom, affixing comments to the bystanders, calling one a lawyer, another a witness, another a stool pigeon, and the like. He was at times so active that the treatment of prolonged baths was executed; and the hypomania so verged upon a true mania that the committing physicians felt themselves entitled to take the extreme step of actually committing him to hospital by procedures of the probate court.

After his discharge from the hospital he remained "on visit"; that is, on the books subject to recall for a year. He got his picture in the newspapers at one time by desiring to enlist in the marines as a water boy who had had plenty of experience. He said that as his name was Marino he ought easily to get into the marines. (Of course the name Marino is fictitious and the very characteristic maniacal pun which the boy made was actually a good deal more complex than the form we offer.)

The case was closed by the social service some eight months after his first appearance at the hospital although, as above stated, his name was carried on the books of the hospital for a year. At the expiration of the eight months it would seem that the great wave of overexcitement which had been punctuated by the various adventures mentioned was now, for the time at least, well over. Perhaps Joe will appear again in another phase of mania or possibly even of depression if our diagnosis of cyclothymia is a correct one. No doubt previous experience with Joe will allow for rapid and accurate decisions concerning him should he become once more a "bad actor."

Hours spent by	Medical record, 14 pages
	Social record, 17 pages
Physician, 8½	Social work:
	Visits, 13
Psychologist, 0	Interviews at hospital, 1
	Telephone calls, 8
Social worker, 25	Letters, 5

Sailor who became overactive. Had been given to "excited actions."

Case 85. The following is Robert MacPherson's story as recorded by the social worker, when she interviewed him on the wards :—

"The patient is a nice-looking boy with a very pleasant manner, which, however, seems to become rather suspicious at times. He is twenty-three years old. He was born in Philadelphia. The family came to Boston when he was a baby. When he was three years old, his mother was taken to a state hospital, and he and his younger sister were placed in some sort of institution at that time. His sister developed pneumonia and died. Patient's father took him at that time, and patient has lived with him since then until a year ago. Patient says his father has never worked very steadily, that he is a drinking man and so was his father before him. His father is now about sixty years of age. He is not a man of much education and patient thinks maybe he was jealous of him because he got so far ahead of him. He thinks his mother was quite educated. He does not know how old she is, as she will never tell him. She is now in a state hospital where he goes to see her. She seems all right but at times if she becomes discontented or something happens to upset her, she is liable to create quite a disturbance.

"Patient went to grammar school, then to a high school of commerce where he graduated, and also graduated from an evening high school. Then he went to a commercial college for two or three years but he did not finish, as he did not like the course. While he was still going to school he worked with Weston Brothers as a clerk (his father works there as a packer). He also worked at the Plymouth Publishing Company and ushered at the Lexington Theater. At clerking he would make about three dollars a week and at ushering he earned fifty cents a performance; however, he thinks the latter is 'a poor way to earn money.' When patient started work regularly, he started in at the National Sugar Company where he earned nine dollars a week. Then he worked at the American Electrical Company, earning fourteen dollars a week; later he worked for the Standard Insurance Company at eighteen dollars a week. He was two years there and he says he knows enough about insurance not to want to take it out.

"When war was declared he enlisted in the naval reserve; he was never called and so secured his discharge August 21, 1917, but reënlisted in the United States coast guards. He was on a revenue-cutter. About July, 1918, he was sent to a naval hospital where he stayed a month. He was circumcised there. He was discharged in August, 1918. It was about this time that his mental trouble began. He became more ambitious, attempted things he had never done before and led 'sort of a wild life.' He had saved up about seven hundred and fifty dollars and he purchased a Big Six Buick. He says that is enough to show he was 'out of his mind.' He would invite everybody to ride and would 'kick them out' just as quickly. He sold the magazine, *The Puritan,* and because he was in uniform he made quite a lot of money and he spent it just as quickly. His father 'kicked him out.' After his discharge he became a four-minute man and it was while he was speaking in different theaters that he was advised to go to the Fenway School of Oratory. There he met a Mrs. Reed. They offered to give him lessons and after a time Mrs. Green (who was also connected with the school), Mrs. Reed, and Mr. Reed (who was a tea salesman) all 'vamped' him, so that he went to live with them. He says he will do anything that they tell him to do. Patient later went to work with the United Importation Company. At first he was a checker. Later he started the follow-up system and soon established a department of advertising. When he started he was the only one in the department, but now there are six and he is the head of the department. His salary is only twenty dollars a week; but he made more on the side in business deals in connection with the firm. He says he has made as much as ten thousand dollars at one time, but he does not often make these sales. Patient wants to get into the foreign department and wants to get down to South America. He speaks some Spanish which he studied in high school and has made arrangements to study Portuguese with the son of a former ambassador.

"Patient says that he has recently become interested in purchasing automobiles again, and he thinks that maybe it is because he has been doing these things that they got him into the hospital, but he intends to sue whoever was responsible for having him 'shanghaied' here. Patient already has four motor cycles, a motor boat, a sail boat, a deer skin, and a bear skin, which he purchased through the company and which he intends to have made into gloves and a coat. He doesn't know how much he has in the bank. He has been looking up Buick roadsters and on Saturday he repeated 'the same sort of stunt' that he had done before, just after he was discharged from the navy.

"At that time he took two girls out riding in his car, drove them out a mile and then stopped his car in front of a garage and made them all walk home. On Saturday he asked the same girl to go out with him in the roadster, which he was trying out; he drove her over to the garage, where he made a deposit on the car; he left the car there and took her home in a jitney. Saturday night Mrs. Reed asked him to lend her four hundred dollars. He thought this was very queer as she had never made such a request before. The more he thought the matter over the queerer it seemed, so he took a suitcase and decided to go back to his father to stay with him for a while. He promised to let them know when he got to his father's, so he telephoned them and they asked him to come out. He and his father went. He says that while they were there, he noticed that they kept a pretty close watch on him. A Dr. and Mrs. Foster arrived, who were evidently friends of the Reeds. Dr. Foster started talking to him and seemed to draw him out, but he was perfectly willing, so he talked ahead. The doctor said that he had a car to sell, and invited him to come riding with him, so they went and he was brought here to the Psychopathic Hospital. Patient says that 'the same stunt was pulled' on his mother twenty years ago and it is no wonder that she is still in a state hospital. He knows that there is something wrong with her now, but his father has never told him what happened twenty years ago. He would like to know about it as he thinks there may have been 'some crooked work.'"

This somewhat highly colored story if taken with a grain of salt gives a fairly accurate account of Robert's experiences between the time of his discharge from the navy, in the summer of 1918, and his stay in this hospital, in the fall of 1919. He was very talkative and active, getting into difficulty with the other patients. He had no marked outbursts of excitement but was continually restless. His hypomanic condition made indefinite hospital care necessary and he was transferred to the same state hospital where his mother was a patient.

Before enlistment Robert had worked in an insurance office and lived with his father, who helped out with his expenses, so that he had been able to save about seven hundred dollars. He had shown average ability in school but had been more interested in athletics than in studies. At one time he was engaged to a girl who broke the engagement on account of Robert's "excited actions." He did not show any great or deep regret over the affair. He was always full of energy; in the habit of having his own way and rather self-centered. He was neat in his personal habits and did not show peculiarities of conduct up to the time he left the navy. His attack of excitement began about a month before his discharge.

Hours spent by	Medical record, 14 pages
	Social record, 5 pages
Physician, 3¼	Social work:
	Visits, 0
Psychologist, 0	Interviews at hospital, 2
	Telephone calls, 5
Social worker, 4½	Letters, 5

Enlisted; gassed; discharged. Became restless, talkative, moralistic. Voluntary patient.

Case 86. Clarence Adams was gassed fourteen months after his enlistment and, after passing through several hospitals in France, was discharged four months later in the neighborhood of Boston. He took a few months' vacation and then during the hot weather of early summer held a clerical position in a large mill. One day he fainted on the job and gave it up. He held several other positions for short periods but was overactive and could not concentrate. His family then sent him to the woods, by a doctor's advice, in company with a man companion. After some weeks his companion felt that he was not improving and brought him back to Boston. When he was admitted to the Psychopathic Hospital he was restless and talkative. He took pleasure in reading the Bible and instructing the patients from it.

Adams was now twenty-six years old. He had had several attacks previously, the first four years before, when he became absorbed in the stock market and speculated recklessly. At this time he became "moralistic," according to his brother, and made efforts to bring together his parents who had been separated. After he had been in this condition a year the family sent him to a private hospital for mental diseases, where after five months he recovered. Once or twice after this he resorted to the same hospital for short periods. Adams had made a rather brilliant record in school and after entering college he had done well for a year. During the second year he became "dissipated," contracting gonorrhea. He was in the second month of the senior year when he went into the army; and he returned to college and got his degree. During his term of army service he did very well, so far as can be learned.

From the Psychopathic Hospital (where he was a voluntary patient) he went of his own accord to a near-by hospital, as a further period of hospital care was advised.

Hours spent by	Medical record, 14 pages
	Social record, 6 pages
Physician, 3¼	Social work:
	Visits, o
Psychologist, o	Interviews at hospital, 1
	Telephone calls, 3
Social worker, 3¼	Letters, 10

SECTION X

PSYCHONEUROSES

Cigar-maker with psychoneurosis. Financial worries: dislike for his trade. Family adjustments. Different forms of psychotherapy. Individualization.

Case 87. In one of the great Atlantic seaboard hospitals (which shall be nameless) there used to be an out-patient department diagnosis *Judaism,* although the diagnosis Judaism was probably a sly Caucasian hit at the frequenters of the clinic. There is some basis for the idea of a preponderance of psychoneurotics amongst Jews. But, inasmuch as the Jews have the excellent habit (from the mental hygiene point of view) of very speedily resorting to physicians for their ills, the statistical preponderance of Jews in many Atlantic seaboard clinics is perhaps deceptive. There may be as many Caucasians of different varieties that fall victim to psychoneurosis as there are Jews. It would be difficult to point out anything really differential in the psychology of the Jew.

Maurice Eastman was a Russian Jewish immigrant, forty years of age. He came on his own initiative to the Psychopathic Hospital complaining of indigestion, stomach trouble, constipation, frequent urination for months at a time, year-long headaches, and what he summed up as nervousness. In point of fact various doctors told him he was a victim of nervous instability, nervous prostration. He had evidently been coached by physicians to know that "it was all foolishness." He said he was always worrying, always afraid (that the children would be killed, that there would be accidents while he was asleep). He was unable to control his thoughts. He had what would almost amount to a symptom in itself; namely, an intense and analytic interest in his case. He slept well, in fact he always felt sleepy and tired, but even more tired on rising. He knew that he ought to "cheer up as there was nothing the matter," but he could not. He had read an account of the Psychopathic Hospital work in the Sunday newspaper. Later interviews showed that he was worried over his physical condition, over family finances, over increase in the number of children (there were now five ranging from twelve to two years), over his domestic relations and over practice of self-abuse which he thought had affected his health.

Here is a sufficiently characteristic picture of a psychoneurotic with many features suggestive of the obsessive or psychasthenic. We omit further medical details, insisting merely, by the way, that the above picture, although characteristic, can be found in a variety of other mental diseases than the psychoneurotic group. (Particular cases of that sort may actually prove to be syphilitic and greatly improve by antisyphilitic treatment.)

Eastman was forthwith placed for some time under the care of a student in psychology who had made a special study of the methods of psychotherapeutic suggestion. (This sort of technique can still well be studied in Bernheim's excellent old work, *Suggestive Therapeutics,* as well as in sundry newer works of Bernheim that carry out the early ideas of Liébault. The patient acknowledged great improvement by the suggestions offered, in periods of one-half to three-quarter hours, and apparently was genuinely much improved for a time. Besides the "talking cure," he was made to read popular works on psychotherapy. The patient thought he was better because he had learned to check his thoughts. He got to reading many books on psychology and on suggestion. He practiced abstinence from sex intercourse for eight months at one time so that the family should not increase too rapidly.

However, he continued to have troublesome symptoms and feared he would become insane. He had obsessions of several sorts (when he saw a knife he wanted to stab somebody with it; upon looking from a window he wanted to jump out). While these psychotherapeutic efforts at persuasion were going on, occasional hospital visits (at the same time patient was taking hydrotherapeutic treatments there), the domestic adjustment had to be made. The mother was an unusually intelligent, thrifty woman, adept at cooking and sewing. Eastman himself, although he had gone to work at the age of eleven in Russia, had picked up a fairly good education, knew several languages, and read some philosophy. He hated his cigar-making trade although he earned good wages thereat. The family income was just enough to meet current expenses, left no margin for clothes, and allowed only tenement-house life on a shabby street, overcrowded with very poor neighbors. It is clear that several of these domestic, economic, and social features cannot easily be met by psychotherapy, either of the simple "Cheer up" or "Forget it" kind or the more elaborate and subtle practice by the student of psychology in Eastman's case. There was a social (family) problem as well as the individual one. Possibly it is the social problem both superadded to and lying deeply underneath the individual problem that has caused physicians to fail in the past to effect cures in many psychoneuroses, despite the fact that a very perfect individual psychotherapeutic technique was being thoroughly carried out. It is an error of the psychiatrist and the psychologist to rest profound faith in arm-chair methods of psychotherapy. It is great merit of the medical social worker in general and the psychiatric social worker in particular to have shown the faults of this arm-chair method taken by itself. Meantime the social worker must not fail to acknowledge the extraordinary results of some therapy *in camera,* such as the amazing results of hypnotism in selected cases and the equally amazing results by psychoanalytic treatment of patients reporting from time to time in the consulting room of the psychiatrist. Our tiresome old formula, *Circumstances alter cases,* is the only true formula to apply to the whole field of psychiatric social work.

If there is anything which this book stands for it is plainly the individualization of the diagnosis and treatment of psychiatric cases. The adherents to one or other method of psychotherapy (such as hypnotism, psychoanalysis) are rather apt to overdraw their statistical values in any psychiatry. The social worker has to steer her way very carefully betwixt these various statistical prejudices of the enthusiastic adherent of some method that is a perfect success in some cases. It is as requisite for the psychiatric social worker not to cry up the wares of a particular kind of psychotherapeutist, as it is for the psychiatrist himself to bear in mind that there is more than one way to "kill a cat." Of course, when one is in Rome, one must do as the Romans do. In a large part of France during the war, hypnotism was officially forbidden as a method of treatment for those psychoneuroses familiarly termed "shell-shock." Nevertheless, elsewhere in France and in other belligerent countries, hypnotism was being employed in *some* selected cases with positive and even startling results. The modern formulations of psychotherapy are not so many decades old that they will not be greatly molded and revamped before the last word is said. When all is said on the matter, however, the doctrine of the treatment of the individual *as such* remains the common possession of all forms of psychotherapy.

After all the psychiatric social worker does not by virtue of contacts with psychopathy become a psychiatrist. The fact that she may know more about individual details and technique of family adjustment than the psychiatrist, does not cause her to have sound ideas concerning the central psychopathic figure in the family under adjustment. In the same sense the student in psychology employed in the case of Maurice Eastman might have been wasting his own and everybody's time by perfectly correct technical endeavors in treating a man with many of the same symptoms which Eastman possessed who should *happen to be not psychoneurotic* at all. One of our Psychopathic Hospital patients who had been regarded for five years as psychoneurotic is described in *Neurosyphilis;* he was actually syphilitic and the patient plaintively inquired why it had taken so long to establish a diagnosis. Neither the social worker nor the psychologist can be expected to avoid pitfalls such as that case presented. On the other hand, it is just as certain that the psychiatrist has neither training nor time to execute the family adjustments undertaken by the psychiatric social worker. Nor has a psychiatrist often the time and perhaps the temperament to execute persuasive therapy in its best form. Indeed, we are sometimes tempted to think that different types of psychotherapeutist will eventually prove necessary for different types of psychopathy, just as different sorts of automobiles suit different temperaments. All of which is another example of our constant insistence; that is, that *psychiatrists as psychiatrists are not social workers or psychologists,* and that neither of these other types of workers is likely by training or temperament to be able to swap places with the other or make more than snap diagnoses in the psychiatric field.

The medical measures adopted in Eastman's case (persuasive psychotherapy) ceased after a time, as all the internal adjustment that could be made in this way had apparently been accomplished. The man was apt to be irritable and unreasonable at home. He would complain of the children's noise which prevented him from reading; he complained that his lot was harder than that of other men in like circumstances, as he was more intelligent (this was true) than the average man. He had the advantage of having no bad habits to interfere with his being a good steady workman. The treatment carried out for a period of some six years now finds him much better adjusted to his lot in life. No other form of work could be found for Eastman that would bring him as high wages as cigar-making. As the family was after all not destitute it proved impossible to get supplementary relief by means of loans, such as might have been put into effect for certain indigent families. The wife and children were getting an annual vacation through the settlement house and a vacation was now arranged for Eastman himself. He had not had a vacation in all of his adult life. He helped with the work of the Men's Club, and from time to time pieces of work were secured for the wife who was a clever needle woman to supplement the family income. Eastman still hates his work.

Hours spent by	Medical record, 2 pages
	Social record, 35 pages
Physician, 4	Social work:
	Visits, 20
Psychologist, 6	Interviews at hospital,
	Telephone calls, 19
Social worker, 70	Letters, 18

GIRL OF 15 YEARS

1913

SOCIAL CONDITION

Hard Work
No Recreation
No Training
Insufficient Income
Feeble-minded and Inebriate
Father
Family Discord

MENTAL CONDITION

Hysterical Convulsions
(2 in one month)

1915

SOCIAL CONDITION

Light Work
Recreation
Trade Training
Adequate Income
Home with Sister

Separation from Family

MENTAL CONDITION

Hysterical Convulsions
(3 in past year)

Girl with hysterical convulsions. Father feeble-minded and alcoholic. Psychoanalysis. Social investigation. Prolonged social treatment. Cure or alleviation.

Case 88. Sadie Strauss was a seventeen-year-old Russian Jewish girl, a case of hysteria whose cure or alleviation could be variously claimed at different times by psychiatrists or social workers. Perhaps neither the psychiatrist nor the social worker should claim too much, since the hysterical trend may be ingrained and persist for years. For some years, however, there have been no clear or striking hysterical outbursts, and only traces of that excessive fear reaction which some of her human sisters often seem a little proud of—that is, fright at a mouse. As it takes more than one swallow to make a summer, so it takes more than one case to break the general medical conception or prejudice: *once a hysteric always a hysteric.* In passing we make remark that it would seem that the war experiences with shell-shock will probably serve to break down this old conception.

There is still another older conception of hysteria as an "aristocrat" amongst the functional diseases, that is as markedly hereditary. Concerning heredity in Sadie Strauss, we can find only that the father is perhaps somewhat feeble-minded; possibly his low mental level is really acquired, *i.e.,* alcoholic. Sadie herself was determined by the psychological examiner to be normal. She was deft with her fingers, but did not prove very resourceful in the tests for planning and analysis. She was very "suggestible," but got easily discouraged and seemed more than normally fatigable. Her measurement by the Binet Scale was 11 4/5 and by the Point Scale 11 7/10.

Menstruation began at twelve. Sadie went to work as soon as the fourteen-year law allowed and was working on piece work in a mill earning from six to seven dollars a week for fifty-four hours' work. After a painful menstruation she one day collapsed, feeling a lump or stone in the stomach. She was taken to the hospital, then home again and back to the hospital, where there was a seizure of pain, screams, laughter,

335

and unconsciousness. She was then brought to the Psychopathic Hospital. It appeared that she had fainted two or three times in the last few years.

The psychiatrists could find no abnormal sign upon physical examination either on the motor or the sensory side. In an attack she rolled from side to side on the couch, held an arm or leg in the air, was sometimes stiff, sometimes quite relaxed, but always apparently somewhat conscious, occasionally assuming a silly expression, sometimes attitudinizing, sometimes pointing as if hallucinated and quite mute. She did not bite her tongue or void urine. This particular attack was slight and took place during an interview for the purpose of psychoanalysis.

Psychoanalytic conversations finally turned up news of an early childhood episode. The child had been terribly frightened by having to undress, one night when alone, her drunken father. This episode may have developed sex-consciousness prematurely or it may have provided "buried" memories that could operate after the manner of the Freudian mechanisms. In conversation it developed that the girl dreamed of a dark man in a white garment who chased her. The man's hands were her father's, but his face was like the face of a man who was the first dead person she had even seen. This psychoanalytic discovery might have been supposed to work, as such discoveries sometimes work, by the so-called method of psychical "catharsis" to effect an immediate cure. That is to say, if there was a "buried memory" of this infantile sex experience, then (according to the theory) talking it out will relieve the effects of the repression. It is not entirely sure that the memory in question was buried in Sadie's mind. At all events she had some eight attacks of pronounced hysterical nature after the supposed catharsis.

Perhaps it will not do to quarrel with the psychoanalyst concerning his therapeutic results, and no doubt a large share of the effect in Sadie Strauss' case is to be awarded to the psychoanalyst. Nevertheless it is to be pointed out that a routine social investigation would bring out very promptly information concerning the Saturday night debauches of the father. A good deal more was found out by such investigation than the psychiatrist or psychologist could discover from the armchair. The father was in point of fact brought to the clinic and

proved to be feeble-minded. Supervision of his life yielded
definite improvement in the family condition, although he
fell from grace and once got into the house of correction.
There were many more than merely the medical and temperamental problems in the Strauss situation. Clothes were provided for Sadie, so that she could go to the trade school for a
year. The family needed Sadie's wages and could not clothe
her. They were too proud at first to accept such help but were
eventually persuaded. The patient then made her home with
her sister; vacations and recreation were arranged for; more
or less regular reporting to the out-patient department was
made a habit, and medical encouragement was there doled out
to her.

Two and one-half years after her initial appearance at the
hospital Sadie was married. She had matured visibly and was
now capable of much better self-control. Attacks had long
since stopped. Her husband was a man of a very good sort,
and the case could appropriately be closed. Her husband said
that he gave his wife pretty things and let her have her own
way in household matters. Outside of hospital time, some of
the social workers attended the wedding.

Hours spent by	Medical record, 18 pages
	Social record, 40 pages
Physician, 17¾	Social work:
	Visits, 44
Psychologist, 1	Interviews at hospital, 24
	Telephone calls, 37
Social worker, 107	Letters, 11

*Voluntary patient in state hospitals from time to time.
Cyclothymia: sex obsession. Industrial adaptation.*

Case 89. Joseph Fangillo, forty, has been three times a
voluntary patient at the Psychopathic Hospital and has also
spent some time at the hospital's suggestion at one of the state
hospitals also as a voluntary patient. His history shows that
he had also, at the age of thirty-four, been a patient at one of
the state hospitals.

He has received a number of diagnoses but he is probably
best classified as a psychasthenic. He had recently gone into

the liquor business and rightly or wrongly felt that his affairs had been going downhill ever since. Besides there had been the Billy Sunday campaign and there was the national prohibition movement. In addition to ideas touching money, he had some obsessions about sex. He thought that he had an uncontrollable sexual desire and interest and felt that he would be tremendously excited if he saw the pictures of women or if he came at all in contact with them. He complained, too, of his eyes although there was no objective evidence of eye disorder.

If we regard the diagnosis of psychasthenia as correct then it is plain that the medical and social contacts with Joseph Fangillo will mean much. His five different hospital experiences have all been as a voluntary patient. In fact, the last four hospital stays have been part and parcel of a single psychasthenic phase out of which he appears now to have passed, aided by the direct influence of counsel and family adjustment between himself and his wife effected by the social service. The wife is intelligent and devoted but needed a great deal of encouragement since she was living upon the family savings.

If our present diagnosis is incorrect and he is actually in some sense a cyclothymic patient, then so far as we are now aware the thing which will bring him out of a given phase is rather the curative power of nature than any medical or social efforts of any description. However, it is clear that if Fangillo is a cyclothymic and the course of his disease is, as the phrase is "self-limited," nevertheless the social service contact with the wife and the counsel to her with respect to her adjustment to her husband's psychopathy would mean a great deal.

This case has not been intensively handled by physicians at any time upon any specific line of psychotherapy such as psychoanalysis. The sexual obsessions above mentioned may date from a specific occurrence which conversation might at last unfold. The psychoanalyst and, for that matter, all kinds of therapeutists, would hope from all cases of psychoneurosis for a fundamental cure by the process of so-called reëducation or rationalization. Without entering the debatable confines of the psychoanalytic question, it is plain that where the diagnosis is so in doubt as in this instance, proceeding to elaborate reëducation upon sex lines or upon other lines of character development would be very time-consuming from the standpoint of the patient himself. If the patient is a cyclothymic, then he is likely to emerge with absolute normality after a time in any event. If he is a psychasthenic, at all events he has the record of having emerged with perfect normality from the previous attack and his psychasthenia may itself be of periodic or cyclic nature. (It is well for the lay as well as the medical observer to bear constantly in mind that cyclothymia is not the only mental disease which is cyclic.) Accordingly, for better or worse, no special psychotherapy has been undertaken other than that involved in the routine social service contacts by competent and intelligent social workers, familiar with psychopaths of various sorts.

Fifteen months after we first knew him Fangillo was able to take a position in the stock room of a large firm with which he is offered a good prospect of advancement. He made the choice of this position rather than a better paying position offered by a former employer because he felt that the larger firm promised a more stable future. Now, a year later, he is still working for this firm and beginning to realize his expectations.

As a detail of social service technique, it may be remarked that Fangillo was gotten a temporary job with a certain firm through the efforts of a worker who was doing special work on the industrial problem of the psychopathic employee. The employer said that he liked to get workers from social agencies because a good deal more was known about such workers than about the ordinary run of applicants for employment.

(See also Appendix A for the social record of this case.)

Hours spent by	Medical record, 26 pages
	Social record, 21 pages
Physician, 7½	Social work:
	Visits, 11
Psychologist, 1	Interviews at hospital, 13
	Telephone calls, 13
Social worker, 23½	Letters, 6

Industrial accident. Traumatic hysteria. Compensation questions.

Case 90. Dennis O'Donnell was sent to the hospital by the Industrial Accident Board. He had gotten a number of fractures, especially of the arms. X-ray examination failed to show that he had any fracture of the skull. After his fall he was treated for a time in the company hospital, went home at his own request, and in the space of three months began to do some work again, though he was not very successful at any kind of job. He left for a distant state but did not work there for some eighteen months. His left hand was weak. Heat and noise disturbed him greatly in various factories where he tried to work. The family had accumulated many debts and he was much worried about these. His memory had been very poor since the accident. He was a very quiet and contemplative sort of man. He said that his hand felt weak and this was verified by test, but besides this it was found that he had a complete anesthesia of the left side of the body with deafness in the left ear and even some visual disturbance in the left eye. Yet at the same time the reflexes were not different upon the anesthetic side from their condition on the right side of the body. The arm muscles were not atrophic. On the whole there seemed to be no evidence of any organic lesion to account for the weakness or the anesthesia.

The diagnosis was one of *traumatic hysteria* which, to quote from the hospital report, is "a very real disease and so far as we can see would justify compensation."

O'Donnell had been paid after his accident nine dollars a week for four months and later for six months at the rate of ten dollars a week. This compensation was discontinued by the Accident Board which felt that the man's condition was due more to alcohol and syphilis than to the accident. After seven months' delay O'Donnell was admitted to the Psychopathic Hospital upon the representation of his lawyer. The lawyer was unaware that the patient was working all this time. Four months later O'Donnell was offered a sum of five hundred dollars as a lump settlement to cover unemployment. This sum O'Donnell is not willing to take but says he has not the funds to contest the case. In war times he earned about thirty-four dollars a week but after being a patient at the Psychopathic Hospital he could not get this thirty-four-dollar-a-week job and is now working at fifteen and eighteen dollars a week in a factory.

Perhaps this case will serve as well as any to indicate the very doubtful question of social-service technique that arises in industrial accidents. Probably the question of syphilis raised by the board is to be answered in the negative; at all events there seems to be no evidence of syphilis of the nervous system as a cause for the symptoms shown. Nor had there been any history of alcoholism for a period of some fifteen years, although before that time O'Donnell had been alcoholic. It would seem wise for O'Donnell to report from time to time to the out-patient department. There is always a question whether the advantage of counsel afforded by the hospital is countervailed by the loss of self-reliance which some men might feel through having to resort to a hospital.

Hours spent by	Medical record, 21 pages
	Social record, 15 pages
Physician, 5	Social work:
	Visits, 1
Psychologist, 1	Interviews at hospital, 7
	Telephone calls, 15
Social worker, 9¾	Letters, 18

Machinist in aviation suffers from traumatic hysteria after blow on the head.

Case 91. Walter Nelson enlisted at twenty in the naval reserve, during the spring of 1917, and in the fall was assigned as a first-class machinist in aviation. While he was working on a plane in a tent hangar during a windstorm, the tent blew down and he was hit by a pole across the back and head. He was unconscious for half an hour and in the hospital three days with weakness and backache. There were no other symptoms at that time. Two weeks later he was among volunteers accepted for foreign service, but the party was not sent at the expected time and Nelson was very much disappointed. After this he became shaky and excited and was sent back to hospital. He went home for a Christmas furlough and was not well enough to return to duty at the end of his time. He seemed to his family to be "far-off, hazy, in a trance" and "had to be cared for like a child." He worried for fear people would call him "a slacker."

After a month in the naval hospital, he went back to duty but was still somewhat dazed and confused. He wrote his family that he was afraid of being court-martialed for having done some of his work wrong and asked them to send him poison to take. In the spring he was discharged for physical disability. On his return home he was advised to come to our out-patient department. He said that he felt "dopey" and changed since the accident, that he had very little interest in anything. Reluctantly he told of having a fear after the accident that he had been cursed by a young woman with whom he had had sex relations for a short time, (he had a friend who had been cursed by a young woman), and said he dwelt on this thought constantly. His condition was diagnosed as *traumatic hysteria.*

In a month he had improved slightly and in another month was much better. In six months under the influence of treatment, including massage, hydrotherapy, suggestion, tonic, and light work, he was much more cheerful and animated and able to work three-quarters time. He had given up the obsessive idea of the young woman's curse and was showing steady improvement.

Hours spent by	Medical record, 5 pages
Physician, 4¾	Social record, 1 page
	Social work:
Psychologist, 0	Visits, 0
	Interviews at hospital, 3
Social worker, 1½	Telephone calls, 0
	Letters, 0

Feeble-minded soldier discharged for hysteria. Married a prostitute to reform her.

Case 92. Martin O'Hara was sent to the hospital by the court charged with indecent assault upon a six-year-old boy in the hotel where he was working as janitor. He denied the charge, the child admitted previous knowledge of perverted sex practices, and it was never determined whether O'Hara was guilty.

He was twenty-nine years old and his mental rating by the Point Scale was 11.8. At the age of twelve he had run away to sea and spent a few weeks on a fishing boat. His father would not let him go again to sea so he started to work and held countless odd jobs in theaters, amusement parks, and circuses. He never liked to loaf and when work was not to be found he would go up to the Maine woods. After war was declared he tried to enlist and was rejected because of bad teeth. A year later he was drafted and became sick in camp during the trial gas attacks. He was sent home for a rest and soon after discharged from the service with the diagnosis hysteria. He was suffering then with gastric pain and vomiting and a slight tremor of the head. These symptoms disappeared after a while.

He went to work and in a few weeks married a girl whom he had known for several years. He said that he had known she was sexually promiscuous, but that he had always treated her with the greatest respect and loved her devotedly. They were married in a pool-room where he worked, by a justice of the peace. That same night he returned to work and continued to work until midnight so that he might get double pay. The girl went to stay with her parents that night. The following day he discovered she had a six-months-old baby, and after inquiry he was forced to the conclusion that the father of the child was actually unknown. He forgave the girl for the deception and wished to live with her, "to reform her," but she left him and continued to live as a prostitute. Both she and the baby were syphilitic. He had never lived with his wife since the marriage.

Under the excitement of these events the tremor had returned. When he left the hospital after nine days he still had it, although at times it disappeared entirely, especially when he was interested and intent upon what he was doing. Later when he came to the out-patient department he would sometimes tremble violently but at other times would appear quite composed. He went to live with his parents and made up his mind to secure a divorce from his wife. After some months he felt able to work and got a job.

He is beginning to feel strong and cheerful again and the tremor is less marked and comes less frequently. He says that although he knew a good deal about his wife, before he married her, he did not know "half of it" and he is no longer in love with her. He has worried a good deal over being dependent upon his parents, who have no surplus income, but now he feels fit to maintain himself.

Hours spent by	Medical record, 25 pages
Physician, 4½	Social record, 12 pages
	Social work:
	Visits, 2
Psychologist, 1	Interviews at hospital, 3
	Telephone calls, 23
Social worker, 5½	Letters, 0

Drafted soldier discharged for physical incapacity. Psychasthenia. Improvement.

Case 93. Joseph Levenson was drafted in the fall of 1917 (twenty-five years old) and discharged in three months for physical incapacity. When he came to the out-patient department six months later he was complaining of insomnia, lack of appetite, and pains in his head and back. He claimed that discipline and the rigorous winter had caused him a physical collapse.

On the theory of a possible developing of acromegalia, an X-ray picture of his head was taken; but it showed nothing abnormal. The diagnosis was psychasthenia. In four months he had made definite improvement and was planning part time work.

At first a marked increase of symptoms occurred when he was told that he ought to get to work. He was living with a devoted family in a good home. He undertook a course in salesmanship, and at first he was unable to sit through the classes on account of his pains. He would stand it as long as he could (for about two hours) and then stretch out on a table or chairs until he felt able to go on again. After a time he could sit through the seven hours of the school day by relaxing for a few minutes now and then. At this time, even after three months of treatment, he could not walk much. He said once he thought he could never "bear it and live" but now he knew he "had it in him" and could "look forward happily to the future." Later on he had a plan for starting a provision store of his own if the Red Cross would make him a loan; but this was decided to be an insecure investment. Levenson then got a position as salesman in a meat market. He works full time and is improving, though he still suffers from pain and weakness.

Hours spent by	Medical record, 5 pages
	Social record, 5 pages
Physician, 4	Social work:
	Visits, 3
Psychologist, 0	Interviews at hospital, 3
	Telephone calls, 12
Social worker, 3½	Letters, 0

PSYCHOPATHIC PERSONALITY

IN A WOMAN TYPESETTER, 28

1915	*1916*
Inebriety	No Alcohol
Insufficient Income	Adequate Wages
Non-support of Mother	Contributions to Mother
Family Discord	Away from Home
Friendlessness	Companionship
Lying	No Lying
Fabrication	Slight Fabrication
Suicidal Attempt	Cheerfulness

SECTION XI

Psychopathic personality. Typesetter, sickly, unhappy, unpopular, discouraged, attempted suicide. Trained to be self-sustaining. Psychiatric social work. Many workers on the case.

Case 94. There is much discussion as to the meaning of the term "psychopathic personality." Whereas in one sense every victim of mental disease shows effects in his personality, the effects by the same token require psychiatric social attention even if the victim have brain tumor. The term has come to be used for many forms of usually rather slighter mental diseases than those which receive more definite designations as belonging to well-defined disease entities. Possibly the term being briefer and smoother is theoretically better than the term "constitutional psychopathic inferiority." But the latter term has been worked into sundry official documents, and it is to be feared we shall have it with us for some decades and until a greater definition of the whole topic of psychopathic personalities shall occur. According to one group of thinkers every psychopath, and especially every victim of psychopathic personality, is practically *sui generis;* that is to say, has a most highly individualized and specialized make-up of soil and taint. Nor does it do any harm to insist upon this ultra-individualism in diagnosis and treatment, as it practically comes up in the clinic. According to other authors there threaten to break out in the group of the psychopathic personalities sundry subgroups. One of these formulations was made a special study of by the former Chief of Staff, Dr. H. M. Adler, at the Psychopathic Hospital. It is mentioned in greater detail in the summary. Perhaps as valuable a statement as any general statement can now be concerning these personalities runs to the effect that the victims are to some extent infantilistic. Some of the per-

347

sonalities are a little infantile along the line of their emotions. These are likely to belong to a group with hysterical trend. Others show more or less childlike obstinacy and episodic over-reactions to ordinary stimuli, recalling effects in certain children. Some cases seem to represent enormous exaggerations of particular instincts and are given to wandering, to special types of sex activity and the like. Possibly some alcoholics may be regarded as weak of will in the direction of psychopathic personality, so that alcoholic mental diseases cannot be set down as directly and proportionately due to their alcoholism.

Harriet Farmer was not at all feeble-minded; in fact tests at intervals of two years showed that she was making a proper improvement to test. Let us take occasion to insist, however, that not seldom the selfsame psychopathic traits do occur in morons or other subnormal persons. We did not have to face in the Farmer case the lack of judgment characteristic of a moron.

Harriet was certainly an average scholar and indeed read much good classical literature. Twenty-eight upon her first contact with the hospital, she had been for two years very alcoholic, not infrequently drinking alone. She had also been untruthful and unreliable; she told scandals about a priest; told of mistreatment by her family; and made up stories about the attentions of men to her. Harriet was rather talkative and aggressive with people with whom she came in contact. Church club members did not want to see her at the club. At home she was lazy, slovenly, and thoughtless. She lay in bed late and expected her mother and sister to sew and wash for her.

It was discovered that her father died of general paresis; her mother was also treated for many years for syphilis which she had contracted from Harriet's father. The girl herself was short, slight, pale—the so-called wiry type, rather unattractive, possibly anemic, and with bad teeth. She came to the hospital after an attempt at suicide, which attempt was made a day when nothing at all unusual had been noticed in her behavior. She had been at times depressed at menstrual periods, but there had at this time been no depression. She had lunched with her mother, who a few hours later was notified that paris green had been taken by Harriet. Harriet said she had originally bought the paris green for plant insects. She had taken it feeling discouraged with her life and with the poor physical condition of her mother.

The psychiatrists found her practically negative in every respect. Even anemia was found to be not present. Psychiatrically nothing abnormal could be found beyond the provisional diagnosis "manic depressive" suggested by some observations. She clearly was not committable. As for a motive for suicide, a somewhat curious history transpired. She had put her name and address in a candy box and had gotten up a correspondence—"object matrimony"—with a man who turned out to be sixty-five years of age and otherwise ineligible. This episode appears to have helped her to think that there was nothing left for her in life. There had, of course, been considerable pecuniary trouble in the family. The two brothers had married and were no longer able to help the family. The parents had been separated when Harriet was eight years of age.

After a month's observation the determined diagnosis was "not insane, not feeble-minded—psychopathic personality." Harriet has now for some years been under pretty continuous observation by the social service. After a period of some two and one-half years she was so compensated or adapted to life as to require little aid. During this period of two and one-half years a rather intensive type of social work, supported by medical consultations, was carried out. The psychiatrist's general recommendation was that a good deal more variety in life was necessary. It was the task of the social worker to secure such variety and to make changes in her living and working arrangements before she should get stale. It was arranged that she should live away from home, and in the house where she lived she now began to make girl friends after a fashion which had been quite unknown to her before. The other girls liked her. Exercise, diet, and bathing became systematic. Menstrual difficulties were discussed with women physicians at the hospital. She stopped drinking and ceased to mention suicide. She no longer told out-and-out lies and the tendency was represented for the most part by exaggerations or slight perversions of the facts.

From time to time she became discouraged and made various complaints, apparently fearing she was "to be put away." But these spells of bitterness were transient and left her with her usual friendliness. She began to have a number of different suitors and went walking with them and took meals at hotels and dairy lunches with them. Harriet very gladly appeared at the clinic for social workers and told her story in an approximately correct and engaging fashion. The experienced social worker is apt to say, "Why this sort of thing is just what every social worker has to deal with!" We are far from denying that such is the case. We hold that statistics of medical social workers will probably show that practically one case in two of all intensively studied medical social cases will turn out to be in some important way psychiatric. If such commentary means to argue that psychiatric social work is unnecessary *as a specialty,* just because psychiatric social cases are so frequent that every social worker has met them, then we should be compelled to decline to follow the argument. One of two conclusions, and we hold that both conclusions, can be drawn from this state of affairs, namely: First, that instruction in social psychiatry should be given to every medical social worker; second, that there should be specialized training to develop specialized psychiatric social workers.

It seems to us that the amount of personality study required for the diagnosis of Harriet Farmer and the amount of personal adjustment required would mean that there must be in the world a group of specializing psychiatric social workers. Many medical social workers are by temperament unfit for psychiatric social work, or at all events not as well fitted as are others. It is also, we believe, going to be held that all social workers whether medical or non-medical ought to be given psychiatric training of some sort. It would be hard to show convincingly the extraordinary change in Harriet Farmer from the unsociable, pallid, unattractive girl, with rather a bitter outlook on life, to the competent, self-supporting, physically much improved, rather pleasing coöperative girl with a normal set of outlets along all of the main social lines.

Too much and too little can be made of the so-called personal relation between some one individual therapeutist and the patient. The slogan "individualization" is often taken to mean that there should be in the ideal a *one-to-one correspondence* between the social agent and the social patient. It is true that many effects, especially in the field of alcoholism, are gained in this manner. But individualized treatment is not necessarily, or as a rule even possibly, the treatment *of* one individual *by* one individual. We do not need to paraphrase Lincoln by saying social treatment is treatment *of* an individual, *by* an individual, and *for* an individual. Treatment is as often, and perhaps always should be, the treatment of all the individuals in a given family—*each individual taken as such*. The individualization of treatment does not refer to carrying all of the measures up to one head. There is a certain democracy in social treatment, the advantages of which have not been sufficiently preached. In the case of Harriet Farmer, for instance, although two social workers not trained in psychiatry had failed to make proper contacts with her personality, yet after the Psychopathic Hospital contact was made the *social treatment of Harriet was carried out by not less than six social workers of various temperaments, who nevertheless all succeeded in aiding the development of Harriet's character* with its consequent stoppage of drinking and bitterness. There were also four physicians more or less intimately concerned with the case.

Of course what Harriet did was in some sense to personify the entire Psychopathic Hospital and to consider herself under its auspices. This relation is by no means uncommon, nay, perhaps, is the usual one. The hospital with its medical and social officers becomes a sort of religion with the patient. No hospital run under what we are sometimes tempted to term "regular-army" regulations can become a religion with such patients. If the social workers were suddenly removed from the institutions, the chances are that a patient of this type would not return to the hospital more than once.

There is a certain uniqueness about this psychopathic hospital relation with its patients which stands out in sharp relief against the "borrow-no-trouble" attitude of the old-style institutions for the committable insane.

(See also Appendix A for the social record of this case.)

Hours spent by	Medical record, 41 pages
	Social record, 55 pages
Physician, 5¾	Social work:
	Visits, 76
Psychologist, 2	Interviews at hospital, 16
	Telephone calls, 50
Social worker, 150	Letters, 14

Son of an educated Belgian family. Wanderer and irregular worker.

Case 95. Louis Sand, the son of a Belgian professional man, was twenty-eight years of age, an immigrant, upon a rather irregular allowance from his father. He had spent time in twelve different states during five years, working here and there for a few weeks or months at factory or farm work. In fact he had made eighteen changes from one place to another and had borrowed small sums of money here and there. He spent much of his time looking for work and reading. He had the ambition to take courses in engineering and had had some college work in Belgium. There was no language difficulty since he spoke and wrote English fluently. It was thought he was a victim of Ménière's disease—one ear was growing deaf and he was dizzy.

Sand never became a house case at the Psychopathic Hospital but was immediately left to the social service after his coming on his own initiative to the out-patient department. Some loans were made to him which he came back from time to time to pay. Nine months after the first observation he was found a position with an engineering firm which he held for some four months and was taking a correspondence course in the general topic. The case was accordingly closed. However, Sand began to feel restless, wrote appealing letters to the social service telling about lack of will power—his desire to get back to Belgium. The case was accordingly reopened by the social service and work was secured for him in new places. He gave the visitor a sum of money which was put in the bank for him, a nasal operation was performed, and new lenses for his glasses were gotten for him. He then left for a distant state.

Sand, although he desired to return to Belgium, was ashamed to go until he had made good in America. He had no friends or associates with persons of his own educational level. He talked a good deal of his interest in books and in music, but these interests proved to be superficial. He had not rationalized his relations with women, affecting refinement and chivalry on the one hand, on the other hand resorting to masturbation. He had a shell of ambition with apparently little power behind it. Perhaps he is to be classed as a sort of constitutional inferior, inasmuch as the disorder or defect is particularly one of will. If we were asked for a single phrase for him, it would be hypobulic. Hypobulics no doubt require the social worker and the physician to act more as mental splints than in any other definable way.

Our Belgian correspondence concerning Sand shows that he had been as unsuccessful there and weak of will as he was here. What is to be the outcome of his Ménière's disease, if that be the correct diagnosis? No one can say, but Sand is going to keep in touch with the Life Extension Institute, whose examiners will no doubt trace the further effects if any of the aural condition.

Hours spent by	Medical record, 13 pages
	Social record, 25 pages
Physician, 5¼	Social work:
	Visits, 11
Psychologist, 0	Interviews at hospital, 27
	Telephone calls, 30
Social worker, 43¼	Letters, 30

Child of a thief and a prostitute; brought up by charity. Psychopathia sexualis.

Case 96. An interest was taken in Theresa Beauvais by a lady who had lived in the town where Theresa was born. Theresa's father was a professional thief and her mother had been a prostitute. Theresa herself had already entered upon this life and was in the poor house when her townswoman found her. When Theresa at fourteen had learned the dangers of pregnancy, she had stopped promiscuous intercourse and begun masturbation. Theresa never tried to conceal her life or habits and a psychoanalyst who saw her said that as there was nothing repressed, psychoanalysis was superficial. Besides, she was rather unintelligent or at all events looked so. (She later tested at 15½ years by Stanford-Binet and by Point Scale as 17.5, accordingly probably not at all feeble-minded.) Although unintelligent-looking she made a very good general impression and was well liked. She had studied in an academy for some years but had not finished her work.

She was observed at the Psychopathic Hospital and finally

regarded as a case of psychopathic personality, though a question of psychoneurosis and a question of dementia praecox had also been raised. She was found to be abnormally sentimental and somewhat dramatic in her attitude toward her delinquency. She seemed rather to enjoy making an impression upon the maids and nurses with details of how bad she had been and the things she had undergone. She was, however, on the whole, fairly truthful. She said that she could not control herself with respect to sex relations. (There was a history of absolute promiscuity for a period of some three months before admission to the hospital.) Amongst the psychopathic personalities there are, no doubt, a number of cases of *psychopathia sexualis* and amongst these a form called *satyriasis* to which Theresa may belong, but of course that designation does not afford much information as to prognosis or treatment.

She had, ten months before admission, started learning to be a nurse and after her discharge from the hospital she was placed as a ward maid in a hospital where she stayed three months. She there had sex relations with an employee who talked of marrying her but had trachoma and was in general unreliable. The marriage was accordingly discouraged. She then got work in mills for short periods, refusing to room in a girls' boarding house, disappeared from view for a fortnight, and then telephoned that she had become a maid in a questionable lodging house. Then she was brought by the police to the hospital again. This was six and a half months after her discharge from the hospital. It transpired that she had been living with a sailor who had forsaken her. She had shown odd conduct, going out two days in succession with her hair down, moccasins on her feet, and a coat over her shoulder, returning exhausted and (by her own story) confused. There was also a spell of screaming and she was picked up by the police sitting on a doorstep. The diagnosis of psychopathic personality was again made.

After discharge she was put to work in a mill and made to live in a very good boarding house for working girls. She talked about taking a fresh start, yet within two months she was found to be pregnant and was sent to a maternity home where there was a miscarriage. She now went to work in a professional man's family near by and actually took full responsibility for his house during his wife's illness. She stayed

there eight months. She had been found to have a positive
Wassermann test with the serum and was receiving treatments
weekly. After a trip to the hospital for such treatment she
failed to return to her working place. About six weeks later
an officer of her maternity home met her on the street. She
said that she had been living as a street-walker and resorting
to masturbation constantly. Sent to another hospital for
syphilitic treatment she ran away six weeks later, was found
again and returned in a few days and again discharged. After
further hospital treatment in another hospital she, two months
later, took another job in a mill and a pleasant room in a good
lodging house was arranged for her. She was interested in
her work but was slow in learning the trade. She was easily
discouraged. She kept in close touch with the social worker
but had spells of being inaccessible and almost antagonistic.
She grew tired of her factory work and a position was found
for her as nursemaid to care for a semi-paralyzed woman.
She was pleased with her new position and was very hopeful
about her future.

Very soon she entered into sexual relations with a man living
in the same apartment house, whom she had met in the hall-
way. She left her position in a few months and made plans
to go to New York with another patient, Bertha Greenwood
(case 10). Bertha, however, weakened and telephoned anonymously to the social worker about the proposed trip; so that
Theresa was intercepted and persuaded not to go. She was
found to be in need of hospital treatment for gonorrhea. In
the end an operation was necessary. While she was in a convalescent home, she expressed gratitude and affection toward
the social workers for the care she had received from them,
but insisted that she wanted "complete independence." In
spite of her desire to work in a factory and live in a lodging
house, she was persuaded to take a more sheltered position in
housework.

Such hypersexuals as Theresa are pathetic figures. Aside
from the hypersexuality, a girl like Theresa may make an
excellent impression and we have letters about her ambitious
although not brilliant school work, her interest in church affairs
and the general esteem in which she would be held for months
at a time. We must remember in particular the skill and
fidelity which she showed in the professional man's family as

above noted. The sex instinct must be thought of as somehow standing out in relief against a pretty normal background
of the other instincts. It is, perhaps, a considerable achieve-
ment that these cases are now considered examples of Morbi
rather than of Vitia. The entire attitude of the world to
morbid hypersexuals must be naturally different from the attitude toward the sexually immoral. Sometimes it seems that
these frequent social diagnoses, "immorality," ought to be replaced with some other diagnosis, since from time to time immorality is made to cover some psychopathic hypersexuals like
Theresa. Yet the psychiatrist would feel a great deal more
comforted could he advocate a special treatment of hyper-
sexualis. An artificial menopause by X-ray often seems a bit
over vehement, at least as routine treatment.

Hours spent by	Medical record, 47 pages
	Social record, 51 pages
Physician, 9	Social work:
	Visits, 46
Psychologist, 2	Interviews at hospital, 13
	Telephone calls, 86
Social worker, 84	Letters, 24

*Family known to thirteen social agencies. Mixed marriage:
marital discord. Outbursts of temper: assault: arrest: probation. Border-line psychopath.*

Case 97. The showing of social "symptoms" (factors and
phenomena) in Leon Blumer was by the card-catalogue as
follows:—

Social symptoms:
  Outbursts of temper
  Assault
  Marital discord
  Arrest
  Probation
  Insufficient income

Social diagnosis:
  Family dissension

Analyzing by forms of evil shown we find provisionally:

Medical—nothing; possibly family discord, outbursts of temper, and assault on wife mean something psychopathic.

Educational—nothing; insufficient income possibly due to language difficulty?

Moral—family discord, outbursts of temper and assault (if not fundamentally psychopathic).

Legal—arrest; probation.

Economic—insufficient income (language difficulty?).

We can easily dispose of the language question. Blumer speaks English, rates 14 years psychometrically, and gives the impression of being fairly intelligent. Blumer had married at twenty a Nova Scotian Protestant girl. This marriage may have been due to bad judgment, but there are perhaps no eugenic principles well established enough to speak against a Caucasian-Semitic crossing.

A Malthusian argument is possible. There were nine pregnancies in ten years. Blumer was a salesman earning from twenty to thirty dollars a week. The family income was insufficient. Advocates of birth-control might use such a situation to point a Malthusian moral. But insufficient income would never by itself have led to assault and arrest, nor would Blumer on the basis of insufficient income alone ever have appeared at the Psychopathic Hospital.

Yet, *mirabile dictu,* the family was known to *thirteen charitable agencies.* Quarrels began soon after marriage. Children had been placed out for years. The wife broke up the home repeatedly. As a rule the different agencies were consulted on account of the marital difficulties (sometimes for children's health, once for financial relief).

There the situation stood. Even our own social service let the social diagnosis stand at family dissension. Our orderly analysis by forms of evil clarifies the issue, if it does not solve it. The issue is moral *versus* medical at bottom. Racial miscegenation is not yet to be conceded an error. The legal difficulties are plainly secondary to whatever underlies the outbursts of temper. The economic straits of the family might have been material for dissension, not its adequate cause.

Let us examine the medical situation. To the offhand observer Blumer had himself well under control. He readily admitted his quarreling, but said he did not know whether his wife or the general situation at home irritated him most. He was rather emaciated and proved to have a pulmonary tubercle on one side (he now was thirty years of age).

It was further found that he had had gonorrhea at seventeen and had at some time acquired syphilis (positive serum test first at twenty-eight).

The wife appeared normal and enlisted general sympathy amongst the agencies. Her husband was sent to the Psychopathic Hospital by one of these agencies in the fourth year of the marriage to see whether there was a psychopathic basis for the marital discord. But neither feeble-mindedness nor frank mental disease nor a milder psychopathy could at that time be determined.

It is the same today: tests and observations fail to prove mental disease or defect, though they do give a definite medical, though non-psychiatric, background for the increasing temperamental difficulty. Discounting early sex irregularity, mixed marriage, and a possibly fundamental overirritableness as not proving psychopathia either alone or together, we can still see the value to the court of thinking about Blumer as a *medical* case. If his difficulty is essentially moral, nevertheless there will inevitably be something medical to do.

But what is a *moral* case? By classifying a major group of evils as *Vitia,* we do not explain the nature of *Vitia.* The medical urge is to make *Morbi* of all *Vitia* forthwith. That decision would lead to nothing practical. There is a certain proportionality between Blumer's bad conduct and the complication and duration of his domestic difficulties. Disease does not so nicely proportion causes and results. There is no doubt a strong moral element in Blumer's plight, whence we may probably infer an improvement by training and by guidance in the future.

Thus we must leave Blumer himself scientifically unresolved. But it is plain that much of value to his family has been brought out. The family syphilis question must be answered. The tuberculosis yields some indications. Next time Blumer appears in the Psychopathic Hospital, further progress may be made in the deep-lying temperament matter. We cannot rid ourselves of the suspicion that we deal with a border-line psychopath.

Hours spent by

Physician, 4½

Psychologist, 1

Social worker, 3½

Medical record, 35 pages
Social record, 2 pages
Social work:
Visits, 1
Interviews at hospital, 1
Telephone calls, 2
Letters, 7

Psychopathic boy enlisted in the navy: discharged after pneumonia. Sick and "nervous."

Case 98. Word came from a neighbor in Francis Corcoran's home town: "The less said about him the better. If he would go to work as the other boys in town have done, he might be a help to his mother." The mother is a neurotic, hard-working woman, who is taking boarders to support the family through the father's illness. The severity of our correspondent's judgment of this nineteen-year-old lad might be moderated if she knew that the physicians at the Psychopathic Hospital found him to be a *person of constitutional psychopathic inferiority suffering from nephritis and possibly from pulmonary tuberculosis.*

He was sent from a public health hospital, where he had been under treatment for his physical condition, because he was "nervous," had "attacks of depression," and "could not keep from telling lies." He told many yarns about himself, among them the story that he was a student at the Harvard Medical School. He explained that he wanted to get in to see the operations at the hospital and thought he would be admitted if he were a medical student. After telling the doctor in the public health hospital a number of contradictory fanciful tales, he later came to him to admit the falsehoods, saying that he had just "realized" what he had been doing. He said that he felt a force that compelled him to tell extravagant stories and to do things that he did not mean to do, such as walking the streets until one o'clock in the morning.

Corcoran was disabled, nine months after his enlistment in the navy, through exposure on transport duty and sent to a hospital with lobar pneumonia. He was discharged after fifteen months in the service. He went home for a while, and then came to Boston to enter a business school. He had done rather poorly in school. He had entered high school at fifteen but had left almost immediately. After a few weeks' study in Boston, he got nervous and discouraged and resorted to the public health hospital. He was advised to return there for further physical building-up.

Hours spent by	Medical record, 14 pages
	Social record, 1 page
Physician, 3¼	Social work:
	Visits, 0
Psychologist, 1	Interviews at hospital, 3
	Telephone calls, 3
Social worker, 3	Letters, 0

Orchestra-player drafted. Sergeant in the band. Gave out in camp.

Case 99. From flute-player in a symphony orchestra to band sergeant in a military camp proved a change too severe for the endurance of Manuel Giordani. As a boy in Italy he had been allowed to stay at home instead of being apprenticed to a tailor, doing odd jobs and studying the flute. When he was seventeen he came to America, and by playing at summer resorts earned enough to study music during the winter, until he had attained a position in a first-rate orchestra. He was drafted when he was thirty and was quickly made *sergeant*. The life was rather hard o him because he was not used to active physical exercise, but he liked it.

Sometimes he would have to play almost continuously from morning to night. One day after the band had been away from camp playing nearly all day, the sergeant remembers that he was tired and had a feeling of uneasiness and timidity. He went past his station and started to walk back along the high-road until an officer in a motor picked him up. He did not sleep well that night and the next day after a cross-country race felt exhausted in the evening. He could not sleep and in the morning got up and went to his old barracks where he thought it would be quieter, so that he might get some sleep. He was found in a confused state lying on a bed spring, and sent by a physician to the base hospital. He was afraid something was going to happen to him, and was excited and very talkative.

In this hospital he was normal in behavior, but very worried because he feared he would lose his standing if it were known that he was discharged from the army because he was "crazy." It was the opinion of the medical staff that his mental disturbance was not of the nature of a psychosis, though they were not able to determine exactly what type of disorder he had suffered from. Four months later Giordani was playing in a summer hotel, and wrote that he was quite well.

Hours spent by	Medical record, 27 pages
	Social record, 1 page
Physician, 4½	Social work:
	Visits, o
Psychologist, 1	Interviews at hospital, 3
	Telephone calls, o
Social worker, 1½	Letters, 2

Draftsman who thought people laughed at him. Given work alone, his earnings doubled.

Case 100. Henry Allen made a very high mental test, being especially good in construction puzzles. He had come to the hospital as a voluntary patient in a depressed frame of mind, feeling unable to do his work. He had been sleeping poorly. He was fifty years of age and was physically quite negative except for tremors of the tongue and fingers. He complained of headache, aches in the bones, shortness of breath, and general weakness, but there was no physical basis determined for these particular complaints. He said that people laughed at him and said things about him in the office where he worked and that they had been doing this for years. In fact, he had really for years been worrying about this attitude of his fellow workers but had kept on in the office up to a fortnight since.

We found Allen a most instructive case from a certain industrial, vocational aspect. He despised the constructional details in his work and rather wanted to do designing. Of course the details in designing would, no doubt, have been as elaborate as the details of the constructive work; apparently it was the matter of an attitude adopted by Allen to the general nature of his work rather than to his mechanical capacity in it. It was as if he wanted to be more of a figure in the whole office by doing designing rather than constructive detail. As the other workmen so constantly talked about him (as he thought) he did not want to work in a large office with many looking on. He felt he had worked only up to about twenty-five per cent of his efficiency because he had not been rightly placed in the office.

The hospital diagnosis remains at psychopathic personality but very possibly we should regard this patient as tending towards the cyclothymic (manic-depressive) constitution where he belongs in the depressive group. According to his own story he has been somewhat blue all his life. The self-accusatory trend is a characteristic of such cyclothymics. Very possibly his idea that he was being persecuted by fellow workers would transform itself upon analysis into a form of self-accusation nor does the story of the whole case suggest anything paranoid, that is, looking in the direction of the persecutory delusions of a schizophrenic.

Allen's case came up for particular consideration at a meeting of employment managers at the Psychopathic Hospital. It was at that time suggested that he ought to work for a firm large enough to employ a number of designers so that he might be given the work he liked, rather than merely constructive detail. It was also suggested that he should work alone in an office. These suggestions have, in a measure, been met by arrangement with an employer who has given him greater and greater responsibility in his work. Short notices and pressure upon him for rapid work are avoided. He is earning now twice as much as before. One of Allen's letters to the social worker will tell the story.

"MY DEAR MISS HALL:

"Your inquiry with enclosure from my sister has only just reached me, owing to an error made in forwarding at the post office.

"My conscience has reproached me many times of late for my apparent discourtesy in neither reporting or calling at the Psychopathic and letting you know what had become of me. Owing to the exigencies of Mr. Anderson's work, in part, and more perhaps because I knew you were on your vacation, I waited at first to get myself adjusted, and lately have had so much given me to do it has taken all my time and energy to accomplish what was expected of me. I am working very smoothly and getting a good deal done, but only by close application. I am not just ready yet to form an opinion as to how it will work out for me. Expect to get together with Mr. Anderson on his return from the South in a few days and see if I cannot get things adjusted more satisfactorily.

"The conditions the work demands are speed, effectiveness, and thought. The two latter I can supply but not the former, so my problem with myself and with him is to reach a compromise which I hope in fact must work out. One cannot work for Mr. Anderson without being put on their mettle, even when, as is certainly true, he is one of the kindest and in intention considerate of employees, and always interesting.

"For reasons best known to himself he has established me in my own office or work room at considerable present expense to himself. His work would be considered by a designer or landscape man as of a very choice and charming character. It is, or should be, all beautiful. Just how I shall measure up to the opportunity we will have to wait and see.

"Personally I feel that I have benefited by my stay at the Psychopathic and the difficulty of concentration which I once mentioned to you seems no longer to exist in my work. Will you please remember me very kindly to Dr. Reed, Dr. Patterson, Miss Dean, and the others?

"In closing I can only say that I am not sure yet for reasons more readily said than written, whether or not the work, as it is coming to me, will prove the work that I should wisely endeavor to hold. I am trying it out in the most matter-of-fact and sensible way I can and am reserving my final opinion.

"When it has developed a little farther, I may want, if I may do so without imposing unduly on your time, to talk over conditions as they develop. For no matter how ideal the nature of the work may be I am by no means sure that ultimately to be pinned down as closely to a drawing board as I have been will become impossible—physically I am waiting to see.

"I trust that your vacation has been very beneficial to you and that you have returned to your profession refreshed for the work which I am sure is as exacting and trying on the social workers in some ways as it is helpful and beneficial to the people you help.

"Trusting you will pardon the length of my letter and my delay in writing, I am   "Very sincerely,
                                    "HENRY ALLEN."

"P.S. It has occurred to me that what I have written of my work may suggest to you that I am being unduly confined. It is true for the time being, but I think I shall remedy it without difficulty; and add this lest you should think it wise to write Mr. Anderson on the subject, for I know it is part of your profession to look after the patients when they need it. In this case there is nothing but will adjust itself. And it is all incidental to getting started, so while I have written to you frankly I shall be quite as frank with Mr. Anderson and can instantly make it right, and I do not know how he would take a suggestion from the staff while I am certain he will from me. Probably you wouldn't think of it in any case. But I have such a warm regard for the intelligent work you are doing at the Psychopathic I am sure you would do it unless you knew there was no need!

"If there is any further information I can send you at any time, I shall be only too happy to do so.

"H. A."

It is a question whether it would not have been wiser to have Allen overcome his fear of working in a large office. Possibly if we had regarded his condition as cyclothymic or an obsessional one, it might have been wiser to try to break up the obsession by counsel and the initiation of new habits. Where we are dealing, however, not with besetting ideas so much as with a habitual and self-accusatory gloom, it is not likely that "rationalizing," or idea upsetting, psychotherapy would be much in point. Here again, as in the case of Arthur Morton, the differential diagnosis between the depression of psychoneurosis and the depression of a constitutional cyclothymia becomes a matter of extremest importance to the victim of the depression which is aided by rationalization on the one hand, and no doubt by abstention from psychotherapy of the argumentative or persuasive sort on the other.

Hours spent by	Medical record, 18 pages
Physician, 4½	Social record, 38 pages
	Social work:
	Visits, 2
Psychologist, 1	Interviews at hospital, 20
	Telephone calls, 10
Social worker,	Letters, 19

BOOK IV

What is man, that Thou shouldest magnify him,
And that Thou shouldest set Thy mind upon him,
And that Thou shouldest visit him every morning,
And try him every moment?

Job, Chapter 7, Verses 17, 18.

EPICRISIS

The **descriptive task** of this volume is complete. The body of the text presents a set of **social cases chosen from psychiatric material to illustrate the theory and practice of social work.** The first three books present the practice of social work inductively, to the end that the student may almost unconsciously gain an insight into the underlying principles of diagnosis and treatment in social cases. To be sure the reader will find scattered amongst the case-descriptions in all three of these books numerous theoretical remarks. But in Book IV these scattered remarks concerning theory are to be united into a body of principles. At the outset of Book IV we shall offer statements of an exceedingly general nature, designed to align this work with others bearing on the various arts and sciences that have come to be termed sociological.

RELATIONS OF SOCIAL WORK TO SOCIOLOGY AND PSYCHIATRY

There is not much in books on sociology, ancient or modern, that touches even the theory of social work. **Works on sociology** since the establishment of the theory of evolution **have treated mainly the relation of the family taken as a group to the community also taken as a group.** That both the family group and the community group are sets of individuals, no sociologist ever denies. Indeed some sociologists proclaim that the unit of sociology is and must be the human individual. But we believe it is fair to say that modern sociology is in the main a theory of the relation of human groups to one another rather than of the relation of the individual "soul" to its fellow or fellows in daily life.

Certain it is that the sociology books rarely present any case material after the manner of the present work. Yet there is much to be said for building up a new sociology from the bottom. If we are to build thus from the bottom, we must certainly begin with **the relations of man to man, woman to woman, and man to woman,** whether those relations are by blood, by marriage, or otherwise. What has been done by jurists upon domestic and personal relations is not only meager but in part doubtless quite false, being founded on the very partial insights obtainable by Bench and Bar. Many of the situations that we have described above will suggest dire need of logical analysis of personal relations with a deeper insight and a less general point of view than the juristic one. This new point of view and insight we can only in this work faintly indicate. We conceive that social work will some day pass, in the form of more or less definite principles, into a great body of sociological theory. The new sociology will in our opinion be, not merely a theory of human "groupism," but a theory of the relation of individuals to each other. Though the student of social work can today find little or nothing to his purpose in sociology books, he should not despair. He is himself recording facts that will go to make up new sociological textbooks of the future and give the theory of human group relations its proper fundament in a theory of human individual relations.

In one sense this volume is a collection of cases of social maladjustment. The whole of **life,** according to Herbert Spencer, is an adjustment—**a continuous adjustment of inner to outer relations.** Roughly speaking, we look to the psychologists for a study of the innermost of life's inner relations. Perhaps it is not astonishing that we should find the sociologists beginning with the outermost of life's relations, namely the group relations of the family to the community. But the history of the mental sciences in recent years shows that the psychologists are beginning to study man's inner relations as they touch society (witness books like McDougall's *Social Psychology*) and that the sociologists are beginning to write books that endeavor to carry society back to certain springs of action in the individual mind. In short we can see signs that the mental sciences are beginning to study not merely life's inner relations *as such* and life's outer relations *as such,* but also the adjustments of interrelations of the two. Now the social worker stands in the practical center of these adjustments, so far as they concern the relations of man to man. The contributions of the psychologists and of the sociologists are still as separately visible to the readers of books on so-called social psychology as the separate flows of the Missouri and the Mississippi for a long time after their junction. We are now inductively building up the facts for a true social psychology (or shall we say *psycho-sociology?*), which is to be something new in which the contributions of psychologists and of sociologists will no longer be separately recognizable as such.

Adaptation is the key word of much of the psychology, sociology, economics, and political science of the nineteenth century. Adaptation and maladaptation are the key words of our own branch of practical or applied sociology called social work. The human mind is no doubt the most exquisite of the adjustments of which the nineteenth century talked so much. But the supreme organization of man's mind has its penalty. That penalty is the ease of its maladjustment and maladaptation. Man builds up outer relations quite as complex as his own inner ones. There are frequent flaws both in the psychic interior of man and in his environment. These flaws, whether in the shape of initial lacks, or of acquired losses, or of mere twists without lack or loss of constituent elements, can hardly be made good without extraordinary effort, conscious and unconscious, on the part of man. These efforts we term efforts at reform, reconstruction, rehabilitation, readjustment, readaptation.

The **fitness of the environment** to life has been affirmed with great strength and skill by the modern sciences of chemistry and physics (witness such works as those of L. J. Henderson on the *Fitness of the Environment* and the *Order of Nature*). Yet the fitness of man in his environment, or the fitness of the environment to man, is a **very general and loose adaptation** rather than a special and precise one. Whether it is the generality of the laws of environmental fitness or whether there is some other reason, we have no point to bring in this work; but it is obvious enough that human maladjustments do occur precisely on the plane in which life's inner relations meet the outer ones. Man perhaps shows the defect of his virtue. He has high sensibility and a delicate responsiveness to his environment. He finds most ingenious ways of shunning obstacles. But he finds equally ingenious ways of contriving new obstacles, along with the devising of new ideas, practical and theoretical. To use a homely figure, man is often in the plight of an adventurous cat, which has climbed a tall tree with admirable audacity, but finds herself quite unable or unwilling to climb down. The order of events is (a) the existence of a perfectly good general adjustment of life's relations, (b) the development of specific maladjustments between those relations, and (c) the social necessity of readjustment amongst the relations. The social worker cannot be responsible, as social worker, for the integrity or the interior perfection of the minds of the human beings dealt with. Again the social worker cannot be responsible for the status of all the outer relations which are indispensable to life.

The duty of the social worker lies in the plane of adjustment and of readjustment between the human mind and society. Modern social work undertakes consciously to effect readjustment, so far as possible, in all concrete human cases in which the vital relations, inner and outer, have become mutually disorganized. Society has come to regard itself as more and more responsible for the cure and the prevention of all human maladjustments. The man who takes a serious view of human life and human society on the one hand may seek to promote man's "welfare" or on the other hand he may prefer to think in terms of man's increased "efficiency." In either event the serious student of social adjustments is looking towards concrete betterment. In a practical age, and with the inevitable memories of the Great War, the student of sociology grows weary of abstractions, generalizations, and universal formulæ, such as dogged the world's footsteps before and up to the year 1914. Modern social work finds the prevailing after-war spirit identical with its own familiar spirit of reconstruction. For decades, doubtless, the world will be in a frame of mind to repair and restore rather than to build uncertain novelties upon shifting foundations. Social work has in fine come into a perfectly congenial atmosphere. Social work can be at the same time as charitable as it likes and as efficient as it likes.

Just as man is more complex and less stable than other forms of life, so inside man himself is **man's mind more complex and less stable than all else he possesses.** Man's mind is at the center and crossing of all those inner relations which Spencer defined as requiring adjustment to the outer world. If modern social work demands readjustment of man to his environment, not to say of the environment to man, then it is clear that the specialist in social adjustment must find his chief aid and mainstay, but also the greatest bugbear and stumbling-block, in this selfsame highly sensitive, highly unstable mind. Inside the developing specialty of social work there is now unfolding with great speed and surprising precision a new type of social work called *psychiatric*.

Psychopathology and psychiatry are respectively the science of the mind diseased and the art of mental healing. Psychiatric facts and observations are what constitute that practical specialty of medicine known as psychiatry. Psychiatry is a practical branch of medicine. Sometimes its theoretical side is given the name psychopathology. Psychopathologists are theorists that describe and explain what we scientifically know or think we know concerning mental diseases. For example, William James, besides being a psychologist (that is a theorist dealing with the normal and general aspects of the mind) was a psychopathologist (that is a theorist dealing with morbid aspects of mind); and the interested reader will still find in James's larger *Psychology,* published in 1890, a majority of the important facts concerning the general theory of mind and concerning its morbid aspects. Indeed, the general reader is perhaps safer in the reading of that older work than in the somewhat precarious plunges he might readily make in the current magazine literature. But, although James was a psychologist of the first rank and a psychopathologist amongst the most competent, he would not have claimed to be a psychiatrist. To be sure James bore the M.D. degree; but he was not a practitioner of medicine and therefore not in the fullest sense a psychiatrist. The interested layman must never confound theory with practice, chemistry with dietetics, physics with bridge-building, psychopathology with psychiatry, the theory of mental disorder with the practice of the cure and prevention of mental disease.

The layman is drawn by a mysterious yet perfectly legitimate attraction into **the field of what used to be called insanity,** but which we now like to spread out into the field of mental diseases and defects. Time was when insanity was somehow in the same breath attractive and repellent. On the whole the mind diseased was a forbidding topic. Nowadays the situation is altered. To be sure, there are in various receptacles contrived by the philanthropic and self-insuring state governments a certain number of legally insane persons, a great many more in the urbanized states of Massachusetts and New York than in rural and unorganized states. Of course what the civilized state is here doing for the chronic insane is in itself a kind of social work which makes for betterment in the state. But the benefits for the state at large are rather negative than positive, and only in states of an advanced civilization is there much coördinated effort, by special treatment, by medical and social teaching, and by well-conceived researches, to the end of directly helping the victims inside asylums and their families at home. Which means to say that the highest type of social work, both general and psychiatric, is seldom found upon the planet. Still, in the most urban portions both of our Atlantic seaboard and in parts of the interior, where the need is most urgent, successful social work, both general and psychiatric, is being carried on. The phrase "experimental stage" can no longer be properly hurled at this work. The blue-prints of it have, so to speak, been manifolded. Committees like the National Committee for Mental Hygiene are forwarding the work throughout this country. But for years to come the work of such committees in many states and communities must be limited perforce to that perfectly crystallized form of social work frequently known as "state care of the insane."

In the first part of this work we have called attention to the distinction between public endeavor and social endeavor, contrasting the public and social **spheres of influence** with the more personal and individual sphere. Practically we no longer term social work that special portion of the community's task which has been taken over by organized government and reduced more or less to thumb rules, which are perfectly good rules unless interfered with by the exigencies of the public treasury, real or imaginary. There is a good deal in the public (that is organized governmental) service which the social worker, operating from voluntary agencies, cannot touch or modify. The social worker then has to operate, as the military men say, "through channels." Nevertheless, the voluntary agency is often able to flick the wheel of officialdom. The fit of government and law is, we are almost inclined to thank Heaven, not a close fit. The legal order and the administrative order are general rather than individual in their application.

There is a wavy line separating the public from the private (where we mean by "private" either social or personal considerations, not yet reduced to rigid rules and regulations). There is also a wavy line between social considerations on the one hand and personal ones on the other.

The successes of public health and preventive medicine it is no part of the present work to restate. Public service is one of the most successful things, so far as it goes, that man has accomplished. The theory of sanitation passed smoothly and efficiently from a set of considerations bearing on such matters as sewage and other sanitary concerns to another far more delicate set of considerations bearing on infection and bacteriology. The public health movement is now passing into a phase in which personal hygiene is coming into sharp focus. The mental hygiene movement is about to fuse with the rest of the doctrines of public health. An important part of mental hygiene is a public affair. In the same state governments that were developing departments of health, another movement was quietly going forward for the so-called "state care of the insane." This program is well-nigh complete, so far as the legally insane are concerned. The models for state care have been laid down. In several parts of the world public service has done practically all that our knowledge now allows for the group of unfortunates known as the chronic insane.

But the **chronic insane form a comparatively small group** of unfortunates. Psychiatry, as almost any case in this book will prove, is luckily no longer limited to the classification, care, and treatment of the *legally* insane. For every insane person now confined in a state receptacle, it may be suspected that there is another almost or quite equally insane person outside brick walls who might very appropriately be interned at once for his own sake and for the state's sake. Laws for the temporary reception and care of such suspects have been placed on the statute books of a few of the most civilized states. In some of these states special psychopathic hospitals have been built and equipped for their care and specialized treatment, study and investigation. The data of this book intend to bring to the layman and to the social worker special information concerning mild, incipient, and dubious cases of mental disease, which we shall come to know either as mild instances of various well-known mental diseases or else merely as psychopaths (*i.e.*, not subject to diseases of a well-known and definite character— as it were unspecified cases).

But the aim of modern mental hygiene is much more ambitious. How can the tasks of modern mental hygiene be defined? It is plain that, if our analysis of "spheres of influence" in Book I is correct, mental hygiene might well deal with (*a*) the establishment, maintenance, and improvement of various public, legal, and administrative institutions and relations, (*b*) the encouragement and improvement of various voluntary and private agencies for the betterment of social relations and the molding of society's opinion on these matters, and (*c*) the establishment of new facts and devices for improving man's individual relations, particularly the very interior relations of the man to himself.

The mental hygienist of the present day, whether he be a psychological theorist, a specialist in mental tests, a psychopathologist with theoretical interest paramount, a practical psychiatrist, or an educationalist specially concerned with high or exceptional talents or with the "ungraded," wants to spread a gospel about mind much wider than the crystallized doctrines of medico-legal insanity, the newer knowledge about the "temporary care" (psychopathic hospital) group and the out-patient group of mental diseases and effects of a more or less mild nature. The ambition of modern mental hygiene is to spread its point of view over the entire field of the mental sciences and arts, wherein sociology and economics look especially accessible. Not only the insane, not only the psychopaths, but also the eccentrics and the very slightly subnormal are topics for modern mental hygiene. Nor, as above hinted, would mental hygiene object to considering the supernormal person and the person with specialized capacities as within the range of its point of view. We may mention again the work of William James, this time pointing out how in his *Varieties of Religious Experience,* published in 1903, he utilized his vast psychological and psychopathological equipment in the study of what he sometimes termed the religious ·"geniuses." It is worth while insisting that the psychiatric approach does *not* mean calling everybody crazy or even a little bit crazy! James himself went to extraordinary lengths in his chapter on "Religion and Neurology" to refute this idea. James's acid test of psychopathology did not destroy the golden geniuses of religion. When, therefore, we say we want to apply the psychiatric insight to practically the entire human world, we are not at all asserting or suspecting that the majority of human beings are in any sense psychopathic. We believe that more of the psychiatric point of view will be of great service to the world, as well in domestic as in political life. Just as James gave new viewpoints concerning the religious ecstasy, and just as Hippocrates and Galen before him were physicians who made the most extraordinary contribution to our knowledge of temperament, so we hope by the spread of the mental-hygienic point of view and the point of view of psychiatric social work to aid the common man and woman to deeper, practical insights into everyday questions.

METHOD OF APPROACH

We shall now try to describe in a few sentences and in the most general way the somewhat novel method of approach adopted in this book.

There has heretofore been no special treatise upon psychiatric social work. There is in fact no comprehensive treatise upon social work in general. Accordingly this book has perforce to include much that may seem entirely non-psychiatric. We do not seek to describe comprehensively the technique of social diagnosis or the technique of social treatment. The general features of the technique of social diagnosis have been ably catalogued by Miss Mary E. Richmond in her work on *Social Diagnosis*. Comprehensive studies upon *Social Treatment* are rumored to be in preparation, and the experiences of decades, from the first philanthropic endeavors up to the more scientific procedures of present-day social treatment, may then become available for the growing group of general social workers. It is not our design to anticipate future formulation of the methods of social treatment or to repeat the systematic chapters of Richmond, so far as they deal with mental hygiene and psychiatry. We have carefully reviewed Richmond's work and found to our surprise that fully half of the social cases presented by her are cases with a strong mental hygienic or psychiatric flavor. What this signifies can be discerned if we remember that Richmond's selection of cases was a purely random selection, made for the purpose of illustrating different forms of technique of social diagnosis. The collection was in no sense designed to display the importance of psychiatry in social work. Reading between the lines we can reasonably conclude that a much higher proportion of the Richmond case collection would turn out upon closer study to be cases involving mental hygiene in its broadest sense—cases, that is to say, that illustrate the importance of considering mild character defects and perversions, mild but important temperamental distinctions, and the like. Rising from this sort of analysis (and any case collection of social work, so far seen by us, will point the same moral), we are tempted to inquire whether after all psychiatric social work is not merely social work in general with special emphasis upon its mental hygienic features.

We conclude that the present case collection is perhaps comprehensive enough to amount to a case collection demonstrating in the rough the main principles of *all* medical social work. We bear in mind that the great medical inspirer of the development of medical social work, Dr. Richard C. Cabot, has for years insisted that the supreme values of medical social work lodge in the diagnosis of human character and the care and treatment of social patients in the light of our knowledge of their character. A chief aim of medical social work must always have been recognized, more or less vaguely, as a sort of character-building, a labor with "sick souls" as well as with sick bodies, a labor inevitably interrupted by all sorts of temperamental handicaps. Even where no such handicaps stood out in silhouette form upon the history of the patient, still even the more positive forms of character-building would need to take account of fundamental, temperamental, and character traits. This insistence by Dr. Cabot upon the centrality of character-building in social work took the right line. But in those days the modern psychiatric point of view had not arrived to deal with the subtle differences amongst men as to their temperamental deviations and slight eccentricities of character. The tendency of eighteenth-century individualism had been to the thought of general ethical principles common to all men. When the eighteenth-century individualism died away to be replaced by the statistical average man of Quételet, and when Quételet's *Physique Sociale* was supplanted or made over by the evolutionary ideas of man as a species, there was outstanding a certain overgenerality of view, a certain opinion as to desirable conformities of human beings, old and young, male and female, married and unmarried, white and black, to some norm or model.

Nowadays we are beginning to look more at differences than at resemblances of human beings. Individualization is the war cry. But the warp and woof of the argument for individualization depends on actual case material. This case material can, we think, be supplied nowhere so well as in the wards and out-patient departments of psychopathic hospitals. To the end of making character ultimately better, we now proximately look at the mild psychopaths, eccentrics, and "deviates" of psychiatric clinics. We are often eloquently reminded to become "masters of our fate" by the utilization of our very handicaps themselves. Grail-hunters, according to available legends, had sundry dragons to slay by the way. The strength of Sir Galahad was as the strength of ten, not merely because his heart was pure, but because of his righteous exercise of soul and body in the leaping of obstacles and the destruction of evils. In point of fact, social work did not lose in moral fervor by taking on the more scientific form of seeking social justice rather than a more or less refined alms-giving. But whether with the philanthropist you are giving gifts, or whether with the social worker you are paying society's debts, —in either event you are a dealer in morals. Even the bare aim of efficiency, which causes our legislatures year by year to appropriate more and more money from the tax levy, has a moral motive. The watchdogs of the state treasury, with whom we are so familiar, have their ears to the ground of morality, of social justice, and of such altruism as the community may afford. Yet withal, it must be insisted that the ideas of character-building, of masterhood of fate, of the utilization of one's handicaps, of old-time philanthropy, and of modern social justice are moral ideas derived from the general stock of such ideas to be found in everyone. Up to recent years the leaders in social work, like their predecessors who called themselves philanthropists, **took their ideas of morals and of moral development from the general stock rather than from any special studies of the moral status and outlook of their patients, taken as "persons," "individuals," or separate and distinct "souls."**

We are entitled to claim for psychiatric social work that it employs not only the general stock of human ideas about character, but seeks with some success to employ the new point of view of mental hygiene. Possibly that point of view can best be intimated in a single word by the term **individualization.** It was the reproach of older medicine, as it was of the educational, legal, and economic orders of our own day, that the human unit was not treated as a whole.

The late Professor James Jackson Putnam was one of the earliest physicians to point out the necessity of treating the **whole man** rather than parts of man, such as heart, liver, or kidneys taken as separately subject to disorder. Man seemed to the analytical pathologist of the last century a heap of viscera, in which systems such as digestive, muscular, nervous, respiratory, and excretory were to be found. Especially in the last decade of the nineteenth century, the "skin and its contents" (as the slang medical phrase runs) began to be tied together once more through the central nervous system, composed, as was discovered, of countless enormously long interconnecting strands, the so-called "neurones." Then followed in the first decade of the twentieth century another process of tying organs together. These new ties were chemical ties; that is, the so-called "chemical messengers" or "hormones," which flowed through blood and tissues from the glands which made them to the organs they were designed to stimulate and control. Thus, by the second decade of the twentieth century, even the analytical pathologists were ready to see in disease and health combinations where they formerly had seen separations, syntheses where they had formerly seen sundering, and all sorts of remote effects which had formerly lain quite unsuspected.

It was as if a traveler had suddenly by the break of day become aware of great numbers of telegraph lines, great quantities of railway trackage, in a landscape which had in semi-darkness seemed to him quite barren and wild, and had become aware of a vast transportation system of highly artificial products capable of entirely altering the scene. The men of science had in short by their own endeavors come to see new unities of body and mind and were once more able to work conscientiously with their colleagues in social tasks. Analytical men of science are thus now able to work again with the rest of the world on the platform of individualization. What may be called the **neurone set-up** of man, that is, his nervous framework in the finest sense, is clearly a very individual affair, and the **hormone set-up,** that is, the special and intimate construction of man in certain vital chemical ways, must needs be also a very individual matter. The individualization of man, as we now look at him in the second decade of the twentieth century, is individualization to the second power, or to the cube, of what it could possibly seem in the third decade preceding ours, the decade in which so many extraordinary discoveries in bacteriology were made. If it were worth while to drag the argument out at greater length, we could point out the obvious increase in individualization in the processes of education and even somewhat in those of law and economics. That the time is ripe for individualization of morals can hardly be doubted. That the technique by which the world shall achieve this individualization of morals is mental hygienic technique, we that write this book are persuaded. The resulting distinctions are not medical distinctions, but purely and simply moral ones. In the field of education it is a matter of familiar history that Madame Montessori derived her special ideas for the education of normal persons from the study of the methods used for the feeble-minded. So it is with the new insight into morality which the study of the mild mental disorders is beginning to afford. The resulting ethics will be ethics for the normal individual. The dynamite of disease may serve to split out building stones. The acid tests of medical study may display the true moral structure of normal human beings. **Psychiatric social work can establish and is now establishing new principles for social work in general.**

The time may come when medicine can be forgotten and hygiene alone maintained. Then would be the golden age of keeping well rather than of getting well. Likewise psychiatric social work may (theoretically) disappear and leave the everyday problems of financial relief, of legal aid, of standardized moral training and of perfectly systematic education. But, even if such a golden age without disease is ever to develop, the chances are good that the study of medicine in its broadest sense would be an indispensable factor in the gilding process. Individualization is very properly the war cry of today. Pathological method will have much to do in establishing the principles of that individualization upon a sound basis. That portion of pathological method which deals with the diseases and defects of the mind, especially **the mildest psychopathies and the faintest eccentricities,** will carry the banner of individualization to the farthest point now visible; namely, the confines of the mind of man. We have already begun to study with delight and profit the nature of geniuses and of exceptional persons with special abilities. The varieties of moral and religious experience are being levied upon in the literature.

Even the legal order, which has been so terribly general in its plan for securing the interests of man, has begun to raise the cry of individualization; witness not only various theoretical assertions of this trend, but witness the jurists themselves and also the pleasing vogue of a book like that of Dr. William Healy upon the *Individual Delinquent*—a book founded upon case descriptions.

Lastly, even in the field of economics, a book like that of Taussig on *Inventors and Money Makers* serves to show how far the idea of individualization may penetrate a field devoted for decades, or practically since its initial survey, to the "average man." Social work, as plainly shown in the case descriptions of this book, touches all these fields of education, morals, law, and economics, and must naturally share the effects of that increase in individualization which all of these great departments of knowledge and practice are showing.

If we concentrate attention upon the medical division of the field of social work we cannot fail to see that the individualizing trend must be greatly strengthened by modern developments in medicine, upon which the analyses of medical social workers must depend. If we further concentrate our attention upon the psychiatric division of the field of social work, we cannot escape the conclusion that here at last we find the very pitch and apex of individualization. Landscapes and habitats extraordinarily differ. Races and people differ still more extraordinarily. Human bodies show differences obvious to the casual eye, and their contents such as livers, kidneys, and other glands, must show even greater differences than the environments of their owners. When we take into account the interconnecting filaments of the nervous system and the special qualities of the various chemical messengers uniting the different parts in the body with one another, we perceive that the resulting unities are capable of still greater differentia-

tion. Leibnitz pointed out that no two grass blades were alike.
He called his discovery by the extraordinarily obscure name of
the law of the identity of indiscernibles. Well! if two grass
blades must perforce be different, two brains interpenetrated
by the highly specialized bloods and juices must be capable of
still greater differences than mere grass blades could display.
From this line of argument our main claim will stand out;
namely, that **progress in the psychiatric division of social
work will inevitably bring progress in medical social work
as a whole.** This progress in medical social work as a
whole must react upon the more general non-medical
parts of social work.

What are the relations between psychiatric social work and
other fields of social case work? Logically, all portions of
the field of social case work are intimately connected. Practically, there are at least three divisions of social case work, if by
"practical" we mean divisions defined by the existence of a
corps of special workers limited by training, experience, and
interest to each special division. On this practical ground we
may thus distinguish (a) a field of general social case work,
(b) a field of medical social case work, and (c) a field of psychiatric social work. We here limit consideration to social
case work as distinguished from the broader fields of community work. We speak merely of that total field of social
work that deals in one way or other with the individual, either
in his public or social or personal relations.

The point of view of (a) the general social case worker
derives historically from the older philanthropic point of view
and is still largely founded upon the necessity and desirability
of the so-called "poor relief" and the economic establishment or
reëstablishment of the family. (We must insist that every
social case worker, whether general, medical, or psychiatric,
has the family point of view ingrained in her training and imbedded in her practice; the point in the text refers to the predominance of the economic point of view in general social
work, pivoting, as it so often must, upon the total wage intake
of the family and its proper distribution or supplementing.)

The point of view of (b) the medical social worker derives,
not so much from the older philanthropic point of view as from
modern developments in medicine. The medical social worker
has her economic interests indispensably, for she also pivots

her work upon the family. But essentially the medical social worker has in mind the restoration of the health of the family and of its individual components. Some of the pioneers in medical social work have been general social workers who had become convinced that medicine must be their particular target. But other leading medical social workers, even at the outset of its development (see Ida M. Cannon, *Social Work in Hospitals*), were persons theretofore quite untrained in the economic aspects of social work, who became medical social workers *de novo*. There was, to be sure, a fortunate union and mutual adaptation of economic and social interests from the beginning of the development of medical social work; and there are signs of an equally happy reaction running both ways between general and medical social work.

The point of view of (c) the psychiatric social worker derives from the modern developments in mental hygiene. Elsewhere in this book we have sufficiently insisted that psychiatry (that is, the art of mental healing) is in one very definite sense a branch of the practice of medicine but we have pointed out with equal emphasis that psychiatry has far broader contacts with the world than with medicine alone. We have pointed out that mental hygiene is in some ways a much broader topic than medicine, touching education, ethics, the legal order, and economics, to say nothing of science, art, political science, religion, and philosophy. Practically, moreover, the field of psychiatric social work would never have been developed in its present form, had it not been for the labors of the mental hygienists, amongst whom we must count not psychiatrists only but also psychologists. Psychiatric social work is accordingly not alone a logically separate division of social work but also practically a separate division, as defined by the existence of a type of specially trained worker and as defined by the history of the movement itself.

It is plain that the field of (a) general social case work stands logically somewhat farther apart from (b) medical social work and (c) psychiatric social work than (b) and (c) stand apart from each other. Indeed, it might be claimed that psychiatric social work is nothing but an important subdivision of medical social work akin to such subdivisions as the tuberculous, orthopedic, heart, syphilis, and pediatric subdivisions. In fact, this claim has been made by some workers, though nowhere supported by a thorough logical and historical argument. The observer must bear in mind, however, that, if we are talking logic alone, the public-health movement ought to carry in its front lines the banner of mental hygiene. Public health officers and specialists in preventive medicine ought to have developed mental hygiene divisions as logically and as practically as they have developed their work in sanitation, bacteriology, and in later days personal hygiene. But the public health movement has never taken the "person" on so broad a basis as the individual "person" of mental hygiene. Whatever the public health movement ought to have been or ought to have become in relation to mental hygiene, the facts are against anyone who should claim that mental hygiene is historically an outgrowth of public health. So it is with the movement for psychiatric social work. The movement is derived from psychiatric clinics, psychopathic hospitals, out-patient clinics for mental and nervous diseases, mental hygiene societies, and kindred mental hygiene units of the community. Perhaps it has been better so. The man interested in sanitation, bacteriology, and the simpler devices of so-called personal hygiene is not apt to be a person profoundly interested in social relationships and their adjustment and readjustment. The person interested in economic relief and primarily in the solution of the comparatively simple problems of the tuberculous, the orthopedic, the "heart cripple," and even of the sick child, is not a person who is apt to give due weight to educational, ethical, and legal sides of her problem, having in mind adjustments which transcend the wage intake and the bodily health and comfort of the sick person.

Now it is perfectly true that to solve the problems of the lame, the halt, and the blind, or of the tuberculous, or of the child sick-of-body, the bigger and more complex social adjustments are more and more coming to be regarded as indispensable. In the terms of the *future* history of social case work, we may safely predict that the psychiatric point of view will react upon the general medical point of view in case work. The very same thing is happening in the field of medicine regarded from the standpoint of the physician. The general practitioner of medicine in every parish is inevitably busy with psychiatric problems, though he may not think of them as such. Psychiatry is a branch of medicine every whit as general in one sense as is the general practice of medicine itself. The nervous system penetrates every part of the body and the mind influences every diagnosis, every prognosis, and every therapeutic procedure in medicine. Nevertheless, it will be a number of years before the general practitioners become equipped with the psychiatry they need. So it is with psychiatric social work. Psychiatric social work is bound to influence medical social work, and, in fact, all forms of social case work. Just as the general practitioner of medicine would greatly benefit by getting into his head the main facts about psychiatry, so the medical social worker will equally benefit by absorbing the new principles of psychiatric social work. Logically the two fields of medical social work and psychiatric social work present aspects of resemblance and aspects of difference. Historically the two fields present separate lines of development. Practically, even at the present day we must insist that psychiatric social work is by no means a specialty coördinated with pediatric or orthopedic social work, but presents a body of principles applicable alike to all the subdivisions of medical social work.

The new theories of social work or practice must soon effect changes even in sociology as a whole. Sociology as a whole has run perhaps too much to a schematic and general account of supposed evolutionary laws of the nature, structure, and development of society. In this general account of society's evolution commonly called sociology, the individual is very likely to get named on page one but not to figure extensively in the table of contents. We claim then that, by beginning with a study of the individual in his finest and most delicate deviations from the normal, we are starting an inductive study which if carried through sedulously will react upon sociology itself and therefore upon political science, economics, ethics, and the rest of human interest. Let no reader say that this is an elaboration of the obvious. The inductive method has been on the cards since the *Novum Organon* of Francis Bacon, but inductive progress toward a completer sociology has *not* begun with the individual and especially not with the individual as delicately dissected out in mental disease.

We have arranged the case studies of this work in a certain formal way. For the most part, however, we have presented them so that each stands upon its own feet. Nor do we think that the data have been essentially modified by the process of analysis to which they have been subjected. The narratives are chiefly drawn from "intensive" cases in our hospital files rather than from cases of so-called "slight service." The data presented are condensed to even far less than one-tenth of their original extent, with the omission, however, of no important link in the narrative, taken as a narrative. The book might thus be read purely at random and each case regarded as a source of texts. We have constructed the index to the book in such manner that many of these texts or special maxims can be studied in particular cases, even where no attempt has been made in the summary to unite the cases to demonstrate particular precepts.

The object of dividing the case descriptions of the book into three main parts was a purely practical one. In Book I we sought to show the main spheres of influence which are brought to bear upon social cases in civilized communities where (*a*) government and (*b*) systematic voluntary social agencies and (*c*) special methods of handling the individual are highly organized. Book II is devoted to a much more individual analysis of the social cases from the standpoint of the various troubles, difficulties, maladjustments, or evils that they present. The analysis of Book III is a medical analysis and gives some slight idea of the varieties of social diagnosis and treatment of cases falling in the more generally recognized groups of mental disease and defect.

THE METHOD OF BOOK I: SPHERES OF INFLUENCE

The principle upon which the seven cases of Book I are presented may seem a novelty in social work. The triple division of the spheres of influence under which social cases fall, viz., public, social, and individual, corresponds with categories of the legal order as developed by Dean Roscoe Pound. Dean Roscoe Pound's forthcoming work on *Sociological Jurisprudence* will soon unfold a logical view of the bases of this triple division. We may be pardoned for remarking more superficially upon the division in these pages. The usual distinction between "public" and "private" is still of practical value, despite the unclear line which may separate public from private duties and responsibilities. The term "public," as we under-

stand Dean Pound, might well be restricted to the operations
of organized government, which is, of course, a part of society
taken in its broadest sense; but the operations of society taken
as a whole are essentially non-governmental, not yet organized
into state affairs.   In short, there are a great many of the
most important concerns of society which are not acknowledged
to be public in the sense of governmental affairs.   They remain "private," although they affect social groups.   In default
of a better term for the non-governmental operations of social
groups, Dean Pound, as we understand him, proposes to use
the term "social."   Social operations in their widest sense
would then include governmental operations as well as numerous others.   Whenever we are talking about governmental operations, however, we shall almost inevitably want to distinguish them as such, and we may appropriately use the term
"public" for these more fixed, solid, and rigid products (fos-
sils) of the social development of bygone days.   Dean Pound
developed these distinctions in a discussion of the interests of
personality derived from a reinvestigation of the so-called
"natural rights" of man.   Into that deep discussion we do not
care to penetrate.   We simply adopt this suggested nomenclature for the agencies and other spheres of influence that come
in contact with our cases.   From a practical point of view the
social worker must soon concede the influence of public agencies
in this special sense of organized governmental agencies.   The
fixity, solidity, and rigidity of the public service may be a
virtue or a fault as the case may be, but in any event nobody
is more clearly aware than the social worker of the existence of these obstacles or leverage points of the public
service.

But we also distinguish between the "individual" and the
"group."   We have come to see that individualization is a
leading trend, not only of modern social work, but of most
departments of human knowledge.   The old distinction between "public" and "private" is accordingly no longer able to
serve our best purposes.   We need to build up the idea of the
private into the idea of privacy as opposed to public or governmental responsibility—privacy in the sense of what James
called "the warmth and intimacy" of the individual man.

Thus an ancient distinction was: public *vs.* private.   Another
very plain distinction is: group *vs.* individual.   We now have

to combine logically these two distinctions and the results are
as follows:

$$\text{Group} \begin{cases} \text{Public} \\ \text{Social} \\ \text{Individual} \end{cases} \Big\} \text{Private}$$

For practical purposes we can then distinguish the interests of
our cases as **public, social,** and **individual.** We shall never
forget that in the present state of advanced civilization in the
communities where social work flourishes, no individual and
no social agency can fail to be affected by the public service in
some fashion. But public servants can and do forget that
their responsibilities, although strictly limited by law, organization, and regulation, are surrounded by conditions in which
the responsibilities of social groups are numerous and also in
some respects paramount. Neither the public officer nor the
social worker should forget his duties to the individual as such.

The social worker, standing as she does midway between
public service ˙on the˙ one hand and the ideal of individual
service on the other, must not remain aloof from both. She
can often imagine a procedure far superior to any now afforded
by the public service for the forcible handling of a given case,
yet she finds the public sphere of influence paramount.
She must bow to the public service. Her recourse is so to
stimulate social opinion that it shall become public regulation.

Looking in the other direction, the social worker may often
find a situation in which she feels that some family group or
neighborhood group would be greatly benefited by a particular
invasion of individual rights and a particular interpretation of
the interests of this individual running counter to his desires.
Persuasion rather than compulsion must here be her aim. This
persuasion may not be hers to attempt or to carry through;
that persuasion may be the duty of some physician or other
adviser. The middle ground occupied by the social worker
between public service and individual desires and rights is a
position of danger. She stands in that middle ground, untram-
meled by the laws and regulations of the public service and
beyond the control in essential ways of the physician. So far
as law and medicine are concerned, she is on rather neutral
ground. In critical and limited phases of her work she is, to
be sure, governed and guided by judge and physician, but she
has every chance to push on to crises and limits that may not

be necessary and may not represent the "one best way." She is, as has been remarked, a sort of **professional or intensive layman.** It may be that a judge or physician would do no better in her place amongst these non-legal and non-medical problems; but, if she pushes her non-legal and non-medical problems into the legal or medical zone, she is likely to be charged with causing difficulties when she has merely shaped their course toward the only available beacons. Can there be any doubt of the importance of securing men and women of the highest grade for social work? Is it not clear that they must understand the main principles of the interrelation between medicine, education, morals, law, and economics? There used to be much discussion as to what might be given if we could turn the problem around. Define what constitutes a psychiatric social worker—the "points" of such a worker would then correspond with those of the so-called "educated" man. Elsewhere we give a summary of such "points" as practical experience seems to agree upon.

So much then for the *raison d'être* of Book I. It will be noted that there are seven cases in Book I. When three terms, such as **public, social,** and **individual,** are combined in eight ways, the eighth combination (logically speaking) is that situation in which all three are absent. Accordingly we find that to illustrate all existent combinations, public, social, and individual, we need but seven cases. Book I also serves as a sort of general introduction to the whole topic, and we have placed in the discussions of the seven cases of Book I a few general remarks that apply to the remainder of the volume as well. But what we especially hope to drive in by the contentions of Book I is a wholesome respect on the part of the social worker for the problems of the individual *as such* and for the problems of public service *as such*. If she does not like all aspects of the public service of the present day and if she is dissatisfied with the medical and other knowledge of the psychic interiors of her patients, she must not kick against the prick of judge and administrator in public matters or act as a substitute for the physician or other adviser upon matters depending upon medical diagnosis. There are certain interests of personality to be secured by the legal order and by the public administrator. There are certain aspects of personality which are to be handled, so far as they can be handled, by the best expert advisers obtainable. The task of the social worker, and especially of the psychiatric social worker, remains a morally heavy task—the task of utilizing the fixities and fulcra of public service and at the same time the delicate and elastic values of the expert in personality. Couched in these terms one might think the psychiatric social worker or any social worker must be something celestial. We can only point to the relative successes and instructive failures of the cases presented in this book to show that there is no celestial claim but only a purely practical and human claim made for these workers. If all expert work in the adjustment of personality seems to be rather atmospheric and if the public service seems to some of us at times to have become a solid immovable mass then we must thank the social worker. She remains liquid. She is the ideal being, a universal solvent. She proves herself to be a useful intermediary in whatever field her path finally arrives.

Whereas the considerations of Book I seem more novel than they actually are, the arrangement of data in Book II is actually the most novel feature of our work. How far the division of the troubles, difficulties, maladjustments, and evils of society into five groups is a sound, enduring division, it is hard to say. This is not a textbook of sociology. We claim a purely practical applicability for our subdivisions. The data of these cases were not secured under the headings so presented. Since the collection of these data and the completion of this work the divisions of the so-called Kingdom of Evils have begun to be practically used in social work by many workers connected with the state institutions for mental diseases in the Commonwealth of Massachusetts. Practical lectures upon these classifications have been given, and the active workers have brought their data to the conferences for discussion. The divisions seem to work out in practice. Surely some division of data is better than no division.

Heretofore social case records have often proved to be nothing more than ill-digested narratives, with vast accretions of facts hardly analyzable by any person save the original collector of the data. The case worker familiar with her case might in the end be able to give a fairly competent account in narrative form of her case. Of course the self-consistent narrative may actually miss the point. We have frequently seen maladjustments set down to the score of ignorance which were actually due to feeble-mindedness; sometimes (though seldom) feeble-mindedness has been erroneously suspected. To call a purely moral defect psychopathic is a slant which psychiatric social workers early in their practical work may fall into. To call clearly psychopathic phenomena immorality is a prevalent fault amongst laymen, many physicians, and very many public servants. To charge any or all of these difficulties up to the account of poverty is perhaps the commonest flaw in social analysis in the world at large. Just as the "economic factor in history" was so greatly the rage some decades since, so the economic factor in personal life has been greatly overdone. To be sure it does not take the data of mental hygiene to demonstrate that poverty is not the main cause of social trouble. Social work, before it had attained the psychiatric range, had long ago proved to its own satisfaction that much more was wrong than mere economics. In fact progress from philanthropy to social work was no doubt largely due to the growing appreciation of the fact that giving alms or financial relief did not go far to solve social problems.

THE METHOD OF BOOK II: KINGDOM OF EVILS

The method of Book II is no less practical than that of Book I. Book I treating spheres of influence over social cases presented the cases in their social matrix, as confronted by the social worker looking for practical results in a workaday world full of necessary and unnecessary obstacles. The compulsions of government, the suggestions of the voluntary social agencies, and the intimate lines of attack upon personality were reviewed in the seven possible forms of their combination. Book I thus endeavored to teach the social worker that no layman can set himself up against the power of government and law with any hope of success in the concrete instance. On the other hand, we perceived that it was the social worker's duty, if she found her patient's trouble intimate, individual, and personal in its nature, to swing the whole policy of treatment at once to the physician, to the teacher, to the spiritual guide, or (often the best plan of all) to the man himself. But how is the social worker to pull apart all the concrete particular and special facts and surmises about the patient, to the end of judging whether the patient is best given over to physician, teacher, moralist, or back to himself? It is the province of Book II to try in a somewhat novel manner to give the social worker a practical method of analyzing the facts available.

It has been found possible to present this method of analysis in Book II in the form of thirty-one cases. We pointed out that the three spheres of influence discussed in Book I could mathematically be combined in eight ways, or practically in but seven ways, since the eighth was the null class in which all three elements were absent. The five great groups of what we term the Kingdom of Evils must likewise mathematically combine in a limited number of ways, namely in thirty-two; but again the thirty-second combination would be that combination in which all five groups of evil would be absent. Thus, after we had sufficiently described thirty-one instances of evil, (that is, in the combination in their various ways of five forms of evil), we might reserve the thirty-second compartment for some absolutely normal person, if there be such, who had never undergone any form of evil whatever! It is very convenient to work with *five* forms of social difficulty rather than with four, with six, or with seven. Had we been dealing with *four* major groups of social trouble, we should have been able to get on with but fifteen combinations, that is, with the mathematically possible sixteen combinations minus one. If we had practically found in our social case analyses *six* forms of evil we should have been compelled to describe in Book II no less than sixty-three cases, for the purpose of illustrating all possible combinations (sixty-four minus one). And if the world had been still more complex and had yielded up *seven* kinds of trouble, our exposition in Book II would have had to contain no less than one hundred and twenty-seven cases (the one hundred and twenty-eight mathematically possible combinations minus the null case in which all seven kinds of trouble were by hypothesis non-existent!).

We must eternally insist that **such analyses** as we make in this volume, and particularly the analyses of Book II, **must be made after all the facts are in hand.** By no means do we lay down any principle to the effect that the practical social worker shall practically collect the case data in the order in which these data are later to be analyzed. It might be signally unwise to fly at the situation with questions concerning health, educational status, moral trends, legal entanglements, before the worker had got in hand the main facts about the economic level of the case or of the family. There must be a proper technique of approach for every case as to the collection of the data. Some points and categories in this connection are offered in Richmond's *Social Diagnosis*. We offer in this book no especially new points as to the technique of the collection of social data. Especially with psychopathic cases the application of any rigidly set method for the collection of the facts might prove injurious, not necessarily to the patient himself, but to the accuracy and speed with which the data are collected. There are some facts which only the extraordinary authority of the courtroom is likely to extract. There are other facts which a judge, however learned, can never hope to unearth by the tools at his disposal. Again it is most obvious that there are many facts that only physician or pastor in consulting room or vestry can obtain. Experience also abundantly proves that there are many facts that physicians and pastors, or even both together, cannot by any means secure. Some of these facts the social worker, especially the woman worker, can elicit by methods which cannot, or at least in this place cannot, be described. And we are quite ready to admit that some facts cannot be dragged out of some patients by wild horses. That experience with mental cases, stretching over a period of several months or years, gives the professional social worker far more insight into the technique of quickly securing the intimate facts most useful for the patient's successful treatment, cannot be denied. It is on this account that we elsewhere in this summary insist on the importance of placing in the practical portion of every social worker's training a certain amount of experience with mental cases. We shall also point out that to give the proper basis and background for the interpretation of such experience with mental cases, the ideal curriculum of every social worker (*whether or not* the worker is going practically into the field of psychiatric social work) ought to contain a strong didactic part dealing with mental diseases and defects and including the mild psychopathies, eccentricities, and deviations from the normal. Dr. G. L. Walton some years ago endeavored with more or less success to get the term *degenerate* replaced with the term *deviate*. Not only was Walton's new standpoint theoretically well based, but there was much practical wisdom in these suggestions by the genial author of *Why*

Worry. For it is much easier to persuade or convince an everyday person that he is perhaps a little deviate than to show him that he is a little degenerate! In short not only would the mental hygiene of the social worker be improved by a study of mental cases as they practically occur in everyday life, but so also would benefit accrue to the mental hygiene of everybody else.

Let us picture the social worker returning from the day's work in a reflective state of mind. Let us suppose that the social worker is thinking over all that is now known as the result of, say, twenty-five hours of contact first and last with the case and its surroundings. In describing the method of Book II in a practical way to elementary workers at the outset of their training, we have sometimes recommended to them the following simple device. Let the worker count off upon the fingers of the left hand (the hand conveniently for our present purpose called sinister) the facts as conceived. Upon the *thumb* let there hang the diseases and defects of the patient and of related members of the family, in fact all more or less non-hygienic features of the situation, including very particularly *even the slightest mental disorder or defect.* Secondly, upon the *index finger* let there be suspended all the forms of ignorance which the patient and the persons around him exhibit, so far as these affect the situation; and let these data include, not merely lack of education, language difficulties and the like, but also all positive misinformations and errors of point of view, so far as these are of intellectual origin. Upon the longest or *middle* finger let there be strung whatever there is of moral defect (of course *not* psychopathic and *not* merely a matter of ignorance), including all sorts of vices and bad habits and many of the so-called sins of theology and common sense. Upon the *ring finger* there may be placed all sorts of legal entanglements, whether in the nature of crimes and delinquencies on the part of the patient or on the part of his associates, whether actually subject to court review or potentially so subject. There remains the *little finger* upon which to dispose all such matters as pauperism, poverty, and other forms of resourcelessness. It is the province of Book II to show cases combining all these forms of social trouble in various ways. If it were quite certain where the trouble of each concrete case should be classified, the task would be relatively

simple. For example in practice many social workers are inclined to ascribe to ignorance much that ought to be called
feeble-mindedness. Elsewhere we have given other instances
of the improper placement of concrete facts in these groupings.
Practical experience goes a good way towards abolishing these
errors of the social worker. The didactic part of any curriculum can never be counted on to prevent such errors. Frequent
conferences are necessary to keep the workers on the right track
during their practical experience.

Book II shows the advantage of considering social facts in
a definite order. Everybody will concede that some order is
better than no order, and everybody knows that a brief list can
be borne in mind better than a long list of categories. We do
not want to dogmatize about our plan. The future may well
yield up a better order for the consideration of social facts;
but we are inclined to prophesy that social work, so far as it
remains a systematic and scientific affair, will surely cling to
some order rather than no order in its analysis of the facts
in hand. Again the social work of the future may provide
a quite different list of categories than the fivefold list of evils
discussed in Book II; but we are inclined to predict that the
final list chosen by the perfected art of social work will not be
a long list of categories, and probably not much longer than
our own fivefold grouping. The very fact, which was pointed
out above, that *six* items would require sixty-four separate set-
ups of social fact to illustrate the possible combinations of the
six items, means that the social worker would find her sixfold
load too great to bear.

Be it remembered, as developed a little further on in this
summary, that oftentimes the difficulties are not merely separate items added to one another to form a mere heap of separate facts, but that in numberless instances the evils multiply
themselves into each other in a bewildering way. Let the social
worker think for a moment of the extraordinary complications
which may ensue when poor moral training is combined with
psychopathic trends. In the body of the book we have abundantly demonstrated the production of social difficulty of this
higher order. A patient combining in himself the effects of
poor moral training and the effects of psychopathic tendencies
may fall into such a status that neither measures of moral
reform nor the procedures of medical treatment will serve to

remove any important fraction of the trouble. For such intimate complications of combined moral and psychopathic trouble, the experts of the future will be required to find combinations of moral and medical training and treatment not yet dreamed of.

We must acknowledge, too, that the perfect art of social work might well in the future shorten the list of categories. There is a widespread tendency amongst social thinkers to regard immorality and crime as forms of disease. We believe that no serious philosopher of the social life is today willing to concede that either vice or crime is in the bulk ready to go over to the group of diseases. The **Vitia** and the **Litigia** are not soon, if ever, as a whole to go over to the **Morbi**. (We do not deny that many instances of so-called **Vitia** really belong in the group of **Morbi**. But that is a matter of erroneous diagnosis in the given instance, and not a matter of scientific reclassification of **Vitia** as **Morbi**. And a like argument holds for various **Litigia**. It is worth incidentally considering that the jurists ought increasingly to admit that many of their **Litigia** or conditions of being "at-law," would be thoroughly resolved if the medical and mental aspects of one or more parties in the case were to be recognized. Nor are signs lacking that, with the tremendous increase of the idea of individualization in at least the criminal part of the law, the jurists will come to see the point of psychiatry.) But we must theoretically allow the possibility of the telescoping of our list. If the list could be telescoped by so much as the subtraction of one item—for example, the item of poverty and the like (what we here call **Penuriae**), there would be but sixteen major combinations of the four remaining great items rather than the thirty-two which form the basis of our studies in Book II of this volume. With the unlocking of great and increasing amounts of energy from the universe by modern research, there can be no doubt that pauperism, poverty, and other forms of resourcelessness, here termed **Penuriae,** are undergoing a decline slower than we might wish but faster than some congenital pessimists readily acknowledge. Someone, the other day, claimed that the science of the last few hundred years, and especially of the last century, had blessed the human being on the average with an amount of energy equal to that of, say, some thirty body slaves (the analysis presumably took into account the great reservoirs of electric, chemical, and thermic energy which we see displayed about us so profusely, though perhaps irregularly, in the great cities). Every social worker, like every other good citizen, should support with all that is in him the cause of scientific research, to the end that more and more energy be unlocked from the infinite quantities available to man. A doubling of the amount of energy unlocked in the last few hundred years ought to diminish the tale of the **Penuriae** to a very visible degree. Available slave power in non-human forms would bring back at least the memory of the Golden Age.

For the moment, no social worker can hope to put the **Penuriae** out of mind or to lose contact with any other of our five categories of social evil. To be sure, in large sections of the American community there is less and less evidence of the effect of raw ignorance or of the result of any other forms of the group that we have called **Errores.** Literacy rules in many communities and illiteracy is a problem that can be far more readily surrounded, it would seem, than the problem of the vices and bad habits (**Vitia**) or of many forms of disease; for example, cancer and mental disease. It has been a matter of curious observation with the authors how relatively few instances of the pure and uncomplicated effect of ignorance could be found in the Psychopathic Hospital material which lies at the basis of this book. Language difficulties were of course frequently in evidence. The misdeeds of quack doctors and their advertisements turned up now and again in the shape of misinformation distinctly hurtful to our patients. Some instances of the evil effect upon the intellect (as well, of course, as upon the morals) of the movies were discovered in certain patients. Sundry housewives had plainly not been taught the rudiments of good housekeeping by their parents or guardians, and extraordinary success in their social treatment was found to follow the education of these patients in very simple procedures. Education serves to remove the bodily filth characterizing sundry immigrants, so that the members of the filial generation look with genuine horror on habits of the parental generation. We are willing to acknowledge certain prejudices born doubtless of our special experience, and one of these prejudices runs in the direction of assigning not quite so much weight to the virtues and importance of education as its worthy devotees are likely to assign. We here allude to education in its narrower, intellectual sense, rather than in the broader usage of education to cover moral as well as mental factors. Our prejudice runs to the claim of far greater value for moral training than for intellectual teaching. It has become a commonplace with many modern observers that the senses are easier to educate than the emotions are to train. The senses are after all a somewhat simpler affair than the emotions; for the latter dig very deep into the "skin and its contents." Those, however, who observe the wonderful results of animal training whether by the technique of terrorism or by the technique of tact, can only be optimistic as to the powers of man to form character. Man can no doubt form character more easily than he can reform character. Man can build and turn his temperament in a variety of ways far more easily than he can reform and divert his temperament after its dilapidation or distortion.

Up to this point we have argued that some arrangement of social facts was better than no arrangement, that a short list was superior to a long list, and that a further abbreviation of our present list was devoutly to be hoped for but hardly to be expected. Let us now ask the further question, Is there a warrant for terming the present list of five forms of evil a sequence rather than a list? If some order is better than no order, why do the forms of evil listed as we list them fall into this particular sequence? The particular sequence we have adopted is a much more doubtful affair than the principle of the sequence itself. The social thinker might well accept the principle of the sequence of evils in this book without wanting to adopt the order chosen. Why should the social worker, it might be questioned, always begin with the topic of disease? Why not begin with the topic of morals, or the topic of poverty, as being the prime logical factor in the particular case in hand? Of course nobody will doubt for a moment that psychopathic hospital material by and large demands and must demand prime consideration for disease. Indeed it is plain that medical social work as a whole demands prime consideration for disease, if only because the patients that come up for social treatment are sick patients. But, the general social worker may inquire, why, in the non-medical and non-psychiatric field, should the consideration of disease so inevitably come up; and why in particular should we think of disease in the beginning rather than in some subordinate place? There are a number of good reasons that we might adduce for our choice. For example, we might claim that the social worker who fixes her mind on the illiteracy in the social situation so frequently forgets the feeble-mindedness or slight subnormality of her patient (or even of several members of the family) that all sorts of effects get erroneously laid at the door of ignorance rather than of mental defect. If a social worker gets firmly fixed in mind at the outset of her work some apparent instances of the effect of ignorance, she may never during the rest of her social work be able to forget that initial concrete instance. She gets dazzlingly in mind the idea of education for all, thinking that education will solve every problem of apparent ignorance as well as every problem of real ignorance. But if this selfsame social worker raises the question of feeble-mindedness or subnormality in the situation she faces, she will time and again be rewarded with a point of view entirely new to her; that is, with a medical and mental point of view, which as a child and in her youth she had no means of grasping.

Again, there are still social workers who have their minds fixed on pauperism, poverty, and other forms of resourcelessness (in this book summed up under the term **Penuriae**) and leap to the explanation by defect of wages or compensation of all the difficulties in the case. We hinted above, this idea was no doubt the idea in the minds of the earlier philanthropists. Although no doubt the early workers in the field of social science in our country recognized that not all history could be given an "economic interpretation," yet the supporters of philanthropy were perhaps more informed with the idea of helping out the resourcelessness of their less fortunate brethren than penetrated with the ideal of consciously altering the entire hygienic, educational, moral, and legal orders. Financial relief is today so much more obvious than legal aid, moral training, intellectual teaching, and medical care, that not a few workers virtually stop in their minds with the idea of monetary aid for their problems. At least we can help out with money, is their feeling. With money we can get for our sick ones proper medical care. As for education, that is now largely a matter of public service. How barren and abstract seem the suggestions for moral training and legal counsel that we have to offer! There is no doubt a certain truth at the bottom of this idea of primacy of so-called "poor relief" in social work. We are all aware that even in the advanced community where a charity organization approaches perfection, there are very many instances in which pauperism or severe degrees of poverty fail to get duly met. Such situations in rural communities can almost be left to the uninstructed neighbor. In the urban community, the organization of charity is, so far as poor relief is concerned, undeniably a statistical success in places. (We do not here refer to any questions of the general raising of the wage level or of other methods than wage-control for establishing the entire community on a higher terrace of wealth and resourcefulness. We can only hope that in the end the slumless condition of certain of our middle western towns and cities can be made to extend the world over, perhaps by the process of scientific investigation, for which the National Research Council, developed in our country during the war and paralleled by similar organizations in several belligerent countries, so boldly and efficiently stands.) But we are entirely sure that the social worker who leaps to the idea of poor relief is rather apt to get breathlessly impaled thereon. She is apt to remain quite incapable of giving due emphasis to the possibility of these other factors, of disease, of ignorance, of immorality, and of legal entanglement, as whole or partial causes for the outstanding poverty. We felt compelled practically to place the **Penuriae** at the bottom of our sequence of evils.

Assuming that the **Penuriae,** that is, poverty and other forms of resourcefulness, may well be placed at the bottom of our sequence, is it not possible to argue that some other group than the **Morbi** (diseases) ought to be placed first? Certainly not ignorance, as was above argued but—and here we approach the crux of many faulty points of view, to our thinking—would it not be wiser to consider any given particular bad social situation as probably the effect of immorality or of bad habits, rather than of, say, disease? Should not the **Vitia** head the list? Everybody who has passed through childhood at all recently or has the childhood experience vividly in mind, knows and feels the immense and almost universal values of moral training, and almost everybody finds in his life a smaller or larger trace of some great moral mistake touching some portion of his life. Most of us, as the years travel on, get a bit of cynicism or a slice of fatigue about *our own* possible reformation of character. But we see various persons about us whose characters are undergoing a transformation and we are irresistibly led to think how these neighbors of ours might rather cleverly be reformed by simple devices, and how many of them might have their characters built and molded anew with the proper models for imitation and the proper tools of training in hand. If our neighbor gets drunk we think of him as probably addicted to a vice— the vice of inebriety. We do not at the very first inquire whether he has not some character defect or is not the victim of some early misapprehension as to the values of a little wine. If the neighbors' children write impossible legends on our backyard fences, we are apt to regard the children as vicious, and we do not charitably trace out the ignorance of their parents or even the feeble-mindedness of parents or children. We feel that the perpetrators of these vices, these "sinners," ought to be morally trained or reformed. We know instances of the successful training or reformation of just such persons. We run to the hypothesis of immorality, vice, or bad habits forthwith, and practically on a basis of our own experience. We see in these "sinners" precisely ourselves, and—charitably or maliciously, according to our natures—we would like to have these persons given what in our American slang is sometimes termed a "course of sprouts." Now "sprouts" is a most optimistic term for the plight of our neighbors, who may be in no condition to allow the new growth of moral ideas by reason of mental twist or lack, by reason of mere ignorance of the socially good. Now it is plainly most uncharitable and itself well-nigh a form of immorality to charge up vice and sin to a mentally defective or merely ignorant person. It is the charitable and right thing to raise the hypothesis in every serious case of social maladjustment whether the center of the situation may not be medical (and often actually psychopathic) or mental (in the sense of misinformation on the part of the supposedly sinful or immoral person). It is assuredly not more "insulting" to charge an alleged sinner with disease, bodily or mental, than to charge him with vice or sin. To be sure, the layman when he thinks of disease is rather apt to think of *severe* disease, and when he thinks of moral defect, he is apt to think of *mild* defect. This is no doubt because he bears in mind only his own *severe* diseases and only his own *mild* moral difficulties. In short, the average citizen thinks of disease with a feeling of terror, and of vice with a leaning towards exculpation. He thinks of himself as just a little sinful and of his neighbors as equally excusable.

But whether this ethical account of the average citizen's attitude on these matters be a correct one or not, there is to our minds no doubt in the world that the serviceable formula for the social worker to bear in mind is to think of each social situation as possibly bearing within it a kernel of disease, especially of mental disease, and particularly of the mildest forms of mental disease known as temperamental deviations and mere eccentricities. If the social worker analyzes her situation from the standpoint of these contained kernels of mild mental deviation and eccentricity, she will gradually lose the terrors associated with the idea of insanity, and will more and more adopt the attitude of William James, which we discussed at length at the beginning of this summary. She will get the psychopathological point of view which the keen spirit of the late Carleton Parker, himself not at all medical in training, got from his practical contacts in living amongst laborers and miners. Carleton Parker, though an economist, got the point of what might be termed the "psychopathic interpretation of history" as opposed to the long famous "economic interpretation of history." Nor will the reader of this book mistake our meaning when we use the phrase "psychopathic interpretation of history." We do not mean an interpretation of history as a product of psychopaths. We mean that history (at all events, the history of our individual instances of maladjustment) can best be interpreted by the **technique which starts from the outset to observe the minor deviations and variations, the differences and the contrasts, rather than the similarities and the analogies that so fill the mind of the observer of "averages."**

There will, we think, be far less objection to our ordering of other factors than the ones just discussed; namely, the ordering of **Penuriae**, the **Morbi**, and the **Vitia**. If a man is not in full possession of his bodily and mental health, it is just a little idle to discuss at length the quantity of his knowledge and the quality of his wisdom. But if a person is not mentally healthy and reasonably well informed, no doubt inquiries as to his moral turpitude are a bit futile. Again, if we do not know a man's health, education, and morals, how can we adjudge the nature, cause, effect, and manner of extrication of his legal entanglements? Finally, if we do not know the medical data, the educational status, the moral tendencies, and the civil standing of the man, how can we sensibly talk about his economic level?

We assume that the reader is now thoroughly convinced that **some order in social case analysis is better than no order**; that **a short list of categories is better than a long list**; and that **our sequence has a good deal to recommend it,** both from the practical standpoint of psychiatric and medical work, and from sundry more general standpoints. But a more general question may be raised, Why do we advocate the analysis of evils at all? Why discuss liabilities instead of assets? Why discuss negatives instead of positives? We might answer and remain content with the answer, that it all amounts to the same thing, and that what looks like a remainder is as a matter of fact a sum. Or again, we might answer that much depends upon the point of view. That is, we might say that some persons like to analyze from the side of evil, and others like to analyze from the side of good, and that we are writing for those who prefer in the first instance to slay dragons rather than to seek the Grail. No doubt we should be on very safe ground if we claimed the existence of these two temperaments; the temperament of the dragon-slayers and the temperament of the Grail-hunters. Moreover, we might point out that the dragon-slayers have perhaps in the past secured as many Grails as those who started Grail-hunting from the first.

IV

COMPARISON OF THE KINGDOM OF EVILS WITH OTHER SCHEMES
OF SOCIOLOGICAL ANALYSIS

Our attention has been called to **a formula of Malthus,** resembling in its categorization **our own grouping of the evils.** Malthus, like his father (a friend and executor of Rousseau) was in a sense a perfectibilian. He thought that societies tend to happiness but have been checked by miseries due to an increase of population. He showed that the positive checks to the increase of population were **war, vice, crime, disease,** and **poverty.** Four of these five Malthusian checks upon the increase of population roughly correspond with four of our own categories. It will be easy to show, we think, that war is in itself by no means a category quite so simple as any of the other four. No doubt also Malthus would have been happy to acknowledge that ignorance was a great cause of an over-increase of population. Indeed Malthus or any other theorist, following Socrates, might well feel that ignorance lay at the bottom of several of our own categories. Population sometimes increases, sometimes decreases. It would be equally easy to show, we think, that either the Malthusian five categories or our own might be as capable of decreasing population as of increasing it. To claim that the increase of population or the decrease of population is in itself an evil is something like the claim that superficial thinkers might make that war is an evil. It is indeed unwise to assert that any condition is or is not intrinsically an evil. It is far better to weigh observed conditions or factors in the light of a set of categories like the ones suggested.

Malthus, it will be recalled, used the phrase **"struggle for existence" in relation to social competition.** Here again is a phrase that suggests that a given condition can be set down as essentially an evil or as essentially a good. The idea that the struggle for existence was not all happy was repugnant to sundry theologians, when Darwin gave reflected luster to Malthus in his new contentions concerning evils. On the other hand it would seem that German thinkers, say of the Ernst Haeckel stripe, might well find the struggle for existence in no sense an evil, but think it rather a good.

It seems to us that **this concept of the struggle for existence also will greatly benefit from an analysis** of what might be called its **evil constituents.** We might find that the pathology of the individual was a negligible factor in that development. We might find the struggle for existence a function of intellectual development in different species and describe it in plain terms in an attractively simple fashion. We might note the moral values of the struggle for existence or again the vicious effects of centering one's life upon mere existence. We might study law and order in its lowest terms (insect life) or work upon the human level, and again find components of a constructive and beneficent nature and components of a destructive, maleficent nature. The field of economics would also blossom under this double analysis. Darwin believed that the struggle for existence greatly aided man and that his rapid multiplication was largely responsible for his success in the world. He fully conceded the values of these moral influences that in the end supersede the simpler factors. Still, even upon the moral level, Darwin was inclined to depreciate measures which would reduce the natural ratio of increase for man. On the whole, he took an anti-Malthusian view of man's multiplication in the world. A blanket view of the evils or of the excellence *in toto* of increase or decrease of population within prescribed limits is, no doubt, apt to be an erroneous view. The analyst will benefit himself and the world if he clearly conceives in his own mind whether he is analyzing for forms of evil or for forms of goodness in the heap of factors that he sees before him. Having made his major decision as to whether he is studying the negative, privative, and destructive factors or the positive, additive, and constructive factors in his world, the analyst will further benefit by an orderly approach in his study of particular situations.

The five checks of Malthus upon the increase of population which we found so nearly to correspond with our own five categories were, no doubt, not original with Malthus. Many of his arguments were derived from thinkers like David Hume, Adam Smith, and Montesquieu. The same set of **categories** with various additions will be found **amongst modern writers.** Thus Small classifies the interests of man under six headings; namely, *health, wealth, sociability, knowledge, beauty, rightness.* It will be observed that these six categories fairly well correspond, though in a different order, with our own five categories.

We have omitted any craving for beauty and its lack of satisfaction from amongst our categories, not because it is non-existent, but because to the practical adult ugliness seems not to be a primary or highly important evil in the world of social difficulty. Small himself can find hardly more than a paragraph of ideas concerning the beauty interest of man; he quotes from Schiller and is virtually done. There seems to be no completed esthetic theory amongst philosophical doctrines even at the present day. The majority of the esthetic dissatisfactions which we have found in our social case work can rather readily be placed amongst the *Errores* as matters of misinterpretation or misinformation; in fact that Platonic theory of beauty which reduces it to a kind of harmony is a theory very consistent with the practical placement of the ugliness evil in our group of *Errores,* but in any event the esthetic dissatisfaction is at the present day wholly upon a practical level of investigation. Small quotes from Emerson's essay on *Resources* an interesting passage which we give below, a passage which also omits from its categories the esthetic. This is the more remarkable as Emerson was doubtless more a *littérateur* than a philosopher or at all events was a *littérateur* of first magnitude.

Ross has quarreled with Small's groupings on a variety of grounds. He sees the main interests in man, hunger and love, as specific demands of man, not at all to be covered in under the designation, "desire for health," and points out that health is more of a *sine qua non* than an object of desire as an end. Concerning the latter point we would commend the placement of health first in Small's series of desires—a placement analogous to our own placing of the *Morbi* at the head of our own list. Furthermore we would take advantage of Ross's critique of Small to point out that, when the morbid side of nutrition and of reproduction comes into view, Ross's objection to Small's grouping to a great extent falls away. We may not regard hunger and love as items in our health program, but when there is disease affecting nutrition and reproduction, certainly these particular categories do imperatively cry for attention.

The **desire for wealth** (Ross again asserts) is not a primary desire but depends upon a still more fundamental operation of the ego (so-called *egotic* desires of Stuckenberg) ; but, if we approach the wealth or economic question from its negative and privative side (*i.e.,* from the standpoint of what we had termed the *Penuriae* or resourcelessnesses) we shall find that by changing our point of view we have escaped this particular critique. The desire for wealth may not "differ in principle," as Ross says, "from the lust of lordship over persons (power), or lordship over man's admiration (glory), or lordship over man's judgment (influence)"; but where there is absolute resourcelessness, the very ego itself is hindered in its progress. Resourcelessness hurts life, as one may say, more than increasing resourcefulness helps life. This is at least true on any particular level of attainment. By setting the mind on the sort of Grail that some men take wealth to be, we may miss various dragons of resourcelessness that could be readily slain.

Ross objects to Small's category of **sociability** on the ground that the craving for companionship is one sort of thing and an eagerness for appreciation quite another\sort of thing. But again consider this phenomenon of sociability in its negative form (as one might say, dissociability). The craving for no companionship amounts to an almost psychopathic trend of seclusiveness,[1] or is at all events a vicious attitude or bad habit which helps neither the race nor the individual. Again an absence, like an excess, of desire for appreciation would form an important attitude of viciousness or a bad habit sometimes developed in degree or kind almost to the point of mental disease.

Concerning Small's categories of knowledge and rightness, Ross makes no particular objection. We can see, then, that, in general, Ross's strictures concerning Small's categories can be readily avoided by change of point of view from the analysis of those interests as positive to an analysis of them in their negative or privative form. Had Small taken the pathological view he would, we think, have uncovered rich leads in the analysis of society.

The passage from Emerson mentioned above is at the end of his essay on *Resources* and runs as follows:—

"But the one fact that shines through all this plenitude of powers is, that, as is the receiver, so is the gift; that all these acquisitions are victories of the good brain and brave heart; that the world belongs to the energetic, belongs to the wise. It is vain to make a paradise for good men. The tropics are one vast garden; yet man is more miserably fed and conditioned there than in the cold and stingy zones. THE HEALTHY, THE CIVIL, THE INDUSTRIOUS, THE LEARNED, THE MORAL RACE— NATURE HERSELF ONLY YIELDS HER SECRET TO THESE. And the resources of America and its future will be immense only to wise and virtuous men."

[1] The name of a familiar symptom in psychiatry.

There are thus five kinds of thing that are essential in the Emersonian search for Nature's secret. But it is interesting to note the order in which Emerson has put the assets of the favorites of Nature. He gives the honorable first and last places to health and morality, but as he sums up the whole situation concerning the resources of America in the future he considers that wisdom and morality are, after all, the greatest aids to the unlocking of the immensest resources of his country. Health he too would regard as indispensable and may on this account put it first amongst the qualities of the race to which Nature will yield her secret. That a race shall be civil, that is a race under government and law—here also is an indispensable rather than an essential from Emerson's standpoint. To be industrious was doubtless also to the New England mind of Emerson a mere indispensable rather than an essential. **Upon the basis of three indispensables, health, civic order, and industry, Emerson builds the more essential science and morals.**

The Emersonian ordering of these five categories is as well thought out as it is sublime in implications. The Emersonian order is, no doubt, the important order leading from the indispensables to the essentials in human endeavor. But, from the standpoint of the analysis of a world run down or of a bad social situation, it may well be that this order is not the best one. Lack of health remains a primary consideration, but ignorance, misinformation, and misinterpretation have far wider scope than the operations of organized law and indeed are found at work in the innermost sanctums of private life, where they destroy morality, render legal advice useless or harmful, and are a prolific source of resourcelessness in themselves.

To be healthy, wealthy, and wise is the desire expressed in an ancient adage. To be healthy is as always indispensable; but hardly any reflective person would rather be wealthy than wise. For our part we are inclined to place education next in order upon the indispensable lower layer of health, not because virtue has really been proved to be knowledge, but because without a healthy and trained intelligence it is impossible to meet successfully the complex moral problems that compose so large a part of the field of social work, not to say of the world's work so far as it concerns the individual.

DEFINITIONS OF THE FIVE GROUPS OF EVILS

We have thought it worth while to set down in a special part of this general discussion some **approximate definitions of evil and its major groups.** Elsewhere we refer briefly to certain philosophical viewpoints about the nature of evil in general. Here our statement must confine itself to a few phrases.

The term **evil** itself seems to be related in root to the words *up* and *over*. *Ev* and *ov* of *evil* and *over* respectively stand very close from the standpoint of those who investigate the origin of words. **Apparently evil carries within itself more the idea of excess than of defect.** This would be the natural view of the early thinkers and word-makers since they would naturally people evil situations with something superadded in the nature of spirits or demons. In fact, in the field of disease itself in relatively recent times there has been a tendency to ascribe disease to an Archeus or an Incubus, that is to something thrown in, as it were, on top of the situation.

By far the **greater number of terms** which we use for evil are used for **positive qualities** although there are a good many privative ones. Thus to be evil (following the Century Dictionary) is to be merely "depraved, bad, wicked, vicious"; or again, to be "harmful, hurtful, mischievous, prejudicial, misleading, boding ill"; or again, "causing discomfort, pain, or trouble"; or again, "unfortunate, miserable, wretched"; or again, "as in reference to misfortune, sorrowful, bad luck, disaster." Several of these terms are positive from one aspect and negative (or privative) from another, but apparently the majority of the words are used in the positive sense. We do not need to take a philosophical attitude towards the existence of evil as such in the world. Even if there were philosophically no evil, still these named conditions would exist to be met in some way or other.

There are also a variety of privative meanings, such as the meaning of being insane, that is of having an "evil head" or again, "unwholesome, of inferior quality, poor, unsatisfactory, defective, unskillful." Evil, in general, is censurable, mischievous, undesirable, painful, disastrous, and the like. It is interesting to note that the term "ill" is the same as the word evil by a natural omission of the consonant "v." We would especially insist that we should not like to have the term evil used for specific evils where it is possible to give it a more exact and specific term such as are to be found under the major subgroups that we describe. The theologians say that the term "evil" is likely to become obsolete. Yet it is used in a number of important places in the Bible. For example, in Genesis we hear of the tree of knowledge of good and evil. In the second book of Esdras the evil is *broken in pieces* and the good created.

It will be, as a rule, a confession of relative ignorance concerning the fact if all we can say of a situation is that it is a bad one, that it is a maladjusted situation, that it, so to speak, belongs somewhere in the *Regnum Malorum.* We must specify further. Our point in speaking of definitions is to insist that the majority of evil's meanings in a practical workaday sense of the term refer to positive rather than to privative badness of situation.

(a) *Morbi: Diseases and Defects of Body and Mind*

As to disease, this term upon its face looks like a privative term for *lack or absence of ease,* and such terms as uneasiness, pain, distress, trouble, and discomfort are synonymous of the term as used outside of pathology. Huxley terms disease as "perversions of normal activities of a living body"; but a question might here turn upon what is normal activity of a living body. Sometimes we try to define disease quantitatively. We seek to show that it means an excess of something or a defect of something. We gather valuable data about disease from the weights and measures of the organs and tissues and the plotting of curves and their reactions. But those same weights and measures and to some extent the curves of reactions may be found in the dead as well as in the living organism of constituent part of the organism.

Another way in which it has been attempted to define disease is, first to describe some norm, pattern or model or structure and function, to which a body and its organs are supposed to conform. Here it is not so much a question of weights and measures of the body and its organs as of the conformity of these weights and measures to some standard set. The standard body and the standard organs that constitute it are developed perhaps by some evolutionary process. The hypothesis would be that that body or organ survived which was of greatest use in the struggle for existence of the species owning such a body and such constituent organs or tissues.

On the whole perhaps it is best to define disease **as an interference with the life of the body or of any part thereof or with the persistence of any activity or function of the body and its constituents.** Thus disease interferes with life of the body as a whole, which lives or dies. But again disease may affect entire organs and, though it destroy them, may not destroy life unless these organs are (as we say) *capital* organs. But the organs are made up of tissues, great portions of which may die and be either partially or not at all replaced by regenerative processes. Herein would be an example of disease and recovery with defect. There are constituent factors of safety in the make-up of the total organism, so that many elements of it may die without death of the whole. Disease may doubtless affect even the smallest cell of the body, though the study of such minute processes of health and disease is a difficult one. But the lay student must not get too much in mind the idea of an organism, an organ, a tissue, a cell in the structural aspects of all things. He must likewise think of disease as affecting function, of the curves of response to certain stimuli as damagingly in excess or in defect. The holding fast to this idea of the functional in disease is particularly necessary in the field of mental disease, where so many of the entities have not been proved to be due to loss of structure.

The difference between a structural and a functional disease is hard to define. We have spoken of disease as an interference with the life of vital units (like the cell tissues or organ) and as interference with the persistence of a given function such as breathing, the heart beat, or the food exchange in tissues. Professor Royce once remarked that almost, if not quite, the total meaning he could extract from the term functional was the idea of reversibility. **A functional disease is,** on this definition, **a disease whose phenomena are reversible to the state antecedent to the perturbing factor.** To ask, then, Is the present situation a reversible one? is often of practical value.

Disease, then, consists of an interference with the life of

living structure or interference with the persistence of functions of those living structures. In the former event there is apt to be something discoverable by the microscope, by the more or less elaborate methods of the pathological laboratory. In the latter event, that is, in the case of the interference with the persistence of vital functions, there may be nothing microscopically to be found; perhaps even theoretically nothing need be found by the microscope in pure perturbations of function.

(b) Errores: Educational Deficiencies and Misinformation

Let us turn to a definition of the *Errores*. Probably we have often spoken of our group of *Errores* under the English term "ignorance." The *Errores* do indeed contain a large fraction of pure ignorance whether in the shape of mere lack of education or in the shape of an immigrant's not knowing the language of the country of his adoption. But **the Errores contain positive as well as negative terms.** A man may be not merely uneducated but actually *maleducated* in that he has been given actual misinformation. So far as the maleducated man is concerned, we may say, *it is no fault of his* (that is, we do not lay it up against any vice or bad habit of his or charge it up to disease). To be sure, his teacher may have been mentally deficient or twisted, or may have been the victim of some vice or bad habit of thought, or may have harbored a vicious design in teaching him certain things. But from the standpoint of the maleducated man himself, he belongs in the group of *Errores* in an analysis of the total situation. His psychopathic or vicious teacher would have to fall in other categories than those of *Errores*. But a still more important sub-group of *Errores* exists. A man may be not merely uneducated or maleducated, but he may be a victim of misapprehension or given to misinterpretation. To be sure, any prolonged trend toward misapprehension or misinterpretation would doubtless throw one into some psychopathic group. Practically there would be hardly any difficulty in determining that degree or kind of error which falls within the adage *"To err is human."* We do find the inexperienced social worker charging up to ignorance, misinformation, and misinterpretation much that belongs in the field of feeble-mindedness. With a little more experience, the social worker, as elsewhere intimated, may swing too far in the other direction and find feeble-mindedness where there has been nothing but lack of education or maleducation. Common blunders and mistakes, as well as logical fallacies of reasoning, belong in this group of the *Errores,* where they do not argue mental disease itself.

When Sir Benjamin Brodie says that much of the evil which exists in the world may be traced to mere ignorance, he is, no doubt, functioning as an optimist. As social workers we must see to it that we hew to the line in both directions. Let us never be content with ascribing the situation for long as a mixture of feeble-mindedness and ignorance. Let us analyze these constituents of maladjustment and try to cure or compensate the one and educate or reëducate the other.

In the dictionaries we can find a number of phrases that indicate the sort of thing that should be included under the *Errores,* such as experience, lack of information, misapprehension, misinformation, malinstruction, no schooling, poor schooling, deception, sophistry, unsoundness of argument, mistaken notions, false belief, delusion (sane), inaccuracy, ambiguity, illiteracy, blunder, misinterpretation. Sometimes the term error is used in a moral sense to indicate a wrong doing or transgression, but to ascribe a sin to a mere wandering from the path is to take away from the sin most, if not all, of its responsibility; it is an over-charitable way of viewing a sin or vice in the eye of the ordinary man.

(c) *Vitia: Vices and Bad Habits*

We now come to that which we shall, no doubt, fail to define thoroughly, namely the group of the *Vitia.* One advantage of the Latin names here adopted is that they are rather more comprehensive than any single English equivalent. Thus the *Morbi* we use to include not only disease in the narrower sense but also defect and anomaly. Again we are using *Errores* not only in the negative sense of ignorance, but in the more positive sense of misinformation and misinterpretation. Again *Vitia* is a term which we intend to use more comprehensively to cover not merely vices but also bad habits. Thus we can see that not merely the most opprobrious vices but also such a bad habit as laziness about brushing one's teeth are to be included under the *Vitia.* There is an extremely long list of synonyms and variants upon the ideas of vice and sin which we do not here reproduce. It will repay the reader to consult a good dictionary and trace down a large number of these conceptions to their final ramifications in meaning. We have not used the term sin to any extent in this book, because we have regarded this term as a theological term and have not cared to venture into the debatable questions of the kinds and degrees of theological sin. Still, in a practical view, we regard most of the sins as falling, socially speaking, into our group of the *Vitia*. Some of them, no doubt, in old times and in certain theological systems of the present day would fall into a field of ecclesiastical jurisprudence (penance questions and the like) and therefore belong in our group of the *Litigia,* but these considerations have nothing to do with the main thread of our argument, which is quite innocent of theology.

A practical question to lodge when one wants to decide whether a thing is a disease, a matter of error (in our special sense), or belongs amongst the *Vitia,* is the following: **Is this factor something I should like to cure** in a medical sense of the term cure? or is it something I am fain to meet by a process of **reeducation?** or again is it a factor subject to some process of **reformation?** We try to prevent disease or to cure it. We try to avoid ignorance and misinterpretation by teaching or by so-called reëducation. We try to train for the moral life or to reform the immoral. The pragmatic question what ought to be done at this point is often the successful step in analysis. If you can't help wanting to reform Tom's character, whereas you want to reëducate Dick's intellect and are fain to cure Harry's mental deficiency, you may find that you are unconsciously on the right track when elaborate final analysis will fail you.

(d) Litigia: Legal Entanglements

As for the *Litigia,* here is a knotty question which presumably none but jurists should strive to answer. It is a nice question whether being-at-law actually or potentially is always an evil. The legal order seeks to secure a variety of interests, many of which are of positive significance to the man or the community. But nevertheless we conceive that being-at-law, whether in or out of court and whether *in esse* or *in posse* is in some sense a maladjustment. Somehow the whole connection of the **law** is that of **a process for securing order where there was disorder.** There may be a legal order which is of purely positive and constructive value to the world. If so we should exclude its processes from our group of the *Litigia.* *Litigia* is a term which is much broader than most terms for legal situations. Its usage accordingly allows the inclusion of arbitration and other processes of law outside of the judiciary. Apparently it is the best term available for the situations we are here attempting to designate. A delinquent falls into this group, but delinquency on the part of somebody else than the patient makes also a situation of *litigium.* There need be no moral attributes (although there may be such) in a controversy against the law. Ignorance is, as we say, no excuse in the eyes of the law, so that one may still be involved in *Litigia* even though one has been ignorant of automobile ordinances. One may inherit legal difficulties as in the celebrated case in Dickens of *Jarndyce vs. Jarndyce.*

Enough has been said to indicate the breadth of this concept of **Litigia,** which runs altogether beyond the considerations even of law books on personal relations and domestic relations. General social work and much of ordinary medical social work may fail to show much sign of the **Litigia,** but the moment one gets into any serious family situation or into any complication of mental disease, there is apt to appear a smaller or larger trace of legal entanglement. The whole concept should be subject to a proper definition. No doubt this proper definition will obtain when sociological jurisprudence has been further developed.

Let us review instances of *Litigia* that appear in this volume. In thirty-five of our one hundred cases legal entanglement of some sort is a major factor of the social difficulty. Minor considerations of legal interest enter into another fourteen cases,—questions of legal commitment (cases 47, 75, 76, 77, 79, 85) ; also matters potentially legal that never developed to the point of legal action, such as instances of illegitimacy (cases 36, 48, 52, 66), non-support (case 78), desertion (cases 32, 74), pilfering (case 25). There are then in this book forty-nine cases of possible interest to jurists. We list below the forms of Litigia presented in these cases :—adoption, case 12 ; adultery, case 8 ; alcohol and drugs, cases 58, 61, 63 ; arson, case 9; assault, case 97; cohabitation, case 81; commitment, cases 47, 75, 76, 77, 79, 85; damage suit, case 7; deportation, cases 1, 5; desertion, cases 32, 74; sex disguise, case 23; divorce, cases 13, 17; forgery, cases 2, 80; guardianship, case 70; illegitimacy, cases 36, 48, 52, 66; juvenile delinquents, cases 20, 31, 65, 84; murder, case 54; neglected child, case 22; nonsupport, cases 4, 37, 78; pilfering, case 25; sexual assault, cases 15, 92; stealing, case 3; technical deserter, case 29; vagrancy, cases 51, 72; "work or fight," case 26; workmen's compensation, cases 11, 19, 90.

(e) Penuriae: Poverty and Other Forms of Resourcelessness

We have insisted throughout upon the fact that our group of *Penuriae* includes not merely poverty in the everyday sense of that term but also all other forms of resourcelessness, which can be defined as belonging to any one of the other categories. A man might be wealthy in the technical sense of a bank account, but be placed in a desert or on an inaccessible island. He would be then resourceless. In the wake of wars such nonpecuniary resourcelessnesses are to be found.

ERRORES

Trust in Inadequate Authority
Force of Custom
Opinion of Inexperienced Crowd
Parading of Superficial Wisdom

It was Roger Bacon (*c.* 1214-*c.* 1294) who dealt systematically with the causes of error; namely, the four Offendicula. These causes of error were: (1) trust in inadequate authority, (2) force of custom, (3) opinion of the inexperienced crowd, (4) concealment of real ignorance by a parading of superficial wisdom. Of these four errors the fourth was to Roger Bacon's mind the most dangerous. The concealment of downright ignorance by a pretense of knowledge was perhaps the cause of all the others. Apparently Bacon had no doubt that some kind of knowledge would be available to everyone. What he feared far more was the foisting upon the world misinformation; he apparently felt that the fourth of the Offendicula, the parading of superficial wisdom, would not in itself produce error had not the thinker been somewhat deceived. Why should one (1) trust in inadequate authority, (2) be overawed by the force of custom, (3) follow the opinion of the unskilled many, (4) be cheated by a pretense of knowledge, if there were not a certain weakness of mind in the recipient of the false ideas. Put another way, the stumbling-blocks to knowledge that Roger Bacon tried to chart reduce largely to a false or weak-willed attitude in the thinker. Overweening authority, the cake of custom, the herd instinct, intellectual fraud, would probably not be effective were it not for a certain frailty of will. In short, to modern analysis the stumbling-blocks of Roger Bacon are at least in a large measure inside the stumbler's mind. The victims of what we might term "raw ignorance" will be fewer and fewer to the close investigator of the causes of error. The *Errores* of our own classification tend to flow over into the *Morbi* in the form of greater or lesser degrees of pathological weak-willedness (aboulia, hypoboulia) or over into the *Vitia* in the form of over-compliances with authority, easy-going habits of thought, following the crowd, facile deception by those who, in modern phrase, are "putting it over." Possibly this tendency of modern science to classify the obstacles to knowledge under the heading of mental or moral disorder rather than as plain errors due to ignorance, misinformation, or misinterpretation will explain why we find in our social patients so little that unreservedly flows into the group of *Errores*. We quote Sir Benjamin Brodie to the effect that the world's evil might largely be traced to mere ignorance—this we might grant as also the truth of the formula "virtue is knowledge." But ignorance and other obstacles to knowledge turned out so frequently to be inborn or acquired mental disorder or character defect or ingrained moral defect that Sir Benjamin's formula sounds to the modern ear a bit hollow.

Francis Bacon (*c.* 1561-*c.* 1626) has yet another fourfold classification of the general causes of error in the human mind. He laid them down so as to clear the path for the introduction of the new method of science which he was to advance. The doctrine of fallacies appears in final form in the *Novum Organon* as the four *Idola*. The first of the *Idola* bears some resemblance to his namesake's stumbling-blocks,—the opinion of the unskilled many; these are the *Idola Tribus*, idols of the tribe, fallacies to which the human race is one and all subject. But for that matter it would seem that all of the Offendicula of Roger Bacon might well be put under the tribal fallacies of Francis Bacon. When we looked at the second kind of *Idola* of Francis Bacon we saw how much more modern is the point of view of Baron Verulam. The *Idola Specus*, the idols of the cave (probably here is meant the hollow of the skull), are fallacies that depend upon the individuality of the particular man. Apparently, for his namesake and predecessor, everybody in general is more or less subject to identical stumbling-blocks. For Francis Bacon the individualities of men stood out. Under this head the Baconian practical rule for avoiding individual tendencies to error runs as follows : "Let every student of nature in general take this as a rule, that whatever his mind seizes, dwells upon with particular satisfaction, is to be held in suspicion." Whereas Roger Bacon sees ignorant men, trust in inadequate authority exerted from without, Francis Bacon sees clearly the error of trusting overmuch one's own internal authority based upon his mental or bodily construction. The psychopathic personalities that appear so frequently in this volume are pronounced instances of subjection to the *Idola Specus*, or idols of the cave, of Francis

Bacon. Of course we suspect that these "Idols of the Hollow of the Skull" are somewhere dependent upon peculiarities of the brains contained within the skull or upon peculiar influences streaming in upon those brains from the rest of the body. It is clear that the classification formulated for the Idols of one's brain pan must be our familiar war cry in all forms of mental hygiene—"individualization." If we are to adjust inner relations to outer relations, as Spencer contends, for a perfect life, we shall be compelled to hold sharply to it when the inner relations themselves are defective. What a rigid aspect the notion of "cure" takes on when by "cure" we compromise all the individualizing processes of adjustment entailed by the individual peculiarity of man!

The third class of Idola were the *Idola Fori,* or Idols of the Market Place. These errors or fallacies Francis Bacon contended arose from the influence exerted upon the mind by mere words. This class of Idola corresponds somewhat to Roger Bacon's stumbling-blocks of the parading of superficial wisdom. How many empty formulæ exist in social work, not to say also in the work of physicians and of public servants, that ought to be classed in the Baconian Idola Fori! Book II presented at length cases that illustrate a variety of formulæ of social difficulties in a series of cases. The cases run, for example, all the way from that of Rose Talbot (case 8), in which all five forms of social difficulty were presented to the five instances (cases 34 to 38) in which one class only of social difficulty were found. Now in point of actual practice the social worker is altogether too much inclined to classify a given case as one of disease alone, or of ignorance alone (or other form of error), of legal entanglement, or of poverty alone. This tendency may simplify the keeping of social record books but it does not comport with the actual situation in point of social fact. It is a tendency that belongs with the *Idola Fori,* or Idols of the Market Place, in the Baconian sense, to fall under the spell of this particular error,—to classify under but one head. How simple social work would be if cases all fell smoothly into place as cases to cure merely, merely to reëducate, or again merely to reform, to supply with legal aid, or to compensate in any monetary sense!

Let us call especial attention at this point also to that group of cases in Book II which exhibits simple binary combinations of two forms of social difficulty. If we should consider the simplest case of medical social work—namely, a case which showed but two factors say, (1) need of orthopedic splint, (2) need of money—possibly these two needs could be separately met. Possibly the granting of financial relief would forthwith settle the question of getting a splint. In such an instance the primary social difficulty might well turn out to be poverty. Whilst the orthopedic need might be a very remote and secondary phenomenon. But suppose we have a combination of poverty with such a weak will disorder as lack of ambition. Let us suppose this lack of ambition is not psychopathic. Then it is obvious with half an eye that the dole-giving is not going to settle the problem. Yet to quote Richmond's *"Social Diagnosis,"* there was in charity organization work "at first no accepted program of treatment other than the giving or withholding of relief." Here and there advanced agencies formed more thorough programs of what could be done; but in the earlier days these were carried out with difficulty against the main current of charity activity which ran strongly toward dole-giving. These two instances may suffice to raise the important point that we shall learn more and more about social work if we study merely binary combinations of social difficulty. That is the combinations of *Morbus* with *Error* or *Morbus* with *Vitium,* or *Morbus* with *Litigium,* or *Morbus* with *Penuria,* or *Error* with *Penuria,* or *Vitium* with *Litigium, Vitium* with *Penuria, Litigium* with *Penuria.* The cases of binary combination (cases 24 to 33 inclusive) in Book II of course present only a simple indication of the possibilities of each of the five main groups. A vast deal of work must be done when we get into the main outlines of social work entailed by a study of binary combinations. When two social difficulties are loosely associated with one another, so that each may be simply and separately treated, social work will be relatively easy. But when two difficulties are multiplied into one another social work will be relatively hard.

To continue with our remarks upon the four classes of Idola, according to Francis Bacon we find the fourth and last class to be the *Idola Theatri,* or so-called Idols of the Theater. (The theater here means the speculative or "theorizing" mind and does not refer to theater in the ordinary sense.) The victims of this class of Idola are those who force nature into empty, abstract schemes and want to explain existing conditions by mere definition. Again there are those that leap to general conclusions by too few experiments, or again those that work in an imaginative way by the overuse of analogies. This particular type of error is one which the theorists of social work must take to heart. The existence of these Idola of the speculative mind is the best reason for our having chosen to place the case material of this volume at the outset rather than as merely illustrative material. We have tried to analyze some of the cases available to us, with the richest display of facts and most intensive social treatment, and to deduce from these data certain general principles. If the reader dissents from the principles he has the recourse of going back to the facts. Moreover, as the cases are for the most part still alive and both capable of investigation and willing to tell their stories, we shall in the long run be able to test the validity of our own conclusions by the test of time.

THE PROBLEM OF EVIL

Although we have drawn the analysis of this volume upon a classification of the social evils taken in their broadest sense, we cannot pretend to be competent in the theory of morals or to write a textbook of ethics. No doubt the historical development of the idea of medical social work (and naturally of its related branch psychiatric social work) are, in the New England community in which we write, greatly influenced by the philosophical work of Professor Josiah Royce upon the problem of evil. Professor Royce's work upon evil as well as upon social consciousness and later upon the logical theories of order have unquestionably prescribed some of the most important lines in Dr. Richard C. Cabot's development of medical social work and in our own additions to the concept from the field of mental hygiene. We have been compelled to choose mottoes for the four books from Job. The initial paper in Professor Royce's *Studies of Good and Evil* deals with the problem of Job. The problem of Job, according to Royce, is the problem of unearned ill fortune. Whatever evil is, Royce is most cordially of the opinion that it is a "distinctly real fact, a fact just as real as the most helpless and hopeless sufferer finds it to be when he is in pain." Elsewhere he speaks of

another view, "that essentially pernicious view nowadays somewhat current amongst a certain class of gentle but inconsequent
people—the view that all evil is merely an illusion and that
there is no such thing in God's world." Good and evil, according to Royce, do not exist as opponents but merely as exclusive agents side by side in experience. A longer account
of this view runs as follows :—

> "Taking a wider view, one may observe that the greater part
> of the freest products of the activity of civilization in cere-
> monies, in formalities, in the long social drama of flight, of
> pursuit, of repartee, of contest and of courtesy, involve an
> elaborate and systematic delaying and hindering of elemental
> human desires, which we continually outwit, postpone, and
> thwart, even while we nourish them. When students of human
> nature assert that hunger and love rule the social world, they
> recognize that the elemental in human nature is trained by
> civilization into the service of the highest demands of the
> Spirit."

A briefer formula is as follows :—

> "It is impossible for one to know a higher good than comes
> from the subordination of evil to good in a total experience.
> Love of moral good is the thwarting of lower loves for the
> sake of higher organization."

It will be seen that, according to Royce, "the eternal world
contains Gethsemane."

This point of view of Royce's is the point of view of the
so-called philosophical idealism ("your sufferings are God's
sufferings"). It is obvious that the considerations of the present volume do not depend in the slightest upon any philosophical view whatever. Even if we should run with the "essentially pernicious view" which regards all evil as an illusion, we
should nevertheless have to grant the existence of the illusion
as a distinctly real fact. The illusions and delusions of the
sane we should be inclined to place in our group of *Errores*.
We should regard those who identify diseases, sins, crimes, resourcelessness with the delusions as unwise persons who have
made singularly poor use of some of the formulæ of philosophical idealism.

In the course of writing this volume we have met sundry
persons who have denied the existence of evil under that name,
maintaining that evil is an illusion or an error. We have

wondered whether they were not all unconsciously identifying the genus with the species and abolishing the *regnum malorum* with its subgroup *Errores*. We are the more inclined to draw this conclusion from our observation that these verbal destroyers of evil are ordinarily turned to the hypothesis that the illusions and errors, or surrogates of evil, are to be destroyed by "taking thought," by adopting certain beliefs and sometimes by the plain anodyne of forgetting. Even the so-called Christian Science may fall back upon establishing sanatoria, thereby conceding that there is a special form of error needing hospital treatment. Christian Scientists also would be righteously incensed if their opponents should charge them with not encouraging morality or the legal order. If the representatives of sundry movements for faith cure have been charged with a loss of interest in the problems of poor relief and charity in certain communities, in any event the believers in these cults are for the most part kindly persons as interested in the economic successes of the community as their fellow beings. Accordingly, we repeat, the point of view of the present work does not, strictly speaking, need to take account of any philosophical view of evil, even such a view as that of Christian Science, which turns even disease into a form of error. Perhaps we should concede that the point of view of the ingrained pessimist cannot be the point of view of social work. The point of view of Voltaire or Nietzsche is not the point of view of the social worker, although be it remembered to the credit of Voltaire that he leaves his wretched heroes and heroines at the end of *Candide* working in a garden, and even Nietzsche insisted that the strong were strengthened by evil.

There can be no doubt that the practical social worker needs to have some philosophical and religious views of the nature of good and evil, not alone for the social worker's own personal guidance but for the sake of grasping ingenious arguments which sundry depressed, deluded patients are prone to offer. According to Royce, the first hypothesis concerning evil is that it is nothing but natural phenomena—"dirt of the natural order, whose value is, that when you wash it off you learn the charm of the bath of evolution." The second hypothesis is that evil has a medicinal and disciplinary value. The third hypothesis runs to the effect that all real evils are the results of free finite moral agents. And finally, according to

Royce, the fourth hypothesis of philosophical idealism runs to the effect that the entire world is built on a basis of "inner tension of manifold impulses and interests," which, as he remarks, are not "mere accidents of rather imperfect human nature but must be a type of the organization of every rational life."

Our own study has dealt not so much with the definition of evil as with the classification of the evils as they have presented themselves in the Psychopathic Hospital, a clearing-house for the evils of individual man. Our study has been an inductive one from the concrete facts to a classification of these facts in certain groups. These groups, it appeared to us, might effectively be united in a greater group of evils taken in a more general way. We have thus come upon an idea of the social worker as a person professionally at work amongst all types of evil. The social worker, as we remarked above, must remain a layman with regard to the great special fields of medicine, education, morals, jurisprudence, and economics. But the social worker is a very intensive sort of layman with, some might say, an exaggerated amount of common sense—that kind of comprehensive insight which utilizes the professional specialist without supplanting him.

The Roycean formula of the inner tension of manifold impulses and interests within our natures goes a step further than the Spencerian formula of the adjustment of inner to outer relations. In the first place Royce calls attention to the existence of tensions within our own make-ups, and in the second place he seems to define ethics in terms of the relations of the interior tensions. We have had abundant cause to observe a practical truth in our patients of this hypothesis of interior tensions. But the world's evil, even according to Royce, is not confined to the inner life of a man but has spread through the universe. Certainly in that part of the universe with which we are dealing; namely, society, some sort of tensions have been found to prevail. But can we conceive that the analyses of the present work do not hang upon the comparative richness of the Spencerian or the Roycean formulæ concerning relations in the universe? The cases here presented are presented on a practical level and the workers who worked with them have as a rule paid no heed to philosophical questions.

But the social worker must not think that because she is practical she is inevitably just like everybody else in her point of view toward the world. It would seem that the social worker possesses a special temperament. At least the medical and psychiatric social workers have a greater interest primarily in the destruction of evil than in the construction of good. When such workers rationalize their attitudes they say to themselves that by destroying evils they are helping to create, or allowing to be distributed, goods, but the temperament which sees evil as the proximate task of destruction and good as the ultimate goal is nevertheless a temperament. And it is a temperament that not everybody possesses. It would seem that there are **dragon-slayers** and **Grail-hunters**. There are those who prefer to be St. George and others who would rather be Sir Galahad.

It is doubtful whether the decision to be one or the other is always a conscious or rational one. Those of us who are informed of the spirit of medicine or medical and psychiatric social work, or of nursing, or of the probation officer and the like, are wakened up in astonishment to the fact that there are perfectly good citizens in the world who prefer to put diseases and other forms of evil entirely out of mind. Nor can we set down these persons who are not interested in evil as merely materialistic. Often they prove perfectly admirable seekers after a Grail of one kind or other. The devotees of religion, wizards of scientific invention, and the artists, do not have, as a rule, any interests that might be termed **malecidal**: they are not built for the destruction of evil, nor should we wish to swerve these zealots of the Grail from their goal. In fact the Grail-hunting temperament in its highest development is next to impossible to divert. We had best not waste our time and theirs by offering wares of social work to the inborn Grail-seekers. But there remains a great mass of people whose parental and filial, and especially whose maternal, joys give them the fundaments of social interest. From amongst the common people we shall draw many of our best workers if we can interest them in the social task, and if we can believe that through evolution habits of destruction are deeply imbedded in all of us. Let us point these destructive powers in the direction of evil. That is the essence of strategy underlying this particular kind of social work. In our task of persuading

the everyday citizen that his proximate task is to destroy evil
we have a number of points in our favor. If he replies that
he would rather do good than merely undo evil we can reply
to him "What after all is the good which you would like to
do?" The chances are that his first response would have to
do with getting rid of some near-by evil. We can point out
to him that evil is very easy to perceive about us. **Evil is
easier to perceive than good is even to conceive.** Perception was ever easier than conception. We see evil all about
us. We do not need to make elaborate conceptions or interpretations of the evil that is at hand. Again, evil is not only
easier to perceive than good to conceive but evil subdivides
very readily into plurality of evils. The good is rather apt
to remain a unit or to subdivide itself far less readily. The
farmer has sick cattle. It is plain that they must be cured or
for their own comfort be killed. But suppose the farmer tries
a program of construction. Shall he breed for beef or for
milk? The plot thickens at once. If we look into the vocabulary for words descriptive of good and evil respectively, we
are certain to find in most languages a far larger number of
words dealing with evils than with the goods.

Evils can thus be seen about us (and be items for destruction) far more readily than the goods. It is obvious too that
evil gets more clearly into the mind than does good. For
whatever evolutionary reason this is so we do not delay to discuss, but there is something insistent, pricking, sensationally
painful about evils. They attract our attention more readily
and are on the whole more definable than goods. Finally, as
above insisted, concerning our relative powers of destruction
and construction, we men are built more for destruction than
for construction, or at all events are more used to the destructive processes in our daily lives. We should, therefore, take
advantage of this ingrained destructive trend and endeavor in
the *first instance* to destroy definite concrete, and observable
evils rather than try to construct indefinite, abstract, hardly
conceivable good. Let the proximate task of evil destruction
be accomplished and the ultimate task of constructive goodness will shortly follow. The formula might run **"Get the
Grail but first slay the dragon."** These are perhaps the
main arguments to the hypothesis of evil's primacy in the
realm of social tasks. We are entirely certain that various

readers of the Grail-hunting group will persist in misunderstanding our program. They will not distinguish a technique that deals with proximates from a program that runs towards ultimates. We conceive that social work is a kind of human technique of proximate nature whose lines are laid down in the interest of ultimate good.

We have been bold enough to borrow mottoes from the book of Job. We have taken care to take them from the words of Job himself rather than from the words of his friends. These friends, however, skillful in rhetoric, would perhaps not prove the most successful of social adjusters. Without undertaking elaborate analysis of the endeavors of Job's friends, for which we are entirely incompetent, we are nevertheless inclined to assert that the world has made a considerable advance upon the ethical situation depicted in Job. Job said that his error remained with himself, that when he cried out of wrong he was not heard, that there was no justice, and that the hand of God had touched him. He thus made an almost complete analysis of his plight, finding concrete evils in most of the departments we have discussed. Is it too much to say that the spirit of civilization, the spirit of Christianity if you will, has shifted the universe of evil at least by a few units? That the land of the shadow of death could contain any sort of order hardly entered Job's mind. It was to him the highest of rhetorical flights to think of the weighing of his calamities. In all these respects the modern world has gained a plan of attack which Job's world certainly possessed not.

Finally as to the motto with which we have introduced Book IV, the nineteenth century by its researches has served to magnify the interest of man, if not yet to offer a perfect technique for preserving him. Remarks like these are petty enough beside the terror of the facts. We do not find the social worker irreligious; but if the social worker were at the outset irreligious, she speedily comes to a sufficient solemnity —the solemnity of the interrelations of the deeper things in mind and morals.

Thus we conclude certain generalities about the evils. By the very order of presentation of the material in this work we have intended to show that our work ran from observed details upward to more or less tentative general statements, and not at all from any preconceived principles downward to the facts. Our study, as we have repeatedly maintained, is inductive and not deductive. In point of fact the observations made were made in the first instance without any grouping of the evils and the maladjustments whatever. It was only when we came to put our work together that we found our material grouping itself in the way most elaborately presented in Book II of this work. We think some such classification presented in some order on the principles of this work will maintain itself in future social work; but whether it does or not, the materials for this particular analysis were not collected with these categories in mind, but were collected with the general principles of psychiatric social investigation in mind.

APPLICATIONS OF THE FIVEFOLD CLASSIFICATION OF EVILS OUTSIDE THE FIELD OF SOCIAL WORK

Our fivefold classification of evils, to which Book II is largely devoted, is a classification that might be applied with great generality to vast areas of phenomena **outside the field of social case work.** It is beyond the province of this volume to discuss these wider applications, though the entire social problem would plainly profit thereby. We shall confine ourselves to two instances of the possible application of our method of orderly approach to the classification of difficulties of whatever sort. Let these two instances be the Great War and bolshevism.

Is war in itself an evil? The Crusaders and the American Revolutionists might well resent the charge so far as it concerned their own aims and duties. Yet they would be compelled to grant the unfolding of numerous evils in the train of crusades or revolutions. To our minds the assertion that war is *an evil* is logically far less accurate a statement than that war entails *evils*. War entails a plurality of evils. What, now, are these evils? We think they can readily be distributed amongst our five groups, though some might desire that we add a sixth miscellaneous group for troubles not specifically listed as disease, error, vice, legal difficulty, and poverty. In the wake of war comes disease and pestilence. Educational systems crumble in war time, vicious attitudes abound. The legal order is assailed. Poverty reigns.

If every analyst of reconstruction were to catalogue the

evils of war even in this rough manner, he would greatly assist in the definition of every post bellum task. Reformers with but a single nostrum would have no preferred standing in political councils, whether amongst government officials or amongst the voluntary associations of the community. An eventual combined development of health programs with educational programs would be assured. The representatives of the church, the lecture platform, and the theater, as shapers for better or worse of community morals, would find themselves shoulder to shoulder with the representatives of government and law. In particular, nobody with an economic panacea would be allowed to run wild without competition amongst theories of reconstruction. To split *evil* into such great rough groups as our chosen five of *evils* would represent an advance in social reconstruction hardly to be hoped for in an era of single-track minds. Yet there would be a place in the sun, a true locus for the single-track minds in the pragmatic attack upon each of the evils taken separately and distributively by some single specialist—a specialist, as you might say, in the slaying of a particular variety of dragon. The higher speed and the greater safety can no doubt be attained upon the single, switchless track, and the straighter the better. In short, the trouble is the ancient trouble of the many and the one, that is, the determining, amongst a plurality of things to do, the pragmatic unit, the thing that "makes a difference."

We may again insist, as particularly pertinent to these generalized applications of our method of orderly approach, that **the items** in the list **and the order** to be adopted in their **consideration are of lesser consequence than the adoption of some order in the consideration of chosen categories.** Suppose now, that we were to analyze·phenomena of the Great War, no longer from the standpoint of the immediate task of reconstruction but rather from the standpoint of historical analysis to the end of the prevention of future wars. We should be **looking into causes. Here again the method of orderly approach in the analysis of data has value.**

Was there a morbid factor at the bottom of the Great War or, more moderately speaking, were morbid factors at all seriously in evidence? Of course some German propagandists went so far as to describe the French attitude at the outset of the Great War, and at various times when the French refused to treat for peace, as an example of *Psychopathia Gallica.* This *Psychopathia Gallica* was a national revenge-psychosis! One German disputant objected. He noted a responsibility on the part of the Germans to France if France was a national victim of mental disease : France would then have to be pitied! But, seriously speaking, was there, or was there not, a morbid and especially a psychopathic factor in the Great War? Was the Kaiser a psychopath? The lay reader must take note that psychopath means, as elsewhere in this book, not necessarily an insane person in the medico-legal sense of that term. The Kaiser might be a psychopath and, as French writers have for years insisted, have still a degree of responsibility.

But we are not here inquiring about the degree of personal responsibility which might be laid at the door of a psychopathic or non-psychopathic Kaiser. We are inquiring into the causes of the Great War. It would be a nice question to determine whether the Hohenzollerns are in so far eccentric or "off-center" or "deviate" that they have had an essential share in shaping European destinies. There are two views about all such matters which frequently blanket or forestall concrete investigations. There are those who believe in some variant of the Great-Man theory of history. There are others who are equally certain that all big social movements are mass movements, reminding one of the prodigies of the social life of ants, bees, and wasps. It is a question whether the real facts concerning the Hohenzollerns and in particular concerning the now living representatives of this group will ever be examined by psychiatric experts. Great educators, wise philosophers, exalted preachers, profound moralists, learned judges, ingenious advocates, formulating political economists and sociologists, to say nothing of estimable laymen, will claim the right to make this momentous decision. Many decades will go by, possibly a century or more, before we can replace the current interpretations of history with a psychiatric interpretation. Yet until that psychiatric interpretation comes we shall not have tried out one of the likeliest measures of prevention. Who now knows whether both the origin of tyranny and tyranny's fate were not matters of psychopathic interest?

But now let us suppose either that there were no morbid factors or only partially effective morbid factors in the Great

War, shall we not assign the Great War's origin to our group of Errores? Was not Darwinism misinterpreted by German expounders? Was not the German populace misinformed concerning political causes and effects? Did the Germans not proceed upon an erroneous theory of morals inculcated under the influence of the Hohenzollerns, Bismarck, Treitschke, and Nietzsche? Here is a very pretty inquiry, localized in the field of popular education and the general opinion of German society. Did not Willisen and Clausewitz misinterpret the Napoleonic successes and method and supply the German community with nationalistic ideas basically wrong? In this part of our inquiry we should need to abstain absolutely from any considerations of mental disease or of false morals. Should it be inquired whether perhaps Nietzsche was not a psychopath and his *Will to Power* the reflection of a psychopathic pessimism, then our inquiry would run back to the group of *Morbi*. Should we determine that Nietzsche, like his predecessor Schopenhauer, was importantly a psychopath, then our ideas concerning the origin of the war would change and some of our measures for prevention would take into account the necessity of analyzing the claims of a Schopenhauer or of a Nietzsche long before political economists usually think philosophy needs attention. Yet the ideas of a Schopenhauer and of a Nietzsche, let them be as vitriolic and destructive by nature as they list, would perhaps not be dangerous to society if they were not spread by an educational process, either by chance or by design.

If it should be discovered that leaders of German thought for national political purpose deliberately encouraged the spread of the psychopathic ideas of a Nietzsche or a Schopenhauer, then the inquiry might throw back once more to the question whether the leaders of German thought were themselves psychopathic or whether they were merely mistaught by predecessors who were possibly psychopathic, or whether they were persons with a vicious streak. In short, this inquiry concerning the spread of ideas ultimately traceable to a psychopathic origin might lead us at the outset to moral attitudes falling in our group of the *Vitia;* but, at one degree removed and in the second generation of educators, we might find that the total immediate cause of the German attitude towards world domination lay in our second group of

Errores. That is to say, ideas might arise in the group *Morbi* or they might not, but these ideas might be promulgated as misinterpretation, or misinformation by the mistaken leaders of a given generation (belonging in group E), themselves not at all psychopathic (i.e. *not* in group M) and even not at all vicious (not in group V). They would secure our forgiveness "for they know not what they do." But again there might be certain vicious leaders of thought (group V) who would influence a circle of less powerful thinkers (group E), who would spread ideas derived from the vicious politicians, who, however, might have obtained their ideas from psychopaths (group M). The analysis might run in a variety of ways; but our general thesis ought, we think, to be accepted, namely, that analysis under some such groups or categories as we have here chosen would be of the greatest advantage to the world.

It is even possible that the exponents of a peculiar form of legal order might have greatly influenced the origins of the Great War. Men firmly convinced of the values of the German legal code might well regard such code and underlying principles as the real skeleton and support of world civilization. Jurists of this kidney would not be psychopaths. Their ideas would not fall into the field of education, as commonly accepted, nor could we charge their system with being in any obvious way a result of misinformation or of misinterpretation. There is no doubt that the representatives of medicine, natural science, morals, religion, economics, and politics take too little account of juristic developments. And the jurists too are doubtless guilty of groping about in the same way in their own water-tight compartment. Only the sociologists appear to try to encompass all these points of view; yet, even where the sociologists have a wide range and a sure touch, they seem to us to fail to take account in an even and representative way of all these divisions of human interest. This is particularly true of the neglect by sociologists, up to very recent days, of any right view of the importance of the psychopath in history.

Lastly we may consider that **an economic interpretation of history might prove** that the basis of the **Great War** was **economic.** Of course this dictum means very little if we are listening to economists who regard virtually everything in the world as essentially economic in its basis. But surely that proof has never been brought.

Enough has been said to intimate the sure advantage which would follow analyzing the Great War in an orderly way concerning both its origins and its effects. Advantage would accrue if the phenomena of the Great War were analyzed under the *positive categories* of health, education, morals, law and order, and economics. But we contend that the negative and corresponding categories of our five groups would possess a still greater advantage for the analyst.

Let us now turn to bolshevism. It would be of fundamental importance and value, could we discover and disentangle any **psychopathic elements in bolshevism.** Marx was, no doubt, not at all a psychopath. Bakunin on the other hand was no doubt a psychopath. Socialism and anarchism need not be set down as non-psychopathic and psychopathic in origin on account of the nature of the lives of their founders, Marx and Bakunin. Modern anarchists are a little impatient of any attribution of great movements like socialism and bolshevism to *great men* like Marx and Bakunin. They are prone to leap into another category when the argument waxes hot concerning individual founders and to begin to talk about general, economic, legal, and moral or educational tendencies, of mass movements and the like. There is a time for the consideration of these other categories, but we can see that there is a time for rounding up all the psychopathic elements that there may be. Let psychiatric specialists deal to the best of their special knowledge and training with these facts, and let all the facts be considered that might have a bearing on the morbid sides of certain bolshevistic, socialistic, governmental, or capitalist trends. (For in this skeleton of an argument concerning bolshevism we must not be understood to say that the various proponents of law and order and of capitalistic ventures are not also sometimes in an important way psychopathic.) After decades it may be allowable to think of George III as a psychopath. How impatient a politician of the present day would be if an inquiry along this line were made concerning the Lenin who lives today! These are very **sharp tools,** the objector to our program of the psychiatric analysis of present-day politics may urge. But the tools we suggest are after all no sharper than the political tools of terrorism used by a Hohenzollern or a Lenin. Finally the world will learn not to flinch under the application of expert analysis.

But suppose we decide that Lenin and the rest are not psychopathic or not importantly so, **how much of the situation of bolshevism is an educational affair?** How much is it due to vicious or quixotic **moral attitudes?** How much is it due to reaction against certain more or less **false ideas of law and order** and how much, finally, is it due to the **economic resourcelessness** of Russian peasants? We are not competent to offer positive points concerning this analysis, but we are inclined to think that every dispassionate person will agree that the present-day type of analysis of such conditions does not make for clarity. We can see that it is because the analyst continually changes his categories, leaping from positive to negative phenomena and leaping from group to group of each, perhaps making each of his arguments swerve in a particular and favorite direction.

The contentions in the last few paragraphs concerning the possible analysis of the Great War and of bolshevism do not touch the argument concerning the utility of our classification of evils as applied to the individual psychopath. Our contentions do not rest upon a thorough study of historical and political phenomena. We shall be entirely satisfied if the reader regards these contentions as pure hypotheses. The argument will at least serve to bring out into stronger relief the method of orderly approach in the classification of social difficulties as applied in the body of our work.

THE METHOD OF BOOK III: MAIN GROUPS OF MENTAL DISEASES

The cases of Book III are arranged according to their occurrence in the *Major Groups of Mental Disease*. Precisely the same types of patient are presented in Book III as in Book I, which dealt with the *spheres of influence* and in Book II, which dealt with the various *forms of evil*. Our volume is in no sense a treatise on psychiatry. Yet for several reasons the arrangement of Book III is a desirable one. In the first place physicians, both psychiatrists and others, may want to learn what kinds of social work are likely to be most applicable in the major groups of mental disease; and, whereas the account here presented is far from complete, we conceive that the major issues of social treatment of the mental diseases are clearly indicated. In the second place the social worker must understand the larger features of mental disease as shown in the great groups which physicians recognize; even if the social worker's ideas are limited to very rough ideas concerning the prognosis in the major groups of mental disease, she will understand the physician's point of view certainly better than do many teachers, pastors, lawyers, and business men, with all of whom the social worker may have to deal. In the third place the cases of Book III may be used by the reader for the purpose of independent judgment whèther Book I's conclusions on the *spheres of influence* and Book II's conclusions on the *forms of evil* are sound conclusions; for the cases of Book III are presented in far bolder form and with more reference to treatment and outcome than to the technique of authority brought to bear or of diagnostic details.

What are mental diseases? Luckily this is not a textbook of psychiatry and we are not stringently required to offer a definition. For practical purposes the mental diseases are diseases which common consent leaves in the hands of a special group of physicians for diagnosis and treatment; namely, the group of so-called psychiatrists. Common consent means that the medical schools, the medical associations, and the medical textbooks are practically unanimous in conceding the existence of a field of mental diseases, related somewhat closely with the so-called nervous diseases but rather less closely with all other forms of disease. Medical schools have formally recognized, though as a rule very inadequately, in their curricula departments of mental disease or of psychiatry. National associations, like the American Medico-Psychological Association, now the American Psychiatric Association, exist for the purpose of promoting the study of mental diseases as opposed to all other forms of disease. Until recent years these associations have been far from "scientific" in the sense of presenting programs of investigation and research. Although the American Medico-Psychological Association is the oldest national medical association in this country, yet its progress upon lines of research and investigation has up to recent times been singularly slow. The predominance in its programs of administrative and other practical features has, however, one point to commend itself in the eyes of the social worker,—the social worker will find that the practitioner in mental diseases, *i.e.*, the psychiatrist, is probably by nature and training a man especially accessible to ideas of social work. In fact the superintendent of a hospital for the insane and his subordinate officers have often been engaged in a type of work not far removed from social work performed as a rule inadequately from a central office desk and without due emphasis, perhaps, upon the educational, moral, legal, and economic sides of the problem. On the whole, however, the psychiatrists had, by virtue of the very nature of their material, made much greater progress toward "socialization" than had practitioners in other fields of medicine. Many of the underlying concepts of social work are far more deeply imbedded in the mind of the psychiatrist than in the minds of other practitioners of medicine.

Psychiatry is that field of medicine devoted to mental diseases, and psychiatrists are the practitioners in that field. Many readers are aware that the term "psychiatrist" has only recently taken hold of this country. The term "alienist" is still used rather freely by the older generation. There is, to be sure, not much difference between these terms, yet the slight distinction is one which is of the greatest importance to the development of mental hygiene. The situation is somewhat as follows. Insanity and mental disease are not synonymous. Insanity is a legal concept, mental disease is a medical concept. A man is sane or insane or as yet indeterminate as to his insanity. Many hold that there are no degrees of sanity or insanity. A multitude of courts will still be found holding that there is but one degree and but one kind of sanity or of insanity.

On the other hand there are all degrees of mental health and mental disease and there are many kinds of mental disease. Insanity, we may say, depends upon medico-legal decisions. Mental disease is an affair of medicine alone. Sanity and mental health, decided respectively by the law and by medicine, may characterize the same human subjects. But—and here is the definite point—*sanity may characterize many subjects of mental disease. These sane subjects of mental disease* are subject to mental disease, mild or severe, of a kind or degree that does not concern the courts. It would even be permissible to say that no man is either sane or insane until properly reviewed and adjudged by the courts. It is perhaps enough to claim that sanity and insanity are characteristics such that courts decide them within limits of accuracy of courts. Accordingly sanity and insanity are legal, governmental, public matters. On the other hand mental health and disease are matters of individual medicine and individual psychology, and while of familial, district, group, or community interest, they do not necessarily even approach governmental régime. Insanity is a public matter, mental disease a social, family, or personal matter.

We believe that the above statements will be commonplaces in the minds of many, perhaps of most advanced medical men. It is probable that many competent jurists hold identical concepts. It was on this basis that the senior author of this work proposed some years since that the medical specialists, who are medico-legal aids, be given the familiar and appropriate designation, *alienists,* and that the term *psychiatrists* be reserved for those specialists who act as physicians only,—in short that the insanity expert be spoken of as an alienist and the mental-disease expert be called a psychiatrist. In a somewhat revolutionary way the suggestion was at that time made that the records on mental cases might run as follows. (The reader must take note that these suggestions have *not* to any extent been applied practically up to this time and are here offered purely to bring out the existence of *border-line cases of mental disease that are not medico-legally insane.*)

EXAMPLE 1.—"As alienist I consider this person insane. As psychiatrist I consider this patient subject to general paresis."

EXAMPLE 2.—"As alienist I consider this person sane. As psychiatrist I consider him in complete mental health."

EXAMPLE 3.—"As alienist I consider this person sane. As psychiatrist I consider him subject to mental disease; namely, subject to a psychoneurosis of hysterical form."

EXAMPLE 4.—"As alienist I consider this person sane. As psychiatrist I consider him subject to dementia praecox in a mild degree."

EXAMPLE 5.—"As alienist I consider this person sane. As psychiatrist I consider him subject to paranoia of great severity. This mental disease (which I find as psychiatrist) I regard, in this case, as of no public interest (when I review the findings as alienist)."

ALIENISTS	PSYCHIATRISTS
Field: Insanity, The Insane	Field: Psychiatry, the Mentally Diseased
Field: Public, Governmental, Legal	Field: Social, Private, Medical
Field: Opinion for Court Use	Field: Medical, Psychological, and Social Diagnosis and Treatment
Decisions Alternative: Sanity versus Insanity	Decisions Selective: *e.g.*, Syphilitic, Feeble-minded, Epileptic, Alcoholic, Coarse Brain Disease, Symptomatic, Senescent - senile, Schizophrenic, Cyclothymic, Psychoneurotic, etc.
Insanity Implies Mental Disease	Sanity Consistent with Mental Disease of Mild Degree or of Special Type
Sanity: Insanity $= 1 : 0$	Mental Disease of All Degrees of Many Kinds

The hypothetical and indeed utopian reports (Examples 1-5) are made, it will be observed, by a physician who announces himself to be both an alienist and a psychiatrist. No doubt every good physician must, in the nature of things, be a good alienist, since the expert in mental diseases, as a rule, must be an expert in those mental diseases which are, from the legal point of view, insanities. No doubt, too, every alienist (in the narrow legal sense here adopted) ought to be a good psychiatrist. Yet it is still true that many alienists are to be found who have no interest in mental diseases outside the field of the medico-legal insanities, and having no interest (especially no therapeutic interest) therein really never do become psychiatrists in a deep sense. This unfortunate state of affairs will persist in most states until the best available technique for handling border-line cases (namely the psychopathic hospital) is established. We place upon another page in parallel columns several of these points.

As we have throughout insisted, psychiatry is an art, a branch of practical medicine. Yet it cannot be denied that there are many generalities about psychiatry which go to make up a respectable body of theory. Some authors distinguish a special psychiatry from a general psychiatry, the former containing descriptions of separate forms of mental disease and the latter presenting a variety of general statements. The better usage is to apply the term "psychopathology" to the body of scientific theory which has been built up out of psychiatry taken in relation to medicine, psychology, and other mental sciences as a whole. The best usage would define the psychopathologist as a theorist in mental disease and the psychiatrist as a practitioner therein. To be sure every practitioner needs a body of theory to go upon and must therefore be trained in psychopathology. The reverse is, no doubt, not at all the case; and non-practitioners, even non-medical men, have made enormous additions to our knowledge of the theory of mental disease. The lay reader who dips into modern works on the topic of psychiatry will almost always find long sections deal-

443

ing with "general" psychiatry or with psychopathology and will find therein descriptions of, for example, hallucinations, delusions, morbid emotions, and will-disorders taken in a general way and outside their setting in the special forms of mental disease. The lay reader must be warned against transferring ideas from these theoretical parts of textbooks directly to the patients. On the other hand it is rather easy for the lay reader to gain some notion of the special forms of mental disease in their larger outlines. Indeed we have known medical students, social workers, psychologists, and even jurists who possessed more exact ideas about some forms of mental disease than do many general practitioners of medicine.

A word concerning clinical neurology. Medical school curricula, national medical associations, and a variety of textbooks assure us of the existence of a field of *nervous* diseases separate from that of mental diseases. The relations here are a little difficult for the lay reader to grasp. The mind has close relations with the nervous system, and the term *neurology* seems to specify a science of everything nervous. Accordingly the neurologist living up to the Greek roots of his professional title is apt to regard himself as *ex officio* a psychiatrist. On the other hand the psychiatrist in his practical diagnostic work has to use many of the coarser methods of the neurologist and finds himself *nolens volens* in the end a sort of neurologist.

In the Great War the surgeon general of the army developed a division of neurology and psychiatry, and practically no distinction was made between the officers working under this division. In fact, they were often termed *neuropsychiatrists*. Some think that a new art of neuropsychiatry combining the neurological and psychiatric branches of older medicine is to be established. This is not the place to discuss or to define the fields of clinical neurology and psychiatry. After all, both the clinical neurologist and the psychiatrist are physicians and have the same fundamental medical training. Many men unite theoretical and practical knowledge in two fields. The senior author of this work has elsewhere tried to define the present-day differences in these two types of professional men by describing the clinical neurologists as rather more analytical and the psychiatrists as rather more synthetical in their viewpoints. This means to say that the clinical neurologist is on the whole rather more apt to leave his patient a mass of reflexes, and the psychiatrist is rather more apt to talk of his patient in general terms. It is easy to see that each method readily slips into over-emphasis of details or generalities. The middle of the road must be taken.

We pass to a brief summary of the major forms of mental diseases as they occur in practice. It is customary to say that textbooks on psychiatry greatly disagree upon their subject matter. But there is far more disagreement upon terms than upon facts. And there is naturally far more disagreement about details than about the major groups of mental disease. The cases in Book III have been presented in groups which are found in most textbooks of psychiatry. These groups are presented in a special order. We do not here need to argue for the virtues of an orderly approach in diagnosis, since our entire work must be regarded as perfectly hopeless if the reader has not been convinced of the value of the orderly approach as shown in Book I and especially in Book II. The value of order in the world's work is a truism. The orderly diagnosis of mental disease is as valuable a method as the orderly diagnosis of the social factors which we have grouped in this book under the title of the *Forms of Evil*. In fact the impulse to the classification of evils herein adopted was derived from the senior author's work on the orderly diagnosis of mental diseases.

We have thrown our cases into eleven groups, of which the eleventh is a miscellaneous or rag-bag group of mental diseases either severe or mild (but for the most part mild) that do not fit the definitions of the other ten major groups of mental disease. This eleventh miscellaneous group would be of special abhorrence to the old-time alienist limited in his view of mental disease to the notion of medico-legal insanity. The old-time alienist who cannot think of insanity except in terms of internment in an asylum or of testamentary incapacity, cannot readily be got to deal with the psychopathic personalities and other disorders of this eleventh group. It is somewhat as if the general practitioner of medicine should refuse to consider any case of disease which was not bedridden. The eleventh group of the psychopathies, psychopathic personalities, etc., must comprise, it will be seen, many of the cases of mild and dubious mental disease which the modern psychopathic hospital has been especially established to class and treat.

The eleventh group is placed last, because the attempt should be made to class every mental suspect more definitely in one of the preceding groups. Concerning these preceding ten groups, it is worth while to insist that nothing ultimate is claimed either for the number or the nature or the special order of the groups. That some order of disease groups should be adopted for the purposes of diagnosis is highly desirable. That this particular order is the best at the present day is perhaps doubtful. Nor will anyone maintain that this particular order will outlast the decade.

The first four groups in this sequence are of particular social interest. The first group contains the mental diseases due to syphilis, a group of diseases of increasing importance in practical psychiatry and the bridge over which the new associations between mental hygiene and public health will pass owing to the fact that the most concrete contributions to the technique of mental hygiene have been made in this field. Nor can anyone doubt that feeble-mindedness is a leading social problem. Epilepsy, particularly in its milder and so-called "equivalent" forms, is another topic of social interest both because public institutions must always eventually be built for epileptics of a given state and because there are always so many "sane" epileptics who are in no sense asylum cases but are very proper subjects for social work and mental hygiene. Fourthly, alcoholism is, or has been in this country up to the passage of the national prohibition legislation, a most important social factor of mental hygiene. Inasmuch as the group here defined contains the drug addicts (so far as drugs produce mental disease and disorder), the group may, no doubt, always remain of practical social significance.

Though the main reason for arranging these disease groups in this particular order (first proposed in 1917) was the reliability of tests and other diagnostic criteria in the groups, yet the order was adopted with a weather eye to the social values of the groups. If the psychiatrist could be made to consider definitely such socially interesting matters as (a) syphilis, (b) feeble-mindedness, (c) epilepsy, (d) alcohol and drugs, the battle was almost won for a broad conception of psychiatry. If the psychiatrist was compelled by routine to learn whether his mental patient was syphilitic, he was compelled to resort to laboratory methods of a certain refinement. If he took seriously the question of feeble-mindedness, he had perforce to resort to standardized methods of mental testing. If he was to make up his mind about either epilepsy or alcoholism he had to have by him the means of securing a social history. In short, the psychiatrist who should deal scientifically with the questions raised in these first four groups would have to have at his command the services of a proper modern clinical laboratory, the resources of a psychological service, and the resources of psychiatric social work.

It will be known, even to the layman who has had contacts with this field, that the majority of cases in these first four groups are cases of the so-called "organic" type. That is to say, these cases will be found upon autopsy to show serious disorder of the nervous system which can be demonstrated either by the naked eye or by the microscope. In fact the whole table of groups is found to have, roughly speaking, the property of being more "organic" at its upper end and more "functional" at its lower end. But the sequence was not chosen upon this particular basis, but rather, as stated above, on the basis of the reliability of diagnostic tests and criteria. Above all, the lay reader should not conclude that "organic" means incurable or permanent as to symptoms.

The fifth group is a group of mental diseases in which the brain shows demonstrable lesions. It is the "organic" group *par excellence* with the syphilitic, feeble-minded, and epileptic cases removed therefrom. The sixth group is a group of mental diseases in which the brain is relatively normal and in which the cause seems to reside outside the brain in some one or more organs of the body. So far as asylum material goes this group of somatic cases has seemed up to recent times to be limited. The seventh group is the group of the senile psychoses. The remaining three groups deal with topics of great difficulty and of doubtful scientific standing even today. The eighth and ninth groups of the so-called dementia praecox and of manic-depressive psychosis are groups whose distinction is a practical matter of difficult diagnosis almost daily in every hospital for the insane and even more so in psychopathic hospitals. These two disease groups may be regarded as "sister" groups of mental disease. The tenth group is that of the psychoneuroses, with which the reader of the first three books has to become familiar, in striking instances in which mental fac-

tors, operating apparently by themselves, have directly produced mental disorders. So far as we are aware, practically
every psychiatrist of today recognizes the existence of these
major groups or of their most important single representatives
amongst the diseases.

The alert reader may well have inquired long before this
point in our exposition whether a patient may not fall into two
or more of these groups. Let us emphatically say that it is
entirely possible that a patient shall be syphilitic, feeble-minded,
epileptic, alcoholic, a victim of coarse brain injury, a victim of
somatic disorder operating from outside the nervous system
and a senile; that is, a patient may possess characteristics that
fall in every one of the first seven groups. To be sure it may
be better to describe him chronologically. He might be described as a feeble-minded person whose brain lesion was such
as to have produced epilepsy, who had not only acquired syphilis
of the nervous system but had sundry other destructive injuries of his brain and who had, in the vicissitudes of life,
become alcoholic, had developed diseases in the body at large
which had in turn reflected themselves in the patient's mind
and who had at last become senile in such wise that the senile
brain changes were contributing a dementia to the already
complicated picture. To be sure for the present we have no
such case to offer, and such extensive combinations of factors
are, no doubt, rare. But can we continue to catalogue on a
theoretical basis? Is it, for example, possible for a feeble-
minded person to become a victim of dementia praecox? The
answer to this question cannot be given with certainty at this
time; but on the whole there is considerable evidence for an
affirmative answer, and some authors freely assert that dementia praecox may be grafted upon feeble-mindedness. As
for manic-depressive psychosis its phenomena are found in the
majority of mental diseases, which may develop periodical
emotional disturbances; but it is doubtful whether we should
term all such instances of an apparently cyclothymic nature
cases of manic-depressive psychosis. As for the psychoneuroses, no doubt they can develop upon any or all of the bases
above enumerated. But if a case of mental disease exhibits
phenomena that might, at first glance, place him in one of the
lower groups in our sequence, then, in fact, it is the usual rule
to give him the diagnosis of the earliest group to which he can

be found related. This is probably on account of the pragmatic and therapeutic value of so classing the patient.

Let us indicate some of the more important social values of these groups.

Group I, the syphilitic group of mental disorders, is a very important one to the social worker. In the first place the establishment of the diagnosis almost always means the possible suggestion of treatment, which treatment may be relatively expensive and sometimes hard to persuade the patient to take. In the next place, the spouse and children of the neurosyphilitic need examination to determine whether they are not likewise infected with syphilis. If so, they can come before they have developed mental symptoms and in their own interest be treated in suitable clinics or otherwise. It is the task of the social worker to see that this family work in neurosyphilis be carried out. Some of the points in this work have been set forth in a work by Southard and Solomon entitled *Neurosyphilis, Modern Systematic Diagnosis and Treatment* (1917), one whole section of which is devoted to medico-legal and social problems. Some of the cases in this book have been presented again in this work redescribed from the standpoint of social work. This group is the group of the popularly known disease, general paresis, sometimes known as "softening of the brain." Southard and Solomon in 1917 reported that something like twenty-five per cent of their cases of general paresis yielded considerably to treatment. This percentage is higher than other authenticated percentages. Perhaps the lay reader will not be too much impressed with a twenty-five per cent yield of therapeutic successes; but if the layman considers the results in chronic diseases in general and remembers that this disease comes as a rule ten years after the initial infection with syphilis, he will see that such results as twenty-five per cent recoveries are important.

The social values of Group II, of the feeble-minded, are too much in the public eye at the present moment to require exposition here. Not only have the psychologists following Binet produced mental tests of value but these tests have been very widely employed by the more or less competent lay workers and the whole topic has absorbed public interest. The articulation of this problem with the problems of crime and prostitution is well known, not to say overdrawn, in the public prints. Practically half of the prostitutes examined by the White Slave Traffic Commission of Massachusetts turned out to be in some degree feeble-minded.

Concerning Group III, note was made above of the popular interest in the "sane epileptic." Some authors have emphasized the relation of the so-called epileptic personality with its very pronounced egotism and ill-humor. Doubtless in this field there will be much scope for mental hygiene in the future. But the social worker can do the most good by remembering that epilepsy has a large number of subgroups. The formula to bear in mind is that it is much truer to speak of "epilepsies" than of "epilepsy."

Concerning Group IV, the alcoholic group and the drug group, we have at times referred to the special values of the Men's Club as employed for some years at the Psychopathic Hospital in Boston. But the idea is an old one. The Salvation Army has in the past done much good in the rescue of alcoholics from their habits. The victim of delirium tremens is an especially good social risk, as he often coöperates extremely well upon recovery.

Groups V, VI, and VII are of lesser social importance since for the most part the problems that arise therein are either not at all to be settled by social work or else can be settled with considerable ease.

Groups VIII, IX, X (that is, dementia praecox, manic-depressive psychosis, and psychoneurosis) become once more of prime interest to the social worker. Dementia praecox and manic-depressive cases are constantly apt to fall into the dubious position, whether they require interning in an asylum or do not. The relations of the friends to this situation then become critical. Apparently a multitude of adjustments may need to be made in these groups by the social worker. Mild cases of both of these diseases, but especially of the manic-depressive group, often want to go home prematurely and often do go home against the advice of the physicians. The social worker may here become of great practical value. Somehow the laity is rather apt to regard the psychiatrist as a kind of ogre who wishes to get even the mildest and most doubtful psychopathies into his institutional net for safe-keeping or observation. The social worker can help to dissolve this idea of something ogreish in the psychiatrist. Patients recovering from depression (manic-depressive psychoses) are particularly difficult cases to handle. During convalescence these patients are approximately normal; yet at a time when the depression still persists but the power of the will has steadily increased comes the zone of danger of suicide. The patient is still dominated by depressing thoughts but is no longer protected against suicide by the weakness of will which prevailed in the peak of his illness. The relatives need to be convinced that their patient should be retained in hospital a few weeks longer to pass through this zone of will weakness.

Finally nothing in this book has been more convincing than the need of social work in the field of psychopathic personalties, here grouped in the last Group XI.

Now and then from a general social worker comes a request for lists of symptoms by which, supposedly, the different mental diseases may be recognized. Social workers who have dipped into works upon psychiatry can follow us when we say it is not at all impossible to match the symptoms of any disease which we may confront with the symptoms of several diseases as described in the medical books. In fact, the more thorough and accurate the psychiatric textbook, the more likely would be the facts in the particular case to match with the facts in the books as presented under a great variety of headings. It is not alone the tyro, but also the expert, who is amazed to find that all the symptoms in his case can be found, let us say, under the different headings of syphilis, dementia praecox, manic-depressive psychosis, etc. To use the language of medical logic, we can briefly put the situation by saying that in the field of mental diseases, there are few or no indicator symptoms. Any symptom, *e.g.,* mania, depression, persecutory ideas, grandiosity, hallucinations, and so on through the list, may be found alone or even in multiple combination with other symptoms of the list in virtually any one of the great groups of mental diseases.

A good many persons believe that a disease is composed of symptoms, but nothing is more erroneous. The symptom indicates the disease. The disease is an infinite mass of processes and of arrangements. It is a mistake to think that because it can be shown that general paresis has a certain kind of pupillary disorder and a certain kind of speech disorder, and a certain mental state characterized by feelings of grandeur, these three things, disorder of pupils, disorder of speech, delusions of grandeur, in any sense constitute the disease. No symptom constitutes the disease. No group of symptoms constitutes a disease. One rather comforting fact about mental disease is that, after all, there are so few symptoms to a given disease. The most complicated disease that runs through the entire make-up of the person, influences every move of his entire future, goes back to his entire past, will be found to have but one symptom, or two or three, rarely more than ten or a dozen symptoms. These must be, in the nature of things, mere indicators of the situation.

In short there are no indicator symptoms, or what are called in the books pathognomonic symptoms. In medicine there are certain pathognomonic symptoms; thus in smallpox, the pock of smallpox is pathognomonic; it does not occur in any other disease, and you get it when you have that disease. Of course there are some doubtful cases where you cannot make out whether you have got a pock or not of this characteristic sort. The pock of smallpox is so characteristic that we regard it as pathognomonic. The tubercle bacillus in tuberculosis is pathognomonic,—it does not occur except in tuberculosis. But in mental disease we have not any such pathognomonic symptoms that point to any certain disease.

There are a few combinations of symptoms or signs that indicate certain diseases. However, these combinations are probably beyond the range of a person not trained in medicine to use. There may be one or two small exceptions to this in the whole of medicine. A nurse, a layman, anyone can learn to diagnosticate smallpox from the pock just as well and perhaps better than a physician. Just as a man without knowing a thing about engineering says about his automobile "the engine is skipping." The man may not know what to do about it, or he may, without knowing anything about engineering, be able to fix it; so that people can make certain diagnoses which are merely recognitions of things, of data. But when it comes to mental disease this is not so. There are not any simple points by which to recognize it, and its complicated ways are not too easy for the medical mind or for any other mind.

MAIN FORMS OF NEUROSYPHILIS

DIFFUSE NEUROSYPHILIS
  (non-vascular forms of "cerebral," "spinal," and "cerebrospinal syphilis")

VASCULAR NEUROSYPHILIS
  ("cerebral arteriosclerosis," "cerebral thrombosis")

PARETIC NEUROSYPHILIS
  ("general paresis")

TABETIC NEUROSYPHILIS
  ("tabes dorsalis")

GUMMATOUS NEUROSYPHILIS
  ("gumma of membranes, of brain")

JUVENILE NEUROSYPHILIS
  (paretic, tabetic, diffuse)

The problems of neurosyphilis (Group I) are presented in eight cases (39 to 46) at the beginning of Book III. In the book of the senior author written in collaboration with Dr. H. C. Solomon, *Neurosyphilis: Modern Systematic Diagnosis and Treatment* presented in one hundred and thirty-seven case histories, there had already been given sixteen cases of neurosyphilis having medico-legal social interests in the foreground. Numerous other cases in that series also possessed social interest. Case 39 of our present series, Greeley Harrison, was case 9 of the book *Neurosyphilis*. Greta Meyer (case 40), Walter Heinmas (case 41), David Collins (case 42), Archibald Sherry (case 45) were also all cases from the *Neurosyphilis* book, being cases 107, 97, 61, and 38. A whole volume might be written concerning the social aspects of the problem of neurosyphilis. The lay reader must bear in mind that the medical men are apt to term protean the nature of neurosyphilis. **Practically every form of mental disease can be imitated by syphilis of the nervous system.** Lesions produced by the spirochæte in the nervous system are of several kinds and of widely varying degree. In the first place syphilis may affect the membranes that surround the nervous system giving rise to the various forms of meningeal syphilis (both the delicate pia mater that immediately invests the brain and spinal cord and the thicker dura mater that overlies the pia mater are affected by lesions that may be either isolated or widespread). The blood vessels of the brain and spinal cord may be the particular target of attack by the spirochætes and the lesions of these blood vessels may give rise to destruction of the brain and spinal-cord tissues which they supply with blood. Again, when neither the investing membranes nor the blood vessels are severely or at all affected, the tissues themselves may be the point of attack by the spirochæte.

We present upon page 453 the main forms of neurosyphilis as classified for practical purposes in the above mentioned book of Southard and Solomon. Of these six main

455

forms of neurosyphilis we illustrate in the present volume **five** forms. The form omitted from the present volume is the form known as gummatous neurosyphilis, that is a gumma of the membranes of the brain. This lesion is sometimes open to surgical attack and sometimes to treatment by antisyphilitic drugs, such as salvarsan, mercury, and the like; but the problems of the disease would have nothing of special interest from the social standpoint. Diffuse neurosyphilis is represented in this volume by Greta Meyer (case 40). This disease may be a long-standing one. There is no prognosis of comparatively early death such as attends the diagnosis of general paresis represented in our series by Greeley Harrison (case 39), Heinmas (case 41), Collins (case 42), Spindler (case 43). In cases of diffuse neurosyphilis, such as that of Greta Meyer, accordingly the social worker may look for a long history of gradual development, numerous variations, remissions, and an outlook of considerable success in medical treatment. With respect to the paretic form of neurosyphilis, commonly called general paresis, we have brought out in our discussion of Greeley Harrison (case 40) that the **paretic form of neurosyphilis is not necessarily completely intractable to treatment.** We here point out that this point is a most important conception not yet well established in the medical mind. Southard and Solomon felt from their work published in 1917 that intensive treatment had proved to be of the greatest value in a number of cases of general paresis. They felt that they had cured an excellent salesman of forty-six years of age who had suffered from most aggravated mental symptoms. He not only recovered symptomatically but all his tests have been rendered negative and he has remained entirely well and economically efficient for about five years even without further treatment.

Southard and Solomon pointed out also that two or three months of active treatment will often be carried out before any signs of improvement whatever are seen. They concluded that it was **"unfair"** to give an entirely grave prognosis in any case of neurosyphilis until the effect of treatment had been tried. But whatever the outcome of the medical treatment of neurosyphilis in any of its forms, we can hope to prove in the present volume that **social treatment** yields efficient results and **should be carried out even if the medical prognosis be regarded as grave.**

The case of Walter Heinmas is a particular one from the standpoint of the social worker. As we pointed out, the rather obvious motto should be adopted by social workers, namely,— **the families of paretics are the families of syphilitics.** This motto should be followed by action. This action should consist in having the blood serum of each member of the family of the paretic (that is, his spouse and children) examined by blood tests for syphilis. The two children of Walter Heinmas had fortunately been absolutely healthy. The patient himself and his wife had no idea that there had ever been syphilis and could remember no symptoms or suspicions. Mother and daughter were well endowed in mind and general physical health, yet blood tests of all three proved positive for syphilis.

The case of David Collins is particularly valuable for the social worker. The data of this case seemed to show that **neither intense medical care alone nor elaborate social care** alone would ever turn the trick. Neither form of treatment would have been quite justifiable from a practical point of view if carried out alone. Whatever is to be the outcome in the case of David Collins, we must concede that partial or temporary cure by social service methods must be scored for the Collins family. At the present writing we have a history of five years since the first appearance of David Collins at the hospital after his falling into convulsions on the street, and we have a history of three years since the initiation of a period of regular treatment.

Archibald Sherry (case 45) is a very unusual case medically, a case of juvenile tabes, sometimes known as locomotor ataxia. Rather good therapeutic results were obtained for this twelve-year-old boy, although social work was difficult by reason of lack of coöperation on the part of the child's mother.

Harold Gordon (case 46) falls into the group of vascular neurosyphilis (see table of main forms). These cases may be completely arrested by medical treatment leaving a certain incurable but not necessarily incapacitating impairment. The point of these results lodges in the fact that the loss of power on the one side of the body (hemiparaplegia) is due to lesions of blood vessels in the brain, which lesions may be cured completely by antisyphilitic treatment, but the destruction of brain tissue entailed by the temporary or permanent plugging or rupture of the artery cannot be made good. Tissue of the central nervous system, once destroyed, cannot be regenerated. However, the victim of such a disease as syphilitic hemiparesis may recover without excessive impairment, as in the case of Harold Gordon.

Neurosyphilis is then one of the most protean of diseases. The blood test for syphilis is one of the most reliable, if not the most reliable, single blood test available to the worker in mental disease. Inasmuch as syphilis of the nervous system may through its special ways of affecting brain and spinal cord imitate practically every other kind of mental disease it becomes important to eliminate the hypothesis of neurosyphilis from virtually all cases of long-standing mental disease, particularly if this disease occurs in the male sex. It is possible for the nervous system to harbor spirochætes that cause syphilis without yielding any symptoms whatever, at all events for years or even decades. We sometimes find elaborate evidence for syphilis of the nervous system in persons who show absolutely no sign or symptom of nervous disease. But again spirochætes may produce extraordinary effects or produce huge tumor-like masses known as gummata. These gummata are in their practical effects rather more like tumors than like most syphilitic lesions.

Again it would seem as though the process is a sort of siege of the nervous system, the spirochætes affecting certain nerve tracts. This is the case in tabes dorsalis (locomotor ataxia) where the destructive process is largely limited to the posterior tracts of the spinal cord. The form of attack in diffuse neurosyphilis is quite different, as if the nervous system were not so much attacked by siege as taken by storm, and the results are disseminated over a large area. Again neurosyphilis is a simple secondary effect of blood vessel disease which results in the scooping out of huge masses of tissue which die and give rise to so-called secondary degeneration in different parts of the nervous system. These lesions or spirochætes may be overlooked and disappear and the lesions may resemble extinguished volcanoes. Yet again the diffuse process may run on apparently with perfectly fatal results to mortality in a few years both with and without treatment. However, in other cases, as we have insisted, treatment appears to accomplish much. As Southard and Solomon insist, **the prognosis of neurosyphilis is not worse than that of the chronic dis-**

eases in general. The prognosis of neurosyphilis so far as
length of life goes is certainly not bad. Remissions are always
possible though they are not frequent. We found amongst
three hundred untreated committed cases of paretic neurosyphilis five that were capable of self-support and ten more
that seemed normal enough to live at home. The patients were
said to have "remissions." Perhaps the most important thing
for the investigator to bear in mind is this: During a good
part of the early period of the course of neurosyphilis, it is
difficult or impossible to tell the paretic from the non-paretic
forms of diffuse neurosyphilis by any combination or single
observations and tests. In short we should take any diagnosis
either of general paresis (with its outlook that the patient is
going to die in from three to five years) or of diffuse neurosyphilis (with its much better prognosis) with a grain of salt.
In either case, however, it is desirable to proceed along the best
lines of social treatment whatever is to be the outcome of the
neurosyphilitic. In each instance also it is important to remember the other members of the family and to submit them to
blood tests. It would be an important addition to the technique of preventive medicine if the spouses and children of
all paretics were subjected to blood tests for their own
individual interest and in the interest of the health of the
community.

FEEBLE-MINDEDNESS

FIELDS OF INQUIRY

Physical Examination

Family History

Personal and Developmental History

School Progress

Examination in School Work

Practical Knowledge

Social History and Reactions

Economic Efficiency

Moral Reactions

Mental Examination

WALTER E. FERNALD, 1917

We present the topic of **social work** in connection with **feeble-mindedness** (Group II of Book III) in six cases (47-52) in Book III. But the topic has been extensively covered also in Books I and II, more particularly in cases 2, 9, 11, 13, 15, 26, 32, 35.

The social worker must become familiar with at least the generalities concerning the major subgroups of feeble-mindedness from the standpoint of the measurement of their mental levels. American usage counts amongst the feeble-minded (*a*) the idiots or feeble-minded of the lowest grade, (*b*) the imbeciles or feeble-minded of middle grade, and (*c*) the morons or feeble-minded proper. (English usage often employs the term feeble-minded for the morons only.) Modern work seems to show that between the feeble-minded proper or so-called morons and normal persons there is a group of (*d*) subnormal persons measuring by mental tests at a higher level than the morons. If this new definition is established, we shall then count from below upwards, four groups of the "feeble-minded"; namely idiots, with a mental level corresponding to that of infants; imbeciles with a mental level corresponding to that of young children; morons with a mentality corresponding to that of older children before puberty, and subnormal persons with a higher mentality but still a mentality falling short of the normal. It must be granted, however, that the mental tests at present available do not serve to mark out these higher subnormals with perfect accuracy. Indeed the term "feeble-minded" seems to have become much too strong a term to use of many persons whom we can still put down as clearly subnormal. It may be well enough to term imbeciles and idiots simply more and more pronounced examples of feeble-mindedness. It is, however, a shock to the layman's mind to hear persons of but slightly substandard mentality termed feeble-minded. Indeed, when we examine the brains of these subnormal persons, post mortem, we find that they are in general appearance but slightly, if at all, removed from normality.

When we perceive normal-looking brains in subnormal persons (even in morons we are apt to find brains that are not strikingly abnormal in the gross) we are likely to think that, by a slight twist of the wheel of fortune, such substandard persons might possibly be made proper inhabitants of the world, proper voters, and even proper parents. Perhaps a slight variation of the glands of internal secretion might serve to turn the scale! Or the trick might be accomplished, we are apt to think, by a little more intensive education! Meantime it is almost or quite impossible to draw a line between those subaverage subjects that go to make up the group of normals from these substandard persons that we are willing to term definitely subnormal. The social worker remains as much at a loss as does the psychologist. Lawyers and even judges flounder in a morass of doubt when it comes to calling these but slightly substandard subjects "feeble-minded."

Is there a group of (as it were) *superfeeble-minded* above the group of the feeble-minded proper (morons) and far above the imbeciles and idiots? The senior author of this work has sometimes argued for a new term to cover all the forms of feeble-mindedness, including the unnamed slight degree of subnormality that lies above the so-called moronity. The term chosen was *hypophrenic* and the condition of feeble-mindedness of whatever degree may be known as *hypophrenia*. We believe that, if the layman, lawyer, or judge feels quite sincerely averse to calling certain persons "feeble-minded," particularly persons in this subnormal group above the level of moronity, he ought to be far more willing to have the term "hypophrenic" used. Moreover in our public discussion of these cases (particularly in the presence of the patients themselves), would it not be highly convenient to be able to use the term *hypophrenic,* a term which is of unknown insignificance to the patient himself. When a patient who is slightly subnormal and perhaps (as often) is rather acutely conscious of his subnormality, hears himself dubbed "feeble-minded," he has a certain right to feel nettled. We feel that the employment of the term feeble-minded, even for morons of the upper grade and certainly for the subnormals that are above the level of morons, sometimes makes a kind of permanent scar in the patient's mind. We have also seen persons, who upon discovering themselves to be "feeble-minded," have forthwith denied all responsibility for any acts of theirs and given themselves serenely up to behavior which they could very readily and profitably restrain. It is all very well to be, as Dr. Richard Cabot has often insisted, *belligerent in truth-seeking* and in telling the truth, but if we employ the term feeble-minded in a very extended sense, not consistent with the lay usage of the adjective *feeble,* we are not telling the whole truth about our patients. It is worth while to insist upon this little point since so much important psychiatric social work has to be carried out with persons that are feeble-minded.

Feeble-mindedness is of interest to a great number of workers in the world. For example, (a) educators, responsible for the laggards, truants, dullards, "exceptionals"; (b) court authorities to whom the educators' problems in part drift and figure as psychopathic cases, defective delinquents, prostitutes, and the like; (c) eugenists and other persons interested in heredity who are inclined to advocate segregation in institutions or perhaps even sterilization of the feeble-minded on the basis that the entire problem is a hereditary one; (d) legislators, to whom of late feeble-mindedness has become the most interesting of social problems.

Under the case of Florence Warner (case 47) we have spoken of conditions under which mental tests must be carried out (absence of fatigue on the part of the examiner and patient; absence of all clouding of consciousness, such as infectious disease, alcohol, drugs, and the like may produce; and the absence of all stupor or dullness of mental faculties incident to mental diseases like dementia praecox).

Florence Warner illustrates the relations of feeble-mindedness to prostitution or at all events to sex irregularity. The White Slave Traffic Commission of the Commonwealth of Massachusetts did indeed find that about one-half of the prostitutes examined for their mental levels turned out to be in some degree feeble-minded. But, even if all or almost all prostitutes were feeble-minded, it does not do for the social worker to think of all feeble-mindedness in women as fatally determining irregular sex life. Further investigations of the lives of feeble-minded persons released from schools for the feeble-minded, after their schooling has been completed, has shown that many frankly feeble-minded persons, even of the female sex, have not fallen into the group of sex delinquents.

Even when feeble-mindedness is present in the sex delinquent it is not always possible to assign prostitution to feeble-mindedness as a cause. The most we can say in this contingency is that a feeble-minded person whose sex irregularities may be due to something quite other than feeble-mindedness may still be *unable to react with proper judgment* to the measures taken to stop the sex irregularity and to divert the patient's interest.

We may also refer to the discussions under case 47 of the differential values of the psychiatrist, the psychologist, and the social worker in the handling of feeble-mindedness.

The case of Bessie Newman (case 48) will be remembered as a very striking family case in which it was psychologically desirable to consider every one of the **ten members of the family** from the **psychiatric** point of view. Amongst all the cases of this work that of Bessie Newman is the one which will perhaps most repay study. The Rosenthal family (case 49) has also shown that three out of five of its members are psychopathic. The case of Bernard Bornstein (case 50) shows how a moron boy in a protected environment could be the support of his family; whereas navy life proved to be beyond his powers.

Beatrice Cellini (case 52) was handled as an out-patient under the social service without ever being in the wards of the Psychopathic Hospital. Reference may be made to the remarks under the discussion of Beatrice Cellini concerning **variations in her moods.**

EPILEPTOSES

Syphilitic

Alcoholic

Traumatic

Encephalopathic

Jacksonian

Symptomatic

Idiopathic

Psychic

Narcoleptic

Borderland

Epilepsy (Group III of Book III) is ordinarily a disease with at least (*a*) unconsciousness and (*b*) convulsions. An attack of unconsciousness alone does not constitute epilepsy and does not in itself prove the existence of epilepsy. Neither would a single convulsion, even though it were very characteristic in its appearance, prove the existence of epilepsy. If, however, the diagnosis of epilepsy is once established through medical observation of several attacks of unconsciousness with convulsions, then it becomes possible for the physician to identify certain **minor attacks** and disorders of consciousness with little or no evidence of convulsions, as epileptic. Accordingly when fainting spells, abstraction, blank feelings, and episodes of loss of memory occur, the physician is very apt to think of the possibility of epilepsy.

Modern work seems to have shown that there is an **epileptic temperament** or personality in which self-consciousness (egocentricity) and inharmony and irritability are found. The epileptic mind seems, on the whole, a little childlike, even when there is little proof of feeble-mindedness. Modern study of *epilepsy* has shown that it is much **more exact to speak of epilepsies than of epilepsy.**

The major or so-called *grand mal* attack of epilepsy consists in a fall with unconsciousness and spasm. The spasm is at first a steady tonic spasm, but there shortly appear interrupted or clonic spasms. Automatic movements follow these clonic spasms. The patient then either wakes up or passes into a deep sleep. On waking the victim feels lame and weak in the convulsed muscles, and his head may ache. There is often absolutely no warning of these attacks though very striking warnings or so-called *aurae* (such as flashes of light, sounds, or smells) may occur and as a rule always in exactly the same form. The muscles are apt to be affected, always in the same order, and the convulsion is then said to "march" in a characteristic way. Tongue-biting and frothing at the mouth are observed, and the patient may involuntarily urinate. It can readily be seen that the social worker who secures the history of tongue-biting or urination in an attack of epilepsy may be contributing most important evidence for medical diagnosis.

It seems to have been proved that the epileptic attack of the nature above described may sometimes be represented by an acute mental attack without convulsion and even without evident loss of consciousness. Such an attack without characteristic features of epilepsy is termed an epileptiform equivalent. The patient may fall into a state of automatism or into a dream-state in which violent and destructive or criminal acts get done, of which the patient will have no remembrance. The crimes of violence commited by epileptics may be of the greatest brutality (see our case 54, Patrick Donovan, who killed his mother). Luigi Silva (case 53) had also been violent and destructive during a fit. The episode in Silva's case followed a heavy drinking bout. Alcohol is clinically known to bring out epileptic attacks.

MENTAL DISEASES CAUSED BY ALCOHOL AND DRUGS

In our account of the pharmacopsychoses, that is, the mental diseases due to alcohol and drugs (Group IV of Book III), we have presented five cases, four alcoholic and one drug (Marian Spring, case 63).

The four alcoholic cases are intended to exemplify the four forms of alcoholic mental disease that come to the attention of the social worker. John Logan (case 58) is a case of acute alcoholism. We may remind the lay reader that **acute alcoholism is not identical with acute alcoholic psychosis.** Of course it is true in one sense that drunkenness is a temporary mental disorder, but drunkenness is not a disease in the sense of an entity with a characteristic onset, course, and duration. Drunkenness is not commonly accounted a mental disease. Acute alcoholism is a term frequently used to cover drunkenness and other comparatively mild mental effects of alcoholism, falling short of our conception of mental disease. Chronic alcoholism is a term used to describe a habit of drinking which, though it may be the basis of a development of mental disorder, is also not in itself a mental disease. Drunkenness and alcoholism, acute or chronic, are conditions, according to present usage, outside the field of mental diseases.

Patrick Nolan (case 59) is a case of **delirium tremens** which may be compared in its symptoms with the case of John Sullivan (case 60) an instance of so-called **alcoholic hallucinosis.** Delirium tremens, the better known and somewhat commoner of these two affections, is a comparatively brief disease whose acute symptoms commonly do not run beyond a week in duration. Alcoholic hallucinosis, on the other hand, is apt to run two or more weeks. Neither delirium tremens nor alcoholic hallucinosis depends for its severity upon the amount of alcohol consumed. Both diseases, as a rule, appear in persons who have long been victims of alcoholism. (Here again it is impossible to assert that the severity of a mental disease can be measured by the duration or extent of the alcoholic habit.)

The distinction between these two diseases is even to the physician far less easy in practice than in theory. The most striking mental difference in the two diseases is the presence of hallucinations of sight in delirium tremens and hallucinations of hearing in alcoholic hallucinosis. Yet even this distinction may fail us in certain cases. The name delirium tremens in itself points to the extreme severity of the symptoms, that is to the existence of (a) delirium and of (b) tremors, and the victim of delirium tremens is, on the whole, a much sicker-looking man than the victim of alcoholic hallucinosis. Of the two diseases, alcoholic hallucinosis is ordinarily the worse one, since the capricious scolding voices readily lead to suspiciousness and delusions of persecution that may outlast the pronounced mental symptoms and reach into the convalescent life of the patient. In fact some of these latter cases during their state of recovery and for long periods after the acute symptoms are over, very strikingly resemble victims of dementia praecox. Moreover cases of alcoholic hallucinosis are not apt to get well so frequently or so completely as victims of delirium tremens.

Michael Piso (case 62) we have used to represent the so-called **alcoholic jealousy-psychosis.** The theory here seems to be that long-continued alcoholism has reduced the sexual power of its victim, who then becomes jealous of the relations of the spouse to some supposed paramour. The case in the text shows a comparatively happy outcome through medical and social effort.

Our case of **morphinism,** Marian Spring (case 63) is, no

doubt, an example of the so-called psychopathic personality, as are many victims of morphinism and cocainism. We count the case as a social-service failure, but the details (note especially the patient's lying) are of interest. Marian Spring also illustrates the tendency of morphinists and other drug addicts to work in groups.

That the reader may obtain some inkling of the conditions in certain other major groups of mental disease, we present in cases 63-68 two instances each of mental disease due to destructive disease of the brain, the disease of the eye indirectly affecting the mind, and to certain complications of old age.

BRAIN DISEASE

It is plain that destructive disease of the brain (Group V of Book III) will, as a rule, send its victim pretty promptly to some hospital for nervous or mental disease, leaving the family problem a comparatively simple one, not as a rule troubled by any special mental feature on the part of the patient himself. The group, a fairly small one in this line of practice, is of no great statistical consequence to social workers.

BODILY DISEASE

As to mental disease due to diseases of the body at large (Group VI of Book III) such as diseases of the glands of internal secretion, typhoid fever, pneumonia, influenza, pellagra, and the like, there are on the whole very few cases, statistically speaking, and still fewer that come under the social worker's care. An exception would need to be made for pellagra in the southern states and no doubt an important piece of social research could be carried out upon the pellagra situation in the southern states. Most important data concerning the culinary and sanitary relations of pellagra could be made by social workers.

We have chosen to illustrate this group by a case of hyperthyroidism, Ethel Murphy (case 66) and one of mental disease due to influenza, Joseph O'Brien (case 67).

OLD AGE

Problems of great interest are associated with social work amongst seniles (Group VII of Book III). Of course it is well known that not all old persons pass into anything like a condition of dementia or evident deterioration. Some authors, it is true, speak of a **physiological dementia** (?) and seem to think of old age as capable of producing mental disease or at least dementia. We must guard ourselves against generalizing in this way. We have chosen two cases which ordinarily would seem a bit hopeless from the standpoint of social work but which proved very amenable to social-service methods. We are under the impression that the psychiatric point of view, if it should penetrate to the homes for aged persons and old soldiers, might prove of singular value in the handling of concrete problems of senescence.

DEMENTIA PRAECOX

The schizophrenic cases—dementia praecox (Group VII of Book III), form a large and important group in the field of psychiatry. Beginning most frequently during adolescence or early adult life and having a very grave prognosis, schizophrenia affords many distressing social situations. This psychosis has two main characteristics: (a) a splitting of the personality (schizophrenia) and (b) a tendency to deterioration. "Splitting" means that there is no longer a congruity between the three psychological elements that form the personality; namely, the intellect, the affective reactions, and the will. The result is emotional apathy, loss of interest in one's family, lack of normal activity, inability to carry out one's purpose. The majority of persons afflicted with this form of disease develop ideas of persecution, believe they are being followed, interfered with, not given a square deal, and the like. Hallucinations are apt to be prominent. These disorders associated with a general psychic decrepitude may necessitate commitment in an institution for the insane. When the disease remains chronic, the patient may continue in an institution for the remainder of his life. The social procedures in the chronic committed cases are relatively simple. It is not, however, correct to assume that no case recovers. Many patients with dementia praecox make fair recoveries and are able to live in the community. Often the defect resulting from the disease is mild in degree. Even so, these patients need guidance and aid, and most of them require some form of social assistance.

The schizophrenic group is brought to the attention of the social worker chiefly, during the early or incipient period of the disease. For months and often for years before a patient has the outstanding symptoms of a psychosis, mental peculiarities, character anomalies, unusual actions, and maladjustments lead to observation by social agencies. Unless an astute psychiatrist sees the patient in this early state, the person is likely to be considered as stubborn, unreliable, delinquent, obtuse, peculiar, or lazy, rather than ill and a proper subject for understanding, sympathy, and help. Many are the difficulties, delinquencies, and misfortunes due to early symptoms of the disease.

Despite the relative impossibility of affecting cures in the disease with our present knowledge, it is surprising how much may often be accomplished to improve the social reactions of these patients by proper social adjustments. Unfortunately much useless effort is expended by social workers in attempts to aid such persons before their disease has been diagnosed.

The symptoms which may be manifested by schizophrenia patients are numerous and varied. In fact, Kraepelin, in his latest classifications, considers seven varieties of dementia praecox and the closely allied paraphrenias. It is obviously not desirable to present the medical points of this complex disease except in a medical treatise. It may be noted that the symptoms result in peculiarities in the patients that lead to a lack of "empathy."

Medical science has not solved the major problems of schizophrenia, *i.e.,* etiology and pathology. As a corollary no specific treatment is known. Every case must be carefully considered, however, from the purely medical side for evidences of endocrine disorder, organic disease, and metabolic disorder, as well as for psychological factors in the life of the patient. Life experience and environmental conditions play an important rôle in the development of the psychosis. So the social worker may have a function in prevention and treatment as well as in social adjustment.

It is important to place schizophrenic patients under care at the earliest possible moment; as it is with any person developing a disease, acute or chronic. Many schizophrenics show character anomalies from early childhood that are suggestive. Among these traits may be mentioned "shut in" personality, inability to make friends and take part in communal activities with zest, supersensitiveness, over-conscientiousness, egocentricity, metaphysical ruminations, obstinacy, phantasy-formation, or day-dreaming. **These characteristics cause such persons to be considered peculiar, eccentric, exceptional, or difficult; whereas they should indicate a careful psychiatric examination.**

Some of the problems of schizophrenia are presented in twelve cases of Book III, cases 70-81. Dana Scott (case 70) is a case of the simplex form, a type that is often undiagnosed. This type of schizophrenia is seldom seen in the institutions for the chronic insane, the victims usually remaining in the community, presenting difficulties to society and finding life a serious problem. Proper environmental treatment met with relative success in the case of Scott.

Ralph Johnson (case 71) is another patient who presented numerous problems to society, which arose, presumably, as a result of his mental state, diagnosed as dementia praecox. Wanderlust, alcoholism, idleness and poverty, hypochondria, hallucinations and delusions, punctuated the life history of this man. Improvement in his attitude and conduct was shown after the combination of medical and social treatment. Persons with this type of mental disease are familiar to social agencies as prostitutes, tramps, almshouse habitués, and dependents.

Paraphrenia is a diagnosis applied to cases akin to dementia praecox, but showing less dissociation of the personality and a slower progress toward deterioration. These cases are relatively rare and present problems similar to the dementia praecox cases. In fact, the paraphrenias are described in a subheading under the schizophrenic group. Manual Rizzo (case 72) is presented as an illustration of this type of disease, diagnosed paraphrenia systematica. (See also case 58.)

The case of Paul Ernst (case 73) emphasized the difficulty in the differentiation of schizophrenia (dementia praecox) and cyclothymia (manic-depressive psychosis) and offers a good lesson in the value of optimism. Hasty conclusions may lead one to a pessimistic inactivity in cases called dementia praecox. It is well to suspect the worst but to act on the optimistic assumption that effort will be repaid. It was so in this case.

The "spoiled child" should always make one suspicious of the possibility of a future psychosis. Nora McCarthy (case

74) was considered a spoiled child. Her later reactions led to a psychiatric diagnosis of dementia praecox. However, with a comparatively small amount of assistance, she learned to get on fairly well.

The usual mistake, especially outside of psychiatric clinics, is not that of making too serious a diagnosis and prognosis, as might be assumed to have been the case with Nora McCarthy (case 74) but, on the other hand, the tendency is to diagnose the early stage of a mental disease as psychoneurosis. A large number of schizophrenias are at first considered psychoneuroses. Clara Goldberg (case 75) received much attention under the diagnosis of psychoneurosis, but after three years of unsuccessful efforts at social adjustment the diagnosis was changed to dementia praecox, and she was put under the care of a state hospital.

George Stone (case 76) calls attention to the difficulty of deciding whether a paranoid individual should be committed. At times such patients are able to get on fairly well in the community under supervision. Stone was unable to get along, however, and had to be committed. George Mullen (case 77) on the other hand, was able to serve in the front lines of the British Army after a five months' stay in a state hospital. His improvement proved to be but temporary, and he had to be committed again after his discharge from the army.

Paul Dawson (case 78) had been a problem from early life. At the Mexican border he "broke" and received a diagnosis of dementia praecox with his discharge. He then became a "difficult case" for his family. Drafted into the army, he was again discharged with the label dementia praecox. He claimed to have "faked" mental disease to get out of the army. Experience has taught that most malingerers are psychopaths and likely to become definitely psychotic. Dawson was considered a real case of dementia praecox. Nevertheless *he made good in the merchant marine.* It is a question how long he will remain well.

Howard Lancaster (case 79) seems to show that environment is an important factor in the development of mental disease. Under civilian conditions he did well but became ill in the military service, recovering when again placed under the conditions of civil life.

The relationship of psychiatry and criminology is depicted

by Major Dobson (Captain Hill, case 80), whose dementia praecox symptoms took, in one instance, the form of forgery. His marriage may also be considered as having a psychopathological basis. It may be assumed that many of his past adventures and his instability were forerunners of more overt symptoms.

MANIC-DEPRESSIVE PSYCHOSES

In many ways the cyclothymic group—manic-depressive psychosis (Group IX of Book III), offers more of interest to the psychiatrist and psychiatric social worker than any other group of cases. The mental disorder called cyclothymia is characterized by occasional attacks with remissions, or intervals of good health. The attacks usually vary from a few days or weeks to a year or more, while the remissions may last for years or decades, or the disease may be limited to one attack. The severity of the symptoms likewise varies from very mild emotional changes to the severest types of mania and depression. The disease is chiefly an affective one, causing pathological exaggeration of the emotions. Depression, with feelings of insufficiency, self-accusatory ideas, difficulty in thinking, and general slowing up of mental and physical activity are present in the depressive stage of the disease. In direct contrast to this are the symptoms of the maniacal phase, feeling of well-being, self-appreciation, exaggerated ideas of one's own power, and mental and physical activity. In the so-called mixed phases of the disease a combination of the symptoms of depression and mania exist. Most of the symptoms are easily understood by a second person, because they are exaggerations of the normal feelings rather than new or "different" or "peculiar" reactions. Hence it can be said that one's "empathic index" is usually high toward such patients.

Cyclothymic patients do not deteriorate. No matter how severe the symptoms, how long the attack lasts, or how frequent the attacks may be, there is no resultant dementia. And as may be expected if this statement is true there is no pathological destructive brain lesion.

The hospital for mental patients is only a temporary refuge for the cyclothymic, if such hospital care becomes necessary at all. Winifred Reed (case 81) spent but a few days in the hospital for purposes of diagnosis during the first seventeen months of her acquaintance with the Psychopathic Hospital, and William Donahue (case 82) has never been an inmate of an institution for his mental diseases. Mild attacks of excitement or depression are frequently not diagnosed, and in the absence of proper diagnosis the patient may be entirely misunderstood and wrongly handled. When one correctly understands Winifred's eroticism as a symptom of the maniacal stage of a manic-depressive psychosis of only temporary duration, sympathy is evoked and proper treatment is available. Likewise one is ready and able to help Donahue over his "grouches" and spells of "lost initiative" on the ground of treating a depressed patient.

Marie Dubois (case 83) is presented as a case of manic-depressive psychosis, having a first attack at thirty years of age and a second at forty. The first attack was one of depression, the second beginning with depression went over into a mild excitement before, recovery. Such a sequence is by no means rare. Her return to the community after a fairly severe attack of mental disease brings into prominence the problem of the complete readjustment that is necessitated. Such a patient must again take her place in a community all too ready to be suspicious of anyone who has been "insane." Friends who comprehend the situation and who can aid are quite essential. The family, even if possessed of sufficient means, are rarely capable of offering intelligent aid. Here the psychiatric social worker is invaluable.

Hypomania falls in the group of cyclothymias. It is a very mild degree of mania. Joe Marino (case 84) developed this condition when but fifteen years of age. Difficulty after difficulty resulted from his overactivity. His activities were rather typical of the hypomanic—frequent changes of position and actions that led to arrest punctuated his useful career. The hyperactivity in Joe, as is typical in cases of hypomania, lasted a comparatively short period, and then he settled down. During the period of excitement, however, he was a very difficult problem, and, as during a large portion of his disease he was able to live outside of the hospital, one can see the great need for some oversight in order to steady him.

Robert MacPherson (case 85) is another example of the hypomanic condition. When the excitement is mild enough, the overactivity that is characteristic of this state may lead to useful accomplishments. This, of course, is not the rule, but at times patients are seen who are more successful during this period because of the lessened inhibitions. They may be more capable as salesmen. They execute their ideas without further thought. MacPherson made more money during his hypomanic state than he would have made had he been normal. However, he squandered it with great abandon. Frequently patients in this condition, as well as patients in the early stage of general paresis, will squander their possessions and run up debts, as well as spoiling their reputations by fast and lascivious living. From this point of view, if from no other, it is very important that recognition of this condition be made early, in order that the patient may be prevented from performing foolish and dangerous acts.

Two main characteristics of the manic-depressive psychosis, namely, repeated attacks and complete recovery, are well illustrated by the case of Clarence Adams (case 86). For the rest his case shows the same type of problem as the two preceding cases.

A word should perhaps be said about one important social complication of the depressive phase of the manic-depressive psychosis. This is the *potentiality of suicide.* While it is quite possible to supervise maniacal patients outside of the hospital, despite their tendencies toward fast living and delinquency, it is much more dangerous to handle a depressed patient outside of the hospital. Although the symptoms may be mild and the patient quite willing to sit about the house, and so may be easily cared for, it is an exceedingly risky matter to leave the depressed patient at home and in the community because of his great tendency to suicidal attempts. It is for this reason that one is prone to advise hospitalization for the depressed case until recovery is quite complete.

METHODS OF PSYCHOTHERAPY

HYPNOSIS

Verbal Suggestion
Fixation
Fascination
Various

SUGGESTION (WAKING)

Verbal
Drug
Apparatus

AUTOSUGGESTION
DISTRACTION
TERRORISM
INFLICTION OF PAIN
PERSUASION
WILL TRAINING
OCCUPATION THERAPY
ISOLATION
PSYCHOANALYSIS

Various classifications have been offered for the cases that fall under the general heading of psychoneuroses (Group X of Book III). A fairly generally accepted and workable classification is that which divides the psychoneuroses into cases of (*a*) neurasthenia, (*b*) psychasthenia, (*c*) hysteria, and (*d*) anxiety neuroses. These various cases were placed together in a group called psychoneuroses on the assumption that there was no definite underlying organic pathology to explain the symptoms. The mental attitude or psychological condition is supposed to have a prominent place in the development of these conditions. The diagnosis is usually difficult. It must be made only after a careful physical examination which rules out bodily disease. Neurasthenics are usually considered by the laity as imagining numerous organic diseases. They feel tired and worn; complain of peculiar sensations in their heads and inability to concentrate; and are apt to fear many types of disease. Psychasthenia may be considered as something of a psychological anomaly. Under this diagnosis are placed those people who are known as worriers and doubters, who have many fears and obsessions, who often have difficulty in thinking clearly and logically, becoming "mixed up" as they often say. This condition is usually present from early life, but is subject to exacerbation of symptoms. The hysterics are those patients who present numerous symptoms, such as paralysis, blindness, deafness, mutism, convulsions, sensory disturbances, in fact, almost any symptom without evidence of organic disease. The anxiety neurosis is characterized by a condition of anxious fear, which may overcome the patient at any time.

Patients suffering from one form or another of the psychoneuroses are very common at all medical clinics, and are usually the despair of the physicians. Finally they make their way to the psychiatrist, possibly after months or years of treatment in the general clinic; possibly after having numerous operations in the attempt to relieve symptoms which it is later believed were dependent upon a mental state rather than upon a visceral pathology. Only in the severe exacerbations of their symptoms do these patients become inmates of a state hospital for the care of mental cases. During a large portion of their disease they remain in their homes, frequenting physicians' offices or dispensaries. Occasionally an outbreak of marked symptoms may lead to residence in a state hospital. As a rule, these attacks last only for a short period, and they are not at all frequent. It is more usual for those patients who can afford the expense to go to a sanatorium for treatment of a "nervous breakdown." A modern psychopathic hospital will treat numerous examples of these cases.

Patients of the psychoneurotic group are patients *par excellence* for psychotherapy. Under efficient psychotherapy must be considered all those factors that affect the mind and life of the patient. Among these should be included the patient's environment. It is generally conceded that the experiences of a person and the conditions under which he lives have much to do with the development of a psychoneurosis. Therefore it is logical that efforts to improve the general environment, habits of life, and living conditions, must have a valuable place in any psychotherapeutic treatment. In conjunction with whatever form of treatment, psychotherapeutic or organic, is applied to the patient, the shaping of his living conditions is very important, and this work must fall, in large part, upon the social worker.

Maurice Eastman (case 87) is presented as a case of neurasthenia, and shows in a degree how much can be accomplished by intelligent social work.

Sadie Strauss (case 88) manifests a fairly typical hysterical condition, and is a good case in point to show the value of social work in addition to formal psychotherapy. The assistance in ironing out the family difficulties was certainly of great value to the psychiatrist in aiding him to get results by his analysis. It is pointed out in the case history that the information obtained by the social worker of the home conditions and environment of Sadie was a valuable addition in giving a rounded view of the case.

Joseph Fangillo (case 89) received the diagnosis of psychasthenia. A hyperconscientious individual, prone to doubt, finding decisions difficult, he had upon such a background at least five acute exacerbations of symptoms. From all of these he recovered fairly satisfactorily, but during a large portion of the period of convalescence he lacked sufficient force to hold himself in line without outside assistance. He had to have someone reassure him. The aid in obtaining work was very important. The family also had to be assisted over the difficult period of his "nervous breakdown." Maintaining the family in good condition was an important aid in the recovery of the patient.

Cases of *traumatic hysteria,* that is, cases in which the hysterical phenomena follow upon an accident, are always open to the suspicion of malingering on the part of the patient in order to obtain compensation. It is quite true that in many of the cases improvement is delayed until the financial settlement is accomplished, and the physician handicapped in his treatment until this matter is adjusted. Something of this matter is brought out in the case of Dennis O'Donnell (case 90) and the question is brought forward concerning the value of social-service assistance in the case.

Another case of traumatic hysteria is that of Walter Nelson (case 91). This man developing an injury during his service in the Aviation Corps, fell to the lot of the social workers of the Red Cross, and presents a similar type of difficulty to that of Dennis O'Donnell.

Hysteria very frequently develops upon what is considered as poor soil or constitutional inferiority. The early history of Martin O'Hara (case 92) certainly showed enough instability to make one consider him pretty poor material. Under army conditions he apparently broke down with what was considered to be hysteria. Upon discharge from the army, he was better, but after running into a very unsuccessful marital experience, his symptoms came on again. This case might be used to show the importance of environment on the appearance of symptoms of a hysteric nature. Assistance to Martin in adjusting his life was followed by improvement of symptoms and an ability to care for himself again.

Another illustration of the effect of environment on the production of psychoneurotic symptoms is brought forward in the case of Joseph Levenson (case 93), who developed while in the army symptoms considered sufficient to make a diagnosis of psychasthenia. Much social work was expended

upon this patient in attempts to find him satisfactory occupation, with a more or less satisfactory result.

Most of the cases of the psychoneurotic group must be considered as potential patients during a large portion of their
lives. Improvement and retrogression alternate. Unfavorable conditions of life are likely to lead to renewed difficulties,
so that these patients represent a fertile field for continued
work and are likely to be known to the social agency year
after year. Nowhere is this service more valuable or necessary, and **social adjustment is nearly always essential** before the physician can get very far with his treatment.

DUBIOUS AND SPECIAL PSYCHOPATHIAS

The last group (Group XI of Book III) includes a pot-
pourri of cases that fit in none of the preceding ten groups.
Among the cases that would fall into this group may be mentioned prison psychosis, sense deprivation psychosis, folie à
deux, litigation psychosis, paranoia, monomania, psychopathia
sexualis, psychopathic personality, and a number of undiagnosed cases. Most of the cases bearing these diagnoses are not
legally committable. They are, rather, individuals with peculiarities, eccentricities, and psychological anomalies. Living
in the community at large, as they usually do, they are likely
to be the victims of one difficulty after another. Their peculiar
mental reactions are rarely compatible with success in life.
Social agencies, courts, and reformatories are frequently confronted with the problems that these persons present. Comprehensive understanding of these people necessitates a psychiatric knowledge and insight into their disease conditions.

Possibly the most frequent of all these types is that spoken
as the psychopathic personality or the constitutional psychopathic inferior. Military experience showed how numerous
are individuals of this type. Many of the conscientious ob-
jectors, malingerers, and deserters fell into this group. They
have in common a personality defect, which usually works
against the best advantage of the patient leading him into a
continuous series of difficulties.

Previous to the military experience, the feeling was that the
vast majority of cases of psychopathic personality or constitutional psychopathic inferiority were of the female sex. This

was largely due no doubt to the fact that it was sex delinquency that brought many girls to the attention of social agencies and public authorities. The characterization of "defective delinquent" was usually given to these girls, and every social agency was familiar with this problem.

A study of defective delinquency was made by Dr. Herman M. Adler. Some of his ideas were published in an article entitled, *A Psychiatric Contribution to the Study of Delinquency.*[1] A brief review of Dr. Adler's paper will illuminate the subject. He calls attention, first, to the six groups of psychopathic personalities described by Kraepelin: the excitable, the unstable, those with psychopathic trend, the eccentric, the antisocial individuals, and the contentious individuals. Dr. Adler states:—

"It is clear that we are dealing with a group of individuals who are so nearly normal that it is only in the course of years and by the effect of cumulative evidence that they appear in any way different from the average.

"There are two main factors to be considered. The one is the intelligence of the individual, his ability consciously and logically to direct his conduct. The other is the emotions. . . . In health the two are well integrated."

As a result of his experience with a group of defective delinquents, Dr. Adler believes that they can be classified somewhat more simply than Kraepelin has grouped them or at least that a simpler classification may be offered as a working basis to understand the reactions of these individuals. He says:—

"I propose to classify the individuals who present mental or social difficulties in three groups. These groups are understood to be meant as symbols for unknown quantities rather than as explanation or precise definitions. The three groups are, in the first place, the group in which the intelligence is found to be below the lowest normal level. This is called the group of *defectives* or the *inadequate*. Into this group fall the feeble-minded, the 'Oligophrenias' of Kraepelin, the end states of dementia praecox, and of other deteriorating psychoses, of presenile, organic dementia, and so forth.

"The next group, *emotionally unstable,* includes individuals who have average intelligence or better, but who show in their

[1] Adler, Herman M., M.D. In *Journal of the American Institute of Criminal Law and Criminology,* Vol. 8, No. 1, May, 1917, pp. 45-68.

conduct and in their careers the predominating influence of the emotions. They are moody, changeable, impulsive, and in general it may be said that their conduct itself does not correspond to their beliefs, or intentions.

"The third group, the *paranoid*, includes individuals of average intelligence or better in whose careers the emotional influences are of secondary importance, but whose main difficulties are a result of mistakes in logical thought processes. The well-known characteristics which are exhibited in extreme form by the paranoid psychoses, these individuals show often to a degree which falls just short of a delusional state, egocentric ideas, and prejudices. Everything that occurs about them is referred to themselves. Their first reaction is to determine what effect any extraneous circumstance may have upon themselves. They are selfish, vain, arrogant. If they feel in optimistic mood, they are contemptuous of others. If depressed, they are resentful. Though this is a trait of their intellect, it does not necessarily interfere with their intellectual abilities, and these people are often very efficient.

"These three groups can be separated only theoretically. There are many cases that are composite, so that their characteristics fall into two or into all of these groups. Thus, few paranoid individuals go through life without strong emotional reactions which often lead to social difficulties. Similarly, the emotionally unstable will, especially during paroxysms of rage or depression, often exhibit paranoid symptoms. The defective group may show paranoid tendencies and emotional instability.

"The distinction lies rather in the behaviour of the individual as observed in the course of years than in a definite quantitative difference to be observed at a single examination. The introspective psychologist will attempt to determine in each individual by psychoanalysis or other means what the mechanism of the disturbance is. He may succeed in doing this, and still be unable to predict the future course of the individual.

"The behaviourist psychologist will not lay too much weight on the results of a single examination by whatever method, but will lay more emphasis upon the history of the case, and the previous experiences of the individual and, above all, upon the reaction of the individual to certain test situations during a period of observation. This behaviourist method offers the hope of a short cut in dealing with these individuals."

Dr. Adler then gives some considerations of a practical nature upon which to base the care and treatment of such people. We quote:—

"In every given case of delinquency or social difficulty it should be determined whether the difficulty is chiefly due to inadequate intelligence, to emotional instability or to paranoid disposition. Nothing can be gained by endeavoring to increase the intelligence of a mental defective. Nothing can be expected from an attempt to change the personality of the paranoid individual. A great deal can be accomplished, however, in controlling the emotional instability of those whose chief difficulty is the result of such instability as well as the emotional difficulties of the paranoid and defective group.

"Classification such as the one suggested in this communication is, of course, entirely too simple to completely satisfy all the demands in the individual cases, and it is to be hoped that this classification may be altered and amplified, or perhaps completely reconstructed till finally a working method may result, but even now, without general information of the subject, such a simple scheme as this one proposed has served not only to keep the ideas of the examiner grouped in orderly fashion, and this to prevent disorderly and unclear thinking on his part, but it has actually appeared to be of benefit when it was applied as a basis of therapy in these cases."

A variety of character defects was shown by the twenty-eight-year-old Harriet Farmer (case 94) who, after a history of unreliability, a long period of fabrication, alcoholism, and inability to make her own way, came to the attention of the Psychopathic Hospital as the result of a suicidal attempt. She clearly fitted into the group of psychopathic personalities. The outcome of the case showed how much improvement a character of this type is capable of making when handled by social workers guided by psychiatric knowledge.

That the type of hypoboulic (weak-willed) individuals who despite a sufficient modicum of intelligence are fated to be failures because of their defect is illustrated by Louis Sand (case 95). A Belgian of considerable education, with the best intentions in the world, with ambition but without power of concentrated effort, he had wandered from place to place. Such might be considered the classical type of constitutional inferior.

The case of Theresa Beauvais (case 96) should be a liberal lesson to the moralist and social worker. Sexual immorality in this girl is explained on the basis of a hypersexuality which might be characterized as falling into the group of psychopathia sexualis or into the larger group of constitutional psychopathic inferiority. Her promiscuity is to be considered rather as a symptom of a disease than as a pure moral deflection. With a background of exceedingly poor heredity (father a professional thief, mother a prostitute) and as vicious an early environment as could be conceived, one is justified in expecting a rather poor social result. Theresa certainly showed enough evidence of instability, will defect, and emotional outbreaks to justify a diagnosis of psychopathic inferiority or psychopathic personality. Appearances might have led to the conclusion that this girl was a moron, but psychological tests showed her of sufficient intellectual ability. It was rather in the sphere of affectivity and will that the disorder lay. It is quite important to keep this idea in mind; namely, that the affective life and the will are often more important in determining the social reactions of an individual than the intellect alone. One cannot avoid the assumption that it would take more than the ordinary amount of will-power to overcome the sexual desires of such a hypersexual individual, and one would be expecting too much if one hoped for a great deal of steadying of such a person after adult life had been reached and many pernicious habits had been formed in youth, but one should have sympathy for this girl as a victim of disease rather than as merely vicious. One arrives at this conclusion from a psychiatric study of the whole life of the patient.

The value of the psychiatric attack on a patient not necessarily markedly psychopathic is discussed in the case of Leon Blumer (case 97). Pseudologia fantastica, or pathological lying, falls under the general heading of the psychopathic personality or constitutional psychopathic inferiority. It is usually associated with other evidence of character defect or psychopathia. A person afflicted with this type of abnormality is certain to be considered a "difficult case" and pretty thoroughly disliked by those with whom he comes into association. This was indeed the fact with Francis Corcoran (case 98).

The results of a constitutional inferiority may only be brought about under the stress of circumstances. Manuel Giordani (case 99), a flute-player, got along well enough in civilian life, but under the stress of military training he had a psychopathic upset which resulted in his discharge from the army. Back in civilian life, he again succeeded.

Until his fiftieth year Henry Allen (case 100) had been considered from the results of his work, merely as a not very efficient constructional designer. A personality study at the age of fifty by a psychiatrist brought out the fact that he was of a melancholy disposition, unhappy in his work because he believed he was being made fun of by his fellow employees. He disliked the type of work he was doing and considered himself only twenty-five per cent efficient, and felt that he was physically ill. Considering Allen from this point of view, it was possible to change his working conditions, encourage him and give him a type of work that was more to his taste. Whereupon he developed greater efficiency and was able to earn twice as much as previously. This type of analysis has great prospects from the vocational-guidance standpoint, and can add to the efficiency of the individual both to the benefit of himself and of the firms employing him.

RECENT APPLICATIONS OF MENTAL HYGIENE

MENTAL DISEASE IN THE GREAT WAR

Military experience in the Great War brought out many cases of mental disorder, and showed the large part that the psychology of individuals played in their adjustment to military conditions. Twenty-five cases are submitted in this work to illustrate, in part, some of the problems with which the military service, the public health service, and the Red Cross have had to deal.

In any large group of men, it is of course evident that all varieties of mental disease will be found to occur, and among the four million men in the American military service, there were of course all varieties of mental disorder and difficulty. The term "shell-shock" which grew up at the beginning of the war from the experience of the English has led to great confusion in terminology. Originally applied by the British to cases of mental disorder, mostly of the type of psychoneuroses, under the misapprehension that these conditions were the effect of high explosives, it has been used variously to include, on the one hand, only the pure psychoneurotic manifestations, and, on the other hand, to include all types of mental disorder. This matter has been treated in full detail in a book recently published by the senior author under the title, *Shell-Shock.*

The Great War brought out a large number of cases of psychoneurotic disorder, to which a great deal of attention has been paid. The American Army treated these cases abroad, in large measure, at base hospital number 117, known colloquially as the "Shell-Shock Hospital." A description of these cases is very adequately presented in a book by Schwab and Fenton, entitled, *The Psychology of Conflict.* On the whole it may be said that there are no new problems rising out of the psychiatric cases occurring in the military service. Many of the mental difficulties would have occurred to the same patients in civilian life. However, the fact that they did occur in military service has added a very natural sentimental interest, which would probably not have been accorded these same patients had their difficulty occurred during ordinary peace times.

A new interest in mental disease has been awakened and this is particularly true in Great Britain, where a veritable renaissance has occurred. This has been one of the subsidiary benefits of the war. The American Red Cross has established psychiatric social units throughout the country, and the problems that confront these psychiatric social units, as will be seen by a perusal of the war cases herein described, are in no particular way different from psychiatric social problems of our civilian population. It is, therefore, proper to employ the same technique, medical and social, in the handling of the war neuroses and psychoses that is applied to the civil cases. As will be seen, many of the military cases have been turned over to civilian hospitals.

One feature that is present in the military cases, which is not often found in the civilian ones, is that of pecuniary compensation. When the mental disorder "did not exist prior to enlistment" and occurred "in line of duty" it has been generally held that the patient is entitled to compensation for disability. The situation in this regard is similar to that which would hold for tuberculosis or any other chronic disease.

Seven of the eleven psychotic groups that have been described are exemplified by the twenty-five patients having relations with the military service.

Carl Spindler (case 43) and Thomas Scannell (case 44) were patients suffering with syphilopsychosis. Carl Spindler was transferred to a civilian hospital with a diagnosis of general paresis. Symptoms of this disease had developed while he was in the service, but the syphilitic infection which led to the development of paresis was acquired long before entering the service. Nevertheless, it is often assumed in these cases that the government is somewhat liable in the way of compensation, the argument being that the mental symptoms developed during service, they were not present prior to enlistment, and that possibly these symptoms would not have arisen had the patient not undergone the hardships of military life.

Thomas Scannell was probably a case of juvenile paresis, that is, he had the symptoms of general paresis which had developed from congenital syphilis. He was being cared for by the Red Cross. Here, again, the same question would arise as to whether or not the government was responsible for his care on the grounds that his mental enfeeblement had occurred while he was in the military service.

The problem of feeble-mindedness was much diminished in the army by the psychological testing and the rejection of feeble-minded individuals by the neuropsychiatric division. Despite this, many feeble-minded were in the army, and it was held by many that for certain work behind the lines the feeble-minded had a very definite place. However this may be, there were numerous examples of the feeble-minded in the army. The navy and the marine corps were not so careful to eliminate individuals of low mental status.

Thomas Fuller (case 9) had had a bad record in civilian life. It was felt that this was largely the result of his mental retardation, his mental age being only 9.2 years. Despite this fact, he made good in the marines, and even rose to the rank of corporal. The obvious reason is that under proper supervision a person of inferior mentality may be a very valuable worker.

It does not follow, however, that all feeble-minded individuals make good under the type of supervision given in the army or navy. Bernard Bornstein (case 50) did fairly well in civilian life, earning between fifteen and twenty dollars a week, but was quite unable to succeed when he joined the navy. His mates plagued him and he was such a misfit that it was necessary to discharge him. The feeble-minded individual is likely to be unreliable, and when this is markedly the case, he cannot be of course fitted into the discipline of military service.

The sort of difficulty that a feeble-minded individual may get into in the army is well illustrated by the case of Howard Driscoll (case 51). His army record was sprinkled with A.W.O.L.'s and after his discharge from the army he was sentenced to a reformatory. He returned to the army during the war, where he got into difficulty by leaving his post for four days because he got angry. He did not receive the treatment that would ordinarily be accorded to a normal individual, but was given his discharge as a feeble-minded person. Supervision will be necessary for this man throughout life and he would probably be best served if he could be put under the paternal care of an institution.

One of the important pieces of neuropsychiatric information that came out of the army experience was the frequency of epilepsy in the community at large. In our series four cases of epileptic psychosis are presented in patients who came within the purview of the military service. John Manaos (case 29) was arrested for not properly filling out his draft papers. In prison he developed a clouded mental state, and at the hospital the diagnosis of epilepsy was made. Upon this finding, of course, the charges against him were dropped, as it was felt that he was not a responsible individual.

Charles Lovell (case 55) was given his discharge from the army because of epileptic attacks. The epileptic phenomena occurred for the first time while in the army service in the cases of Frank Wayne (case 56) and John Bristol (case 57) Wayne had been a weakling throughout his life, was recognized as somewhat simple-minded, and incapable of hard work. Under the stress of the army, the seizures of epilepsy made their appearance, and after discharge he was, of course, a subject for compensation. John Bristol, on the other hand, had been a very healthy and stalwart individual, serving on the police force before his enlistment, and being athletic instructor at camp. For some reason, seizures began after typhoid inoculation, and have continued with great frequency to the present time. He is, therefore, another subject for compensation, and has been obtaining assistance from the Red Cross in securing work that he is capable of performing.

The types of manic-depressive psychosis will have to be considered. In a general way, it was considered before the war experience was at hand that the conditions of the military service would produce a great many cases of manic-depressive psychosis, and that the individual who had had a psychosis would be very likely, indeed, to break down.

Robert MacPherson (case 85) developed a hypomanic condition which was probably the cause of his discharge from military service.

On the other hand, Clarence Adams (case 86) had had psychotic symptoms from which he recovered before entering the service. He did very well, being at the front and being gassed without having any return of his symptoms. After his discharge, while in civilian life, he again developed psychotic symptoms which led him to the hospital. It is indeed to be borne in mind that the change from the military back to civilian life is quite a severe shock at times, and it takes a considerable amount of ability to make a successful and easy change.

Dementia praecox cases were frequent enough during the war, and are still occurring as a problem in men who have been in the service. If there is one feature that might be considered as somewhat different in the military cases from those in civil life, it is that the prognosis of soldiers who were apparently schizophrenic was much better during the war period than in the usual prognosis of this type of case as seen in civil life.

Of the war cases described in this book, five had the diagnosis of dementia praecox. Kevork Ardinian (case 26) was never actually in the army, but was picked up under the "Work or Fight" law after which it was discovered that he was really a victim of dementia praecox.

George Stone (case 76) had done well in the army, where he had won the *croix de guerre*. After his discharge he developed a psychosis which was diagnosed as dementia praecox, and while outside of an institution he gave a good deal of concern to the Red Cross.

Howard Lancaster (case 79), on the contrary, developed his mental symptoms while in the army and did well when he returned to civilian life. Whereas George Mullen (case 77) was much like Clarence Adams (case 86). Mullen was committed as a case of dementia praecox in 1915, but was discharged. He joined the English Army, where he did well, and was given an honorable discharge after being wounded. On his return to civilian life, he developed a psychosis which brought him into an institution with the diagnosis of dementia praecox.

Major Mark Dobson (case 80) would have been in very serious difficulty for forgery had his condition not been recognized as dementia praecox.

The cases in the psychoneurotic group were very frequent throughout the war. Abroad they came chiefly under the acute manifestations of shell-shock. The cases as seen in America, following the war, or during the war among those patients who had not been abroad, were very much less dramatic.

James Bailey (case 7) developed neurasthenic symptoms

following a street-car accident. These symptoms did not give him very much difficulty, however, until he was at camp, when they became quite manifest, and led to his discharge.

A good example of traumatic hysteria is presented by Walter Nelson (case 91) who developed his symptoms following a blow on the head by a tent-pole which blew over in the wind. His symptoms were those that one ordinarily sees from the same type of injury in civilians, but, occurring while he was in the aviation service, it was distinctly a psychoneurosis occurring in the military service.

Martin O'Hara (case 92) had had evidences of hysteria before his army experiences. He was discharged from the army for physical disability, and after getting into an unpleasant marital arrangement, developed his hysterical symptoms again.

The picture of neurasthenia was not an infrequent one in the military service. An example is given in the case of Joseph Levenson (case 93).

The constitutional psychopathic inferiors presented themselves to the military surgeons in considerable numbers, and their vagaries will be before the people who deal with returned soldiers for many years to come. Francis Corcoran (case 98) had been a ne'er-do-well all his life. After his military experience, he became a burden to the public health service, and will probably remain a "case" for many years. Paul Dawson (case 78) had been discharged from the army for mental disease, both at the time of the Mexican border affair, and during the Great War. He claims that in both these instances he malingered. As a rule it is true that individuals malingering mental disease are really the victims of some form of mental disease. Whether or not Paul Dawson was a case of dementia praecox, as some considered, or of psychopathic personality, it is hard to state. At any rate, he did not fit into the conditions of military life.

From the standpoint of the psychiatric social worker, the military man may be of interest not as the main actor in the drama, but as a subsidiary. Thus, Elliot Calderwood (case 22) who was thought to be more sinned against than sinning, as he had been deserted by his father, a soldier in the Canadian Army. Nora McCarthy (case 74) was the fiancée of a soldier and was pregnant. Her mental difficulties arose after his departure for France, and were to a large degree patched up by marriage after his return from overseas.

MENTAL HYGIENE OF INDUSTRY

There are at least forty-two cases in this volume that have interest from the standpoint of the new mental hygiene of industry, a movement which we conceive may prove of primary value in the general social situation of the world. But we also know that it will be difficult to persuade either the theoretical psychiatrist or the practical industrialist that he **must build his sociology or his practical plan of meeting the economic unrest, from the very bottom, namely from the individual.** The standpoint of theoretical sociology and likewise the standpoint of practical industrialism has interested itself in man's movements rather than in the individual. Modern sociology feels Herbert Spencer too much of an individualist, yet some sociologists note with alarm the generality of sociologists. Ross says: "How futile is the endeavor to establish laws of succession based on the parallelism in all societies of any special development (*e.g.,* domestic or political) taken in its entirety. The error here lies in taking too large a unit of social life." Tarde also is right in saying, "This attempt to confine social facts within lines of development, which would compel them to repeat themselves *en masse* with merely insignificant variations, has hitherto been the chief pitfall of sociology." "Even the keen-eyed Marx," says Ross, "opposes to a social Past dominated by class struggle a classless, strifeless Future under the collectivist régime." But he does not come down upon the individual as the true bottom factor. "The individual," says he, "is a true factor," but he goes on to identify individualism with the "Great-Man" theory and says, "There is little of value in the Great-Man theory, which sets up a Hero for each epoch or movement and subjects multitudes of men through centuries to the spell of his purpose or ideal." He continues, "We cannot take the *individual* as our unit." Groups, relations, institutions, imperatives, uniformities are five units favorably considered by Ross who says "They precede the individual and they survive him; nevertheless they have all risen at some time out of the actions and interactions of men. To understand their genesis we must

ascend to that primordial fact known as *the social process.*"
From our point of view we rather hold that these social products can best be studied by analyses of interactions of men
starting even in the simplest groups. This point of view is as
true in industrial psychiatry as in other situations.

We found that many of our patients who were started on
an industrial decline were competent and even excellent workmen, and that with a little assistance in adapting themselves
to their employment and an explanation of their condition to
their employers, they could be refitted into industry. This
led at once to the idea that similar methods of understanding
and assistance might keep other employees from falling into
the condition of hospital patients, and further to the thought
that mental hygiene, necessary for the psychopathic employee,
would be beneficial to all persons in employment to the end of
promoting their efficiency and personal satisfaction. A committee was formed in 1914 to carry on a special investigation of the subject, on which psychiatry was represented by
Dr. Herman Adler and industry by Robert Valentine. A special social worker for psychopathic employees was engaged,
and men patients between the ages of twenty-five and fifty-five
were selected for the study. In addition to the cases assisted,
industrial histories over a period of five years have been secured for two hundred and fifty cases. The continuation of
this study until 1920 was made possible by contributions from
the Committee of the Permanent Charity Fund, Incorporated,
Boston Safe Deposit and Trust Company, Trustee.

As an outgrowth of this work, the Engineering Foundation
of New York, in 1919, undertook an investigation of the possible applications of psychiatry in industry. The term "mental
hygiene of industry" was devised by the senior author to include the contributions of three fields—psychiatry, psychology,
and psychiatric social work. Four papers were written as a
result of this inquiry.[1]

One of our anchor cases, Henry Loyal, steamfitter (case 4),

[1] Southard, E. E., M.D.: "The Movement for a Mental Hygiene of Industry,"
   Mental Hygiene, January, 1920. Also *Industrial Management*, February, 1920.
   —— "The Modern Specialist in Unrest: A Place for the Psychiatrist in Industry,"
   The Journal of Industrial Hygiene, May, 1920. Also *Mental Hygiene*, July, 1920.
   —— "Trade Unionism and Temperament: Notes Upon the Psychiatric Point of
   View in Industry." *Mental Hygiene*, April, 1920.
Jarrett, Mary C.: "The Mental Hygiene of Industry: Report of Progress on Work
   Undertaken under the Engineering Foundation of New York," *Mental Hygiene*,
   October, 1920. Also *Proceedings of the National Conference of Social Work*, 1920,

was a productive, competent, skilled worker and for the most part fairly steady in employment. The irregularity in his employment was due to his mental disease, his psychopathic personality with its periodical waves. He should not figure in the turnover analyses.

The Portuguese laborer, John Manaos (case 29), epileptic, was an irregular worker and brings up certain problems of epilepsy which every employer of labor should bear in mind. On the one hand epileptics are prone to exhibitions of extreme irascibility and bad humor from time to time. On the other hand they are often of a strongly religious cast exceedingly faithful in work, as shown to the most casual visitor at institutions for epileptics where even the so-called insane are under proper conditions made to work ably and willingly.

The nickel-polisher, Luigi Silva (case 53) is another epileptic unable to work in a community but finally successfully put to work on a farm.

The chemist John Logan (case 58) was a most steady employee and most valuable to his firm. In fact his firm was willing to allow occasional absences due to his alcoholic attacks. There can be no doubt that these occasional alcoholics would be greatly benefited if the plants employing them would call upon consultant psychiatrists for analyses of these often very valuable men. In fact such alcoholics might be saved almost completely for the community.

The salesman Paul Ernst (case 73) was a victim of periodic disease, manic-depressive psychosis (at first thought to be a case of dementia praecox).

The waiter William Donahue (case 82) had always been irregular in employment. His irregularity was no doubt due to the same cause as that operating in Paul Ernst. Another type of irregular worker is found in Louis Sand (case 95) who was a rover and had worked during five years in as many as twelve states, having originally wandered from Belgium where he had been well educated and came from a good family. We, however, likewise were unsuccessful in keeping him at a job for more than a few months.

There may be more types of irregular employment than here illustrated. We have seen instances of the periodic disease, manic-depressive psychosis, and of the permanent disease epilepsy, both of which may lead to irregularity of employment due to the mental disorder. Especially in the case of manic-depressive psychosis will it be true that mild attacks of depression hardly visible to the lay observer may lead to the throwing up of a job and to premature discharge. Some of these are amongst the cleverest workmen and the fact that they figure at all in the turnover is probably on the whole a great loss to industry. We have seen instances of periodic alcoholism (the laity is familiar with these cases under the name of dipsomania) and have called attention to the sales values to industry of some of these men. Indeed employers are fairly familiar with the necessity of letting these men have their sprees. We have become familiar with the rover or victim of wanderlust, a tendency perhaps allied to that shown in the psychopath Henry Loyal (case 4).

Alfred Mack, the packer (case 6), was one of our industrial successes. A man, it will be remembered, made better than he was to start with. His physical disability was removed and his alcoholism stopped. He has since remained a steady worker and one of the best employees in his plant. We might count the case of the woman who lived as a man, the factory worker Julia Brown (case 23), as another instance of alcoholism with certain complications of character, who after social treatment became a competent and trusted worker in her plant.

The real estate sales agent, John Sullivan (case 60), had a bad attack of alcoholic hallucinosis but was encouraged to discontinue alcohol and did so. He was advised to return to gardening and did well at it. Another alcoholic, Patrick Nolan (case 59), returned to work after D. T.'s that lasted ten days. He has since discontinued alcohol. National prohibition will tend to solve many of these problems but we must not be too optimistic concerning the relief of all problems of alcoholism by prohibition. We do not here refer to the possibility of getting alcohol illegally. We refer rather to the fact that alcoholism when it reaches the psychopathic degree or comes out in a psychopathic way is perhaps permitted to do so by some hereditary taint or acquired soil in the nervous system. We may look now for the pure illustration of such hereditary taint or acquired soil in persons who can punctuate such taint or soil by drinking.

The industrialists must be interested particularly in cases of disability from a functional neurosis, that is theoretically an always curable disease. The laundry worker, James Bailey (case 7) was apparently saved from permanent disability due to hysterical paralysis. The cure was slow.

The roofer's helper Lewis Goldstein (case 11) made a slow recovery from an industrial accident, but there were economic complications in the Goldstein case. The shipping clerk Mark White (case 16) was industrially disabled from a psychopathic condition that dated back to an accident. He was restored to industrial efficiency under social treatment, as was also Hamilton Green (case 18). John Flynn (case 19) was one of complete disability following traumatic neurosis. He was given work of no great difficulty—made slow improvement and after two years was restored to full efficiency. The machinist Dennis O'Donnell (case 90) had a psychoneurosis following an industrial accident. There are a number of problems in the O'Donnell case; owing to the new economic conditions of the war he is able to get higher wages in his new job than before.

David Collins (case 42), the paretic machinist, had to have money raised for his treatment and his wife also had to be put under treatment. The child, fortunately, when examined as to its blood serum, proved negative to syphilis.

This is not always the case as the special work of H. C. and M. H. Solomon, working in the Massachusetts State Psychiatric Institute, under the Interdepartmental Social Hygiene Board, has shown:

"Figures for the two years 1917 and 1918 show that the social worker dealt with 301 families of syphilitics, of whom 70 per cent reported to the hospital for examination. In 40 per cent of the families every member reported. Among these families 579 individuals were desired for examination. Sixty-nine per cent were actually examined and an additional 10 per cent came but were not examined for special reasons.

"As a result of this examination of families, much undiscovered syphilis—both conjugal and congenital—is found. Of 394 individuals examined, 21 per cent showed a positive Wassermann reaction. Of those found to need treatment, 51 per cent were treated at the hospital and 40 per cent were referred elsewhere for treatment." [1]

A very interesting and complicated case of psychoneurosis was the case of the cigar-maker David Stone (case 24), who

[1] Solomon, Harry C., M.D., and Maida H.: "Social Work and Neurosyphilis," *Social Hygiene Quarterly*, January, 1920.

was handicapped by a fear of open spaces. He has now recovered from this fear and works regularly at good pay as an insurance agent. Herman Simonson (case 27) also had his employment changed. He had a neurosis from which he made slow improvement. He was originally a clothes-presser and has now become efficient as a porter. The plumber Daniel Griffin (case 34), unable to work for six years as a result of psychoneurosis, was treated for a year and a half and will not yet go out alone. He has become far more active about his house and hopes are entertained that he will finally become able to work again at his trade. The machinist Ralph Johnson (case 71) was another rover and was suicidal. Under treatment he has become a steady workman.

An especially interesting case was that of the architect Henry Allen (case 100). Allen imagined unfriendly attitudes on the part of the employees and did not want to work in a large room full of fellow employees. He has now found a chance to work by himself and is doing well. The cigar-maker Maurice Eastman (case 87) was a neurotic in employment quite distasteful to him. With encouragement and occasional vacations he has been kept at work steadily. A man in the liquor business, Joseph Fangillo (case 89), had a breakdown. He was gotten into the state hospital under voluntary commitment. It was his second time in a state hospital. He has now recovered and has gone to work. A typesetter, Harriet Farmer (case 94), attempted suicide. She was at odds with her family and friends, was in poor health, and was earning low wages. Under treatment she became self-sustaining and has even been advanced in her work.

We have attempted to give in this volume all the manifold psychiatric suggestions that come from industrial accidents. We conceive that industrial accident boards all over the country should make increasing use of psychiatrists, expert medical men, but especially of the psychiatric social worker. The Industrial Accident Board of Massachusetts has to our knowledge in numerous cases got most important results from such social investigations.

That the high-grade feeble-minded person, or so-called moron, may make a good worker is shown in a number of cases. Take for instance the elevator operator Thomas Fuller (case 9). Fuller was even promoted to be corporal of the marines in war time. The army authorities are not too sure that they want to get rid of all their morons, some of whom may do very good work in menial tasks that the more normal soldiers balk at. The moron Agnes O'Brien (case 13) whose trouble was complicated by hysteria was finally made self-supporting in factory work. The laborer Rosenthal (case 49) was another moron with psychoneurotic complication, and might in fact have been figured amongst our accident cases since his symptoms date chiefly from an accident. He is now a perfectly steady and capable worker.

Whilst writing this volume we have heard of an up-to-date industrial firm that is adopting the policy of establishing a school for its morons. Such a policy is to psychiatrists encouraging since it follows the lines of Séguin and Madame Montessori.

No doubt almost every employment manager would hesitate to employ a known syphilitic. Let us, however, call attention to Greta Meyer (case 40), a case of cerebrospinal syphilis; that is to say, syphilis affecting several parts of the nervous system in a more or less diffuse way. Mrs. Meyer, after her improvement under medical treatment with salvarsan, became a social problem which could actually be closed and referred to the voluntary division of the service after a period of a year.

Another syphilitic case is that of David Collins (case 42), a machinist, a victim of general paresis; that is to say, a disease whose duration seldom runs beyond three to five years from the onset of symptoms. Many social workers and perhaps a majority of employment managers would regard such a man as hardly worth the expenditure of an extraordinary amount of time, and no doubt more time might well be placed upon other members of the family than upon the syphilitic. Still, an examination of the records of David Collins shows that he was made industrially competent and was even promoted to a job as foreman. Consider also Harold Gordon (case 46), a victim of syphilis in that form which is characterized by paralysis on one side of the body due to a destructive lesion of the brain. The medical outlook for Gordon is one of persistent paralysis on the side affected so far as this fails to be improved by orthopedic means and by the methods recommended by Dr. S. I. Franz of Washington. Gordon is now working regularly at his trade, that of steamfitter. We single out these three cases of Greta Meyer, David Collins, and Harold Gordon as illustrative of three of the major groups of syphilitic diseases of the nervous system, each with a different outlook as to duration and impairment. Application of the best methods of social work secured surprisingly good results.

The jail-bird group of psychopaths would doubtless be scouted as potential employees by many employment managers. Plain jail-birds might be regarded as bad enough; crazy ones would be thought impossible. Consider, however, the elevator-operator, Alfred Stevens (case 25) discharged for pilfering. After recovery from depression this elevator-operator became one of the best employees in another plant. We were also able to secure for Ignatz Simanski (case 33), a forger, something like a good future. He was a capable workman and was gotten work by us after his discharge from the house of correction. It is to be sure doubtful whether Simanski was at all psychopathic. Ordinarily he might have been handled by some agency for discharged prisoners. However, he got into the Psychopathic Hospital's hands through the suggestion of a layman and on the basis that he might possibly be a victim of psychopathic personality.

We are also afraid that after approaching the matter from a psychopathic point of view, most persons would be disposed to look with suspicion upon such a person as the mill worker Julia Brown (case 23), who lived for so long as a man. Nevertheless with proper measures of social work, Julia Brown has become a competent and trusted factory worker. No doubt her mental twist is a profound one. "The inner relations" of such a person are hard to integrate; or shall we say that there is integration of grotesque independence in Julia Brown to start with? At all events it has been found possible to adjust the "outer relations" of the environment in such a manner that this particular psychopath is getting on well. Almost equally hard to deal with is such a matter as the fear of open spaces exhibited in the cigar-maker David Stone (case 24). Yet Stone has recovered and is now working regularly at good pay as an insurance agent.

Perhaps such interior difficulties as those of Michael Piso (case 62) might be regarded as still more difficult of adjustment. Piso had illusions of jealousy that interfered with his employment; but as his jealousy was made to subside (or shall we say, as the jealousy subsided of itself?) Piso went back to work and got his wages raised.

Another apparently disconcerting fact is the long duration of disability in some cases, which seems to argue that little enough can ever be done. But consider the case of the plumber Daniel Griffin (case 34) who is a psychoneurotic and had actually been unable to work for six years. After a year's treatment he has become more active about his home, although up to date he is not willing to go out alone.

We now turn to an analysis of the *family interest*s in the industrial cases which we have just summed up from their standpoints as individuals. Certainly twenty-three out of forty-two industrial cases of this volume are cases with the family problem in sharp focus.

Consider the case of Henry Loyal (case 4). Here was the family problem of non-support with marital discord. The wife was sick; one child had chorea; the second tuberculosis; the third required special feeding; one daughter was a sex delinquent. Every member of the family was an object of special attention. Industrial rehabilitation of Henry Loyal meant happiness to at least six separate persons. We are inclined to think that the non-psychiatric social worker would have taken the Loyal family situation as not particularly psychiatric. The questionnaires concerning deserted families, gotten out by various social agencies, do not bring the psychiatric question into sufficient relief. It would have been easy to dismiss Henry Loyal as a "degenerate." Particularly Mrs. Loyal, his wife, the sex-delinquent daughter, and the choreic child, that is at least four of the six members of the Loyal family, should be more or less constantly under psychiatric review.

Alfred Stevens (case 25), the elevator-operator discharged for pilfering, had his case complicated by the situation reverse to that of Henry Loyal, since Stevens' wife left him taking their child, a child to whom Stevens was greatly devoted. Upon Stevens' recovery from his depression the family was reunited.

Martin O'Hara (case 92), a loafer, presented another story of family problem. He had been recently married but never lived with his wife. He found that she had had an illegitimate baby. The medical problem was one of hysteria on the part of O'Hara. No doubt the hysteria was on the basis of psychopathic personality, from which O'Hara will not recover. The problem of social work will be a chronic one.

More or less continuous *financial aid* had to be granted in a number of cases. Lewis Goldstein, a roofer's helper, during his slow recovery from an industrial accident had to be helped and the health of his wife and children made the whole situation difficult,—practically difficult, however theoretically simple enough.

The case of John Flynn (case 19) resembles that of Lewis Goldstein; Flynn required two years of care before he could be restored to full efficiency following his complete disability from traumatic neurosis. The Flynn family also had a number of sick children to care for.

David Stone (case 24), the cigar-maker who feared open spaces, was also another case not of individual disease alone, since through the process of his becoming industrially competent ran also the problem of supporting Stone's family and steering his wife through illness.

Paul Ernst (case 73), the excellent salesman who had been discharged after a manic attack, had an income decidedly insufficient for his family. Assistance was given the family in the form of clothes and vacations for the children. One of the nine Ernst children also had chorea. The social worker had to contend with Ernst's rather natural worry about the family finances.

Hamilton Green was psychopathic with a mother to support and the Green family had been in receipt of aid from public funds. The improvement in Green's mental disease permitting work regularly abolished the problem of public aid.

Ignatz Simanski (case 33) showed in some sense the opposite situation since he was making financial demands upon his sister who was only able to support herself with difficulty.

The health of the child of the divorcee Agnes O'Brien (case 13) had to be considered and the second (illegitimate) child had to be provided for in public custody.

Nathan Rosenthal (case 49), a laborer, was a moron with psychoneurotic symptoms dating from an accident. The Rosenthal family first came under observation through the examination of a son—another example of the rather frequent uncovering of family problems through the resort to a mental clinic of some psychiatric case. The Rosenthal family entirely was put under social care. Work was procured for the father. The mother was given suitable encouragement. The son was placed under supervision. Meantime the family had an insufficient income.

Another special problem of advice was offered by the case of Maurice Eastman (case 87), the cigar-maker whose trade was distasteful to him. The family problem proved a long one. The fact that the family was inclined to maintain a high standard of living made the small income seem more than ordinarily insufficient. Aid with clothes was given. But more particularly a specialized kind of encouragement and advice had to be given with relation to the children's education. The Eastman family showed the usual Jewish ambition for the children's education. All the children were bright, and there was even an indication of special talent in one or two thereof. The problem of the right kind of encouragement for the education of a psychoneurotic is a psychiatric one. Of course we may say that not even psychiatrists find always the right way in such a plight. Yet, perhaps the psychiatrists should have more to say in the premises than some other person exempt from any knowledge of psychoneuroses whatever.

That the industrial problem could not be treated in and for itself successfully and that the ordinary non-psychiatric view of the family problem would be decidedly insufficient are points illustrated also in a case like that of Harold Gordon (case 46). Here there had been cohabitation with a woman probably psychopathic.

Paul Dawson (case 78) separated from his wife, failed to support her and was perhaps a case of dementia praecox. He had always worked irregularly and under our care could not be got to take a job. However, upon being drafted he made an allotment to his wife. Upon his discharge he went into the merchant marine.

Other cases of family interest amongst the industrial group are those of Herman Simonson (case 27) with a wife and six children and wife's parents in Russia dependent upon this clothes-presser; Nathan Blumberg (case 37), a case of non-support in financial difficulty, confused about his affairs, separated from his wife; John Logan (case 58), the expert chemist whose wife was at first afraid to live with him but upon advice and encouragement kept up the home; Patrick Nolan, a laborer whose family was dependent upon his wages and who was gotten to return to work after recovery from delirium tremens; the jealous teamster Michael Piso (case 62), whose family required material aid and also the care of health of the wife and children; the paranoid case of George Stone (case 76), whose delusions were not severe enough to permit his being committed to a state institution and who wandered about not working and threatening his wife; Joseph Fangillo (case 89), whose illness ate up his savings so that his wife might be maintained; the industrial-accident case of the machinist Dennis O'Donnell (case 90), where there was an economic problem of the family and the problem of advice to the wife.

We have added up the more striking problems amongst the twenty-three family cases in our industrial group of forty-two and find that no less than eighteen of the twenty-three cases yielded acute economic problems for the family as well as for the industrially disabled patient. When the non-psychiatric family case worker approaches such a case as a purely family problem she has unquestionably in the past been inclined to regard the psychopath as an unfortunate additional complication. We submit that the treatment of these family cases with the psychopath as the primary target of attack is the rational strategy of the present day. Nine of the twenty-three cases show degrees of sickness in the wife or children. The medical social worker will no doubt give proper attention to these physical sicknesses; and perhaps the medical social worker from her hospital community experience may exhibit an advance in social attitude upon that of the philanthropic family case worker of a former generation. But here again we are inclined to say that the data of this book proved that the standpoint of physical health, valuable as it is, is very frequently not the central problem. Let the central problem of the psychoneuroses or other mental diseases in the father or mother be properly treated and the problems of sickness on the part of the wife and children will get solved upon comparatively small lines. But if we try to solve the problem of sickness of the non-psychopathic spouse or children upon a purely health basis the psychopathic difficulty in the parent will be apt to run on indefinitely. (See particularly such a case as that of Henry Loyal, case 4, or Nathan Rosenthal, case 49, or Maurice

Eastman, case 87.)   There were nine cases also of marital discord.   Marital discord is perhaps a purely primary and moral difficulty, though we are not aware that any proper statistics on this point of marital discord with relation to psychopathy have ever been collected.   The point of this volume largely turns. upon our considering every case of social difficulty as possibly in the first instance medical, and perhaps psychopathic. This point, as we repeatedly insist, is not grounded upon statistical frequency of mental disease amongst cases of social difficulty; we do.not feel that there are anywhere in the world proper statistics on this matter.   Our point is that every instance of social difficulty should. first or last receive consideration as possibly a medical matter.   So with these nine cases of marital discord.   In the Loyal (case 4) family the wife was possibly slightly psychopathic although the big problem of non-support was unquestionably grounded in the psychopathic personality of the husband and father.   Nathan Blumberg (case 37) was separated from his wife after a quarrel, but we do not here find evidence of mental diseases on both sides of the family.   The discord in the case of Michael Piso (case 62) was unquestionably due to this teamster's delusions rather than to any attitude on the part of the wife.   Likewise with George Stone (case 76).

There were two cases complicated by illegitimacy of a child. Agnes O'Brien (case 13) had an illegitimate second child. Martin O'Hara married a wife with an illegitimate baby. Agnes O'Brien illustrates one problem of illegitimacy in the fact that she was a hysterical moron whom we should not regard as too responsible for the fact of illegitimacy.   On the other hand the wife of Martin O'Hara was as far as we know not in any sense psychopathic.   As with the questionnaires regarding non-support, so with the questionnaires regarding unmarried mothers; we do not find that these questionnaires take sufficiently into account the possibility of feeble-mindedness on the part of the unmarried mother or father.   We have not the slightest doubt that the problem of illegitimacy will have a flood of light thrown upon it by intensive study from the psychiatric point of view.

To sum up concerning the family interests in the industrial group of cases, we must emphasize the fact that first, each industrial case must be handled upon its merits as a psychopathic case; second, the members of the industrial psychopath's family must be treated socially like the members of any other family case group; third, the treatment of such a family case group containing a psychopath as a central figure should not be treated as a family unit (that is, from the ordinary standpoint of the family case worker dealing with the situation largely from the economic side); fourth, the point of view of the ordinary medical social worker (that is, the point of view which takes into account the physical health of each member of the family), is an inadequate approach, good so far as it goes but missing the psychiatric point. Cases of industrial disability might well seem, even to the educated layman, primarily cases for economic handling from the standpoint of the so-called family case work. Yet the educated layman who should think that this primarily could be handled by financial aid alone would fall far short of the ideals of the present day. Let us emphasize as ever that both the family case worker and the medical social worker do their best as moral advisers in these situations. But the kind of moral advice they are equipped by nature and training to give needs supplementation by psychiatric training if the best results are to be obtained.

The moral advice given by the worker untrained in the contrast of temperament and the peculiarities of the different major forms of mental diseases and defects is but too apt to follow some particular slant of the social worker's own nature and experience. She is but too apt to try to make the family as a whole and the central psychopathic figure conform to some set ideal of action. It is these industrial cases that bring very acutely the combination of diseases, moral defect, and economic disability. The formula of these cases is rather apt to be M. V. P., to use our abbreviated terminology. That is, we find in these cases some examples of the morbi, some examples of the vitia, and some examples of the penuriae rolled in one.

Our complaint as to the shortcomings of the present-day social work is that too great emphasis may readily be laid upon economic disabilities (penuriae). Furthermore, even if the hypothesis of disease (morbi) is brought into the foreground we find that the morbi are taken in a physical sense rather than in a mental sense; the medical social worker is not sufficiently a psychiatric social worker. With respect to the vitia, our chief complaint reduces perhaps to the charge that the non-psychiatrically trained person is but too apt to think that all men conform to or fall short of certain standards of morality, whereas the psychiatrically trained person is apt to see many types of moral shortcoming following the lines of temperament and the psychiatric worker suspects that there has been too great emphasis upon the uniting of moral standards in the human race as a whole.

All moralists admit that the moral situation (that is, the situation which considers good and evil, right and wrong) involves voluntary activity—a point handed down from Aristotle. "The agent must know," say Dewey and Tufts, "what he is about; he must have some idea of what he is doing; he must not be a somnambulist, or an imbecile, or an infant." They go on to say that such unformed or deformed personalities exhibit voluntary activities and in moral activity they may show character or herein necessarily be viewed morally. Now this standpoint may be perfectly well chosen from the standpoint of voluntary moral life (we are inclined to concede even this point, to grant it for the sake of argument), but the standpoint is assuredly not well chosen if we are trying to evaluate the vitia; that is, tell just how far the acts formed are immoral acts and how far they are the acts of untrained or immature persons or how far they are actually psychopathic. In short, we feel that the study of morals will greatly benefit from psychiatric analyses. But this point takes us far out of the immediate range of industrial interest. The most prominent difficulties in the handling of family situations of industrial disability is the tendency on the part of persons without a psychiatric training or experience to deal with families upon a purely economic basis or upon a basis of mere physical health.

OUT-PATIENT SERVICE

Some patients resort upon their own initiative to the out-patient service (for example, Ethel Murphy, case 66, and Jeanette Burroughs, case 68) and are then, if desirable, readily persuaded to enter the hospital wards. William Donahue (case 82) came of his own initiative to the out-patient department and never seemed to need treatment in the wards. Maurice Eastman (case 87) was treated as an out-patient only by psychotherapeutic means. And though Eastman's troubles seemed to require at least three types of worker and much individualization, yet ward treatment never came in question. Louis Sand (case 95), the roving Belgian immigrant, remained also an out-patient case throughout a long and rather intensive social treatment.

Shall mental treatment be carried out in hospital beds or in the out-patient department? Many states still possess no means of treating mental cases in adequate out-patient departments, such as those provided for example by Massachusetts and New York. Yet the establishment of such out-patient departments should be easily brought about in forward-looking states, since it must be apparent to the most fiscally-minded legislators that **out-patient departments are cheaper to run than hospital wards.** It is obvious that many patients can be got in for out-patient examinations who would not readily consent to come even as *voluntary patients* who stay in beds. The values of out-patient department work are shown in the majority of our cases, first from analysis of their reports thereto through the follow-up work after they have been released from the wards. But a number of cases are particularly interesting from the standpoint of the values of the **out-patient department mental examination.** Consider Bessie Silverman (case 21). This Jewess came herself upon her own recognizance to the out-patient department of the hospital to find out the degree of her mental capacity. Bessie, it will be remembered, was that case of disharmony between ambition and ability who was bent upon somehow going through college.

Emma Marburg (case 30) came to the out-patient department through the advice of another patient. She was unable to hold out any longer on account of her fatigue and worry.

Some cases are treated with success as out-patients only; compare Beatrice Cellini (case 52), who came of a family known to at least twenty-four social agencies. The diagnosis in the Cellini case could be rendered with apparent safety without resorting to the hospital wards.

We may properly use these cases to prove the independent value of out-patient services and dispensaries for mental cases. Yet, we must not forget that where an out-patient service is a departmental service and lodged in an imposing hospital structure surrounded by evidences of intensive medical, educational, social, psychological, occupational, and nursing work, the effects gained are not purely those of the out-patient service *per se*. The out-patient service in this sense is under the auspices of something big, complex, almost sacred, ever in the eye of the patient as a vista of resources for help.

We have spoken of imposing structures. The state hospital structures whether of the Bastile type or of the more modern scattered cottage description (sometimes, we regret to say, like a lot of small Bastiles!) will no doubt ever remain forbidding to certain types of mind in difficulty, which will be entirely willing to visit the out-patient department of a psychopathic hospital or the consulting room of a mental hygiene society. These values are very delicate ones to estimate. The consulting office specialist cannot quite see how his type of patient could willingly resort to any form of out-patient department, if he could possibly get the money to resort to a private medical consulting office.

Yet there are certain types of men and women that seem to abhor private consulting offices and much prefer public contacts. Again there is a certain class of persons who are effectively drawn under observation by the state and local mental hygiene societies whose rooms are found in office buildings and may be resorted to without fear of observation at the door or in the corridors. Another type of patient is drawn to the modern psychopathic hospital divorced in construction and in its practical associations from the district state institution. The Psychopathic Hospital in Boston has without artificial stimulus an out-patient department that usually runs to the number of fifteen hundred per annum. It would be entirely impossible, we venture to say, for any district institution primarily for the committable insane to show such a record—a record partly founded in the public recognition of especially trained physicians, psychologists, and social workers to be found therein, but more effectively still in the good effects advertised from neighbor to neighbor as shown by returning patients. We doubt whether any institution not primarily constructed for the voluntary class of patients and for the so-called temporary care group of non-committable patients, will ever draw from the community so important and extensive a group of out-patients.

The scope of this work does not include a special discussion of methods of **psychotherapy**. We give upon another page the main methods of psychotherapy mentioned in textbooks (a list drawn from *Shell-Shock and Other Neuropsychiatric Problems,* 1919, by the senior author). **The adjustment of man to himself is not primarily a function of social work** and we are prepared to admit that there are numerous cases of complete adjustment of man to himself altogether outside the field of social work. The works of Janet are filled with instances of such interior adjustment by the psychotherapeutists. We may call attention to several cases in our group.

Daniel Griffin (case 34) was a case in which there were many psychogenic factors; that is, factors of mental diseases that took their rise from troubles inside the patient's own mind. This was the case of the man who did not work and never went out in the daytime for a period of about six years. A psychotherapy by persuasion was adopted. Another instance of this is that of Louis Sand (case 95). And Maurice Eastman (case 87) should be carefully reread by the reader interested in psychotherapy. This man had been coached by physicians to know that his disease was "all foolishness"—an instance in which psychotherapy may defeat itself. He was given a sort of talking cure by a psychologist in the Psychopathic Hospital and was made to read popular works of psychotherapy. We shall not repeat the remarks under this case concerning the fact that psychiatric social work is not psychotherapeutic in the full sense of the term (at all events not in the medical sense of the term), and is decidedly not competent to decide upon the respective values of the different forms of psychotherapy listed in the chart (page 481), especially upon the values of such methods of psychotherapy as hypnosis and psychoanalysis. The spheres of influence of the psychiatric social worker as of any social worker are decidedly not either the public or the personal spheres. The social worker cannot take the place of the judge or public administrator and must not feel irked by her inability to act as a substitute for the public servants. As we have repeatedly said, she must use the public service as fulcrum. But it is even more true, though perhaps less obvious, that the psychiatric social worker cannot replace the physician in the most intimate and personal matters of treatment.

The reason why this is not too obvious to every psychiatric social worker is that everybody is aware that the methods of psychotherapy grade very gently over into methods of conviction and persuasion, in short of suggestion, as employed in everyday life. Every father or mother, brother or sister—everybody who has served in any dominant way in relation to some human being—is aware of his or her suggestive powers. It is very natural therefore for the psychiatric social worker to fall victim to the belief that she might solve the problems of suggestion in her psychopathic patients as well as the physician. She knows that she can in fact exert certain suggestive powers under certain conditions of time and place that the physician can exert. She·has in mind certain successes in conviction or persuasion as exerted upon given cases in her experience. Yet mutual adaptation of the interior relations of the mind to one another under psychopathic circumstances is not at all easy. Suggestion is easy but the right suggestion is difficult; when we examine the life histories of certain patients we find them a succession of layers of suggestions like the layers of paint in certain ancient canvases. Universally the human mind is a little more like water-color painting than one in oils, so that it is often impossible to eradicate the earlier impressions by fresh ones. Armed with new knowledge about suggestion and plied with the histories of successful adaptation by psychotherapeutic means, the youthful social worker may be inclined to enter where the psychotherapeutist would hardly dare to tread.

Is it wiser to let the public service adjust its own environmental services, gradually molded into proper shape by improvement in communal opinion, and to let the specialist in psychotherapy pursue his own difficult course of the mutual adjustment of inner relations without undue interference by the social worker? To be sure communal opinion about improvements in the public service will never acquire greater strength than when supported by the concrete facts supplied by the experienced social worker. By the same token the psychotherapeutist may be unable to make his weighty decisions (whether he or she act by conviction or persuasion, terrorism or the velvet glove, hypnotism or psychoanalysis) only in virtue of some little special indication that the social observer has recorded.

PSYCHIATRIC SOCIAL WORK

HISTORY

In the development of a new profession, from time to time new interests come to the front, dominate the scene for a while, and gradually become assimilated into the body of experience. A new branch remains upon the main trunk, and at the same time the parent stem is strengthened. This process is the current history of psychiatric social work. In the multiform activities of social work, gradually taking shape in a new profession, there are found many traces of interest in mind as a primary factor in social life,—the keynote principle of psychiatric social work. St. Vincent de Paul's efforts to relieve the sick poor, among the earliest attempts at organized social work, had for their object "to teach the poor to be provident for themselves," as well as "to point out to them sources of employment." Cicero considered the mental effect of alms: "We must take care that our bounty is a real blessing to those we relieve, that the claims of gratitude and justice are preferred to mere compassion, and that due regard is given both to the character and the wants of the recipient."

The aim of all modern social work has been to build up character. Nevertheless, until recently, there has been no systematic attempt to study character by exact methods. Social work has not heretofore attempted to apply the mental sciences to understanding of the individual. "Common-sense" methods have been relied upon in estimating personality, and "trial-and-error" methods in solving mental problems. While the world is far from possessing a science of character, there is a certain amount of knowledge derived from the mental sciences, psychology and psychopathology, that can be applied to advantage in dealing with human beings. Even a small amount of scientific knowledge may afford a large amount of practical value. The benefit to the individual, whose difficulties are better understood by reason of some bit of science, may be incalculable.

This new branch of social work known as psychiatric social work is a new emphasis rather than a new function. It has grown out of ideas and activities that already existed in scattered forms. A similar situation is found in the development of medical social work during the last fifteen years. The new emphasis upon attention to disease and care of health spread rapidly in general social work, until now the idea of using scientific methods to maintain health is part of the equipment of every well-trained social worker. Theory, to be sure, is ahead of practice, as it must always be, and social work has far to go before it can be said to be making 'the best use of medical science; but the principle of a medical point of view is established.

At first social work was dominated by the economic point of view. Economic features of social disorder are most conspicuous (food and shelter are the first obvious needs), and therefore receive first attention. Moreover, the social worker's special contribution to social problems is knowledge of the environment (the social worker is a specialist in environment), and here also the outstanding features are economic. Again, the origin of systematized social work in "poor relief" put economic considerations in the lead. But just as the medical point of view came to the front and was assimilated, so at the present time the psychiatric point of view is in the foreground and is in process of being absorbed into the movement.

The history of psychiatric social work is the focusing of various recent influences leading to **more attention to the mind in social practice,** under pressure from psychiatry demanding **more attention to social needs in medical practice.** In social work, among these trends, one that stands out prominently is the increasing insistence of the family welfare group upon better understanding of motives and more exact methods of arousing interest and purpose. In the children's agencies, there has been growing a sense of the need of applying child psychology in the education of young wards. Agencies caring for the unmarried mother have come to recognize the primary importance of mental conditions in these cases. Psychiatric clinics established in connection with courts (of which Dr. Healy's clinic in the Chicago juvenile court was the forerunner), and in connection with prisons and reformatories (such as the clinic started by Dr. Glueck at Sing Sing prison), have given impetus to the psychiatric interest in social work. From medical social work came another influence in the insistence of Dr. Cabot that social work was essentially the development of character under adversity.

In medicine many definite trends may be seen that have contributed to the present development of psychiatric social work. A very explicit statement of the need of social work in the practice of psychiatry was made twenty years ago by Dr. Theodore H. Kellogg, superintendent of a hospital for mental diseases, in his *Textbook on Mental Diseases:* "Insanity practically is loss of the power of conformity to the social medium in which the patient lives. This power is regained in convalescence gradually, and it is a part of psychotherapy to furnish a normal personal environment to which the patient is to practice adjustment;" and again: "The physician who has conducted a case of mental disorder through all the vicissitudes of an acute attack to perfect recovery has a final duty to perform. There are to be laid down definite rules of life, points in physical and mental hygiene, suggestions of the best way to meet social and business difficulties, and advice as to domestic relations." It was some fifteen years later that systematic provision began to be made for seeing that these "rules of life" laid down by the physician were actually followed by the patient. It was thought that the physician could perform this function of social readjustment and many hospital superintendents and physicians did so to the best of their ability. Others were beginning to see the possibility of specially trained lay workers for this purpose.

Meanwhile psychiatrists were coming into closer association with social workers. It is of some interest that at the first meeting of the National Conference of Social Work (then the Conference of Charities and Correction), in 1874, the first subject considered was "The Duty of the States toward Their Insane Poor," in a paper by a state-hospital superintendent; and the subject of "insanity" figured largely in the programs of the early years. A section on feeble-mindedness and insanity was created and in 1917 became the mental-hygiene section. Another medical influence, which no doubt gave considerable impetus to the development of psychiatric social work, was the growing appreciation of physicians in general hospitals of the value of the social service, and the experience of psychiatrists in mental clinics of these hospitals that the assistance of social workers became indispensable.

The chronology of psychiatric social work down its main line of development, social care for cases of mental disease, begins with the Society for the After-Care of the Insane in England, which as early as 1880 was engaged in giving friendly supervision to patients discharged from hospitals. The first attempt in this country to employ social work in the care of patients with nervous and mental disorders seems to have been in the Neurological Clinic of the Massachusetts General Hospital in Boston in 1905, when Dr. James J. Putnam, who was in charge of the clinic, secured the assistance of a social worker, Miss Edith N. Burleigh, and personally trained her for the work. A year later a social worker was placed in the psychopathic wards of Bellevue Hospital, New York. The New York State Charities Aid Association was a leading influence in developing this field through its Committee on Mental Hygiene, which in 1910 appointed an "after-care worker" to supervise patients discharged from two of the state hospitals of New York. The first social worker to be placed upon the payroll of a state hospital for mental diseases was employed through the influence of this Committee in 1911, by the Manhattan State Hospital, New York, where she had previously been engaged upon salary paid by the Committee. Two years later, 1913, two Massachusetts hospitals, Danvers State Hospital and Boston State Hospital, each added a social worker to the staff.

The same year the Psychopathic Hospital began to organize its social service. Although the original plans provided for a social service, the work was not regularly started until a year after the hospital was opened. The ideas of the Director concerning the introduction of this new agency into the institution are expressed in some notes written a year or two later:—

"The social service movement seems to be waxing fast, although not fast enough for its problems. Personally I seem to have been greatly influenced by some of Professor Royce's earlier ethical papers touching the social 'consciousness' so-called, by Professor Putnam's contentions, and by the point of view of Professor James which culminated in his marvelous address on *The Moral Equivalent of War*. Then came brief but uplifting observations of the Social Service Department of the Massachusetts General Hospital under the leadership of

Miss Ida M. Cannon. After the establishment of the Psychopathic Hospital, I began to get light from a group of persons
interested in social service, among whom, besides Miss Cannon,
I should especially count my colleague Dr. W. P. Lucas, Mr.
Michael M. Davis, and Miss Katherine McMahon.

"My own ideas are derived from many sources. The need
of a social service in the new Psychopathic Hospital became
obvious at once when the plans were tentatively begun in 1909-
1910 and the obvious need was expressed in so many words in
the State Board of Insanity's report of 1910. So far as I can
remember, space was reserved for social service in the very
first of the plans from which the eventual plan was developed.
To be sure, many physicians who were shown the plans affected astonishment at the large space assigned to the out-
patient work as a whole, and there was almost no general
appreciation of either the whole out-patient work or its social
service constituents. These critics are now easily won over
by the practical results obtained."

We claim no novelty or originality for the social work of
the Psychopathic Hospital, but rather, we would claim to have
created **the part that the social worker is to play in the
mental hygiene movement** and to have given it a name—
psychiatric social work. The bases of this new division of
social work are the principles common to all forms of social
case work. It is the application of old methods in a new field.
It will, we expect, develop some new methods, which will in
time be applied in the older fields. In the new field there was
need of bringing to a focus existing trends, of defining functions, outlining requirements of special training, and giving
the whole a distinctive name.

The Great War had an important influence upon the spread
of psychiatric social work. It was clear to those who had seen
the importance of social service in civilian hospitals that psychiatric social workers would be needed for army hospitals.
But there were only a handful of social workers with this special training in the whole country. Plans to enlarge the capacity of the training course at the Psychopathic Hospital were
proceeding when it was found possible to combine with Smith
College in a course, given in 1918-1919, under the auspices of
a committee of the National Committee for Mental Hygiene.
Similar courses, conceived as emergency measures or as permanent developments of the curriculum, were offered by other

schools in New York, Philadelphia, and Chicago. In Canada a similar course was given at Toronto University. Fifty-odd graduates of the Smith College course went into army hospitals or Red Cross organizations. The pioneer piece of psychiatric social work in the army was done in the neuro-psychiatric hospital at Plattsburg, by Miss Margherita Ryther, who had been for some years social worker in the Neurological Clinic of the Massachusetts General Hospital, Boston. The need for social service in any program for adequate care of neuropsychiatric cases among soldiers was demonstrated. This principle established in the army hospitals has carried over into the public health hospitals. The Red Cross in connection with the public health service and the Veterans' Bureau are now endeavoring to develop a complete organization of psychiatric social work for the care of ex-service men with neuropsychiatric disabilities.

The effect of psychiatric social work upon general social work came into focus in a surprising way at the National Conference of Social Work in Atlantic City in May, 1919. There was suddenly a realization in many quarters that psychiatry's contribution to general social work ought to be made available. Dr. Cabot spoke of the new force, "new, not in name, but in efficiency and energy—which has come into social work—the force represented by psychiatric social work. In thirty years I have never seen anything so important as the irruption of psychiatric social work into social work." The idea is now widely accepted that social case work calls for psychiatric knowledge and the psychiatric point of view. It remains to find ways and means to enable social workers at large to get what psychiatry can offer. A number of means are at hand,—the best perhaps are the summer courses in social psychiatry offered by certain schools of social work. Evening courses may be arranged. Brief extension courses as an introduction to the subject are offered by some schools, with clinics to demonstrate types of mental disorder. Reading helps, but the literature of social psychiatry is mostly in the form of detached articles. In Boston, a group of twenty-five executives of social agencies and leading social workers formed a class to study with a psychiatrist, who was familiar with their field, the best means of applying psychiatry in social work.

To avoid confusion of terms, it may be well to state here

that *"social psychiatry"* is not used as an alternate for *"psychiatric social work."* Psychiatric social work is the special form of social work in which psychiatric knowledge is particularly required. Social psychiatry is an art now in the course of development by which the psychiatrist deals with social problems. Social psychiatry is a branch of psychiatry and a special kind of medical art. That part of the knowledge of psychiatry which has a bearing upon social problems is given to social workers in courses named social psychiatry,—that is, the essentials of psychiatry from the standpoint of social work. The special preparation of the psychiatric social worker should consist not only of courses in social psychiatry but also of practice in social work with psychiatric cases. The inclusive term mental hygiene is used to cover the activities of psychiatrist, psychologist, the psychiatric social worker in promoting mental health wheresoever.

ORGANIZATION AND FUNCTIONS OF THE SOCIAL SERVICE AT THE BOSTON PSYCHOPATHIC HOSPITAL

Some account of the development and organization of the social service of the Psychopathic Hospital may be suggestive to similar departments in process of formation. Any scheme of organization is a growth determined largely by local conditions, and therefore may not be suitable to transplant. There are, however, some fundamental principles and practices common to all similar institutions, in regard to which experiences may be exchanged with profit. The psychopathic hospital and the state hospital for mental diseases will differ in the organization of their social service as well as of their medical service; but both types of hospital will have common features in both medical and social work. This account is by no means intended to present a model form of organization. The system here developed, however, works on the whole with reasonable effectiveness, and most of its fundamental principles and chief devices we would recommend with confidence.

The question of the proper organization of the social service depends fundamentally upon whether a hospital is regarded as a community institution, in which medical and social departments coöperate, or as a medical institution controlled and directed by physicians with social assistants. This question of organization arises irrespective of the question of functional control and direction of social work in a hospital. Besides the question of immediate direction (or supervision) of the social worker's activities, there is a question of the right administrative relation between medical work and social work. The position taken by a particular hospital on this point affects the development of its social service in both frank and subtle ways. A confused policy on this point leads to misunderstandings and retardation of the work of the social service.

At the present time most of our hospitals are acknowledged medical institutions, primarily for the treatment and study of disease, and they are administered by medical men. Therefore the social work should properly be subordinated to the medical work, the physician employing social assistants and relying upon their special skill (without attempt to direct a form of practice in which he is not trained) to promote the medical work. As the horizons of medicine widen, it is conceivable that the hospital of the future may be a social institution, administered by men of sociological-medical training. The community no doubt will more and more demand that the hospital treat the whole man, that the treatment of disease aim at complete social adjustment, and that the hospital go outside its walls to prevent disease.

At the Psychopathic Hospital the social service was organized to assist in the medical work of studying and treating mental disease. Its function of assisting in treatment was construed in the broadest sense to mean (a) restoration of capacity for normal living, or (b) provision for greatest possible comfort. The out-patient department and the social service have developed with close interrelations. While many social-service cases first receive attention on the wards, the greater part of the work is of course with patients in the community. The medical and social aspects of out-patient treatment for nervous and mental disorders are so closely interwoven that they can hardly be discussed separately. An occasional case may be free from social complications and call for treatment by the physician only. Also, in an occasional case the physician may find that the root of the difficulty is social and may leave the case in the hands of the social worker. In most cases, medical treatment is supplemented and reinforced by social care. The efforts of the social worker in such cases must, of course, be definitely designed to contribute to medical treatment.

For the best results, social work should be immediately under social direction, but the practice of the social worker in every case must be strictly in accordance with the doctor's ideas for the patient; and if in any case a conflict of social and medical interests arise, the medical decision obviously must prevail; since the treatment of a mentally sick person is primarily a medical problem. This relation between medical and social work is sometimes not understood by observers, who see the large amount of responsibility borne by the social worker in certain cases that the physician sees infrequently, and who do not realize that the physician has delegated responsibility to the social worker to carry out social treatment in conformity with the medical plan.

A routine social examination for all admissions was our ultimate aim,[1] but was impossible with the number of social workers available. Therefore the expedient was adopted of relying upon the physicians to report cases in which social work was required. About one-fourth of the cases referred by physicians are likely to be cases where a history is required for medical diagnosis, but social care is not required. (See cases 54 and 72.) The physician is apt to look upon this function of the social service as its most important duty, since his primary responsibility to the patient is to endeavor to make a correct diagnosis. In a sense it is also the primary responsibility of the social worker to contribute to this object, which is the hospital's first duty to the patient. Equally important to the social worker, in addition, is the welfare of the patient in the community. Moreover, the benefit of careful diagnosis can be secured in many cases only by painstaking, thorough social care. The social worker, engaged in social treatment, is bound to feel a sense of interruption if histories for medical diagnosis cause deferred attention to social cases. The success of social treatment may depend upon timeliness, steadiness, persistence, or close application; and emergencies continually arise when least expected. No matter how thoroughly the social worker recognizes the importance of the medical-social history, she cannot feel the same enthusiasm that the physician would feel

[1] From Annual Report of the Director, Psychopathic Department, Boston State Hospital, 1915: "Of course with a properly increased staff, we should like to secure a social examination for every patient on admission."

in devoting a day's work to it, while perhaps neglecting work that is her own immediate responsibility. This is especially likely to be true if the significance of the history turns upon some fine medical point. Therefore it might be more effective to have certain social workers give their time wholly to getting medical-social histories.

Individual case work is the nucleus of the department. Since it was impossible to treat all cases with thoroughness, on account of an insufficient number of workers, a distinction was adopted between "intensive" and "slight service" cases based upon the degree of responsibility for social care assumed by the department. In the intensive cases the social service attempts to assume responsibility for making a full inquiry into the social condition of the patient and his family and endeavors to secure the largest measure of social well-being possible for both patient and family. The "slight service" cases are those in which assistance is given without inquiry beyond the apparent facts or responsibility beyond the immediate service. (For examples of slight service cases, see cases 39, 41, and 67.)

An attempt was made to estimate the staff of social workers needed to cover the case work. There is no direct precedent or definite standard for determining how many cases one social worker in a psychopathic hospital can carry, but by a comparison of the experience of the Committee on Mental Hygiene of the New York State Charities Aid Association and that of other agencies doing somewhat similar work, it was estimated that one social worker could take in a year one hundred and fifty cases for investigation and miscellaneous services or could care for about fifty patients a year under supervision (that is, ten under treatment at one time for an average period of three months each), so that a social worker engaged in both investigation and supervision would average one hundred cases a year.

Not every patient will require the care of the social service. In a city with well-developed social agencies, about twenty-five per cent of admissions may be already in the care of other social workers, and about twenty-five per cent of the patients appear not to require social care, the majority being patients committed to hospitals, who have no one dependent upon them or whose families have already become adjusted to their mental condition. Others have families able and intelligent enough to do for them all that can be done; a few are unmarried persons who habitually wander, so that it is impossible to keep in communication with them. So it is possible to estimate roughly that for every two hundred admissions a social worker will be required for individual case work. The additional functions of research and teaching will call for additional workers.

The expense of the social service of a psychopathic hospital considered from the standpoint of efficient hospital administration (with the object of restoring patients to competency as far as possible) has yet to be carefully estimated. We have a few notions on the matter. (See also case 71.) The saving of expense to the state in the prevention of crimes by psychopathic individuals through social supervision cannot be calculated; but special instances indicate that it may be considerable. Through the care of social workers many patients who would become a charge upon the state are kept at home, either self-supporting or maintained by relatives. During our first two years' work at the Psychopathic Hospital, twenty patients, who by all indications would otherwise have required institutional care, were kept in the community through the activities of the social service. Averaged at a saving to the state of one year's maintenance each, these cases showed a saving of $5,200 which was more than the amount paid by the state in salaries to our social workers during that period. As three of these patients, who were insane, were returned to relatives in their native countries, the state was probably saved in their cases many years' support. So that, in relation to the state treasury, the department was then more than paying for itself.

In systematizing the case work, the social service borrowed a number of devices from the organization of the medical service, when Dr. Herman M. Adler was chief of staff. Workers and students are divided into *"groups"* (the *"head of the group"* being the most experienced worker on that duty), and cases as referred are assigned in rotation to the groups, record being made on a *"rotation sheet."* The head of the group is responsible for assigning the case within her group in the best way to get the work done promptly and well. A worker (or advanced student) is assigned each day to duty as *"visitor for the day"* to receive inquiries and deal with emergencies and to attend to certain routine duties. The whole staff meet every morning for the first half hour for discussion of cases. On the fourth day after assignment new cases are presented in summary with an analysis of "social symptoms" so-called (factors of social maladjustment) indicated so far as it has been possible to carry the investigation. Results of social treatment are reported every three months at the "morning discussion."

A method of giving each case worker a *"daily reminder"* of her work for the day has been found serviceable. An explanation of this method and a sample of the card that the social worker receives each day are here given.

August 15, 1916	H. A.
1 day case	George Brown
4 " "	Beulah King
14 " "	John Sheehan
1 month case	Grace Haskell
	Bessie Snow
3 " "	James Johnson
	Ada Jones
Records up to date	

Explanation: Cards are to be marked with a check after the patient's name if the work has been done, and returned at the end of the day to the stenographer. If the work has not been done, the name will be carried forward onto the card of the following day with the number of days overdue indicated.

1 day case, twenty-four hours after assignment.—Preliminary examination to be made, including interview with examining physician.

4 day case, fourth day after assignment.—To be presented at morning discussion.

14 day case.—Investigation to be completed. (If an intensive case, summary to be completed.)

1 month case.—Status to be reconsidered (whether case should be closed or should be continued for advice and supervision).

3 month case.—Summary of results to be made.

15th of each month records to be brought up to date.

30th of each month monthly statistics to be made up.

A procedure for the work upon a new case has been developed as follows:

a. Case assigned by recommendation slip.
b. Assignment noted on rotation sheet.
c. Memorandum slip filled out (see Appendix B, Form I).
d. Examining physician seen.

e. Patient's story obtained by interview.
f. Registration slip made.
g. Entry made on visitor's monthly statistical sheet.
h. Case folder made.
i. Inquiry slip filled out (see Appendix B, Form II).
j. Decision whether to be dealt with as "intensive" or "slight service" case made within twenty-four hours if possible. Otherwise case registered as "slight service," and later if desirable changed to "intensive."
k. Record folder made out on fourth day (for intensive cases; records of slight service cases kept in form of "Notes" only).
l. Case presented at morning discussion on fourth day.

The *memorandum slip* is for rough notes taken from the medical record or obtained from the patient for use in the investigation. It is taken along on visits and filed on return to the office in the folder for the case; so that even before the record is written there will be some identifying information in the folder. After the information contained on the memorandum slip has been copied into the record, the slip is destroyed. The *inquiry slip* is for the purpose of laying out a plan of investigation. As soon as all clues immediately obtainable are in hand, the informants to be interviewed by visit or telephone or to be written to are listed. Others may be added later on, or the original plan may be altered. The inquiry slip is taken along on visits and filed in the case-folder on return. It is destroyed when the investigation has been completed.

The interview with the patient before any steps in investigation are taken is considered important. In addition to the information obtained by the doctor, the social worker needs certain sociological data for the purposes of investigation, such as (*a*) exact names and addresses of relatives, employers, neighbors, teachers, clergymen, friends, who are possible informants; (*b*) resources among relatives and friends that may be a help in social readjustment; (*c*) details about the home and neighborhood; (*d*) exact knowledge of all the members of the family group and other close associates; (*e*) the patient's attitude toward his family and his idea of their attitude toward him; (*f*) the ratio between income and expenditures, and the relation between income and standard of living; (*g*) the patient's tastes in regard to employment, recreation, occupation in leisure time; (*h*) what relatives or friends have most influence with him; (*i*) his own plans for the future.

From the beginning of the department it was considered

important to differentiate clearly between the various functions of the social service. Even when different parts of the work must be performed by the same person, because of an inadequate staff, it is desirable to keep different forms of work clearly separate, so that each may receive its due share of attention and may be in line for expansion. After individual case work, the first duty of the social service that stood out was assistance in the out-patient clinic, and the first assistant secured was the *clinic manager,* whose duties are :—

Executive:
  a. To direct patients to the examiners during the clinic.
  b. To keep in order the records.
  c. To keep statistics.
  d. To see that reports of examinations are sent to social agencies.

Social:
  a. To take the social history of new patients.
  b. To assist in discovering and dealing with the social problems of out-patients.
  c. To see that patients and friends with them understand physician's directions and are able to carry them out.
  d. To act as a go-between for outside social workers and the physicians.

Among other divisions of the social service developed as the opportunity arose is the *follow-up service,*[1] a routine method of keeping informed by a card system of the failure of patients to keep their appointments and inducing them by letter, telephone, or visit to report. This work, besides its clerical aspects, has been found to require fine judgment and the point of view of a social worker, and to show good results in so far as these factors are present in the worker in charge.

The *syphilis service*[2] was developed as a routine system for keeping syphilitic patients under treatment and securing examination of their relatives. Here skill and judgment are obviously required in suggesting to relatives apparently healthy in most instances a blood test for syphilis. Of 579 persons for whom examination was sought in the years 1917 and 1918, 69

---

[1] Boston State Hospital, Annual Report 1917—Report of Director, Psychopathic Department—Follow-up Service by Dorothy Q. Hale, pp. 53-57.
[2] The same—Social Work with Syphilitics and Their Families, by Maida H. Solomon, pp. 57-65.

per cent were examined; and of these 21 per cent required treatment (see cases 41 and 45).

The *Men's Club,* started at the suggestion of Dr. A. Warren Stearns as a means of therapy for alcoholic patients (see cases 6, 58, and 71), proved to be an effective aid in social treatment for men patients with the habit of alcoholism.

The aim of *research* has been kept in view and as far as possible material (records, statistics) has been gathered with a view to possible use in the future in medical and social investigations.

A study of the psychopathic employee in industry, begun in 1914, was continued until 1920, through a special social worker to assist men patients with difficulties of industrial adaptation, and led to an investigation in the mental hygiene of industry conducted by the Engineering Foundation of New York. (See also page 499.)

The principle has been maintained that the search for new truth concerning human beings rests at bottom upon careful study of the individual in action. Research and assistance to the individual in social work are two aspects of the same matter. This seems to be a truism too simple to require statement; but research has become associated with laboratory experiments in the minds of some persons, to such a degree that they are apt to lose sight of the human value to individual patients of social case work that is done with the ultimate object of research.

Plans for special research in methods of social case work were interrupted by the war. Studies of technique of social investigation and treatment by the most thoughtful and experienced social workers to be found are clearly the next step in the development of scientific methods in case work. The psychiatric social service affords unusually favorable conditions for such study,—with psychologist and psychiatrist at hand to give their aid, which is indispensable. Moreover, traits of human nature are more conspicuous and therefore more readily studied in psychopathic patients. Just as principles of education were discovered through teaching the feeble-minded, so we may look for principles of social work to be found in case work with psychopaths.

The department was organized from the start to permit the *training of students,* for we felt a responsibility to prepare new workers for this field. As none of the schools of social work had yet developed training courses in psychiatric social work, we offered an apprenticeship course in which the student gave full time for six months. The term was later increased to eight months, as six months was found insufficient for acquiring even the rudiments of social work and social psychiatry. Several attempts were made to take students on part time for a longer period, but this plan was unsatisfactory, for the interruptions in the students' work increased the difficulties of organization to such an extent that part-time students became more of a burden than a help. From the students' point of view, it was apparent that they received much less benefit from part-time work than from an equal number of days' work on full time. The full-time student is an asset, taking her share in routine duties and after a few months giving valuable assistance in the case work. The presence of students in the daily morning discussion adds greatly to the value of these conferences. The alert, inquiring attitude of the student is stimulating, and the necessity for being definite and clear enough to be understood by the beginner helps to keep the more experienced workers in perpetual training.

Another function of the social service from the beginning has been *public education*—to promote understanding of mental disease and to reduce prejudice against mental hospitals, and particularly to help social workers acquire the essentials of psychiatry. Social workers were encouraged to seek from the physicians an explanation of the patient's condition and needs in every case brought by them for examination. In order to make sure that a correct statement of the examination was filed with the case record in the agency which had responsibility for the patient's care, this verbal report was supplemented by a routine written report consisting of brief summaries of the physical and mental examinations and intelligence tests. Some social workers came to depend upon this report without consulting the medical or social workers of the hospital, although the brief summary of medical findings furnished them was not sufficient in most cases to serve as a guide to social treatment.

The social worker would like a written report giving a full exposition of the case,—the character of the difficulty, the prognosis, and practical measures of treatment. Such a report, however, seems to be so complete that there is still more danger that the social worker will rely upon it entirely without further consultation. And there is danger that misleading or superficial conclusions may be drawn from any written report alone. Moreover, the time required for a physician to write a careful explanation of the case, adapted to the understanding of the particular type of social worker to whom it is to go, is prohibitive in most clinics and hospitals. The time required for a stenographer to make a transcript from the medical record is another matter. It is true that in the present state of education for social work, a report expressed in medical terms will not be understood by all social workers; but in every case the worker responsible has the opportunity to find out the meaning of the medical report. On the whole, the method of furnishing a transcript from the medical record and requiring a personal consultation has seemed best calculated to secure the interests of the patients.

Social clinics have been held every year, sometimes for a particular group (the Boston Conference on Illegitimacy, a Red Cross Institute, classes taking extension courses in social psychiatry at the Boston School of Social Work) and sometimes for social workers at large. A series of clinics for employment managers was also given. The history and the actual patient are, as a rule, both introduced. Patients suitable for demonstration are carefully chosen with an eye to seeing that the patients do not themselves suffer. In the majority of instances the patients are actually helped by the clinic, in that they are made to see the nature of the problems which they present, and yet are not overborne by the legal authority which a court appearance would assert. Some of the most instructive cases, from the standpoint of diagnosis and disposition, are in fact cases of delinquency or suspected delinquency, in which the clinical demonstration is far less of an ordeal than would be an appearance in court. As a rule, from forty to sixty social workers have appeared at the social clinics so far carried on. Amongst these workers will appear, as a rule, persons greatly sympathetic with the patient, and the "third degree" aspect of the meetings is reduced to practically nil. To many patients, instead of being a severe ordeal, the experience is rather agreeable. In many cases it is really beneficial to the patient who is forced by the interest of so many persons to confront his own mental difficulties and is put on his mettle to do the best he can to overcome his limitations. At a clinic for employment managers, one patient suffering from a persistent traumatic neurosis, John Flynn (case 19), was presented and apparently enjoyed the meeting. A few weeks later he sent several of his themes, part of an evening course in English that he was taking at the Trade Union College, for the physician whom he had met on that occasion to see, confident that he had a new friend in the doctor.

SOCIAL CASE RECORDS

Most existing record forms in social agencies are admitted by everybody concerned to be unsatisfactory, either because they do not contain the material they should or because the material they contain is not readily accessible. Notwithstanding abundant discussion, very little work has been done on improved methods of social case-recording. The only available studies of the subject are the work of Miss Georgia G. Ralph, *Elements of Record Keeping for Child-Helping Organizations* and recent books by Mrs. Ada D. Sheffield, *The Social Case History: Its Construction and Contents,* and by Miss Gertrude L. Farmer, *A Form of Record for Hospital Social Work.*

The stage at which a life history was recorded by means of a printed form seems to have passed. Most agencies now have an outline of facts adapted to the particular needs of their work to serve as a guide in recording the social examination. Probably no record system could be devised that would meet fully the needs of all agencies. Within the same agency it may appear economical to use a different form of recording for "slight service" and "intensive" cases. As a rule the record of a "slight service" case reduces itself to a brief memorandum on an index card or a record sheet. It is in the cases where responsibility is assumed for a complete history and thorough treatment that the record problem arises.

While the same form will not meet the needs of all sorts of social agencies, it might seem that the main outline of the facts to be secured would be the same in any case whatsoever under social care. The records of different agencies would vary in the details of some of the subheadings of such a general outline. The children's agency would be likely to go into more detail concerning the developmental history of a particular child than the family agency would need to; the society for protecting neglected children would require details of evidence not essential to the work of other children's agencies; in a medical social service certain items of bodily condition not significant for the general agency might be needed; certain details of mental states bearing upon the mental diagnosis would be found only in the records of the psychiatric social service. In general the social service of a psychopathic hospital requires for its work just such a record as would be needed by a children's agency, the parole department of a reformatory, or a family agency (in individual cases). With certain modifications, a standard history outline for all social records might prove very serviceable. It must always be borne in mind, however, that the value of the record depends not upon the outline but on knowledge of what facts are significant and on skill in obtaining information. Given, however, a skillful and intelligent social worker, a good history outline as a framework for investigation is a helpful support. With beginners and less reliable workers, it is an essential.

In considering social case-recording we are of course thinking of the history of an individual. The so-called "family record" is another thing,—there is the story of the family life to be written. But each member of the family has his own individual history, which has a claim to be separately recorded. Each member of the family must be studied separately in order to understand the family group. And for study of the individuals of the group, individual histories are required. If information concerning the different members of the family is not sorted out and recorded separately, the effect of the record will be very much like a composite photograph. There will be a hint of this or that individual member of the group, but no clear picture. To individualize each member of the family, it would seem to be essential to record his history separately. Certain facts that relate to all members of the family might be referred to by cross reference in order to save space and time. The family case worker would perhaps object that in the process of making individual records the story of the family group life would tend to get lost. It may be that a *summary of the family* would meet this need. We have no claim to offer a solution for any of the perplexities of record-keeping,—we aim here only to emphasize individualization in social case work.

There is hardly a question anywhere today as to whether social records should be or not be,—the case is proved that good records help to make good work. Yet the relative value of a good record system is indistinctly seen; and many agencies question the proportion of time that it pays to give to record-keeping. This depends first of all upon the purposes that the record serves—the ways in which it promotes the welfare of the patient or client.

The *immediate purposes* of the record are to make the history available for use (by physicians, as well as social workers) in a hospital; to save reinvestigation if the case is renewed after being closed; to enable a new worker who must take up the case to understand the situation; and to oblige the worker to think clearly and to make her work definite. Social records serve also the *ultimate purposes* of furnishing material in accessible form for social and medical research; making it possible to study the work of the agency and estimate its performance; furnishing standards for bringing the work of other agencies to a higher level; and affording material for teaching students.

The necessary documents of the record we have found to be:

a. A brief first sheet giving identifying information and facts needed for statistics (see Appendix B, Form I).

b. History (record of the investigation or social examination; for outline see Appendix B, Form II).

c. Treatment (record of the action taken, the current history of the case under social care).

d. Summary of history.

e. Summaries of treatment and results at regular intervals and when the case is closed.

f. Address sheet for addresses in current use.

g. Financial sheet for expenditures or special donations.

h. Correspondence arranged chronologically.

Examples of full records of cases 46, 89, 94 are given in Appendix A; examples of "Summary" will be found in cases 20, 24, 32; and examples of "Results" will be found in cases 31 and 62. The summary of the history is prepared under the divisions of social, physical, and mental history, and results are summarized every three months in the same manner.

In the discussions of social workers there seems to be an uncertainty of opinion as to the nature and uses of a summary. Some look to it for a full presentation of the case, a complete digest of the history, which is recorded elsewhere in the form of interviews and letters. We conceive the summary as the briefest possible statement of the essential facts of the case, following in form the outline used for collecting the data. The judgment of the worker in selecting the essential facts necessarily enters into the summary. A thorough consideration of a case cannot be based upon a summary alone. In our case conferences the summary is supplemented by comments and questions. There have been certain attempts to adapt the fivefold classification of the Kingdom of Evils to the purpose of the summary by using the positive aspects of the evils there comprised as headings for a summary, but this is a mistake; for the fivefold classification is far from being a scheme for the collection of data but is proposed as an orderly method of case *analysis*. The summary is a synthesis of the case, intended to present a vivid picture of the main outlines of the individual's history.

One of the chief difficulties in studying methods and results in social treatment is the lack of information in the record concerning the plans and purposes of the social worker. It is usually impossible to form any idea of what the patient owes to social care and what to "nature." The technique of treatment can rarely be discovered from the record. There may or may not have been a method in the treatment, as far as the record shows. One way of supplying this deficiency is to record at the beginning of the "treatment record" the general plan that is to be followed and to indicate in the periodical summaries of results the modifications of the plan later adopted. Sometimes a social record will go to the opposite extreme and consist largely of the worker's own plans and opinions to the exclusion of information concerning the patient. It is easy to slip into the habit of recording intentions and impressions rather than to make the effort to secure facts.

In order to make a clear distinction between the current history of the patient under care and the social worker's plan and methods in treatment, an effort was made for a time to keep a "treatment sheet" separate from the main case record. (For examples, see cases 14, 17, and 36.) This attempt had to be given up under pressure of work after a short trial; but the device seems to us to offer promise of better study of method in social case work. At the same time it has a tendency to make the treatment more definite and effective, and to stimulate ingenuity and resourcefulness in the social worker. It might be just as well to make the "treatment" entries on the regular record instead of on a separate "treatment sheet," provided the statements of aims and methods were arranged in such a way that they would stand out clearly.

TECHNIQUE OF SOCIAL DIAGNOSIS AND TREATMENT

Concerning the technique of social diagnosis and treatment we do not claim any approach to complete discussion, even of the facts which we note in this book. As a preface to such remarks as we make below upon social technique and diagnosis, we wish to speak of what has been called "family case work" and to make a general remark about it. The unit of interest in social case work, like the unit of interest in social reform and even in theoretical sociology, has often been the family group. "As society is now organized," says Richmond in *Social Diagnosis,* "we can neither doctor people nor educate them, nor launch them into industry, nor rescue them from dependence in a thoroughly social way without taking their family into account. Even if our measures were for the welfare of the individual solely we should find that the good results of individual treatment crumble away often because the case worker has been ignorant of his client's family history." (Richmond used the term client instead of the term patient, which at least in medical social work seems to us preferable.) Briefly put individualization in social treatment unconditionally requires consideration of the family group. Richmond quotes the Swiss neurologist Dubois and the American neurologists Healy and Putnam in support of these contentions with which we must all perforce agree. The following items in the family group relations are discussed by Richmond. The main drift of the family life, what is it on the whole? The important distinction between the united family and the unstable family (especially emphasized by Mrs. Bosanquet in her book *The Family*). The necessity of "seeing the man" as well as the mother of the family and of seeing him at home; the question of the unmarried father; the question of the young couple requiring relief; problems of desertion and inebriety; the wife and mother; the home situation; the family housing; children (here we find the blood relationship and all those undercurrents of antagonism which it implies); the other members of the family group including undesirable relatives. Volumes should and must be written upon these questions of the family group. Of particular value in a study of family cohesions (the united and the unstable family as distinguished by Le Play) will be the psychiatric point of view. Families are said to "arrange themselves along a scale with the degenerate family at one end and the best type of united family at the other." But what is the degenerate family in many or most instances except a family with psychopathic trends in one or more members? Then there are instances like that of Henry Loyal (case 4) of Book I in which, except at times, there was extraordinary close cohesion of a degenerate family. Even in this instance the family "solidarity" proved as social workers have always insisted to be the greatest asset. Another good psychiatric point is the systematic point of seeing husband and wife separately so that each may get an individual opportunity to present the personal view. Where character deviation enters, this point comes out in strong relief. With respect to the unmarried father as well as the unmarried mother, an enormous insistence has to be made according to our view upon the question of greater or lesser feeble-mindedness in the erring parent. If a wife and one or two babies of a young able-bodied man in ordinary times need any service that involves social work, this is a situation that demands the closest scrutiny and to our mind the closest psychiatric scrutiny. Neglectfulness, slackness of such degree as to involve the necessity of dole-giving, certainly need a psychiatrist's attention. "Laziness" is another phenomenon which not seldom turns out to be in some way psychological.

Inebriates would nowadays one and all be subject to psychiatric scrutiny. There is one set of statements that can safely be made about all inebriates. Richmond quotes Neff favorably to the effect that "the treatment of the inebriate can best be expressed in the word individualization." The like can be said of the family deserters, male or female. Perhaps the relation of psychiatry is not too evident in questions of home-making and family housing and many programs of social reform have in the past endeavored to center upon conditions of housing and home-making, which would in part at least derive not so much from economical disability as from ignorance, bad habits, or even mental defect. It is extraordinary what different reports will be rendered concerning some family situations by workers who have the economic view uppermost and by psychiatric workers. As for children, here the work of Healy, as Richmond rightly claims, is far beyond his chosen scope of mere delinquency and points the path of psychiatric social work far beyond the confines of potential crime. The psychiatric worker tends to look at social situations rather than at family groups. The psychiatric social worker finds social situations dominated by psychopaths, by one or more persons whose mental disease or disorder may be extremely mild and entirely invisible to members of the social group in question. Sometimes the remote members of the family group or the boarders and lodgers, and even the neighbors, may have a more penetrating view of what is really going on.

We are more and more tending to insist that each social situation, looked into by the psychiatric social worker, shall be analyzed in the end according to the number of persons involved. This number of involved persons may be small or large. But we almost always find that the number of distinct and separate points of view in each social situation is comparatively small. In a quarrel between a husband and wife there may be two points of view and the social worker may add the third point of view. Whereas the husband and wife are agreeing to disagree within four walls, the social worker may upon analysis advise another policy, that of separating husband and wife for a longer or shorter period. Of course the worker cannot execute any such policy without the consent and approval of all legal, ecclesiastical, and medical authorities engaged; the supposition in the textbook is that the decision of the social worker is supported by these authorities. Or again the husband and wife may have separated and entertain antagonistic views of what the family ought to do, whereas the social worker may leap into the situation with the idea of reunion. The point we here make is that after all the persons in the social situation have been listed (somewhat after the manner of the dramatis personae in plays) the really distinct and separate points of view in the social situation are to be analyzed and listed (just as one might distinguish the principals and accessories in a dramatic cast). We have not consciously adopted this method to any extent in the analysis of the material of this volume, although in effect we have often got practical results,—consider, for example, Henry Loyal (case 4) or Alice Nardini (case 31).

But how shall we distinguish the principals and the accessories and the less important units in the social situation? The psychiatric social worker learns that the family is not the unit of interest for psychiatric social work but finds that the unit of interest is the individual in his group. There will be found one, two, three, four, or perhaps sometimes five, but rarely more than five, human units of interest in social situations. The children may split as to what they want done, some going with the father and some going with the mother. Relatives may take a third point of view separate from that of the father and mother. Sometimes the social worker may enter with still a fourth point of view and so on. But many of the persons listed as engaged in the social situation turn out to be of subordinate importance in that situation. They add themselves in to enforce a little more strongly some particular policy but they are accessories agreeing with the policies of some principal. How shall these principals be defined? They are, we think, non-interchangeable elements in the social situation. They are not merely **associates** like the members of a club but they are **consociates** like the officers of a club that have separate functions not interchangeable with one another. How many separate, non-compatible, non-interchangeable points of view are logically to be found in a social situation? This is the real question which the social case worker must strive to answer. The family is a **consociate group of persons** (as father, mother, children) having separate and non-interchangeable functions. Their intimacy of relation, or, as we may say, their consociate relationship may fall apart, particularly under the influence of something psychopathic in some member of the group. They become mere associate members of the group —that is to say, they are no longer intimately united with one another or even possibly quite antagonistic. Indeed, their antagonisms may be so intimate that they become almost friendly enemies, suggesting mutual antagonism, like two universities

such as Harvard and Yale. These members of the group whose
views simply add themselves into the views of some principals
in the situation are merely *associates* in the situation.   Their
views are interchangeable with one another.   They numerically
strengthen a point of view—they do not determine it.

It is upon these lines that we predict the careful social
analyses of the future will run.   Upon these lines we shall
study more effectively the relations of man to man, man to
woman, and woman to woman, whether these relations are
dual, triple, quadruple, or still more complex.   Throughout all
this study the psychiatric social worker will be apt to see with
great clearness the predominate importance of the psychopath.   But the psychiatric social worker will study each member of the social situation individually, and each from his own
personal point of view, so that there will be no psychiatric
prejudice in the long run.   We conceive that this kind of
analysis has a range much greater than yet afforded by available analyses of the family group.   But we also know that it
would take a long time to reach the confines of the vista.

Discrimination between the **summation of evils** and the
multiplication of evils has been referred to (case 8) as having a bearing upon social treatment.   In one case the elements
of disorder may be loosely combined, heaped, while in another
case they are tightly combined, coiled.   It is important to know
whether we are dealing with *summands* or *factors*.   Evils
multiply into one another.   The effect of hypersexuality and
lack of information about sex lead to more difficulty combined than the sum of the two evils alone.   (See also
Book IV.)   The case of Rose Talbot, intelligent sex delinquent (case 8), gives an elaborate example of tightly coiled
troubles.   A contrast of our first case, Agnes Jackson, with
this case brings out clearly the sum of troubles versus the
product.   The Jackson case is a simple additive case,
$M+E+V+L+P$, while Rose Talbot is a complex multiplica-
tive case, $M \times E \times V \times L \times P$.   In a multiplicative,
interpretative case, if you remove poverty you change the whole
situation; but in the simpler additive case you may send the
patient for various sorts of help to various sources, dealing
with his difficulties one by one.   The case of Elliot Calderwood,
misrepresented "little fiend" who proved quite amenable (case
22), as an example of educational, legal, and economic diffi-

culties, is a case in which the factors of difficulty were not interwoven in any practical sense and could be disposed of in turn,—the misunderstanding with the court set right (L), a home provided (P), education started (E).

Will the difficulty of social treatment vary with the tightness of the coil, or on the other hand will the whole coil unravel quickly when the secret is found? There may be cases for quick treatment, where a single line of action will solve the problem. Cases that are sums of social trouble mean increase of steps to be taken in treatment,—they are logically simple but time-consuming. We cannot hope to do more in this book than suggest the idea of the **social sum** versus the **social product** as a method of approach in social treatment.

Psychiatric social work employs the technique of general social work in so far as systematic methods have been developed in social case work. There exists a certain amount of technique of social examination (usually called "the investigation") that is now generally agreed upon and made available in the literature of social work, and a smaller amount of technique of social treatment, which is fairly definite, although still somewhat tentative. Scientific methods of examination will naturally precede scientific methods of treatment, for although in the development of its practice social work first learned to treat and later learned to examine (or "investigate"), in the development of scientific method examination must necessarily come before treatment. So that the newly created psychiatric social worker finds already at hand a considerable body of systematized experience in examination and a small amount in treatment. Obviously it is the part of wisdom to acquire this technique, which is the accumulated experience of twenty-five years or so of tentative effort toward scientific method. The new psychiatric social worker impatient with the disregard of mental science in the general technique may have an impulse to discount the experience of social workers in the past and begin all over again. Sometimes under the influence of physicians whose acquaintance with social work in the past has been slight, and perhaps on that account unsatisfactory, the psychiatric social worker is inclined to discard the incomplete technique of social work altogether, and to feel a naïve responsibility to create a new profession. But the existing technique is not so much *incorrect* as it is *incomplete*.

The ambition of psychiatric social work should be to modify and add to the general technique of social work new methods developed by special experience with psychiatric cases.

Some of the more conspicuous points at which psychiatric social work may be expected to influence the technique of case work are: (*a*) individualization in both examination and treatment; (*b*) objective accurate observation; and (*c*) training of character through use of the emotions. The subject of individualization has been discussed elsewhere. (See cases 48 and 87, also pages 378 and 379.)

Focusing upon *the individual* soon leads to the recognition of the fact that human beings are infinitely varied and cannot be rated for practical purposes at certain levels of merit. Within the same personality are to be found faults and virtues, abilities and disabilities. This point of view often gains respect for even the most unsuccessful individual. In cases where failure is due to natural causes too strong for the individual's control, the knowledge of this fact will eliminate the attitude of blame that we instinctively feel for misconduct. The question of praise and blame is important for social workers. Undoubtedly much harm is done by the discouragement and loss of energy that blame produces; and praise is obviously an effective therapeutic agent. One of the primary aims of the social worker is to deepen the sense of moral responsibility; a process which is apt to involve frequent expression of disapproval. But it is doubtful whether reproof and blame promote this object. The truth of the matter probably is that reproof or blame as ordinarily administered is compounded of our knowledge of the error and our impatience with it. It is perhaps the tinge of personal impatience that gives blame its unpleasant quality. Many unfortunate psychopaths who have been censured and despised by acquaintances, and often by social workers, when they meet the psychiatric point of view, feel a sense of relief and renewed self-respect and are stimulated to fresh effort. (See cases 2, 4, 6, 12, 13, 52, 98.)

Another product of the psychiatric point of view is the habit of *objective observation*—the study of an individual as he really is, not as we feel that we should be in his place, or as he himself tells us that he is. In social case work we need to know accurately the nature of our patient or client. We do him an injustice if we form a conception of him in terms of our own experience. His own account, though honestly meant, may not be accurate. Through observation of his behavior and reports of other observers upon his conduct, the best account of his character is to be obtained. When we come to the point of trying to understand him, we must necessarily think in terms of our own experience, but the objective study should precede the interpretation. We first find out what an individual is like, and then think how we should feel and act if we were like that. This process of objective study, preceding subjective understanding, simplifies many problems in social work and promotes sympathy. Personalities quite unlike our own when studied objectively become comprehensible.

Training through use of the *emotions* rather than through appeal to reason is a familiar technique of everyday life in dealing with children and in getting our own way. Everyone is familiar with the practice of asking a favor when the prospective donor is in a good humor, and upon the strength of the resulting good feeling after a suitable interval asking another favor, thereby helping to develop habits of generosity in the donor. Such technique seems to be the most hopeful method of training individuals in whom misconduct is the result of emotional instability. In discussing this point we cannot do better than to quote somewhat at length from *A Psychiatric Contribution to the Study of Delinquency,* by Dr. Herman M. Adler (see also page 487), who as chief of staff at the Psychopathic Hospital guided the first efforts of the social service in cases of delinquency:—

"It would seem that by careful training based upon an analysis of each individual—especially from the behaviorist's point of view, considering the past life and career rather than self-explanatory, subjective statements—it would be possible to influence the future conduct of these individuals (*i.e.,* the emotionally unstable). While their fundamental equipment cannot be changed, these people suffer more from the effects of their conduct than from their subjective attitude towards themselves or their environment.

"Thus, as Kraepelin points out, alcohol is an important factor in producing the final downfall. Extravagance, profligacy, sex excesses, bad companionship, and so forth, are the factors which combine to cause the social difficulties. The suggestibility of these individuals, their intelligence and insight, which is usually adequate for their needs, can be made use of in acquiring and strengthening the habits which the individual would never be able to gain if left to himself.

"What is desired, therefore, is a system of mental and emotional exercises for the purpose of habit formation. This might be designated as orthopsychics. This term is further applicable in that a good many of those cases are instances not of disease in the sense of an acquired, deteriorating process, but rather comparable to physical deformities. For the present, our experience in orthopsychics is limited. We have had a few cases in which, after a preliminary survey at the Psychopathic Hospital, a course of training has been applied, which has consisted above all in arousing the interests and appealing to the pleasure-loving side of the individual. It is a well-known fact, for instance, in dealing with wayward young people that even under the most advantageous circumstances and even with the most favorable and friendly environment, the individuals do not do well. This appears to be due to the fact that the emotional impulses are of short duration and leave no strong impressions behind them. Therefore, when the novelty of a situation has worn off, there is nothing to hold the interests of the delinquent and tide over the tedious days of monotonous routine.

"We have proposed in a number of cases (and have carried it out to some extent in a few) to arrange to change the environment of each individual before the novelty has quite worn off. The length of time in which an individual stays in each home varies in each instance, and must be determined carefully each time. We are all so prejudiced by our early ethical training that it is difficult to be perfectly objective in dealing with these people. It is hard to eliminate pedagogic and purely academic demands for that which we consider right. None the less, this must be done, and in every instance, in every disagreement, at every change in the routine of the individual, emphasis must be laid on the fact that it is done from a medical point of view, that is, from a point of view of therapy and help, with kindly feelings toward the patient, and never as a corrective or as a punishment, and above all, never vindictively.

"Education and training, therefore, rather than punishment are the methods that hold out a chance of success. These individuals are not able to learn by experience. They receive the equivalents of punishment in their daily life, which are sufficient to influence the formation of adequate resistance in a normal individual. In these individuals, while they often recognize the full significance of those circumstances in which their delinquencies placed them, their experiences have no corrective influence.

"To punish such an individual, therefore, is to increase his defeat rather than to strengthen his defenses. It is like administering alcohol to the patient suffering from delirium tremens. It is like injecting diphtheria toxin into the circulation of a patient suffering from diphtheria. We may draw a final analogy from immunology in applying this therapy:

"The first duty is protection against the immediate effects of the acute attack. In our cases, this means freeing them from their immediate difficulties, supplying them with food and lodging, helping them to recover from alcohol and drug intoxication, relieving their physical symptoms, curing them of venereal disease, and building up their physical health.

"In the second place, immunization: This is often in the nature of after care, and cannot be achieved at once, but can be accomplished by a building up of the defense habits, by training, and not by overwhelming an already breaking organism with the hostile conditions, but by gradually strengthening their habits so that they will meet the particular unfavorable conditions without fear of breakdown. In the group of emotionally unstable, this offers great hope."

The relation of social worker to patient (or client) seems to be causing the development of a new *professional attitude.* The ideal attitude of the established professions, such as medicine, education, theology, is one of authority and impersonal friendliness. The effective attitude for the professional social worker is essentially the same, but the proportions of authority and friendliness are reversed, and the friendliness is less impersonal. The social worker (except the probation officer) carries no such authority as the institutions of hospital, school, and church bestow, but must rely for prestige upon her ability to help. The friendliness of her relation to the patient, in successful treatment, is of a high degree; for almost immediately she secures an exceptional intimacy with the patient's whole interior and exterior situation. The patient responds to this sudden intimacy by regarding her as a near friend. To influence him throughout the intricacies of social adjustment she must preserve this regard. She must identify herself with him, directing him from his own point of view, giving him the counsel of "a friend" not merely the advice of "an authority." On the other hand she must preserve enough of the element of authority to be a decided and respected influence. This continuous intimate relationship is apt to make the social worker very sympathetic; but even in the most appealing cases she must combine with her sympathy an objective impersonal attitude that will leave her judgment free. When it is said in justification of a social worker "she puts her heart into her work," it must not be forgotten that the patients have a claim upon her head as well. The social worker must find a way to be at the same time a personal friend and an impersonal adviser.

The fact that the social worker stands to the patient in the light of a friend might seem to argue the importance of having but one worker deal with a case throughout the period of social treatment. But this in our experience is not so important as it might seem. A change of workers can be made without loss and may even be an advantage. In any case under long-time treatment, with the changing staff of a hospital, it is unavoidable that there should be several different workers in succession. Some of our most successful cases have had as many as six or seven social workers, and three or four workers not infrequently deal in turn with one case (see cases 8, 32, 94). The success of the transfer of a case to another person depends of course upon the skill of the workers concerned and upon their consideration for the feelings of the patient. In some cases the patient likes his new social worker better, and in most cases he feels it is some advantage to have acquired a new friend. There may be of course some loss in a case where the patient has gradually come to confide in the first worker; but such loss is apt to be overestimated. The bringing in of new ideas and influences through a new worker may be a positive advantage to the treatment.

The patient will feel decided opposition to the transfer if he has formed an excessive attachment to the social worker, but this relationship is not to be encouraged in any case. Another reason for objection from the patient may be that he fears opposition from the new worker in something which he has been allowed to persist in doing. On the whole we believe the best results come from teaching the patient to look upon the social agency or the hospital as the source of help and direction, medical and social, and inspiring him by uniformly considerate treatment to feel confidence in every member of the staff who deals with him. This might appear as a theoretical principle too ideal for application, were it not that it is a conclusion derived from actual experience. We have found the point of view to be of more importance than the personality of the worker (see also case 8).

MEDICAL TREATMENT IN SOCIAL CASE WORK

We do not deal systematically with **medical treatment** in this volume. Hamilton Green (case 18) was an "eye" case—a man with severe astigmatism. No doubt the treatment of the astigmatism is indispensable in the handling of Hamilton Green. Yet it would be improper to think of Green as merely an eye case or of the treatment of his eyes as the essential thing in his case. Good but subordinate effects were gained by **baths** for Agnes Jackson (case 1). In fact, the excellence of hydriatic treatment in cases of dementia praecox has been pointed out by our colleague, H. M. Adler, in his analysis of the effects of baths in different forms of excitement (contrary to expectation, Adler found that better effects of an important nature were secured in cases of dementia praecox than in cases of manic-depressive psychosis). It would be natural to draw **hydrotherapy** into the foreground in this or in other cases with which we are familiar. The baths serve to draw patients to hospitals, and an unfailing stimulus to the size of the out-patient clinic is the establishment of a good hydrotherapy system so associated with the clinic that proper hydriatric prescriptions can be made for systematic treatment. It does not do to scoff against these baths as some observers are apt to scoff. Possibly they are not essential to the treatment of any form of mental disease whatever (always excepting forms of excitement); possibly they are not even indispensable aids in treatment in many cases; but though they may be neither essential nor indispensable in treatment, baths remain important aids to any clinic. Moreover, it must be conceded that the true effects of hydrotherapy have never been scientifically measured by the metabolic chemists or otherwise.

Similarly with **dental treatment** which comes especially into question in the case of Margaret Dolan (case 38) whose dental defects and indigestion complicated a mental situation which was itself the result of a well-founded wrong. Despite all Margaret Dolan's financial trouble and the death of her sister, she recovered with social aid. Another dental case was that of Nathan Rosenthal (case 49). The dental complication was subordinated here also, but this always subordinate influence was still important. Social workers so often ask what the effect of dental treatment is upon mental diseases; owing to the fact that extraordinary claims have been made on behalf of dental work (especially extraction) in cases of mental disease. The public prints have in recent years been full of such claims. The rational answer to this question is that a few cases are marvelously benefited by proper dental treatment. These improvable cases are no doubt those in which pyorrhea or other infection about the teeth is responsible for mental symptoms through a process of septicemia (with bacterial invasion of the blood) or toxemia in which bacterial poisons find their way into the blood. Michael Piso (case 62) suffered extensively from pyorrhea but the dental treatment thereof was only a part of the total treatment of Piso which served in the end to raise his wages and procured relatively complete family adjustment with abolition of jealousy.

Occupational therapy is a means of treatment of the insane in institutions and of psychopaths outside of institutions. In war time groups of occupational therapeutists were trained to get ready for contingencies of disease amongst our American soldiers; and the work of these occupational therapeutists was so good and the outlook for their need under civilian conditions is so well established that the work is likely to be continued. An extensive literature has been built up around this form of therapy. Instances of its employment are afforded by Agnes Jackson (case 1) and Kevork Ardinian (case 26), though both cases illustrate relative failure rather than success in occupational therapy. A successful instance of its use is John Flynn (case 19).

Our group of cases is decidedly not representative of the values of occupational therapy and it would be a highly meritorious work for someone to collect a series of clearly diagnosticated cases of severe or mild mental disease and defect for the purpose of tracing the exact ways in which occupational therapy works in the different forms of psychopathy. For example, the reasons for the relative failure of occupational therapy in Agnes Jackson and its absolute failure in the case of Kevork Ardinian are different reasons and consequently do not have a word to say against the general values of such therapy. We should not forget that in the background of our minds the main value of sending the feeble-minded subject to a school for feeble-minded is the elaborate occupational therapy which he will there secure. Perhaps it is not too much to say that the **theory of occupational therapy will be built up from the work of the schools for the feeble-minded.** Workers in Massachusetts and in the country at large are familiar with the principles of such therapy for the feeble-minded as developed by Dr. Walter E. Fernald at the Massachusetts School for Feeble-minded in Waverly. These methods were first proposed and in part carried out by the eminent early worker with the feeble-minded, Séguin. An effect of the new theory of occupational therapy for the feeble-minded as proposed by Séguin, Fernald, and others is the proposal by Madame Montessori for new methods of education of the normal. We can forbear to insist that such workers as Séguin and Fernald are working along lines more in the interest of the normal than in the interest of the abnormal. These men and all mental hygienists are not making the frontal attack upon education which the teachers of the normal are making; but the flank attack by these mental hygienists may yet prove as successful as the more obvious forms of frontal attack.

Whilst we are talking of occupational therapy it is important to remember also the work for the chronic insane as carried out in the industrial shops and on the farms by victims of dementia praecox and other forms of mental deterioration. Colonies for the systematic development of the working powers of chronic patients have been established by some state governments, either separately or in connection with existent and exceptional units. From this source also it is to be hoped that new theories concerning the fundamental principles of work and industry may accrue. There is hardly any better way to evaluate the excellence of state institutions for the insane than to ask to see the industrial shop work and the farm work of the hospital patients. The best hospitals have efficiency recording devices which stimulate their officers to the securing of higher quotas of active workers and to increase in the number of hours of patient-occupation. Not so much

can be told from striking exhibition of arts and crafts by particular patients as from the statistical story afforded by the
annual reports of institutions. ⹁Occupational therapy is a most
important branch of mental hygiene. The theory of it is incomplete. The value of what has been done is not doubtful.

EDUCATION FOR PSYCHIATRIC SOCIAL WORK

What difference will it make to the world whether we consistently unfold the social side of the mental-hygiene program
and develop a group of **trained psychiatric social workers?**
The functioning elements in the mental hygiene of the present
day appear to be three in number, all indispensable though of
different scope and values. Mental hygiene would of course
be nowhere without the psychiatrist or neuropsychiatrist as
its professional leader. In mental hygiene conditions are the
same as in the general field of preventive medicine and public
health. After all, the things to be dealt with in the present
phase of civilization are'diseases and defects, and the fact that
mental diseases and defects come in question does not mean
that physicians lose their responsibilities or can by any means
hand them over to psychologists or social workers. To be
sure, not all **physicians** have yet seen the light of their duties
in public health and there may be a few moribund **psychiatrists**
that do not see their responsibilities in **mental hygiene.** But
the topic of mental hygiene engrosses the interest of national
technical associations that deal with mental and nervous diseases and plentifully scatters the literature, quarterly, monthly,
and weekly, with propagandist articles of high level. Even
certain daily newspapers carry mental hygiene topics under
the medical banter.

But **let not the physician nor the psychiatrist feel that
mental hygiene begins and ends with medicine or psychiatry.** The recent extensive review of ten years' activities
in mental hygiene by Dr. Lewellys F. Barker shows the almost
universal relativity of mental hygiene, and discovers hardly a
field of human activity to which mental hygiene is not germane.
But the practical relations have so deepened and solidified in
certain places that their intensive values almost outstrip the
extensive relation which Barker so broadly expounds. By
practical relations are meant those above specified in addition

to medical relations; namely, the relations with the psychologist and the social worker.

For the moment it is not our duty to discuss the values of the **psychological examiner** in the field. Those values do not need to be justified. Recent analyses of concrete work in our field have shown that the psychologist can often do more in an hour's contact with the patient than the social worker or even the psychiatrist can do in ten, twenty, or even one hundred hours of contact. The trouble is that the psychologist runs out of technique and method after his hour is up. He can do nothing more in the second hour of contact with a human being with whom he is in sympathy. Accordingly the work of the psychiatrist and of the social worker, though less intensive and powerful during the first hour of contact with the patient, lasts much longer and may in the long run effect far more. Both from the standpoint of prescribing medical or social adjustments and from the standpoint of making these adjustments really work in a compound environment. Let no one, and especially let not the psychiatrist or the social worker, look with contempt or with uneasy apprehensiveness on the work of the psychologist. But the **psychologist** is a scientific rather than a practical person. He **has at his command more the method of a science than the technique of an art.** He differs in his relation to our topic from the psychiatrist and from the social worker, both of whom are primarily engaged in the **practical arts of medicine and social work.** To be sure, the difference between applied science and the technique of a highly advanced art is so very slight that a pragmatist might well inquire whether they were not identical. Now and then a psychologist will be found claiming himself to be a sort of practitioner. He claims to become a sort of social or psychic technician rather than a methodologist at work at the fundaments of things. But on the whole the psychologist remains "-ologist," a man of science, and after he has exactly applied his strict categories in a brief time to the problems of the patient or to the classifications of an applicant for work, his province as a psychologist comes to a sharp limit, beyond which his activities are little more than those of an educated layman.

We trust that in all this we shall not be charged with belittling **psychology** which as a science, and as **in some sense** the deepest of sciences, must in the long run prove **as broad a field as that of medicine or even as the fields of physics and chemistry.** There is nothing that one would like better than to contribute to psychology as a science. Nevertheless psychology contributes method rather than technique, is working at the fundaments and generalities rather than the outcrops and specialties of social work.

What then shall we say about the social worker? In the first place there may be some lingering doubts in the minds of physicians, or administrators, of politicians, of various charitable authorities, whether there is a definite field of social work, but we take it that the National Conference of Charities and Correction, recently renamed the National Conference of Social Work, proves in all its recent transactions that there is a field of social work. It is in point that Isaac Ray, perhaps the greatest of the early American psychiatrists, was one of the founders of the Social Science Association. Nowadays we think more of social arts than social science and it was rather a service to our cause to have the National Conference name itself a Conference of Social Work, though the phrase is at first sight bungling enough. The object of these workers in selecting that title was not that they felt themselves the only workers in the world but that they did not wish to be dubbed "scientific" and, as we in the American scene so constantly say, impractical.

It is entirely clear that **social work is taken** by most of its votaries and propagandists as **an art** and **not as a science.** This, it seems to me, is as it should be. The social worker has in some ways identical aims and purposes with those of the psychiatrist. Both are practical workers engaged in social and medical arts which to some extent fuse and overlap but which in the long run will not interfere with each other any more than the physician and the nurse, or the public-health man and the public health nurse, will interfere with one another. Two psychic bodies can occupy the same place at the same time without breaking any important laws of the world's construction. It is perhaps hard to get both the physician on the one side and the social worker on the other to acknowledge the indispensability of each in a field where a single authority appears to be necessary—the field, namely, of the family disrupted by its central or subordinate psychopathic figures.

Let us assume in this argument that the physicians and the social workers in general agree upon their respective duties with respect to the same *corpus vile*.

What now about the medical social workers? Is not medical social work a very special and limited field within social work in general? Is not social work, the technical or applied side of sociology, an economic rather than a therapeutic field? Will not the bulk of the problem be settled on an economic line? What the statistical truth here is remains obscure. All medical social workers will agree that whatever the statistical truth about mere economics as applied to social difficulty, there is enough to do in medical social work to require a large corps of especially trained medical social workers. There is now in its early years of development an association of medical or hospital social workers, the American Association of Hospital Social Workers, which is to meet an affiliation with the National Conference of Social Work. The medical social workers form, as it were, a neat little trades-union of their own. They do not require laudation or special support from any source. Medical social work has justified itself.

What about psychiatric social work? Every medical social worker should obviously receive a large amount of social psychiatric training in his or her school of social work, and *a fortiori* should receive more and more if the mental hygienists are right in thinking that more than **one out of every two cases of social trouble is a psychiatric case.** Should there not be courses developed in connection with every school of social work that shall give a sufficient fundamental training to social workers in psychiatry to allow them to effect proper contacts in their practice? This is undeniable and we are heartily in accord with a program for giving the psychiatric touch so far as that is possible to every social worker. It is almost inconceivable that social-work courses have not, for a decade past, developed in their curricula lectures and demonstrations dealing with the common, nay universal, phenomena of syphilis, feeble-mindedness, epilepsy alcoholism, and even somewhat concerning the obscure field of the so-called psychopathic personalities.

Of course the social worker might readily get beyond the range of everyday **medical practitioner** in these regards, at all events if we consider the medical practitioner of elder vintages. But this comparison is a bit odious and it is certainly not the duty of those who make the curricula of schools for social work to dampen their ardor just because **medical schools have grievously neglected psychiatry.**

Another question of deeper interest to the close student of mental hygiene is the question whether there ought not to be special schools or curricula that deal with psychiatric social work with the endeavor to produce a special brand of social workers,—**psychiatric social workers.** It is a matter of history that Smith College, with the assistance of Dr. Spaulding, the New York School of Social Work through Dr. Glueck, and the Pennsylvania School for Social Service through Dr. Taft did actually develop courses for training psychiatric social workers. These courses were developed during the war fervor. They attracted and are attracting women as a rule with college degrees with very special interests in the humanities and with a point of view perhaps a bit less economic than the point of view of the ordinary social worker. The infusion of this blood, a little more radical and fiery than the sober reform blood of the type of social worker familiar to us all, no doubt, will have some rather surprising results, but we think the advantages of novelty and freshness of point of view may counterbalance the disadvantage of oversobriety and conservatism.

The comparative youth of sociology, of applied sociology (social work), of applied medical sociology (medical social work), and of the putative new branch (psychiatric social work) entails a certain fluidity of nomenclature at first not unserviceable. Nor would it be necessary or even desirable to fix at the outset a nomenclature for logical compartments of an undeveloped art, as we might thus condemn the art to stasis or bad *culs-de-sac.* We raise the question, therefore, only on the practical ground of whether or no specialists, professional or technical, have been developed or are in course of development in this field of sociology. For, if so, that is, if the new art has found its shoulder-to-shoulder workers, then it is high time to state the principles of their alignment, and the nature of curricula and practical experience necessary for these workers.

We assume that medicine and applied sociology are professions with their professors and practitioners having due recognition in university degrees, M.D. and Ph.D., respectively, and in commonly accepted titles, physician and sociologist. On account of the recency of sociology's foundation, everybody is prepared to accord to many workers without the degree Ph.D. just as good and perfectly equivalent dignity. Nor should such a contention as that sociologists will more and more tend to be Ph.D. bearers be regarded as propaganda of Professor James' "Ph.D. octopus," since everybody is now aware that novelty, in medicine, sociology, or any other branch, is perhaps more likely than not to come from some distant science. Thus the teaching branches of medicine are more likely to get novelty from, *e.g.*, chemistry, or physics, than from their own more limited fields. And the teaching branches of applied sociology are very likely to profit more from anthropology or psychology than from the recognized rounds of sociological research as narrowly conceived, *e.g.*, in the field of social statistics. Perhaps even it might be said that many branches of didactic medicine and sociology would get more food for new thought from each other than each from itself. We are not here talking of the technique of research, but of the sort of training which allows us to concede that such and such a person is entitled to rank as a professional sociologist alongside the physician.

There are, to repeat, persons to whom we accord an equal professional rank as didactic or practical masters of their fields—physicians and sociologists. But every profession must develop apprentices or ancillary workers of various sorts. Thus medicine has developed the nurse. Applied sociology, we make bold to say, has developed quite on the same level— the social worker. One has to be bold For many social workers, perfectly modest as to their own private capacities, have developed a surprising group-consciousness concerning the proper dominance of the ideal social worker in all social maladjustments. This group-consciousness of social workers often leads to a not unwarranted derision on the part of physicians, judges, men of the world. The point here is probably simple: just because not every eminent sociologist is a Ph.D. and because many sociologists prefer to call themselves "workers" (from the American habit of denouncing theory and suspecting all "-ologists" of carrying lugs), many humbler persons conceive that there is no theory behind their practice, no sociology behind their social service. It is as if, on the one hand, physicians seeing that medicine is so much a matter of nursing should announce themselves as a kind of nurse; it is as if, on the other hand, nurses seeing that the physicians are so ignorant of many practical matters should suddenly conceive that nurses were after all a sort of physician. Practically, too, in the present phase of social-service development, social workers are apt to be of a finer grain and a more finished higher education than the majority of nurses, and accordingly the social workers are inclined to develop a feeling of group-superiority to nurses. This attitude is of course a matter of dispute as to its justifiability, but is none the less existent. But we conceive that, unless a person wishes to go to the length of special training of professional grade, he can hardly claim equivalence to a man of professional training. We conceive that professionally trained social workers, of the Ph.D. level or equivalent, will finally admit themselves to be sociologists, albeit applied sociologists. And we hope that further there will be a group-consciousness developed of social workers below the "-ologist" grade with an attitude resembling that of nurses to their work—an attitude, according to temperament, of humble pride or proud humility with respect to their acknowledged leaders, the applied sociologists. Nor should the term *profession* be made a stumbling-block: if nursing is a profession, so ought social work (below the level of sociology) to be acknowledged a profession also: this last is a matter of terms only.

But no two sciences or arts can in these days long exist without fruitful contacts. Pathological and sociological progress have gone hand in hand. Many a physician is, we say, really and by temper a sociologist; many a sociologist develops so deep an interest in, *e.g.*, sanitation problems that he becomes in effect a physician, at least an expert in public health. Social medicine and medical sociology have much in common: either could receive the term **theory of the public health** without special error of definition.

Not to linger over the definition of public health, hygiene, and preventive medicine as against the non-medical branches of sanitary science and art, it is clear that both **social medicine** and **medical sociology** have brought to life auxiliary groups of practical workers, viz., the **public health nurse** and the medical social worker. It is clear, too, that just as social medicine and medical sociology are different in their points of view, so the aides in the practical work of each field are likely to have a different point of view. If the lively growth of the public health nurse group sometimes threatens to engulf the medical social worker (*e.g.,* by proposals that the same curriculum will do for both), the fact is that no such forced union will ever take place, judging by the quality and nature of the persons each field has so far attracted.

Now it is obvious that the public health nurse of today is no better prepared to be an aide to a psychiatrist than the ordinary physician is trained to deal with psychopathic cases. Should there not be a group of nurse-like human beings who should be aides to psychiatrists in much the same sense as public health nurses are aides to the public health physicians? On the other hand, should not there be a special group of social workers skilled in the psychiatric side of medical sociology? Such a trained mental hygiene aide would be then an assistant to the psychiatrist in medical treatment,—a special type of public health nurse trained in the care of mental diseases. She would be equipped with an understanding of social conditions and remedies to the extent that such appreciation of social problems has been found desirable for the public health nurse. She should not be confused with the psychiatric social worker whose function is to assist in social diagnosis and treatment under sociological direction. In short, we think it will be possible to show that the point of view of medicine and the point of view of social work are at bottom sundered from each other, so that the *physician* and the *sociologist,* the *nurse* and the *social worker,* the *mental hygiene aide* and the *psychiatric social worker,* will always remain persons with somewhat separate sentiments. It is worth while to insist that these sentiments though separate are not necessarily opposed to one another. It is even possible that within a single personality a worker can be an effective individualist, on the one hand, and an effective social-groupist, on the other; that one can be both a physician and an applied sociologist successfully; but the success attained will probably be like that in which the right (or medical) hand will not know what the left (or social) hand is doing.

So much for our theory of the future of education for psychiatric social work. The present practice follows a middle course,—the trained psychiatric social worker today is not, as a rule, the applied sociologist of Ph.D. grade, nor yet the practical worker bearing the same relation to sociology that the nurse bears to medicine; but something of both.

The special training courses for psychiatric work now given in several schools (Smith College Training School for Social Work; New York School of Social Work; Pennsylvania School for Social Service) are graduate courses covering a period of approximately two academic years. Such courses approach the requirements for the A.M. degree. There are persons who think that the degrees A.M. and Ph.D. may not reasonably be offered in social work on the ground that such education is practical rather than scientific. Even if it be granted that social work is a form of applied science, there are probably forces at work in a good many universities and colleges•that regard with suspicion all science that has the flavor of practicality.

To meet the demand for social workers for the neuropsychiatric hospitals of the army, the plan of the Smith College Training School of Psychiatric Social Work was conceived by us, in 1918, as a war-emergency course. Intensive courses of instruction were given at Smith College during eight weeks of the summer, and the students were then distributed among four cities—Boston, New York, Philadelphia, and Baltimore —for six months of practice work in various hospitals and social agencies. Some experienced social workers were admitted for the summer course only. The following year Smith College continued the course as a permanent school under the name of the Smith College Training School for Social Work. The length of the course was changed from eight to thirteen months, and training for other branches of social work also was undertaken. The work falls into three divisions—a summer session of eight weeks of theoretical instruction combined with clinical observation; a training period of nine months of study and practice carried on in coöperation with hospitals; and a concluding summer session of eight weeks of advanced study. The summer sessions are held at Smith College, Northampton, Massachusetts. The practical instruction is arranged by placing students with hospitals in different cities, under supervision, locally and centrally, by the staff of the Training School.

This method of preliminary instruction followed by continuous practice was the outgrowth partly of the necessity for training quickly a larger number of workers than could be provided with practice facilities in any one city, and also partly of our experience with an apprentice course given for several years at the Psychopathic Hospital. We found that a student who was on duty continuously, giving full time to case work without the distraction of class work, acquired experience and skill more quickly and more confidently. If the student gives full time in the hospital, is on duty regularly and without interruption, she becomes completely assimilated into the organization and so gains in depth of experience as well as in drill and discipline. Moreover, a student who has received preliminary instruction can from the beginning do more responsible case work. It is doubtful whether practice work with social cases can be carried on satisfactorily along with intensive instruction, for human problems cannot be regulated so that experience will run parallel to theoretical instruction. On the other hand, the concentration of study in two periods at the beginning and end of the practice work permits a high degree of mental application. A thread of theory running through the practice period, in the form of a weekly class, required reading, and preparation of a thesis, serves to unite the two study periods.

The potential student then should in the first place be a somewhat educated person, that is, the possessor of an A.B. degree or else equally well educated by less formal methods than a full college course. She will need both the qualities requisite for all forms of intellectual work and the qualities requisite for all forms of practical work. Further, she must have the qualities that all social work requires—interest in individuals and a liking to follow them into the scenes of their daily lives, an impersonal attitude, the power of intelligent sympathy, a high degree of disinterestedness, and the capacity for sustained purpose. In addition, the special qualifications that the psychiatric social work requires in a marked degree are patience, analytical ability, and capacity for objective observation.

A course in preparation for psychiatric social work presupposes the college branches—biology, psychology, sociology, economics, and government. The content of the special graduate course given at the Smith College Training School includes social psychiatry, the theory of mental tests, the essentials of medicine, social psychology, government as related to social work, organization of social work, and the theory and practice of social case work. Theoretically it might seem desirable to add such a course to a foundation of one year in general social work, where the student would acquire the technique of social case work and a knowledge of the organization of social work. But there is reason to think that the best results are obtained at present by admitting students at once to specialized training. Schools of social work have not in the past given a place in their general training to principles of mental hygiene, so that training in social work is apt to be deficient in the psychiatric point of view, which it is desirable for the student in psychiatric social work to acquire as early as possible.

Principles and technique of case work may be acquired as readily in psychiatric cases as elsewhere. Nor is the experience of the student working on psychiatric cases limited to psychopaths, for all the members of the family come within the field of action.

A NOTE UPON LEGAL ENTANGLEMENT AS A DIVISION OF EVIL

ROSCOE POUND

In civilized society the individual must adjust not only to his fellowmen and to groups of his fellowmen but to the political organization of society and to the legal order. Maladjustments in the latter respect, whether due to fault of the individual or independent of his fault, whether inevitable because of inherent difficulties in the administration of justice through law or remediable by improved and better-operated legal machinery, are *Litigia* in Dr. Southard's sense. Briefly, he means forms of social maladjustment involving contacts with the law. For he conceives rightly that mere involvement in a legal controversy is an evil, and an evil to which we are naturally subject in society quite as much as to disease or to poverty. The legal machine, like any other machine, in the nature of things will operate mechanically, and in that mechanical operation the just as well as the unjust are likely to be caught.

Conditions of controversy and legal entanglement may be aggravated by or may result from some of the other main types of evil. But as disease or poverty or ignorance may be of independent non-culpable origin, so conditions of controversy or legal entanglement may arise quite without fault of him who suffers therefrom. Moreover, whether we turn to the reported decisions of the courts, or to the reports of legal aid societies or to the accounts of actual experience of judicial administration of justice which lawyers have put in the form of fiction, we may find abundant testimony that those who for any reason become entangled in legal controversy may suffer as acutely, without moral fault on their part, from evils not easily separable from our social and political and legal organization as their fellows who are burdened with disease or poverty, or ignorance. In *Ten Thousand a Year* and in *Farmer Bumpkin's Law Suit,* two lawyers have painted in enduring colors what it means to be a party to a hard fought law suit.[1] The story may be told no less vividly from the actual

[1] The effect of protracted litigation in paralyzing the energies and sapping the vitality of a litigant is set forth by Dickens in *Bleak House* and by George Eliot in *The Mill on the Floss.*

563

records of the courts.   No doubt the social worker encounters legal entanglement as a complication in cases primarily involving other evils.   But it may serve better to demonstrate Dr. Southard's point if we look exclusively at cases of legal entanglement pure and simple or cases where involvement in legal controversy is the primary factor.

One may find himself seriously involved in legal controversy, without fault on his part, either as a matter of pure misfortune or as the victim of the culpable action or inaction of others.   In the first category (pure misfortune) four all too common cases may be noted: mistaken identity, circumstantial evidence, the chance that one may be a casual eyewitness of another's crime, and inheritance of a *bona fide* litigated claim.   The case of Lesurques,[2] positively identified by numerous witnesses and executed for a crime of which the event showed he was wholly innocent and for which the real perpetrator was afterwards brought to justice, and of Adolf Beck,[3] twice convicted and subjected to imprisonment for crimes with which he had absolutely no connection upon mistaken identifications by the victims and only saved by the apprehension of the real offender for like crimes committed while Beck was in custody, stand out in the annals of the criminal law.   But Lesurques and Beck were men of a certain social position, of education and of some means.   How many such cases occur where the accused cannot invoke such resources and thereby bring the injustice to light we may but conjecture.[4]   At the very least we must admit a potential danger of legal entanglement through mistaken identity as something never to be overlooked.   How an innocent person may be the victim of appearances and of circumstantial evidence has been a fruitful theme for dramatists and novelists and is continually illustrated in the courts, despite all provisions for careful deliberate trial of the facts and presumptions of innocence.[5]   Less serious, but bad enough, is the condition of the upright and busy or upright but indigent citizen who chances to be an important witness to the commission of a felony.   Mr. Train has told us from first-hand observation what the witness must go

[2] As to Lesurques, see Fouquier, *Causes célèbres de tous les peuples*, III, no. 12; 1 Green Bag, 72.

[3] See *Report of the Committee of Inquiry into the Case of Mr. Adolf Beck*, 1904.   Not only was Beck imprisoned for crimes with which he had no connection, but he lost his property through inability to preserve it while in prison.

[4] For the more notable older cases of mistaken convictions, see Loeffler, *Die Opfer mangelhafter Justiz*, 3 vols., Jena, 1879.

[5] Examples are collected in Hellwig, *Justizirrtümer*, 1914.   For an American case, see *People v. Teiper*, 186 App. Div. 830.   Teiper was acquitted upon a retrial.

through with if he is able to give sureties to appear and testify.[6] If he cannot give security, he is likely to be committed to jail to secure his appearance as a witness and to suffer almost as much as if he had actually offended.[7] But it is quite as possible to be caught innocently in the mill of civil litigation. One type of case is inheritance of a *bona fide* litigated claim. Dickens pictured what this means in *Jarndyce v. Jarndyce,* and the Gaines case in the United States may serve to show how impossible it is for fiction to rival fact. The litigation which occupied the whole of her long life came to Mrs. Gaines as an inheritance in 1813. In 1886 she died at the age of eighty and bequeathed it to her grandchildren, having outlived her children. In 1891 it finally came to an end and the inheritance for which she had struggled all her days came to her heirs. In the meantime the case had been fourteen times before the Supreme Court of the United States and had been fourteen times before the highest state court or the United States Circuit Court on points of sufficient importance to call for reported opinions.[8] The reports are full of cases of which the Gaines case is but an extreme example.[9]

As to the second category (cases where one is the innocent victim of the fault or default of others) at least seven important types are of common occurrence. (1) Cases are legion in which the innocent have been drawn into ruinous litigation because of judicial vacillation. Thus the chronicler of the Gaines case tells us: "The decision in 12 Howard being thus overthrown by this last decision, ruin was the consequence to many who confided in its soundness and purchased . . . on the faith of that decision." [10]

[6] Train, *The Prisoner at the Bar,* chap. 7, entitled, "If the Cook Should Steal the Teapot.
[7] California endeavored to meet this situation by a constitutional provision that witnesses should not be unreasonably detained. Under that provision it was held that a witness might be released on *habeas corpus* after he had been held for *ninety days* and the hearing of the prosecution had been put off repeatedly. *Ex parte* Dressler, 67 Cal. 257. Compare *Ex parte* Petrie, 1 Kan. App. 184.
[8] See Payne, *A Celebrated Case,* 14 Rep. Georgia Bar Association, 219.
[9] E.g., the case of Patience Swinfen, a widow whose father-in-law left her his property as a tardy reparation for driving his son from home at the time of his marriage. Nine years of litigation, involving ten reported decisions, were required to enable her to hold the property. See Burnham, *Some Famous Litigants,* 6 Green Bag, 399, 400-402. For an American case, see *Giles v. Little,* 2 McCrary 370; *Giles v. Little,* 104 U. S. 291; *Little v. Giles,* 118 U. S. 596; *Little v. Giles,* 25 Neb. 313; *Little v. Giles,* 27 Neb. 179; *Giles v. Little,* 134 U. S. 645; *Chase v. Miles,* 43 Neb. 686; *Lincoln Transit Co. v. Rundle,* 34 Neb. 550; *Roberts v. Lewis,* 134 U. S. 153—thirteen years of litigation over the meaning of a gift to a widow in her husband's will.
[10] 14 Rep. Georgia Bar Association 239. Compare: "But in the meantime many whose purses were not long enough to keep up the fight yielded

(2) Again the mere delay which is too common in all litigation, may be aggravated to the substantial ruin of litigants.[11]   (3) One may be involved in protracted and even ruinous litigation through the roguery of a plausible impostor.   The Tichborne case in England, which charged a goodly inheritance with a burden for generations to come, is the classical example.   But the United States may furnish examples of its own.[12]   (4) One may also be the victim of a protracted prosecution based on false testimony adduced to shift responsibility from the guilty to the innocent.[13]
(5) Again one may be the victim of governmental dishonesty and be compelled to spend his days in vain endeavors to procure justice from a state that cannot legally be compelled to pay its just obligations.[14]   (6) One of the most common types is willful aggression which compels him whose rights are infringed to engage in prolonged and expensive litigation whether he will or no.   Thus it often happens that the victim of a malicious defamation or a malicious prosecution must vindicate his reputation and his honor in order to live a human life among his fellowmen.   A striking instance of what this may involve is afforded by the well-known *Jones County Calf Case*.[15]   In that case a farmer who had been maliciously prosecuted by an organization found himself entangled

to judgments in ejectment in the federal court based on the first opinion in the federal Supreme Court, and sued their grantors upon covenants of warranty.   As these grantors had not felt able to continue the litigation, they were compelled to pay damages, although, in the event, they had conveyed a good title."   Pound, *Principles of Procedural Reform*, 4 Illinois Law Rev. 491, 492-494 (referring to the litigation described at the end of note 9).
[11] "Hundreds of causes were remaining to be heard; thousands of suitors had abandoned proceedings, and many were ruined under grievous oppression merely because they were unable to afford the money or the time necessary to enable them to proceed.   Even those who found the means and expended the money and time necessary to get their causes ready for hearing, were kept in suspense for an unreasonable length of time, uncertain whether they were thereafter to be rich or poor; many, from the tardy steps of justice, were unable to form or settle their plans in life, and were kept in a state of the most harassing wretchedness."   Duffus Hardy, *Life of Lord Langdale*, I, 349.
[12] E. g., *Flora v. Anderson*, 75 Fed. 217.   For a sketch (founded on fact) of the position in which innocent persons may be put by a plausible impostor, see Mark Twain, *The Major's Story*.
[13] Those who have studied the case attentively believe the Frank case to be one of this sort.   See Connolly, *The Truth about the Frank Case*, 1915.
[14] Mark Twain has given us a picture of the condition of such a victim in *The Great Beef Contract*.   See Fleischmann, *The Dishonesty of Sovereignties*, 33 Rep. N. Y. State Bar Association (1910), 229.   Compare the twenty-six years of litigation to which holders of coupons of Virginia bonds were subjected, *McCullough v. Virginia*, 172 U. S. 102, and prior cases set forth in the opinion of Mr. Justice Brewer.
[15] *Proceedings*, Iowa State Bar Association (1920), 141-156.

in twenty-five years of bitter litigation and was able to clear his character only through persistence under discouragements which would have worn out an ordinary litigant. (7) Finally there are cases of what may be called parasitism—cases where swindlers and extortioners, who have learned the possibilities of using the machinery of the law as a means of oppression, deliberately involve their victims in legal entanglements, in the confidence (often but too well founded) that they are too poor or too ignorant or too busy to be able to extricate themselves and will thus become an easy prey. The reports of Legal Aid Societies are full of such cases.[16] The innocent man of scanty means but high sense of duty who seeks to help a near relative out of trouble and finds himself caught in the web of litigation, the wage-earner whose wages are held in an illegal attachment in the endeavor to take advantage of his necessities and coerce him into what he is not bound to do, the innocent victim of get-rich-quick swindlers who invests his savings in worthless "securities" and finds himself involved in elaborate winding-up proceedings, the loyal friend or relative who becomes surety for a borrower from an unscrupulous and exacting lender at extortionate interest—all these are but too well known.

It will not do to say that the state provides an elaborate and expensive machinery for administering justice and that the law operates to prevent conditions of controversy with one's fellowman from being or becoming a serious type of evil. Public agencies for preventing or suppressing vice, public health service, public poor relief and public education do not prevent us from recognizing that vice and disease and poverty and ignorance are evils with which civilization must contend. Strife is one of the oldest evils in social history and is the one toward which politically organized society first directed its powers. Yet the legal order has but mitigated this evil. It is by no means abolished. Moreover, the machinery which the state has set up to obviate strife and put an end to controversies has many possibilities of injury for the innocent, the unwary and the impecunious. In part these possibilities of injury are inseparable from legal administration of justice; they grow out of difficulties of proof and infirmities of judgment which are incident to human action. In part they are due to reparable defects in our legal system and judicial organization. In either event conditions of legal entanglement, involved in the endeavor of the state to put down strife, adjust controversies, and administer justice, are not the least of the evils with which men must reckon in social life and of which, therefore, the social worker must take account.

[16] See Smith, *Justice and the Poor*, 9 ff.

APPENDICES

APPENDIX A *

CASE 46

PSYCHOPATHIC HOSPITAL

SOCIAL SERVICE

NUMBER 2004
FILE NUMBER 7938
O. P. D. NUMBER 3562   NAME Harold Gordon †

RESIDENCE Soldiers' Home, Derby, Mass.
CORRESPONDENT Mrs. Bessie Driscoll, 49 Glenwood St., Chelsea
SEX M   AGE 45   COLOR W.
CIVIL CONDITION S   PLACE AND DATE OF BIRTH U. S.
RELIGION P   OCCUPATION Steamfitter
TIME IN BOSTON 45   IN MASS. 45   IN U. S. 45
PREVIOUS ADDRESSES

WHEN KNOWN TO SOCIAL SERVICE 1/16/18
WHEN DISCHARGED FROM SOCIAL SERVICE 7/1/18
REASON FOR BEING KNOWN TO SOCIAL SERVICE Employment
REPORT FROM CONFIDENTIAL EXCHANGE No record

NAME OF FATHER George Gordon
ADDRESS 61 Jackson St., Malden, Mass.
NAME OF MOTHER Jennie Drake
ADDRESS 972 Irving St., Chelsea, Mass.
NAME OF SPOUSE
ADDRESS
NAMES AND AGES OF CHILDREN OR SIBLINGS

ADMITTED TO HOUSE 1/4/17   AUTHORITY Vol.
DISCHARGED 1/10/17   ADMITTED TO O. P. D. 1/16/18
DIAGNOSIS Luetic hemiplegia;   CONDITION
          Vascular lues

SOCIAL SYMPTOMS   DATE 2/5/18
    Cohabitation
    Industrial disability
    Unemployment

SOCIAL DIAGNOSIS Disease   DATE 1/20/18

* These case records are printed as written by the social workers without revision.
† All names used in this record are fictitious.

571

PSYCHOPATHIC HOSPITAL

SOCIAL SERVICE

CASE NO. 2004
FILE NO. 7938

NAME Harold Gordon

ADDRESSES

Patient:

Soldiers' Home, Derby, Mass.
49 Glenwood St., Chelsea.

Relatives and friends:

Brother-in-law, George Price,
12 Newbury St., Charlestown, Mass.

Brother-in-law, Xavier Price,
27 Tuttle St., Charlestown, Mass.

Patient's mother, Mrs. Jennie Gordon,
972 Irving St., Chelsea, Mass.

Patient's father, George Gordon
61 Jackson St., Malden, Mass.

Paternal aunt, 61 Jackson St., Malden, Mass.

Employers:

Mr. Yale,
5½ Glenwood Court, Boston, Mass.

Young & Daniels,
241 East 52nd St., New York City.

Mr. David F. Hyde, F. Q. Crawford Co.,
Quint St., Boston, Mass.

Patient's wife's employer:

Mrs. Howell,
73 Quirk St.,
Chelsea, Mass.

Patient's wife:

Bessie Driscoll,
49 Glenwood St., Chelsea.

PSYCHOPATHIC HOSPITAL
SOCIAL SERVICE

CASE NO. 2004
FILE NO. 7938

NAME Harold Gordon

EXPENSE SHEET

Paid			*Received*		
1/23	Marriage certificate....$ 1.02		2/6	From patient..........$ .50	
1/29	Loan .... .50		5/1	" " 1.00	
5/1	Wedding 11.00		5/10	" " 11.02	
	12.52			12.52	

PSYCHOPATHIC HOSPITAL
SOCIAL SERVICE

CASE NO. 2004
FILE NO. 7938

NAME Harold Gordon

SUMMARY

1918
January 20.
Social History:

Patient is a single American man 45 years old, a veteran of the Spanish War. He lives at the soldiers' home, Derby. There are no expenses incurred there and patient has a little money which he has received from the Steamfitters' Union. Patient is a steamfitter by trade and for 11 years prior to illness worked as such, making approximately $5 a day. In October, 1916, patient became ill and as a result now drags one leg and is slow and awkward on his feet. Patient's mother lives alone on Irving St., Chelsea, having 3 small tidy rooms. She has a small saving of her own. Patient's father was a Civil War veteran. Lives with his sister in Malden, Mass. The separation from his wife was due to the fact that patient's mother wanted him to go to Maine to live with his married daughter. Patient's father refused and, as a result, patient's mother went to Maine without him. She apparently is a difficult woman to get along with and soon friction occurred between her and her son-in-law; as a result she came back to Chelsea and, disliking patient's sister, has refused to go to Malden. She feels that her husband should come to her and says that his pension is being used to help take care of his sister. Patient visits his mother every little while.

Patient has been having sex relations with Mrs. Driscoll, a widow with a daughter 13 yrs. old. She lives at 49 Glenwood St., Chelsea. Patient stays two or three nights a week and Mrs. Driscoll is now probably pregnant by patient. Patient claimed at first that he was married, but later confessed that he was not. Mrs. Driscoll does housework by the day two or three days a week and her brothers pay her rent. Her brothers are wealthy; one owns a machine and is manager of the Hartford Tire Company on Coolidge St.

Physical History:

October, 1916, patient had a shock and was taken to the City Hospital. January, 1917, patient came to this hospital and was under treatment for neurosyphilis and has reported regularly for treatment. He claims to have had syphilis 18 yrs. ago. When patient first came to us he was practically crippled and could not use his arms or legs to any extent. Now he has control of his arms and control of one leg. He must report regularly for treatment.

Mental History:

October, 1916, patient became very dizzy and confused; felt that he might throw himself into a furnace when he attempted to throw wood in. He was admitted to this hospital in January. Shortly after his admission his confusion subsided and there have been no returns of symptoms. Since, he has apparently been a steady worker and faithful, working better, however, as an assistant than when sent off on a job of his own. MN

RESULTS

January 18 to April 18, 1918.
Social:

Patient and woman with whom he had been having irregular sex relations were married February 9, the money for the wedding service being loaned by the Social Service Department. Patient's wife was examined at the Boston Dispensary and suspected of being 2 months' pregnant. Patient's brother-in-law feels that patient's wife has always been a drag on them and they wish they might be well rid of her. Felt that her marriage would merely mean one more person to support. They refuse to assist her in any way if she marries, but later promised visitor that if she loaned money to them they would be ready to pay it back should patient fail, but felt they should at first be made to understand that they must stand on their own feet. Patient and wife have moved to an apartment at 5 Yale Terrace; the rent is $35 a month, but as they do janitor work they receive same rooms for $20. Work has been obtained for patient, F. Q. Crawford & Co., and patient is making between $17 and $18 a week. He has been raised and is now second to the foreman. There is a chance for overtime work with extra pay, but patient tires easily and has not yet done any overtime.

Physical:

Patient reports regularly for treatment and is improving.

Mental:

Patient slowly improving. Feels better and gets tired less easily. He hopes soon to be able to take up his old work as steamfitter. He has had a position offered to him, but felt that he should not undertake it just yet. Patient shows poor judgment, especially in money matters. He has a happy attitude that everything will be all right and will occasionally spend money for a steak and be obliged to borrow money for food the next couple of days. Patient is rather proud of himself for having stuck by his wife and married her. He occasionally will say, "If I hadn't done this for Bessie I need not have worked; I could have stayed at the soldiers' home all my life, they would have had to take care of me." On the other hand patient seems proud of the fact that he is able to support a home and does not want his wife's brothers to think he has any intention of sponging on them.
MN

HISTORY

1918
January 16.

Patient's story: Patient and alleged wife, Mrs. Bessie Driscoll, seen together at hospital. Patient states that he is living at the Soldier's Home in Derby, being a veteran of the Spanish War. He is without any visible means of support. His wife is living at 49 Glenwood St., Chelsea. She has three rooms, for which her two brothers, living in Charlestown, pay $15 a month rent for her. She has one child, now 11 years old, by her first husband. Patient claims he was married about six months ago, but cannot give the exact date or place of ceremony. He is a Protestant, and his wife is a Catholic. His wife claims to be about two months pregnant, at least she has had no menstrual periods for the past two months. She talks of having an abortion, but apparently has no real intention of doing so.

Patient is a steamfitter by trade, having worked steadily for Mr. Yale, 5½ Glenwood Court, Boston, 11 years ago, then going to New York City, working there for Young and Daniels, for 10 years. He returned then to his former employer, where he worked until he was taken ill in October, 1916.

Patient tells of how crippled he was one year ago,—even six months ago,—and how slowly and gradually he has regained the use of his arms, and how he feels encouraged that before long his left leg will be cured.

Names and addresses of friends and relatives were obtained. Visitor promises to look up possible openings whereby patient may make use of his trade without the undue fatigue which would occur were he to resume steamfitting.

Patient is well groomed, pleasing in appearance, affable personality, though somewhat apathetic. Mrs. Driscoll appears nervous, less intelligent, and less attractive.

January 18.

Soldiers' Home, Derby, Dr. Pearson, visited. Informant states that patient has been under their care from Jan. 25, 1917, to the present time. As a Spanish War Veteran, he is entitled, while disabled, to receive room and board free. He receives no pension, but is permitted to leave prac-

1918
tically whenever he requests. Patient as a rule receives a pass for the duration of two or three days a week.

Informant considers patient irresponsible, claiming that he put him on a job to run an elevator, the pay being $8 a month, and patient went off several times, leaving the elevator with no one to man it. This was done in spite of the fact that informant explained to him how embarrassing it was at mealtime to have no elevator in order to assist the feeble men to and from their meals. Patient seemed indifferent, and after three or four months on the job, informant took someone else. Informant states that it will be nearly impossible to find work for a man of patient's type.

January 18.
Impression: Somewhat cynical, but willing to coöperate in any possible way.

January 18.
Employer, Mr. Yale, 5½ Glenwood Court, visited. Informant states that patient was a good worker, steady, no drinking, and that he would take him back to-morrow at $5.50 a day, if patient would come. He states that patient did his best work when he was on a job with others. If given a small job to do himself, informant felt responsible to oversee the job. He stated that probably patient could not take charge of men, but was a willing and energetic and fast worker.

Impression: Informant seemed to have no interest in patient as an individual, but would be interested if patient were physically able to work, as there is a great demand for steamfitters at the present time.
MN/S

January 18.
City Hall visited. No record of marriage certificate is recorded.

January 18.
Alleged wife, Mrs. Bessie Driscoll, 49 Glenwood St., visited.
Informant stated that she had known patient for about two years, and told that she was not married to patient of her own accord. During this time she has been having intercourse with patient, and claims that her standing by him after he had had the paralytic stroke is one big factor in patient's recovery.

Patient visits informant about once a week for a period of two or three days. Informant claims to be without passion, and that patient is very easily excited. Informant states that she does cleaning two or three days a week, which gives her $4 to $5. Her two brothers pay her rent, and their wives give her shirtwaists, and help her out in little ways. She has one child dependent upon her. Her attitude toward her brothers is that they must not know her condition until after she is married, because, as she says, "they look up to me, and know I know better." She states that they are better educated than she is,—that they went to High School and business colleges. She went only as far as the 8th grade, being 16 years old when she left. During her schooling she was obliged to be out long periods of time owing to illness of first her own mother, and then of her step-mother. Her step-mother died when she was 16, and she brought up her two brothers. Six years later she married, and two years later, at the time of her confinement, her husband was electrocuted at work. The brothers take the little girl at times, as for vacations; and once, four years ago, when informant had an operation at the Boston City Hospital for fallen womb. As soon as patient is able to work informant is willing to

1918

marry, but does not wish to give up $15 a month, three attractive rooms, etc., with no apparent means of support ahead. She feels also that patient, who has a big appetite, had better stay at the Soldiers' Home until he gets work. Informant states that patient's mother, living at 972 Irving St., Chelsea, is very hard to get along with. She calls her "an indifferent, old-fashioned Yankee, who cares more for the dollar than for anything else." She states that patient's mother is jealous because she feels that when patient gets to work he is going to give money to informant rather than to her. Patient's mother has a small income of her own which enables her to be independent. Patient's mother was in Maine visiting her only daughter. Her husband refused to go to Maine, and he is now living with a sister in Malden.

Second impression: Informant seemed excited over her condition, not for her own sake or reputation, but because of her family. She appears more kind-hearted and intelligent than at the first interview.

January 23.

Patient's mother, Mrs. Jennie Gordon, 972 Irving St., Chelsea, Mass., visited. Informant has three basement rooms in a congested district, but the rooms are immaculately neat—even the floor looking as if scrubbed daily. Informant is a frail, delicate-appearing woman. She gave for her reasons for living alone that her married daughter's husband in Maine did not really want her, so she thought she would come back to Chelsea. She went to see her husband at his sister's, 61 Jackson St., Malden, Mass., and invited him to come and live with her. This was six months ago, and he has never been to see her. She claims that he is feeble, and is influenced by his sister who wants, and probably needs, his pension of $33. He is a Civil War veteran. She says she does not know whether or not she would live with them if they wanted her to. She has small savings of her own, and realizes that she is entitled to share in her husband's pension.

Patient was spending the day with his mother. He took the "laissez faire" attitude that everything would be all right when he went to work.

Patient walked out with visitor, and was asked what plans he had made about marriage, etc. He promised to see "Bess" and talk the matter over with her.

February 5.

Brothers of patient's fiancée, George and Xavier Price, Hartford Tire Co., 851 Coolidge St., visited. George is the manager and has an office to himself. Xavier very prosperous looking. Informants stated that Mrs. Driscoll had never been able to support herself, and that they had for years paid her rent and given her a little money besides. Stated that they had no use for patient, felt that they did not want him in their home, because they knew that their sister had had a Wassermann taken and felt that sexual relations must have taken place between her and patient. Informants asked if they would back the loan for the wedding fee. Xavier stated that when they made out checks for this month's rent he would put in some extra money. George said he would too, but on second thought they both said they thought it would be better for patient to understand that he could not get any help from them and both refused, stating, however, that if visitor loaned the money and did not get it back they would pay visitor, but did not want their sister to know. They feel if their sister marries it only means one more for them to care for. They want the marriage plans discontinued. Mrs. Driscoll's condition is ascertained and brothers both agree that marriage is the wisest thing.

MN/MCW

ACTION TAKEN

1918

Patient to report at regular stated intervals, at present two weeks apart, for medical treatment. Patient to get lighter work.

January 23.

Employer, Mr. David F. Hyde, Supt., F. Q. Crawford Co., telephoned to. Informant states that he would interview patient in regard to work. Patient sent with note to Mr. Hyde. See letter No. 1. Employer, Mr. Hyde, telephoned visitor. He stated that he would employ patient provided a recurrent stroke was not likely to occur, as they have insurance for employees over a limited period of time, and he did not wish to employ men if the risk was too great. Visitor had informant connected with Dr. Traiser by phone.

January 23.

Patient seen at Men's Club. He states that he is to begin work at the F. Q. Crawford Co. to-morrow, salary $15 a week.

January 24.

Patient's fiancée, Mrs. Driscoll, taken by visitor to the Gynecological Clinic of the Boston Dispensary. Dr. Kellogg examined her. Patient is probably three months pregnant, and is to return in one month. Mrs. Driscoll wants to get married quietly. This costs $16, $11 if announced three consecutive weeks in the church. Application for license made at the City Hall. License may be obtained on the 29th.
MN/S

January 29.

Patient to clinic. Seen by Dr. Traiser. Patient not to return for 3 weeks. Patient said that his work was lighter than steamfitting. Patient promised loan for wedding fee. Patient loaned $0.50. Patient stated that "Bess" had been to Worcester to attend the funeral of her uncle.
MN/MCW

January 30.

Patient to Men's Club. Patient enjoyed himself and talked a good deal of the time. The conversation was on the war and patient reminisced on the Spanish war.
MN/MCW

January 30.

Patient's fiancée, Mrs. Driscoll, visited. Says patient is to be married on the 11th. Is much upset about patient's disregard for money. She anticipates quarrels on the subject after they are married. Said the $0.50 visitor gave him on way to work he spent, saving only $0.05 and expected her to give him money to go to work on next day.
MN/MCW

February 5.

Patient's fiancée's brothers called on. They are willing to help if the sister asks them to help, but feel that patient should handle his own affairs.

Impression: Fair-minded but disgusted with their sister and what has been going on between her and the patient for some time.
MN/MCW

February 6.

Patient's fiancée, Mrs. Driscoll, to hospital. In an upset condition because patient had struck her daughter. Thinks she cannot marry

1918
patient and that it is best for her to have an abortion. Feels that if
patient continues to spend money as he does now that they will soon be
in debt if they are married. Patient advised not to marry if she feels
that way and told of agencies that can help her if she does not marry.
MN/MCW

February 6.
Employer, Mr. Hyde, seen. Employer stated that patient was a good
worker and that he would see that he received a raise. The raise would
be $0.02 an hour, giving patient $0.33 an hour.

February 8.
Coöperative Work Shop, Miss Manson, telephoned to. Promised to
consider the case and have visitor get Mrs. Driscoll some work.

February 9.
Visitor called on Mrs. Driscoll. Mrs. Driscoll stated that patient had
been very kind to her and her daughter and they would be married at eight
o'clock on the 11th.

February 11.
Visitor attends wedding at St. Francis' Church and gives patient check
for $11, wedding fee.
MN/MCW

February 13.
Coöperative Work Shop, Miss Manson, telephones that patient has
received work.

February 13.
A worker in training takes her washing to patient's wife.

February 20.
Visitor called. Patient's wife stated that her brothers had not helped
her out on this month's rent, but that she and patient were saving so that
they could pay it soon. Patient's wife promises to go to the Lying-in
Hospital to-morrow.

March 2.
Patient's wife brings in Steamfitters' Union papers to be filled out
by administrator.

March 6.
Papers filled out by Dr. Phillips, stating patient treated here for
neurosyphilis and under treatment since Jan. 21st.
MN/MCW

March 16.
Wife in. Stated that patient is 2nd in charge of his room. That he
and foreman like each other very much.
MN/MCW

March 25.
Coöperative Work Shop, Miss Manson, telephoned to. States patient's
wife has been in 3 times for work; does not work well, but she improves
each time. She has asked for work for her husband's mother. Visitor
stated what she knows about patient's mother.
MN/MCW

April 10.
Patient in for treatment. Patient stated that he is feeling better and
that family are now living at 5 York Terrace, Chelsea. Have 5 rooms,

1918
electric lights and steam heat, for which they pay $20 a month. Rent is really $35 but they do the janitor's work for the balance. Patient states that he earns about $16.50. He could make more money, but gets tired and therefore does little or no overtime work for which he would get 1½ extra. Patient hopes soon to be able to return to steamfitting, but promises not to do this until the doctor feels it is the wisest and best thing to do. Patient stated that wife will not go to the Lying-in Hospital. She will either go to St. Catherine's Hospital or be confined at home.

Visitor has urged patient's wife to go to the Lying-in Hospital, but she has many friends who have been to St. Catherine's and she can be confined by a Catholic doctor. Patient's wife is persistent in this in spite of the fact that Miss Dean, Supt. of the Lying-in Hospital, says she might have a Catholic priest called in if she so wished.

Patient stated that they had had no help from wife's brothers and that they were not looking for it and did not want it. Said that they were planning to visit them some time, but that they felt that since the brothers owned autos they could take the initiative. Patient working and improving and shows no mental disorder and they are both capable of making their own plans. Patient reports regularly for treatment. $11 to be collected.
MN/MCW

May 1.
Patient in for treatment. Gave visitor $1 on $11 owed for wedding fee. Patient very much pleased with new apartment, but feels they will have to move before another winter as the boilers are not sufficient to give enough heat to the entire building. Patient claims that his wife has the money. He does not know what she does with it, but he is constantly after her to pay the visitor back. He says she is pretty stingy and said he had to pay for 2 treatments in order to get the extra $1 so that we could start in paying visitor. Will try to bring more soon.

May 10.
Patient in. Paid balance of $11.02.

May 13.
Patient's wife in. Patient's wife delighted with new apartments. Feels now that as soon as a few more dishes, etc., are obtained she can invite her relatives to come and see her. They have none of them been to see her since she was married. She wants to have everything fixed up and then invite them. If they refuse, well and good; she won't bother them any more. She seems very proud of the fact that she has never asked them for money since she was married. Informant is 6 months pregnant, but as yet has not felt any life. Has an appointment with a private doctor who will confine patient at St. Catherine's. Will let visitor know results. Informant does not believe she is pregnant. Informant is anxious that husband obtain work in some other department, as she feels that working in the basement is not good for him. She says that he gets very, very tired. As yet they have received no money from the Steamfitters' Union and seem to feel that now they may not. Informant has some money saved up toward confinement expenses, but promises to bring in money for visitor. Visitor urged upon her the importance of this, stating that she probably would have less money rather than more later on.
MN/MMM

May 13.
Patient to clinic. Patient is anxious to obtain new work. He feels that dampness where he is working does not agree with him. Visitor

1918
refers him to Mr. Shackley of the Y. M. C. A. and gives him notes to Mr. Young, Library Bureau, and to Mr. Nason, Simplex Company, Danvers.

June 1.
Case closed: Patient has shown no mental symptoms and seems well pleased, industrious, and able to obtain a new job whenever he wishes to. His wife is expecting confinement soon, has money saved up to see her through, and is insistent upon having a private Catholic doctor and refuses to go to B. L. I. or in fact to any hospital.

Patient reports regularly for treatment and is told to let visitor know if he gets into difficulties.
MN

CASE 89
PSYCHOPATHIC HOSPITAL
SOCIAL SERVICE

NUMBER 2935
FILE NUMBER 11201
O. P. D. NUMBER   NAME Joseph Fangillo *
RESIDENCE 28 Central Ave., Arlington
CORRESPONDENT Mrs. Theresa Fangillo
SEX M   AGE 42   COLOR W
CIVIL CONDITION M   PLACE AND DATE OF BIRTH Boston,
RELIGION C   3/4/1876
TIME IN BOSTON Life   OCCUPATION Bookkeeper
PREVIOUS ADDRESSES Long St., Mat- IN MASS. Life   IN U. S. Life
  tapan

WHEN KNOWN TO SOCIAL SERVICE 1/28/19
WHEN DISCHARGED FROM SOCIAL SERVICE
REASON FOR BEING KNOWN TO SOCIAL SERVICE History
REPORT FROM CONFIDENTIAL EXCHANGE No record

NAME OF FATHER Henry C. (deceased)
ADDRESS
NAME OF MOTHER Nell Bonelli (deceased)
ADDRESS
NAME OF SPOUSE Theresa Costelli
ADDRESS 28 Central Ave., Arlington
NAMES AND AGES OF CHILDREN OR SIBLINGS

Children: Siblings:
  John—13   Mrs. Bonelli—about 50
  Emma—4½   Theresa—about 45
                                Antonio—about 47
                                Mrs. Cavalaro
                                Mrs. Mardini

ADMITTED TO HOUSE I, 1/24/19;   AUTHORITY I Vol., II Vol., III
  II, 2/24/19; III, 4/9/19   Vol.
DISCHARGED I, 2/13/19; II, 4/5/19; ADMITTED TO O. P. D.
  III, 5/8/19

DIAGNOSIS   I. Manic Depressive   CONDITION   I. Recovered
             II. Psychasthenia De-   II. Unimproved
                  pressed
            III. Psychasthenia
SOCIAL SYMPTOMS   DATE 3/1/19
  Unemployment
  Industrial decline
  Worry
SOCIAL DIAGNOSIS Disease   DATE 3/1/19

* All names used in this record are fictitious. In this case an unusually detailed
record was kept, as it was one of a group of cases included in a study of the psychopathic employee in industry.

PSYCHOPATHIC HOSPITAL
SOCIAL SERVICE

CASE NO. 2935
FILE NO. 11201 NAME Joseph Fangillo

ADDRESSES

Patient's telephone:
    Can be reached at Arlington 2640
    Mrs. Giordani,
    28 Central Avenue,
    Arlington, Mass.
Family Physician:
    Dr. Sullivan
    Arlington 1786
Patient's sister:
    Mrs. Bonelli,
    97 Main St.,
    Boston.
Patient's brother:
    Antonio Fangillo,
    Bradbury, Vt.
Patient's sister:
    Mrs. Cavalaro
    Hamilton St.,
    Chelsea, Mass.
Patient's cousin: *Place of employment:*
    Nicholas Tosi,   60 Manhattan St.,
    930 Hamberg St.,   Boston, Mass.
    Dorchester, Mass.
    Tel. Dorchester 946-W
Wife's sister:
    Mrs. Jennie Riley,
    43 Howley St.,
    Roslindale, Mass.
Patient's wife's mother: (Can be reached by telephone of
    Mrs. Costelli,   neighbor in same house—Beach
    10 Victoria St.,   1459-M)
    Boston, Mass.
Wife's sister:
    Bertha Costelli,
    10 Victoria St.,
    Boston, Mass.
Patient's sister:
    Mrs. Mardini,
    Cedar St.,
    Cambridge, Mass.
Patient's sister:
    Theresa Fangillo
    Lives with her sister, Mrs. Mardini.

PSYCHOPATHIC HOSPITAL

SOCIAL SERVICE

CASE NO. 2935
FILE NO. 11201   NAME Joseph Fangillo

SUMMARY

1919
February 12.
Social:

Patient is a man of 42—born in Boston of Italian parents. He completed a 3-year high school course at 15, and then took a year of advanced work there, after which he completed a business course of 6 months.

He then did various kinds of office work, followed by bookkeeping. He was a bookkeeper for the Stratton Piano Company, Boston, for 16 years, starting at low wages and working up to $35 a week.

After being for 2 months in 1911 at the Boston State Hospital, he spent 2 summers on a small farm in Bradbury, Mass., which he has partial use of for $23 a year. Then for a year he was manager at the Marko Café. For the past 3 years he has been one of three partners in a liquor concern which proved fairly successful, each member clearing $1,000 a year in addition to his salary. Patient withdrew from this work before Christmas, 1918, and has been without a position since.

Patient is married, having a son, 13, in high school, and a daughter, 4½, at home. Family rents a 4-room flat in Arlington for $14 a month. The rooms are on the first floor and sunny, neat, and comfortably furnished, and there is a fair-sized garden.

Physical:

Patient's mother died of spinal meningitis. Otherwise the family history is not of interest, except perhaps the fact that patient's brother had a breakdown 15 years ago similar to patient's.

As a child patient had typhoid and diphtheria, and 2 accidents. In one he was run over and his legs were in a plaster cast for 9 months. There are no results now. In the other his head was hit.

He is of strong build and is in good physical condition at present. He has worn glasses since 19 years of age, his eyes having troubled him more than usual of late. They have been treated only by an optometrist who says his vision is low but perfect with lenses. The Wassermanns of his blood and spinal fluid are negative. He admits gonorrhea and soft chancre years ago for which he had treatment.

Mental:

Patient was a good student at school. He was graduated from a 3-year course at high school at 15, and then took a 4th year there followed by a business course of 6 months.

1919

His work at the Stratton Piano Company was responsible work, and patient had the ability to keep the position until 6 years ago. He has always been inclined to worry, however, and about 10 years ago developed a sex phobia, becoming afraid even to meet women on the street. This worried him excessively. He has always been especially fond of outdoor sports and of reading both fiction and books on economics. His wife had urged him to mix more with others although he has not been especially seclusive.

In 1911 he became nervous and fearful, and at the advice of his private physician left work and went voluntarily to the Boston State Hospital where he was given a diagnosis of psychasthenia. While there he had hydrotherapeutic treatment. After 2 months' care there, he was discharged and went to work on his farm off and on for 2 or 3 years.

Patient has always been of even disposition, not moody, enjoying company, though being somewhat quiet. He enjoys his home, children, and reading. He is not sensitive or irritable. He has always been inclined to worry.

Both patient and the Stratton Piano Company agreed that he was unable to return to them. Patient was unhappy while in the liquor business. He found the work and the environment uncongenial. After withdrawing from this in December, 1918, he became worried and apprehensive about the future and felt some former fears return. He attempted to keep his self-control through walks of 10 to 15 miles, but was unsuccessful, became depressed and hypochondriacal. He came to this hospital as a voluntary patient.

RESULTS

February 12 to May 12.
Social:

There has been no income, but patient's wife says most of the $500 saved remains, as she and the children spend about half of the time living with her mother, who apparently stands most of the expense during the visits. Her mother lives in the East End, Boston, and is supported by a son and daughter, both single.

Patient's wife tried work a few nights, dipping chocolates at $1 for 3 hours in a candy factory, but was readily persuaded of the inadvisability of this. She has devoted a large part of her time to visiting patient at the hospital and taking him out for walks.

When patient was last discharged from the hospital, she took Emma and patient to their little farm in Bradbury, but returned to her mother's on his re-admission to the hospital. She has considerable understanding of patient's condition and, though somewhat worried about the future, is making a very brave fight and is always cheerful in the presence of patient.

Physical:

Patient has continued well physically. His eyes have not yet been examined by an ophthalmologist.

Mental:

Patient was discharged from the hospital 2/13/19 much improved, and visited his brother on a farm in Bradbury, Vt. He got along well for a

1919
week, but after an idle Sunday his fears returned and he was readmitted to the hospital 2/24/19. He seemed worse after this second admission, but pulled himself together sufficiently to try his farm at Bradbury, being discharged from the hospital 4/5/19. He worked there outdoors a few days when his old sex phobia returned, and he was so discouraged about this that he returned to the hospital, readmitted 4/9/19. All through his stay at the Psychopathic he has worked hard on the wards, pleading constantly for hard work.

His chief fear all spring has been that prohibition will not be put into effect, and that therefore he has lost out by giving up his liquor business. Although he can reason with himself that he is fortunate at all events to be out of the liquor business, this fear still possesses him so much that he dreads reading the newspapers. In the last few weeks, however, this fear has decreased considerably, and he feels that he has it pretty well under control.

He is very anxious to get well and repeatedly says he will do anything in his power to do so. He frequently asks whether visitor thinks he will ever get well.

On 5/8/19 patient was discharged to the Middlesex State Hospital as a voluntary patient, Dr. Lawson, his examiner, feeling that he would do much better there with the increased facilities for recreation and team-work outdoors.

May 12 to September 30.
Social:
Patient remained at Middlesex until July 14 when he went to live at his camp in Bradbury. His wife and children preceded him there by a few weeks, patient visiting them often during his stay at Middlesex. Patient's wife has canned a quantity of vegetables for the winter. Her family have been frequent visitors to the camp and have brought them food for the family. Patient plans to move back to Arlington about October 1, the rent having been paid all along by his wife's relatives who feel very kindly toward patient as do his relatives also. Both patient's family and his wife's family are superior Italian people of ambition and thrift. Patient's mother-in-law has a large household to cook for, as her single son and daughter, both working, and a married daughter, son-in-law, and their two children live with her, and in addition the patient's wife and children are frequent visitors.

Patient is one of six siblings. The oldest, a sister with whom patient lived several years before his marriage, has several grown children able to support the family without her husband's assistance, who is now a semi-invalid. A brother is on a farm in Brayton, Vt., and two of his sisters live together, one of them married, the other working.

Patient has done his own farm work this summer as well as hiring out to neighboring farmers frequently. John has begun his second year at high school in Arlington and Emma was sent to school for a few days, but is now kept home for a week or two until the family canning is finished at camp and the family move to Arlington for the winter.

Physical:
Patient is in excellent physical condition as a result of outdoor work.

Mental:
Patient improved considerably at Middlesex, doing six hours pick-and-shovel work there a day most of the time and farm work at his camp

1919
week-ends. Early in August efforts were made to get him into the employ of the Gray Motor Company, Dorchester, in the fall, but the employment manager has found no vacancy. The Schuleman Paper Box Factory in the East End, which prides itself especially on its humane handling of its employees and where another patient is apparently very happily placed, stated early in September they would be glad to interview patient. As a result, patient came down from camp a few days ago to visit Schuleman's. They agreed to take patient on any time but patient feels that though they are most considerate the chances for advancement are not large. Patient says he knows "beggars can't be choosers" but says "I would like some place where I could begin work and work hard if I felt that I could learn some useful trade or where I could be sure of advancement provided of course I merited it." This indicates a desire to plan for the future which he has not manifested before.

Patient reports that occasionally he has "fear spells" but much less frequently and of shorter duration. He is full of hope for the future and sure he will be entirely well after getting into new work. His eyes look very bright now instead of apathetic.

September 30 to December 12.
Social:
Early in October patient's family moved to Arlington for the winter but still visited the farm frequently week-ends. The children are in school. Patient remained in the country until the end of November picking apples and coming to market in Boston frequently. The family has on hand quite a little fruit for the winter and patient earned most of the expenses of the summer by his farm work. His wife remains very philosophical.

While in the liquor business, $300 was borrowed from patient, and a brother owes him $700, and a brother-in-law $200. He hopes to be paid some of this soon. He has two $1,000 semi-endowment life insurance policies. Patient's wife returned to candy dipping this fall at $1.25 for three hours in the evening, planning to stop when patient is regularly employed.

Efforts have been made to find patient suitable work through the Y. M. C. A., State Employment Office, Bureau for Returning Soldiers and Sailors, and Bryant & Stratton's. He applied definitely for clerical positions at the Riverside Book Shop and at Schuleman Paper Box Factory. Stratton Piano Company have no openings for patient.

Physical:
Patient's eyes have not been examined as Dr. Jacobs advises no examination for the present.

Mental:
Dr. Jacobs agreed to see patient because doing research in psychoneuroses, and saw patient early in October. He felt patient's diagnosis was between manic depressive depressed and psychasthenia or a combination of both, but that patient was rapidly recovering and soon would be in as good shape as after his attack several years ago. Every three months or so he should report to some psychiatrist to make sure he is not overworking. He says there is no reason why patient should have to try work different from his former clerical work but emphasizes the necessity of patient's having a hobby. His fears are so slight now that they can be disregarded. Patient gives the credit of getting well to his wife. He has been a little afraid of attempting bookkeeping again but has been persuaded to do so.

1919
The Riverside Book Shop felt they could not consider patient, as the work was especially nerve-racking, there being only women among the customers and help and books being behind. They also felt that patient must be rusty at bookkeeping as he had not done any in five years.

The Schuleman Paper Box Factory was ready to consider patient for clerical work but patient felt the chances for advancement were not great enough. When he was finally convinced of the desirability of the job, the job was no longer open.

December 12, 1919, to March 12, 1920.
Social:
Patient and his family spent a few days at Christmas with her relatives. The children received about $35 in Christmas gifts and patient $25 from his farmer friend, James. His brother has paid back $50 but no other debts have been paid him. His wife is still working at candy dipping at $1.25 for three hours. The children were sick at the end of January, John with influenza and Emma with stomach trouble, and patient's wife was tired out at this time. She still keeps up good courage. The relations with the landlady have been a little strained but not markedly so.

Patient did not get a job until February 11, when he has since held a temporary position as bookkeeper at $25 a week. Many agencies assisted in helping to look for suitable work for patient but clerical openings for men have been exceedingly scarce, especially without stenography and typewriting.

Physical:
Patient had a slight cold but has otherwise been well.

Mental:
Patient looked up many openings on his own initiative as well as those suggested by agencies and visitor. On patient's part the following were reasons for not taking the jobs offered: too much responsibility, and not enough chance for advancement. He kept up good courage although admitting more and more discouragement at not being able to get a job. He admits he feels much better since working, and feels sure he will be perfectly well when a permanent position presents itself, efforts to obtain which are now being made.

HISTORY

January 29.
Patient seen on ward.
Impression: pleasant, intelligent, good insight into condition.

Patient says that in his family his brother had a "nervous breakdown" 15 years ago, which seemed similar to patient's present trouble. Brother was worried, broke down; went "up country" where he recovered. Patient did well at school, going through High School and finishing a commercial course in 6 months. He finished the two courses in as short a time as possible because he had little money. He had his commercial training at the Comer Commercial School, Somerville, now out of existence.

Patient has worked as private secretary and for 16 years as bookkeeper in the Stratton Piano Company, a very good position of responsibility and from which he has recently been given a good recommendation.

1919
When he went to the Boston State Hospital in 1911 they would not re-employ him at the Stratton Piano Company on his return.

He stayed out of work for 2 or 3 years, and for one year was manager of the Marko Café, and for 3 years was in the liquor business from which he retired in 1918. The business was fairly successful, each of the three partners making $1,000 a year besides their salary. Patient retired because he disliked the business and because he felt it would be better to get started in another position some time before prohibition comes in July, 1919.

Patient seems to be happily married. His wife has ingenuity and a happy disposition. Of his children, John, 13, is in the high school. Emma, 4½, is at home.

Patient likes to be among people, but he is particularly fond of reading both fiction and books on economics. His wife has urged him to mix more with others and he realizes that one is better mentally when not alone too much. He is particularly fond of outdoor sports, likes farming, walking, etc. He and his wife go out together occasionally in the evening; he seems to have several friends.

Patient says he had children's diseases. At the age of 9 he was run over across his body and in a plaster cast for 9 months. He believes he has no serious results of the accident. Patient has suffered from neuritis for some time. His eyes also have troubled him. He has been to several doctors for treatment, among them being Dr. Baker from the Patton Building. He has been under medical care of Dr. Francis.

Patient says that at the time of his going to the Boston State Hospital he was run down physically and nervously. He went voluntarily and seemed to improve under the treatment of the baths he was given. After leaving there he could not return to his former position and so for 2 or 3 years he lived "up country," renting 2 or 3 rooms and being given all the land he wanted to farm. He improved here and he seemed stronger until suddenly about 2 or 3 weeks ago he felt a "fear spell" come on him; things worried him which he was unable to drive from his mind. He felt that he had made a mistake in leaving the liquor business; that he was not well, etc. He realized that he had to fight this off and for three days he had been taking long walks, sometimes for 18 or 20 miles a day. He suc-ceeded in driving it off but in 2 days it returned again. He could not sleep, but felt he had to be up walking all the time; but even while walking he could not keep himself from worrying. He became discouraged, intro-spective, and disappointed. He went to Dr. Sampson for advice, asking if it were not possible for him to come here. The doctor agreed and patient wanted to come immediately on Thursday, January 25. The doctor per-suaded him, however, to wait until morning. He came here voluntarily without telling his wife or children where he was going.

At present he does not sleep well, but says he is feeling stronger and says he is much better able to control his thoughts and keep himself from worrying. His main desire now is to get strong so that he can be able to take a position, preferably not in the bookkeeping line because of his eyes.

His wife said that if he is not better she will break up the home and go to live with her mother or go to work herself, but he feels that he can take a good position when the opportunity comes.

January 28.
Neighbor, Mrs. Giordani (28 Central Avenue, Arlington) telephoned to. Informant lives in flat above patient's family and has known patient

1919
several years. She says that since leaving Boston State Hospital in 1911 patient has been "fine" until about 6 weeks ago when he said that he felt nervous and that the "same trouble was coming on" again. He was told to mix in more with others and thus he would feel better. He did this; he continued to be nervous, however—he could not keep quiet and seemed to have to keep going all the time. He was a little irritable.

Informant believes patient does not drink. He has complained at times of his eyes. He has always been quiet—has always been pleasant. She does not know that patient has been sensitive or that he has been fearful of enemies or suspicious of friends.

January 29.
Present illness:
Previous to patient's attack in 1911 he had been complaining of neuritis in his wrist. For this he took medicine. He stayed home for a week but found even at the end of that time that he could not return to work. He was advised by Dr. Francis to go to Boston State Hospital, where he did go voluntarily; remaining two months. While there he was given baths, which patient considered most satisfactory treatment. While still at hospital informant used to take him out to walk and would occasionally take him home to spend Sunday. Upon his return home he could not work (even had not his former position been filled). Informant believes he was run down physically at the time. The succeeding summer he spent "up country" on a friend's farm, where he dug and worked outdoors, and where his condition improved. He and informant spent the next winter at patient's sister's home. The following summer he spent again at the farm and in the autumn of that year he returned to work for the first time in two or three years.

Informant feels that the three years patient spent in liquor company have been a contributing factor in his second attack. This business brought him into contact with a much less desirable class of men than he had known when a bookkeeper, the environment about his place of work was not pleasant, and patient did not, moreover, like the liquor business. For some time he had been considering withdrawing from the company and finally did withdraw just before Christmas, 1918. This business worry has been the only matter over which patient need have felt trouble; he had nothing at home to cause him worry.

Patient intended to get into some other form of employment, but on a night after Christmas a "spell" similar to one in 1911 returned, which, according to patient, was much less severe than in 1911. After three days it wore away, for patient said he was resolved to resist it and fight it off. In 2 days, however, it returned, to wear away again. On Wednesday, January 22, patient felt well in daytime but was worse at night; on Thursday night he hardly slept at all and he decided to come here for care at this hospital.

Informant denies hallucinations, delusions, or fears in patient. She says his mind, even at the present time, has always been clear and normal. Patient's nerves alone need some sort of treatment. Informant feels that patient has improved while being here and that in two or three weeks he will be well enough to return home.

February 1.
Dr. Lawson, patient's examiner at hospital, consulted. Stated that patient has insight. Informant has not gone into his sex history, but does

1919
not feel that the reasons for his leaving Stratton Piano Company are of
vital significance in his condition. Patient's prognosis is good. Patient
has initiative and can himself state what work is best for him.

February 3.
Patient seen on ward. Stated that a friend of his has a farm in
Bradbury, Mass. For the use of a few rooms there patient pays $25 a
year. He has gone up there several summers in succession. Patient has
between $500 and $600 left. Has known his wife since she was 7 or 8
years old. "Went with her" about 10 years. For details of patient's work
see "Industrial History" enclosed.

February 4.
Patient's wife seen at hospital. States that she is of a worrying nature
—trying to look on the bright side. Both her children have stomach
trouble from time to time. Her family doctor is Dr. Sullivan of Arlington. Treats them from time to time for gastritis. Patient's wife often
takes the children to her mother's for the week-end, opposite Station 2,
East End. Informant's father is dead and her mother is supported by a
son and daughter who live with her.

February 12.
Place of employment, Stratton Piano Company, 288 Bagley St., Mr.
Dawson and his father seen.

March 15.
Dr. Malcolm, Optometrist, Rice Building, telephoned to. Informant
stated that he has treated patient for several years, the last time being
December 16, 1918. At that time his vision with compound lenses in both
eyes was perfect (20/20) though without lenses was 15/20 in each eye.
Sees no reason why patient could not do any kind of work he pleased as
far as his eyes are concerned. Stated that patient's lenses should be
changed about once a year, though he would like to see patient soon as
he had added a little to patient's prescription on December 16 for near
work and would like to know how this affected patient.

May 24.
Patient's mother-in-law, Mrs. Costelli, 10 Victoria St., Boston, visited.
Sister-in-law, Bertha Costelli, also seen.
Impression of Mrs. Costelli: Looks intelligent, kindly, and healthy,
but speaks almost no English.
Impression of Bertha Costelli: Intelligent, warm-hearted, and exceedingly interested in patient and his wife.
Impression of home: Exceedingly neat and well furnished, up three
flights. The street is a blind alley consisting of tenements crowded closely
together.
Mrs. Costelli cooks for ten people including patient's wife and child,
Bertha Costelli and her brother, both of whom are single, and a married
sister with her husband and two children. Patient's wife is always afraid of
intruding. Informants do not feel that she is, however, Bertha Costelli
stating that the Italians are more sympathetic with their friends in trouble
than other races.
Both patient and his wife are splendid people and devoted to one
another. Informants see no reason why patient should worry. Bertha
regrets that her mother has always worked, having started at the age of 6
on a farm in Italy and refusing to rest now.

1919
May 24.
Patient's older sister, Mrs. Bonelli, 97 Main St., visited.

Impression: Informant is an intelligent, refined Italian, devoted to her family and to patient.

Impression of home: Very neat and well furnished, on the first floor of a tenement house at the better end of Main St.

Patient has always been studious, ambitious, and conscientious. Patient was with informant 4 years before his marriage 15 years ago. He preferred being with informant to living with his mother. Informant sees patient and his family often. At bookkeeping he worked much overtime and toward the last wore 2 and 3 pairs of glasses at a time. Informant ascribes his first illness to overwork. She thinks that now he is in better physical condition than when he broke down 6 years ago.

All the relatives on both sides are very sympathetic with patient. Patient has always made friends easily and had many. Informant would do her share financially if help was needed, but patient's wife's family are aiding at present.

Informant is the oldest child, followed by Antonio who has a farm in Brayton, Vt., and has been recently married. Patient is next followed by a single sister who lives with the youngest, Mrs. Mardini, Cedar St., Cambridge, Mass. Patient has not been overly religious. Informant's husband has not worked in the past 2 years. He was formerly a laborer and insisted on giving his children a good education. Visitor saw one daughter who is a High School graduate and attended Bennett's Business School.

January 29.
Dr. Francis, E. Boston 488-W, telephoned to. Informant says cause of patient's trouble is that he went "sexually wrong" about 10 years ago. Informant would not make more definite statement over telephone except to say that patient was abnormally sexually excitable,—if he saw a female approach on the street he would have to cut down a side street, so strong was his sexual instinct. He brooded and worried over this until it became a mania with him and this was the sole cause of his having to leave the Stratton Piano Company where he had a good position. He was at the Boston State Hospital for a short time and has been better in recent years.

Patient used to be cheerful and optimistic before marriage. Informant says his married life has been only fairly happy, and that recently patient has had great financial worry. His trouble dates from his marriage. In recent years patient has grown coarse and vulgar, contrary to his former personality. Informant feels that the fact that patient had to "rough it" while associated with liquor business was a good thing for him.

Informant says that patient has complained of nervous trouble, having "wandering pains" over body. Informant titled this "neuritis" or "neurasthenia," but believes the pains were psychogenic.

Informant says patient did not have syphilis, but that his worry over his sexual desire is cause of his nervous condition.

January 29.
Wife interviewed at hospital.

Impression: Pleasant, intelligent, self-possessed. Seems to be cooperative, yet at times noncommittal, perhaps desiring to shield patient.

1919
Family History:

Grandparents: Unknown to informant.

Mother: Died at 75 probably of pneumonia—bright, cheerful, of excellent disposition.

Siblings:

1. Sister, Mrs. Bonelli, 97 Main St., Boston.
   About 50 years old. Is well and has several children.
2. Sister, Theresa, about 47. Unmarried.
   Works in box factory. When 3 or 4 years old she had spinal meningitis, as a result of which she lost the sight of one eye and became quite deaf in both ears.
3. Brother, 47. Married. No children. Is well and works in Brayton, Vt., on a farm.
4. Patient.
5. Sister, Mrs. Cavalaro, Hamilton St., Chelsea, Mass.
6. Sister, Mrs. Mardini, Cedar St., Cambridge, Mass.
   Married. Well; good disposition.

Informant knows of no constitutional disease, nor of any mental or nervous trouble in family. Family is normal.

Personal History:

Developmental: Not known to informant.

Educational:

Patient graduated from High School (which was then composed of 3 grades) at 15. Being too small to take a position he spent next year in the "advanced course." He then went to Comer's Commercial School. He seems to have been noticeably bright in school.

Economic:

Patient's work at Stratton Piano Company satisfactory to all concerned.

Marital:

Married 15 years. Lived previously on Long St., Mattapan. Has two children:

| Boy, 13—1st year High School | } | Both children are well and |
| Girl, 4½—fond of dancing | } | bright in intellect. |

Habits:

Patient is not a drinker. He takes only an occasional glass of liquor. Is only moderate smoker. No drugs. Informant knows of no infectious blood disease.

Personality:

Even disposition, not moody. Is fond of company and enjoys people. He has friends in to call and he and informant go out together not infrequently. Is quiet, however; likes to be home with his children and likes constantly to read. Is not sensitive nor suspicious. Is not hot-tempered nor irritable. Patient has always been rather inclined to worry.

Medical:

Informant knows of no serious illnesses. Patient has been at no other hospital beside this except Boston State Hospital. He has been under care of Dr. Francis for several years. No fainting attacks.

ACTION TAKEN

1919
February 1.
Patient seen on ward. Anxious to remain another week to get a hold on himself. Thinks he will be much better off after his stay here and after he gets to work. Says he worries when not working. Is anxious to do any sort of work whatsoever. He had his eyes examined as recently as a few weeks ago by Dr. Malcolm and had his lenses changed.

February 3.
Patient seen on ward. Will stay several days longer.

February 7.
Newcomb's Ink Co., Mr. Pierce, employment manager, telephoned to regarding possible opening for patient. Stated that he had a position which would involve general picking up about the place, which might do for patient. Asked that patient be sent to him.

February 8.
Patient and wife sent with note from Social Service to Newcomb's Ink Company. On his return patient stated that Mr. Pierce had not been aware that the position was already filled by one of the foremen.

February 8.
Newcomb's Ink Company, employment manager Mr. Pierce, telephoned that without his knowledge the position had been filled by a foreman.

February 10.
Patient seen on ward. Stated that he would like to visit his brother on a farm in Brayton, Vt.

February 11.
Newcomb's Ink Company, employment manager Mr. Pierce, telephoned to. He has no openings but will let Social Service know if he has a little later.

February 12.
Patient seen on ward. Stated that his brother is to call for him 2/15/19 and take him to the farm of this brother's fiancée in Brayton, Vt. Patient has felt better since contemplating this. Social Service agreed to think this plan over and talk it over with Dr. Lawson.

February 12.
Dr. Lawson, patient's examiner at hospital, seen. Thinks plan a good idea. Would like to see employer, Mr. Dawson, regarding patient's sex tendencies. Patient has not spoken of this to informant.

February 12.
Patient's wife seen. Took patient out for about two hours to-day as she has done for a number of days.

February 13.
Patient discharged to-day from hospital as he suddenly decided he had sufficient grip on himself to make the plunge now. He will go in a day or two to the farm of his brother. Patient's wife agreed to let Social

1919
Service know how patient gets along. After a few weeks there patient plans to return to Boston and would like Social Service to look for a job for patient in the meantime.

February 25.
Patient's wife telephoned that she visited patient 2/22/19. Found him doing fairly well though he still has "fear spells" at times. He is working hard all day. Has not yet planned on date to return to Boston. Will telephone when she has further news of patient.

February 25.
Patient was readmitted to hospital yesterday, this fact not being known to Social Service or patient's wife at the time of her telephone message.

February 25.
Patient's wife later visited patient. She was somewhat worried over patient's apparent relapse, but is hopeful of a good recovery, and puts forward a cheerful face to patient.

February 25.
Patient seen on ward. Somewhat depressed and disappointed that work has not cured him. Is determined to put forth every effort to get well, but is doubtful whether he will recover. Spent the time in Vermont in doing farm work, cutting ice, hauling wood, etc. On Sunday 2/23/19 patient was idle and had time to worry considerably, and yesterday he was too nervous and excited to work. His brother told him he was a "fool" to return to the hospital and urged patient to "stick it out," but patient felt he could not.

February 25.
Dr. Lawson, examiner of patient, seen. Stated that she will go into patient's sex history this time.

March 3.
Dr. Lawson, patient's examiner, seen. Patient is very depressed to-day and is having hydrotherapeutic treatment. Informant has talked with patient about sex matters. Patient gives no history of anything of the sort disturbing him in several years.

March 7.
Patient seen on ward—very depressed to-day; easily weakening. Knows he should not worry about giving up the liquor business, but has an idea that prohibition may not be put into effect. Realizes fully that the liquor business did not agree with him. Also realizes that his present worry is inconsistent. Has a fear of being sent to the State Hospital. Reassured patient on this point. He is "pining" for good hard work.

March 7.
Superintendent of Nurses, Miss Murray, seen and urged to give patient more work on the wards.

March 10.
Patient's wife seen at hospital—looking more tired than usual. Stated that for the past week she has been working nights at a chocolate factory on Bar St., dipping chocolates at the rate of $1.00 for each night of three

1919
hours, 7 to 10. She was anxious to earn car fares in this way and was getting lonesome at home.

Social Service pointed out other sides to the question; namely, that patient would resent her working now whether or not he finds it out until later, and that her children need her at home, especially as she visits patient at the hospital daily. Also urged against it from the point of view of her own health. Suggested that she think the matter over. She stated she now felt she would not return to work. When asked the name of the firm, she would give no further details than to state that only a few employees work there. Informant did not seem at her ease. Social Service made an appointment to visit at her home 3/12/19 in the morning, and she and Emma will be at home. Emma is now staying with wife's sister, Mrs. Riley, 43 Howley St., Roslindale.

Later, when Social Service saw informant on the ward, informant beckoned in uneasy manner to her to state that she hoped Social Service was not going to visit the neighbors. Social Service stated that they had no intention of visiting neighbors now.

March 10.
   Patient's examiner, Dr. Warren, consulted. Stated that in his estimation patient can do any kind of work; is strong physically and could stand indoor work. Informant is willing for patient to leave the hospital at any time he wants to; the sooner patient starts to work the better. Informant does not know what patient's vision is and says patient does not know what he fears during his "fear spells."

March 10.
   Patient talked with on ward—very depressed; still afraid he did not do the right thing in leaving the liquor business, and that perhaps he should not have settled to the disadvantage of his partners, even though they had previously robbed him. Does not like to think of leaving the hospital soon, as he is afraid he might attempt to make away with himself. Assured patient that he could not expect to be entirely well until after getting to work.

March 12.
   Home visited.
   Impression of home: Very neat, sunny, well-furnished rooms; four in number besides pantry, on first floor of a frame house. Situation on a high hill in Arlington, five minutes' walk from Grant College.

Patient's wife and Emma at home. Patient's wife visited patient yesterday and found him exceedingly depressed. Her courage was good until then, but she has been considerably worried in the last twenty-four hours. Tears came into her eyes easily during the visit. She insisted on serving a little luncheon to visitor, which was well prepared and nicely served.

Landlady dropped in for a few minutes, a very intelligent, kind, neighborly person, evidently knowing the details of patient's illness.

Emma obviously has adenoids, and does not look exceedingly well. She seems bright but quite restless, a very affectionate and winning child.

Patient's wife has given up her work at the factory. She would hate to have to give up her present home, but does not see any necessity of it for several months at least. The rent is $14.00. Family has lived in this house five years—landlady occupying the second floor. Patient's wife left with visitor to go to hospital.

1919
March 12.

Newcomb's Ink Co. visited. Mr. Pierce out. Was shown through factory by Miss Martin, his office assistant, and by one of the foremen, Mr. Gordon. Both stated that they felt sure Mr. Pierce would take patient if he could make room for him, unless he had some plan of his own to the contrary.

The factory is very well lighted and roomy, and the atmosphere is kindly. Miss Martin will let Social Service know in case Mr. Pierce can fit patient in soon.

March 12.

Patient seen on ward. Seemed very cheerful.

March 14.

Patient seen running down the steps from one floor to another of the hospital. His face was beaming and he stated that he is feeling very well to-day. His wife brought his former partner in, with whom patient settled one or two matters on his mind. He has been cleaning windows with the attendants to-day and has spent a good part of the day doing this. Willingly agreed that work was good for him.

March 24.

Patient's wife seen at hospital. Informant says patient was still depressed yesterday and does not feel equal to getting out or seeing an employer. Visitor asked wife to urge patient to go out for a walk.

March 25.

A. F. Gainsboro's employment manager, Cambridge, telephoned to. Informant stated that they are not in need of anything but skilled machinists. He suggested telephoning to the Federal Steel Trades Corporation.

March 25.

Federal Steel Trades Corporation, 83 Auburndale St., employment manager Miss Fiske telephoned to. Informant stated that openings have been very few and she has no suggestions at unskilled or clerical positions.

March 25.

Patient's examiner, Dr. Warren, telephoned to. Informant stated that he still feels patient should soon return to work, and that he has stressed this whenever he talked to patient. Informant has not talked much with patient recently, but will do so soon.

April 5.

Patient discharged to wife and O. P. D.

April 9.

Patient admitted to house as voluntary.

April 10.

Patient's wife seen at hospital. She was disappointed that patient has not been able to hold his own away from the hospital, but feels that a longer time here will eventually set him on his feet.

1919
April 11.
Patient interviewed on ward. He is discouraged over the fact that his fears return as soon as he leaves the hospital. He clings constantly to the hope that his disease will be cured eventually. He tries to keep his thoughts off of himself, and forces himself to read the newspaper, although in so doing he reads the news concerning "Prohibition," and concerning the fact that the new law may possibly not go into effect after all. This worries him, as he feels remorse over the fact that he may have made a mistake in retiring from the liquor business. He is anxious for work and for reading material.

April 15.
Four current magazines sent up to patient.

April 15.
Patient's wife seen at hospital. She goes walking with him every day and feels that he is slowly improving. She is buoyant and full of encouragement which patient seems to appreciate.

April 17.
Patient's wife seen at hospital while she was waiting to take patient to walk. If in the near future patient is considering leaving the hospital again, she will let visitor know.

April 21.
Patient seen on ward. He was pleased with the magazines. Said he read eagerly every word of them.

April 22.
Patient and wife seen on leaving hospital for a walk and told of the return of Miss May, former visitor.

April 24.
Patient and wife reported to visitor before going out for a walk. She takes patient walking several hours a day now. He says this is the only time he enjoys during the day, as it is the only time he is free from fear spells, even when working at the hospital. He still cleans windows daily.

April 28.
Patient seen on ward. He is much improved though still fearful regarding prohibition. He reads the papers daily in an effort to throw off this fear. The farmer on the land on which patient's camp is located in Bradbury has written urging patient and family to move out. He will get the ground plowed and all ready for patient. Patient likes the idea and thinks his wife will go up soon to see about this. Visitor urged that wife do this 3/30/19 and that patient get to work there soon.

April 28.
Patient's examiner, Dr. Lawson, consulted. Informant stated that she has not talked with patient in several days, but that a week ago she advised his going to another hospital, such as Middlesex, to get into a more suitable atmosphere. At such a hospital she feels there is more opportunity for exercise, recreation, and work with "gangs." She does not consider patient in fit condition to work in the community as yet. She had hoped patient would act on this recommendation himself.

1919
May 1.

Patient and his wife talked with visitor before going out for a walk. Dr. Lawson, patient's examiner, has advised his care at Middlesex and told patient she would see Dr. Lang about this. Patient thinks it would be a good thing, as he could do outdoor work under supervision, and he hopes he will be allowed there to frequently visit his country home, Bradbury, near by.

The farm patient visits consist of 20 acres belonging to an Italian who has a frame house there divided up for seven families which he rents to patient and others, all of whom grew up together. Patient pays $25 rent a year, having the use of 2 rooms. He can plow all the land he wants. Patient would consider also being discharged from the Psychopathic Hospital and going to Bradbury, reporting frequently to the O. P. D. Visitor agreed to talk with the doctors about this. Patient says very emphatically that he will do anything in his power to get well.

May 3.

Patien. seen starting out for a walk with his wife. He is still hesitant about going to Middlesex, stating that he is not sure they will keep him outdoors sufficiently. Visitor told him she would write the Social Service worker there, and that as Dr. Lawson had told him he would work there outdoors a great deal, there was no ground for hesitation. Patient agreed to decide by 5/5/19.

May 8.

Patient and his wife talked with in the morning. His wife told him to do whatever he thought best; but he has been considerably hesitant. He had been advised by some one to report to the Middlesex Clinic at the Homeopathic Hospital 5/6/19, where he could personally ask the superintendent what the chances of outdoor work were. He did not go there, however, as he decided to try longer walks daily, his wife reporting to the Psychopathic early in the morning.

Visitor assured patient that Dr. Lawson did not approve of his making plans of his own at present. Patient agreed that she was right, and decided to take a trip to Middlesex to-day with his wife to ask the superintendent about the nature of his care should he stay at Middlesex.

Patient's wife stated that for a number of weeks she and the children have been living with her mother at 10 Victoria Street. Her expenses have been light, consisting of rent in Arlington and occasional food at her mother's besides carfares. She said most of the $500 was still left but would not be definite.

Patient agreed to stay at Middlesex if conditions seemed satisfactory. Later he was admitted to Middlesex as a voluntary patient.

May 13.

Patient's wife telephones that she visited patient as recently as 5/12/19 and found him very contented. He has not yet been put at outdoor work but the weather has not been suitable. Superintendent said he would have to know patient better to decide whether he could let patient off for frequent visits to his farm in Bradbury.

Patient's wife has received a long blank to be filled out regarding patient's mental history. Visitor agreed to help her in filling out the blank.

1919
May 16.

Patient's wife reported to hospital with a blank to be filled out. As she is going to Middlesex to-morrow, visitor advised that she take the blank with her to be filled out at Middlesex. She has taken the children with her this afternoon for a week-end in Bradbury but is returning to Boston after that.

May 23.

Patient's wife telephoned that she found patient doing fairly well when she saw him 5/18/19. She is going up to the country again to-day, planning to stay until the end of next week. John will continue to attend school, living with his grandmother.

May 24.

Patient's mother-in-law, Mrs. Costelli, 10 Victoria St., Boston, visited. Informant invited visitor to supper, but visitor had already eaten. Her daughter, Bertha Costelli, says that Emma needs her tonsils removed because she has great difficulty at night in breathing. Bertha's single brother has just paid patient's rent in Arlington and Bertha expects to pay the rent a little later, as informants do not want patient to give up his home yet. They are not discouraged about patient, although Mrs. Costelli has lost some weight worrying about him.

June 2.

Patient sent a friendly letter by visitor.

June 19.

Patient heard from. The letter was written at his camp in Bradbury where he was spending Saturday and Sunday. He says he is much improved although still bothered with those "fear spells" at times. He was planning to return to Middlesex from the camp. His stay at Middlesex is more satisfactory than at the Psychopathic, as he can work outdoors with pick and shovel and keep busy with other indoor work.

Patient's wife is due in Boston on the 25th to attend John's graduation in Junior High School.

June 30.

Patient's wife reported to visitor at the hospital. A letter to another patient named Fangillo had been forwarded from the Psychopathic Hospital to patient's sister on Main Street for patient early in June. Patient's sister had been busy and neglected to forward the letter to patient. Patient had just heard from hospital asking that the letter be returned. Patient's wife came in at once this morning to straighten out the matter. She is looking well and says she feels well. Patient is constantly improving and is spending the week-ends at their camp in Bradbury. He works six hours a day with pick and shovel at Middlesex and sleeps very well. He is now in the parole ward.

Informant's relatives visit her at the camp occasionally and before long her mother as well as her married sister will stay for some time at the camp. Her relatives bring her food and patient has planted quite a few vegetables which will be maturing before long. Her money is holding out very well and she says she has nothing to worry about. She has not attended to Emma's tonsils and adenoids, claiming that she has been too busy. In spite of visitor's arguments to the contrary she seemed to think this matter should have to be put off until later in the summer or fall.

1919
Emma will attend school in the fall. Informant agreed to keep visitor closely informed as to patient's progress. She has jokingly told patient that the next thing he would worry about would be his future work. Patient told her that he would ask advice from the Psychopathic Hospital when he was ready to work and that he was sure work could be found for him at which he could keep well.

June 26.
Patient's wife heard from. Letter states that she is too busy to come to town for her son's graduation and states that her husband is improving though still worrying somewhat.

July 8.
Patient written to. Letter was sent to reassure patient.

July 29.
Patient heard from. Letter states that he was discharged from the hospital on the 14th of July and that he is feeling much better though still "very nervous and irritable." He is busy with his garden and in the past two weeks has put in thirty hours' work for the neighboring farmers. He expects to stay there until November 1, doing work for the farmers whenever it is available. He expects to improve rapidly now and suggests that visitor may be able to help him in selecting a line of work later. He has not decided what line of work to take up yet. The family are well.

August 7.
Gray Motor Company, Dorchester, employment manager, Mr. J. Sanborn, written to. Letter asks whether informant could place patient in the fall, stating that patient would be willing to start at any type of work, but would aim to work toward clerical work or a combination of clerical and physical work.

August 13.
Patient's wife telephoned. She came to town to do some errands, coming with a friend by automobile. Patient is doing very well. He sleeps fairly well but not yet perfectly. He takes fishing trips and enjoys the farming. When he left the Boston State Hospital the doctors warned him not to leave the country too soon. Informant plans to come to Boston by October 1, probably starting Emma in for a month of school at Bradbury. However, informant may possibly come to Boston earlier, if patient is well enough to come, spending the week-ends at the camp.

August 13.
Jackson's employment manager, Mr. Brown, visited. Informant states that he has but few men on the clerical force and that all the vacancies are filled.

August 18.
Gray Motor Company telephoned to. In the absence of Mr. Sanborn, chief of the education department, word was left for him to telephone visitor regarding patient.

August 21.
Gray Motor Company, employment manager, Mr. Sanborn, heard from. Letter states that visitor's letter of August 8 has been held up pending

1919

their decision concerning patient. At present, they are completely filled up; but if a vacancy occurs whereby they can use him to advantage they will let visitor know.

September 4.
Patient written to. Letter asks patient whether he is ready to start in at work at any time visitor has suitable position.

September 9.
Schuleman Paper Box Factory visited. Visitor attended the "Shop Committee Meeting" which is held every week, all the foremen and executives being present to discuss their needs and grievances. Two weeks before visitor had gone through the factory. There are about 250 employees and the firm prides itself on the fact that they all feel like "one big family." The foremen are called by their first names. Obviously the employees are treated very considerately and they seem unusually happy. Mr. Jones, superintendent, stated he would be glad to have a talk with patient and place him to best advantage in the factory, though he is not sure that the work will lead to clerical work. Mr. Chase, efficiency expert, and Miss Macpherson, nurse, were also talked to about patient. They are all interested in another patient from the Psychopathic Social Service, John Flynn, who has been there two weeks and is giving the greatest satisfaction.

September 10.
Patient written to. Letter describes the factory of Schuleman's and suggests that patient come to Boston soon to see about an opening there even though he may not be ready to stay on in Boston as yet.

Note:
The firm is glad to take employees known to reliable social agencies as they consider that as good as knowing their families. In so far as possible, they employ neighborhood people because the families are accessible.

September 11.
Patient's wife telephoned. She is in town to-day and to-morrow, starting Emma in at school. The family expect to stay at camp three weeks longer. Patient will answer visitor's letter soon. He is doing pretty well. Informant will telephone again to-morrow as she can hardly hear where she is to-day.

September 16.
Letters to patient, addressed Bradbury, Mass., returned unclaimed. They were remailed to patient to Box 13, R. F. D., Bradbury, Mass.

September 19.
Patient writes that he has just heard from visitor. He will be at the hospital on September 22 in the morning. He would come in to-day, but his potatoes are rotting in the ground and he has about thirty bushels to dig immediately. John is going to high school. Emma went to school for a few days, but is now at the camp for about a week until things are in shape for the winter.

1919
September 22.

Patient reported to visitor in the morning, having just come down from camp. He looked better physically and decidedly improved nervously. His eyes were bright and he was full of hope for the future. He occasionally has "fear spells," but he gets over them rapidly and he thinks that when he is at work they will vanish entirely. He has been doing farm work for several of the farmers in the vicinity as well as at his own camp. At present, patient's wife and his mother are at the camp putting up tomatoes. His son John would rather live at home in Arlington than with his grandmother. Yesterday he was out to the camp and returned last night to stay in Arlington. He gets his own meals and the landlady keeps an eye on him. Patient is sure he gets into no mischief and says he is a thoroughly reliable boy.

Patient is ambitious to undertake work which gives promise of advancement. Visitor talked with him about the opening at Schuleman's which in many ways appealed to him. He agreed to go down to the plant at once and interview Mr. Jones, superintendent. He is planning to return to camp this afternoon and will let visitor know result of his interview either by letter or telephone.

September 24.

Patient writes that he had a nice talk at the Schuleman Paper Box Factory with Mr. Jones and Mr. Chase (efficiency expert) and was shown over the factory. Mr. Jones said patient could begin work any time, starting with at least $16. Patient has thought the matter over carefully and feels that though the people there are all very nice the chances of advancement do not look especially bright. He says, "I would like some place where I could begin work and work hard if I felt that I could learn some useful trade or where I could be sure of advancement, provided, of course, I merited it." At the factory. apparently the most he could aspire to was to be a "machine man." Patient asked for visitor's advice, stating that though he knows "beggars cannot be choosers," he does not want to make a false start and have to change again in a short time.

September 24.

Gray Motor Company, Dorchester, employment department, telephoned to. The employment manager, Mr. Sanborn, is away for a few days.

September 27.

Patient written to, stating that visitor would give him more definite advice about his work in two or three days.

September 29.

Gray Motor Company, Mr. Sanborn, employment manager, telephoned to. Informant states that there is no opening there for patient.

September 30.

Prospective employer, Schuleman Paper Box Factory, visited. By invitation, visitor addressed the Shop Committee Meeting on the subject of mental hygiene of industry, explaining her work at the Psychopathic Hospital in particular. The superintendent, Mr. Jones, stated that he would employ any patient visitor sent to him and if there was no opening he would "make one." He was interested in talking with patient the other day. Informant had in mind clerical work for patient to advance to and thinks patient could very soon be placed at such work there, as there is

1919

an opening now. It is informant's custom, however, to have every office employee advance from the factory force. He did not tell patient about the prospect of clerical work, however. Visitor agreed to let patient know just what the probable opportunity was and to get in touch with informant again. The nurse, Miss MacPherson, states that should opportunities, for any reason, at the factory seem limited to patient, there is always a chance of his advancing from the paper box factory to the Schuleman Candy Factory, where there is a large clerical force.

September 30.

Patient written to, giving the result of the interview at Schuleman's this morning and stating that, though visitor did not want to force patient to consider this opening, she felt the opportunities of advancement were very good and the atmosphere there especially suited to patient. Her letter explained the chances of advancement to the Schuleman Candy Factory from the paper box factory.

October 7.

Patient writes that he has heard from visitor, but has not yet come to a decision. He is very anxious to get to work soon, saying, "I certainly feel the position I am in at present." Patient would come in October 6, but he has promised a farmer to pick apples until October 8. Patient will come to see visitor October 8.

October 8.

Patient reported to visitor in the morning, bringing with him a satchel full of apples for visitor from the farm. His wife plans to come to Arlington to stay on October 13, but patient plans to follow her a few days later unless he has a definite job in town before that. He is still undecided about the kind of work he should undertake, feeling that possibly indoor work will be too confining, and that his eyes might not permit of confining work. He stated that he would be glad to see Dr. Jacobs this afternoon for advice about his work and that he would be glad to see the employment manager at the Cole Rubber Company relative to possible employment there later, visitor explaining that the employment department is especially good there. Patient took with him a letter of introduction from visitor.

Patient says that when his mother died she left about $1,000, of which she gave $600 to patient's sister who is blind in one eye, the other siblings receiving about $200 each. As a matter of fact, most of them owed patient's mother at that time so that the full amount of $200 per person was not available. Patient loaned his share to help out and $80 is still due him from this time from a brother-in-law. Patient's brother Antonio, in Brayton, Vt., wrote patient's wife shortly after Antonio's marriage this summer about his marriage. Patient's wife was too busy to write at that time and Antonio has not written patient since. Patient feels friendly toward all of his relatives, but apparently cited these instances to explain that often others were more considerate of one than one's own relatives. Patient feels especially grateful to his friend "Henry" who owns the farm where patient has been all summer. It is not clear how much money patient still has on hand, but he says that he paid most of his expenses this summer from the work he did on the farm. He has on hand a large amount of fruit for the winter.

Patient still has occasional "fears," especially when not busy, but says they are very mild.

1919
October 8.
Cole Rubber Company, assistant employment manager, Mr. Carlton, telephoned to, who stated there is only one vacancy in the clerical department now, which is for a man who is accustomed to figuring costs. There are only three or four laboring jobs open, which are all excessively heavy. Informant would be glad, however, to talk with patient relative to future employment.

October 8.
Patient reported to the hospital in the afternoon to see Dr. Jacobs. Dr. Jacobs states that there really is no "medical problem" as far as patient is concerned. In other words, patient's diagnosis is probably something between manic depressive and psychasthenia or a combination of both, but patient is rapidly recovering. He will soon be in as good condition as after his attack of years ago. Every three months or so he should report to some psychiatrist to make sure that patient is not overworking. Dr. Jacobs feels that there is no reason why patient should have to try work different from his former clerical work and that patient could now hold a responsible clerical position. Patient should have a "hobby," as recreation is quite essential for him. In the past, when at clerical work, patient had practically no recreation. Patient's fears are so slight now that they can practically be disregarded.

October 8.
Schuleman Paper Box Factory, Superintendent, Mr. Jones, telephoned to, who stated that there is temporarily no work open for patient in the office as another patient from the Psychopathic Hospital, Martin O'Connor, is, for a time, doing clerical work there. However informant feels that before long he will need further help and says that at almost any time he could arrange things to take patient on. It was mutually agreed between informant and visitor that patient look around for other openings and if patient was not successful, informant would make place for him at Schuleman's.

October 8.
Patient reported to visitor that Mr. Carlton at Cole's was very nice to him this morning but stated frankly that there was no opening now and took patient's name, agreeing to let patient know should an opening turn up. Patient had a very satisfactory interview with Dr. Jacobs. Patient says he is not as sure as Dr. Jacobs that he can go ahead and do bookkeeping right away, but as Dr. Jacobs says he can, he will try to believe it himself. Visitor agreed to look into other openings which would be distinctly clerical and to let patient know if a good opening was found before he plans to return to Arlington. Patient's wife has said she would gladly go to work to supplement the income. this winter, but visitor assured patient this would undoubtedly not be necessary. Patient left the hospital considerably relieved by Dr. Jacobs' advice.

October 14.
Psychopathic Hospital Staff, Dr. Jacobs, states that patient's eye condition should not be attended to now, as patient would probably not like any glasses ordered now. Patient will probably have another breakdown in about five years.

October 16.
Patient's wife telephoned stating that she has been in Arlington all week, but goes to camp for the week-end to-morrow. Patient will probably

1919

remain at the camp as long as weather permits until a definite opening is found for him. The family are well.

October 23.
   Patient left some apples for visitor at the hospital in her absence.

October 30.
   Patient's wife telephoned that patient will probably return from the farm the first of next week to stay. As to-day is a school holiday in Arlington, informant and the children will go to the camp for the week-end. Visitor stated that several openings had been looked into ·for patient, but that visitor delayed about writing patient until the right opening presented itself. Informant agreed to have patient get in touch with visitor the first of next week.

November 1.
   Federal Employment Office, 4 Cherry St., registrar, Mr. Brown, telephoned to, regarding clerical openings for patient. Visitor had personally interviewed informant during the week regarding openings and had telephoned several times since. There have been no suitable openings for patient.

November 5.
   Patient's wife telephoned that as the weather has been so pleasant patient will remain in the country until next week. Informant prefers to wait until next spring about Emma's tonsils, but agreed to speak to Emma's school teacher about this.

November 17.
   Patient's wife telephoned that patient is still in the country and will remain there for a few days more unless visitor sends for him. He no longer talks of himself, but is planning for the future. He is busy packing and shipping apples. Informant is now housecleaning. She seemed pleased to know that the hospital feels she has done a great deal toward patient's recovery and assured visitor that her family as well as the hospital had done a great deal also.

November 17.
   Y. M. C. A. Employment Office, Mr. Grafton, telephoned to. Informant will keep patient in mind for a clerical position. The coal strike has temporarily pulled down business so that openings are few. Informant asked to have patient drop in to see him when next in town.

November 24.
   Federal Employment Office, 4 Cherry St., registrar, Mr. Brown, visited, who had no suitable openings for patient.

November 28.
   Patient reported to visitor. He came to town to stay on November 26. Patient has been busy bringing apples to town with "Henry," the farmer at whose farm patient stays. They came to market from three to five times a week. Patient is now ready and anxious to get to work, but a little fearful of clerical work. His face clouded somewhat at the mention of clerical work, patient asking visitor whether she thought he could safely

1919

do clerical work. He is insistent that he shall never have a recurrence of his disease. Visitor reminded him of Dr. Jacobs' advice about his work.

His wife has been working since she came to town this fall at a candy factory in the East End, near her mother's home. She dips chocolates from 6:45 to 9:45 P. M. daily at $1.25 for three hours. She did likewise in the late spring before coming to the camp, but did not tell patient about this until during the summer. Patient asked visitor definitely not to tell his wife he had spoken of this. Visitor told patient that his wife had told visitor about her working early in the spring and that now she would doubtless speak of it when visitor called. Patient's wife says she would miss work now if she stopped as she enjoys the companionship of the women there. Financially the family is getting along "O. K." though patient does not know the exact amount left, as his wife manages. He plans to collect about $300 due him from individuals who borrowed from him when he was in the liquor business, and he says his brother-in-law still owes him about $200 from his mother's estate, which he will also try to collect. Patient loaned his brother Antonio about $700 several years ago. At one time patient paid Antonio's board at the rate of $7 a week, giving him from $2 to $3 a week besides. Patient is glad he laid in a supply of clothes a year ago considering the cost of living now. He has always provided in advance when possible.

Patient's wife and children are not insured, but patient carries two semi-endowment policies under the National Life Insurance Company. In case of death a thousand dollars is due from each of them, but before that time, if he lives a number of years, a few hundred dollars is payable in addition to patient.

Patient plans to join either the Arlington or Boston Y. M. C. A. and will look at once into the possibilities. He is determined to have exercise and recreation to keep him well. Patient was given a number of letters of introduction to the Y. M. C. A. Employment Bureau and the State Public Employment Office, where he expects to report to-morrow morning. Patient understands that clerical openings are scarce for men at present and is very glad to have Mr. Boylston, Bureau for Returning Soldiers and Sailors, keep him in mind for suitable clerical openings.

Patient says he is feeling better all the time and finds he is best when working hardest. Only occasionally does he have "fears," but he is able to control them.

November 28.
    Y. M. C. A. Employment Bureau, Mr. Grafton, telephoned to. Informant knows of no clerical openings now.

November 28.
    Federal Employment Office, 4 Cherry St., Mr. Brown, telephoned to. Informant knows of no clerical openings now.

November 28.
    Bureau for Returning Soldiers and Sailors, Mr. Boylston, telephoned to. Informant knows of no clerical openings for patient now, but hopes to have some soon and will let visitor know when he has a suitable opening for patient. He does have openings from time to time into which the discharged soldiers do not fit.

December 1.
    Y. M. C. A. Employment Bureau, Mr. Grafton, telephoned to. Informant sent patient to apply on November 30 at J. K. Hodge's Hay, Grain,

1919
& Seed store in Chelsea, where there was a vacancy at office work at $18. Patient has not reported to informant since. Informant referred to patient as a "nice chap."

December 2.
Patient telephoned that he had been trying to reach visitor for the last twenty-four hours to report. Mr. Brown, of the Federal Employment Office, took patient's name and asked him to report in a few days. Mr. Grafton of the Y. M. C. A. took patient's name and said he would let patient know when he had a suitable opening for him. The only openings the Y. M. C. A. had were suitable really for boys. Patient agreed to report to-morrow again and visitor agreed to get in touch with the Bureau for Returning Soldiers and Sailors.

December 3.
Patient telephoned, stating that he plans to go to the Federal Employment Office this afternoon. He is watching the advertisements in the papers and looking about somewhat.

December 3.
Federal Employment Office, 4 Cherry St., Mr. Brown, telephoned to, who knows of no openings for patient to-day. Patient reported to informant this morning and will report again to-morrow morning.

December 3.
Jackson Commercial School, Mr. Ware, visited, who spoke of an opening at the Riverside Book Shop. Miss Martin there is looking for a first-class bookkeeper to straighten out the accounts now handled by two women, who together are paid $45 a week. Miss Martin would probably pay patient $30 a week. Patient should apply at once, stating that he heard of the opening through a friend. Informant could not recommend patient as he does not know him.

December 3.
Patient's home visited as no response was received by telephone. Patient was home taking care of Emma and George Giordani. Patient's wife went to the Arlington Theatre to the movies, and John, on returning from school, did likewise. Patient felt he could not leave the house until his wife returned, and telephoned the Riverside Book Shop to see whether he ought to apply this afternoon. Miss Martin's sister answered the phone, stating that Miss Martin was leaving for New York to-night. Patient gave visitor's name, which she said she did not know, and asked patient to write her his experience. Patient's wife then returned home and went with visitor to the street car. Visitor agreed to get in touch with the Riverside Book Shop soon.

December 4.
Riverside Book Shop, Miss Martin, visited. She at once asked whether patient had been a patient at the Psychopathic Hospital and then said she had troubles enough of her own without employing someone from there. Visitor then talked briefly on the subject of the prevalence of psychiatric conditions and need of treatment. Informant was then attentive and agreed to look up patient's references, although, she explained, she considered the work "nerve-racking" as all the customers were women and all of the help, except one, were women and the books were behind.

1919
Informant felt also inclined to think that patient must be rusty in book-keeping if he had done none in five years. Informant is leaving for New York this morning and will not be back until next week.

December 4.
Stratton Piano Company, Office Salesman, Mr. Blair, visited as visitor was passing by. Mr. Dawson was not noticed until almost the end of the interview and visitor did not remember Mr. Dawson's name so could not ask for him. Informant stated that patient's work was first-class and that patient was confidential clerk, only one man being over him. Patient knew all that was going on in the office. Informant knows of no openings in the piano line now, but thinks patient's experience would serve him equally well in the lines of furniture or installment work. The firm would give patient an excellent recommendation at any time.

December 4.
Patient seen at the Federal Employment Office, 4 Cherry St., Mr. Brown had no opening for patient then. Patient expects to join the Y. M. C. A. as soon as he is working. There is a swimming tank there but none in the Arlington Y. M. C. A. Patient is reporting to the Y. M. C. A. Employment Bureau, Mr. Grafton, this afternoon, and visitor agreed to look into the openings at the Y. M. C. U.

December 4.
Y. M. C. U. Employment Bureau, Mr. Howland, visited. The bureau places only non-union men and fills no factory or laboring positions. Informant will be glad to see what he can do to find a suitable position for patient and visitor agreed to send patient in to-morrow morning. Informant states that though clerical openings are not abundant they are to be had.

December 4.
Patient's home telephoned to, leaving word for patient to report to the Y. M. C. U. to-morrow morning.

December 5.
Jackson Commercial School, Employment Office, Mr. Ware, telephoned to, reporting developments on the Riverside Book Shop. Informant suggests getting in touch with Miss Martin early next week again.

December 5.
Y. M. C. U. Employment Bureau, Mr. Howland, telephoned to, who was favorably impressed by patient. Informant says he is sure he can find a suitable opening for patient soon. Patient is willing to do selling or clerical work.

December 8.
Riverside Book Shop, Miss Martin, telephoned to. She is sure that she could not take patient on.

December 8.
Bureau for Returning Soldiers and Sailors telephoned to. Mr. Boylston has left, but his successor, Mr. Max, suggested that patient might find an opening at Henley & Coolidge, Accounts Engineers, 350 Rice Building,

1919
as this firm has been advertising for bookkeepers and the bureau has sent one or two candidates. Informant agreed further to keep patient in mind for an opening.

December 8.
Patient's wife telephoned to, asking patient to telephone visitor to-morrow morning.

December 8.
Patient written to, suggesting the opening at Henley & Coolidge.

December 9.
Patient telephoned that none of the agencies have found an opening for him yet. The Y. M. C. A. sent him to a garage at Freeman Square, Chelsea, where a bookkeeper was needed, but they really wanted only a boy for a job.

December 10.
Patient telephoned to. He has found no suitable openings, but expects to through the help of the agencies interested in him. If he needs advice during the visitor's absence until January 2, he will get in touch with the Social Service or Dr. Jacobs. When visitor complimented him on his success in getting well he said his wife deserved all the credit. Patient expects to sell two pianos by Christmas, netting him about $75.

December 20.
Patient was mailed a Christmas card.

1920
January 2.
Patient's wife telephoned to. Patient is planning to see visitor soon. Informant, patient, and the children were with her family several days at Christmas time. Patient has not yet found work, but is not discouraged

January 3.
Patient reported to visitor, bringing a two-pound box of candy as a Christmas gift, which his sister had given him. She works at Young, Cobb & Sanborn and each year gives patient candy. Patient's wife is still working. Patient has made the rounds of the various employment agencies, having added the Commercial Reference Association and the International Reference Association. The only definite positions offered him have been through the Y. M. C. A. One of these positions was suitable only for a young fellow; the other is pending, a position as ledger clerk at $25 a week at Hudson Shoe Polish factory in Mattapan. Patient has applied there and telephoned regarding the opening several times, but each time has been told that no decision has been made. Patient will telephone soon. The last few days patient has felt somewhat discouraged, but has been able to control himself. He has not sold the pianos as yet, as the purchasers find that they are twice as expensive as they thought.
The children received a total of about $35 for Christmas from relatives and patient received $25 from his friend Henry on the farm. Patient's brother has paid him $50 of what he owes. Patient agreed to telephone visitor soon and plans to continue consulting the employment agencies. Mr. Brown of the Federal Employment Office has shown the most interest in him, but he has had no suitable openings.

1920
January 3.
Jackson Commercial School, Mr. Ware, telephoned to. Informant
knows of no openings for patient now, stating that there are less clerical
openings for men now than there were last fall. Informant would be glad
to help out at any time he can.

January 3.
Hudson Brothers, Mattapan, telephoned to. Employment Manager,
Mr. Beers, was out and person answering, apparently in the superintendent's office, would give no information about the firm, but suggested getting
in touch with Mr. Beers.

January 5.
Patient telephoned. He is willing to have visitor use her judgment
about consulting Hudson's.

January 5.
A former Mattapan A. C. worker states that the Mattapan A. C. considers Hudson's factory a very poor place to work. The employees are
underpaid and the girls working there are looked upon as hardly respectable by other working girls.

January 7.
Y. M. C. A. Employment Bureau, Mr. Grafton, telephoned to. Informant states that the outlook in the office line is bad. It is hard to fit
patient in other than clerical position because he has had no experience.
Informant will keep patient in mind, however, and try to place him.

January 7.
Federal Employment Office, Mr. Brown, telephoned to. Informant
offered patient two jobs, both of which patient felt were too far away.
It is not the fault of either informant or patient that former has not
realized before that patient would consider other than clerical work. He
will continue to keep patient in mind, looking out for both clerical and
other openings.

January 7.
Hudson Brothers, Manufacturers of Shoe Polish, Mattapan, visited at
2:30 P. M. The employment manager, Mr. Beers, was out. The telephone
girl asked whether visitor would see some one else, but when visitor said
she would see the superintendent, was informed that Mr. Beers was also
superintendent. The advertising manager spoke to visitor, but said he
could do nothing about the opening for patient as this was up to Mr. Beers.
Visitor asked to be shown over the factory, but the advertising manager
stated that no visitors were allowed as the process was secret.

January 7.
*Bureau for Returning Soldiers and Sailors, Clerical Department, Mr.
Max, visited.* Informant would be glad to talk with patient and try to
place him. He seemed more than willing to advise visitor regarding clerical openings.

January 7.
Patient telephoned to in the evening, asking him to report to Mr. Max,
to-morrow morning. Patient had not found any openings.

1920

January

   Patient telephoned that he reported to the Federal Employment Office, 4 Cherry St., this morning. Mr. Brown told him that though there was labor trouble at Root's patient might find an opening there. Patient applied at Root's and the employment manager, Mr. Fielding, told him to come in again the next morning. Patient asked visitor's advice, but visitor advised against the firm as paying poorly and not giving much promise of advancement for patient. Patient finds it difficult to go all over town looking for a job. He has not reported to Mr. Max, but will do so at once. He answered an advertisement in the *Globe* to-day at a team firm as ledger and trial balance clerk.

January 9.

   Patient telephoned that he reported to Mr. Max yesterday, who was ready to send patient to the Loyal Shoe Company but on finding patient was not an ex-service man felt he could do nothing for patient. Visitor agreed to get in touch with Mr. Max again.

January 9.

   Bureau for Returning Soldiers and Sailors, Mr. Max, telephoned to. Informant did not fully understand visitor's work as predecessor, Mr. Boylston, did not explain it to him. In only rare instances has informant's bureau placed men not ex-service. If patient is interested in a job as chief accountant at the International Optical Company, Lexington, informant would be glad to get in touch with the employment manager there, Mr. Bates, as informant has no service man willing to go out of town to take the job.

January 10.

   Patient telephoned to, explaining the opening at Lexington. Patient agreed to talk it over with his wife and report later.

January 10.

   Patient telephoned that he feels the opening would be too responsible at Lexington and he does not care to break down again. In order to live away from his family he feels he would have to earn quite a large salary. He agreed that there is no harm done in looking into the opening, by correspondence, at least, and thinks the same opening is offered through the Federal Employment Office. Patient is getting discouraged about not finding work.

January 10.

   Federal Employment Office, Mr. Brown, telephoned to. Informant has no openings to-day except the one at the International Optical Company, Lexington. Informant does not blame patient for not being interested in the opening for the reasons patient gave.

January 10.

   Y. M. C. A. Employment Office, Mr. Grafton, telephoned to. The only opening this morning is one as a bookkeeper at $20 on St. Charles Street. Informant knows no further details about it, but feels patient would not consider it as he keeps saying he cannot accept less than $25.

January 12.

   Jackson Commercial School, Mr. Ware, visited. Informant states that there are no openings suitable for patient as all of them combine stenography and bookkeeping.

1920
January 12.
Women's Educational Association, Appointment Bureau, Miss Black, visited for possible suggestions about patient. Informant suggests Wood & Berry Service, 60 Eagle St.; both Miss Wood and Miss Berry were formerly connected with the U. S. Employment Service.

January 12.
Wood & Berry, 60 Eagle St., Miss Berry, visited. Informant states that clerical openings for men are very scarce, but suggested the Underwood Motor Company, Sawyer St., and the City Gas Corporation, as both employing large numbers of male clerks. The latter has taken on night men lately as business is so heavy.

January 12.
City Gas Corporation, North Street, Chief of Collection Division, Henry McMillan, visited. No men are employed in the clerical department and there are now no vacancies in the collection department, though men are working in the collection department day and night. Their pay begins at $19.50. Informant would be glad to put patient's name on the waiting list if patient cares to come in to see informant. Suggested the bookkeeping department on Victoria St. as a possibility.

January 12.
City Gas Corporation, 52 Victoria St., Chief of the Bookkeeping Division, Mr. Grant, visited. Informant states that there are no openings now, but he employs about 50 men at bookkeeping and accountancy. The firm is apt to promote from below but will be glad to see that patient is put on the mailing list.

January 12.
Patient visited at his home. His son John was at home reading and seemed a bright, manly fellow. Patient's wife was out. Patient feels that the landlady has not been quite as cordial to the family since their present misfortune, but admits that relations are not very strained, as the landlady's daughter still practices on patient's piano and patient feels free to use landlady's telephone.

Patient is discouraged at having so much difficulty in finding work, but realizes that many others are in a similar predicament. He grits his teeth in an effort to drive away any fears and has been fairly sucessful. He feels better after talking with his wife or visitor. He agreed to go to the Cole Rubber Company to-morrow morning ready to accept any kind of work. He is anxious to get to work more to have his mind occupied than to get immediate income. Work out of town, such as ice-cutting, he would find very dreary. He admitted the futility of work such as elevator work, however, as he would be no better off on leaving the job than he was on beginning it. To-day patient answered an advertisement in the *Globe* by writing a rubber company who wanted men to learn the business, starting at $23. He applied at Reed's, who needed salesmen, but said 125 applicants applied, most of whom had to be turned away. Patient was not among the first so was not successful. He applied at another place which was advertised in the *Globe,* but on application found that the place had been filled and that about 20 men had applied.

John cooked visitor some coffee and patient served some Italian "ravioli," and custard pie, all nicely cooked.

1920
January 13.
Patient telephoned that he applied at the Cole Rubber Company this morning, but Mr. Carlton there told him that there were no openings. Patient plans to visit the City Gas Corporation this afternoon.

January 15.
Schuleman Paper Box Factory, nurse Miss MacPherson, telephoned to. Visitor explained that patient had not considered an opening there a few months ago because at the time the opportunities there seemed limited to him. In the meantime the patient has had an opportunity to look about considerably and he would be interested to consider an opening there now. Informant agreed to see the superintendent, Mr. Jones, about this.

January 15.
Patient telephoned and was interested to hear of a possible opening at Schuleman's, though he evidently still felt he might have made a mistake in not making further efforts to get a place at Root's, asking visitor whether the Schuleman opportunity was as good as Root's.

January 16.
Patient telephoned that he is home this morning as his wife has lumbago.

January 16.
Schuleman Paper Box Company, nurse, Miss MacPherson, telephoned that both she and Mr. Jones remember patient well and liked him but that there is no opening this week. Possibly there will be an opening next week and informant will let visitor know if there is.

January 17.
Patient telephoned—somewhat discouraged because he has found no openings. He would like to go to his friend Henry in the country in Bradbury to help him chop wood and to consult him regarding openings in automobile factories as Henry is in close touch with some automobile men. Patient feels he cannot leave his children alone at night while his wife is working.

January 19.
Patient telephoned that at Ring's Service Bureau this morning he was told that the John Meredith Company at Milton would take on a number of new men for general factory work. Patient would like to look into this opening and agreed to telephone an hour later after visitor had got in touch with the firm.

January 19.
John Meredith Company, Printing and Lithographing Inks, factory, Milton, telephoned to. Superintendent Guili, who hires the factory help, stated that he will take on a number of new men if of the right sort; that is, having common sense and with good physical strength. The firm manufactures printing ink and the processes are easy to learn. The pay is 52 cents an hour for a 48-hour week. On certain processes after two months the pay is 70 cents an hour. Mr. Guili is not in charge of the office help but connected visitor with Mr. Mills.
Mr. Mills, Chief of the office force, telephoned to. Informant states that he has a number of men in his department earning varying salaries

1920

depending on the responsibilities. He has no openings now, but will be glad to talk with patient and keep him on his list. Should patient want to begin at factory work, he would be glad to try and have him advance to office work when there was an opening if patient were suitable. Visitor agreed to have patient ask for Mr. Mills, on arrival in Milton to-day. Mr. Mills states that commuting would be too hard on patient and that it is somewhat difficult to find a boarding place and very difficult to find a place for a family.

January 19.

Patient telephoned and seemed interested in the possibilities at Milton. The family have a friend in Needham with whom either he or the family could probably live if it was hard to locate in Milton. Patient agreed to go out to see Mr. Mills at once. Patient did not look into the International Optical Company, but frankly feels the work there would have been too responsible.

January 20.

Patient telephoned that he had his usual luck at the John Meredith Company yesterday. At the factory applicants were talked to in a group and told frankly that the work was very trying as they would have to work with all kinds of acids, and with dyes which would color the employee the same as the tint of the dye. Patient says the smell was "awful" and that he could never stand it or the change of shifts. The plant runs on a three-shift basis and patient would have to vary in his shift 8–4, or 4–12 or 12–8. There is only a late afternoon train besides the 1:45, so patient took earlier train, though he was unable thereby to see Mr. Mills, who was away for luncheon. Patient saw Mr. Jackson, assistant manager with the John Rider Company yesterday afternoon. He gave patient the name of a public accountant who might need an assistant. Mr. Jackson is the brother of the man who was in charge of the business school patient formerly attended. Patient will look up that opening to-day.

January 20.

Cole Rubber Company, Employment Manager, Mr. Carlton, sat next to visitor at a dinner of the Boston Employment Managers' Association, and stated that though the factory needs female help it has no openings for male help now. There are, however, a number of men doing clerical work there.

January 21.

Schuleman Paper Box Factory, nurse, Miss MacPherson, telephoned to, who said she plans to see superintendent, Mr. Jones, about an opening for patient this morning.

January 21.

Underwood Motor Company, Sawyer St., Employment Manager, Mr. Johnson, telephoned to. Informant says there are no openings there for clerks and that he has the problem of fitting three of his present book-keepers into general work as they are putting in bookkeeping machines. Informant volunteered to talk with patient about his work. Visitor agreed to send patient to him.

January 21.

Jackson Commercial School, Mr. Ware, telephoned to, who stated that the openings for male clerks grow scarcer and that informant is solicitous

1920

about being able to place some of his students who will be ready in a few months. If patient has any openings at all he had better take them.

January 21.

Patient telephoned that yesterday afternoon he applied at Fletcher & Lothian, Public Accountants, to whom Mr. Jackson referred him. Mr. Fletcher was out, but patient saw his partner, who talked with patient and asked whether patient was willing to leave Boston occasionally for six or seven days to make a trip with the public accountants. Patient told him· he was willing to travel and agreed to come in on January 24 to see Mr. Fletcher. Patient plans to ask Mr. Jackson to telephone Mr. Fletcher on January 24 regarding patient's qualifications.

January 21.

Patient telephoned that he had a pleasant interview with Mr. Johnson of the Underwood Motor Company, but there is no opening there now. Mr. Johnson took patient's name and agreed to let him know if any suitable openings developed. Patient plans to visit Mr. Jackson this afternoon and asked visitor what she thought about his visiting the Gray factory. Visitor explained that the turnover was so small at Gray's that there was but little chance of an opening, but that if an additional visit does not tire him there is no harm done by applying.

January 21.

Y. M. C. A. Employment Office, Mr. Grafton, telephoned to. Although clerical openings are scarce for men, informant has a few such openings right along. The only thing now which would be possible for patient is as an assistant to a public accountant. Informant says that work is quite strenuous at times and dull other times. Patient might find work a strain at the beginning of the year, the busiest time. Informant has two such openings, but has had them some time and does not know whether they have been filled. They are: John J. Seavey, 36 Main St., and Gerry & Co., 38 East St. Each of these pay from $5 to $6 a day with half pay when laid off.

January 22.

Patient telephoned and agreed to look up the positions as assistant to public accountant at once. He will then make the usual rounds of the employment offices.

January 22.

Schuleman Paper Box Factory, nurse, Miss MacPherson, telephoned that both the superintendent, Mr. Jones, and she say there are no openings there now. Both informant and Mr. Jones are very sorry as they remember patient well most pleasantly. Perhaps in a few weeks there would be an opening. Mr. Wells, employment manager at the Schuleman Confectionery Factory, is laying off help at present.

January 22.

Madison Razor Company, Employment Manager, Mr. Mahoney, telephoned to. He states that there are no openings in the plant for men at present. He says clerical openings are scarce for men, but he does not know why.

January 23.

Patient telephoned that he applied to the public accountant, Mr. Bates, but that there is no opening there now. They were nice to patient there.

1920
Patient is keeping up his courage pretty well, but his wife is beginning to get discouraged.

January 23.
   Y. M. C. U. Employment Office, Mr. Howland, visited. Informant said Stratton Piano Company gave patient a good recommendation, but that the firm said patient's doctor had said he could not stand his former type of work again. Informant is willing, however, to abide by the advice of the Psychopathic Hospital. Because of patient's age and also because of scarcity of positions in general, informant has not been able to place patient, but suggested that visitor visit the National Baking Corporation, Mr. Lowney, Manager, who asked informant to have a crippled soldier placed there. This soldier has been doing very well. Informant suggested that visitor get in direct touch herself, as Mr. Lowney generally asks informant for a "hustler."

January 23.
   Federal Employment Office, Mr. Brown, visited. He will continue to try to place patient, but agrees with visitor that the best chance to place patient probably will be through interesting some employer in him personally, as otherwise patient's age usually stands in the way. Informant has allowed patient to look over the cards containing the requests from the employers so that patient will be convinced informant is doing everything possible for him.

January 24.
   Patient telephoned that he did not go around visiting the other public accountant, but applied at Ring's Service Bureau and the Y. M. C. A., also to his friend Mr. Jackson who will get in touch with Mr. Fletcher soon. Mr. Jackson advised patient to send out some form letters to several public accountants applying for positions, which patient will do Sunday. Visitor advised patient to get some work shovelling snow if he was finding the strain of looking for a permanent position discouraging him. Patient seemed inclined, however, to continue his search. Visitor asked whether patient would be willing to consider work in Lawrence and he said he would.

January 26.
   General Anderson Craig, Lawrence, Mass., mill owner, written to, reminding him that he offered to let visitor see some of the Lawrence mills some time and asking whether visitor could do so within a few days, stating that she would like to talk over possible openings for patient.

January 26.
   Patient telephoned that he had just telephoned his friend, Mr. Jackson, who will get in touch with Mr. Fletcher about 11 o'clock this morning. Patient sent out letters to six public accountants whose names and addresses he secured from the telephone book. He will make the usual rounds of employment agencies to-day.

January 26.
   Y. M. C. U. Employment Office, Mr. Howland, telephoned to. In his absence word was left that there did not seem to be any opening at the National Baking Corporation for patient.

January 27.
   Patient telephoned that he has answered an advertisement of the Jenkins Graphophone Company, Dalton, Conn., for general factory work.

1920

The Federal Employment Office had an opening for patient to consider but it required detailed knowledge of the income tax, which patient said he has not kept abreast. He has received three replies to his letters to public accountants, all stating that they need no men.

January 27.

General Anderson Craig, mill owner, telephoned that he could arrange for visitor to see the mills any time this week. He is coming to Boston to-morrow and will meet visitor at 4:30 to discuss the plans of the next day.

January 27.

Howland Business School, 9 Center St., Employment Office, Mr. Fenton, visited. Visitor explained that one of his former students in her employ had suggested that he might be willing to advise visitor regarding clerical openings for men. He stated that though clerical openings for males had been exceedingly scarce for the last six weeks, they have been on the increase and he feels that the high water mark of replacing men by women has been reached and that firms are now putting on men in place of women. He suggested as firms frequently inquiring for help, Burton Tire Company, International Optical Company, Gleason Company, and Lowell, Johnson & Co., public accountants.

January 28.

Patient telephoned that there was an advertisement in the *Globe* this morning for a grocery warehouse man on East Street. From the address patient thinks the firm is Sullivan's. Patient's brother-in-law works for Sullivan's, so patient will look into the opening through him. Patient agreed to look into some of the openings that Howland Business School had suggested and visitor agreed to write the International Optical Company herself as she knows Miss Henderson in the employment department. Patient said he would be willing to move to Lexington if the chances of advancement were good there. Patient seemed interested in hearing about visitor's plan to go to Lawrence.

January 28.

International Optical Company, Employment Department, Miss Henderson, written to, asking whether there would be any opening for patient there and what the living conditions for families are in Lexington.

January 30.

Patient telephoned that he was home most of yesterday as John is ill, having the grippe. He is better, but Emma is sick to-day. If she does not respond to home treatment, patient will call in doctor. Patient received one further reply from his letters to accountants which stated that there was no question but what patient was experienced but that there were more highly trained people available for this accountant's purpose. Patient will try to get in touch with firms that visitor suggested on January 28.

January 31.

Patient telephoned that he has a slight cold but that the children are better. He has received a reply from Dalton, Conn., stating that they cannot place him anywhere. At this point patient said he certainly had "bad luck" and "everything seems to go hard." Last night he came home and told his wife he at last was sure he had a job. Yesterday Mr. Brown of the Federal Employment Office put him in touch with an opening as a

1920
bookkeeper for the Dean Blacking & Staining Company at $25 a week.
This morning patient telephoned the firm and was told that they had
settled everything with their present bookkeeper so that a new one was not
needed. Patient is afraid his age was against him and that the explanation given is not the real one. He promised to rest up this week-end from
his cold.

January 31.
   Federal Employment Office, Mr. Brown, telephoned to, who agreed to
let visitor know later what the real situation at Dean's was.

February 2.
   Patient telephoned that Mr. Fletcher has not yet returned from Providence. Patient's family are feeling better. They called in their doctor for
Emma, whose stomach was affected, though she did not have influenza.
Patient's wife has a slight cold and patient is still about the same. He
plans to stay home to-day. He is answering two advertisements in yesterday's *Globe.*

February 2.
   Y. M. C. A. Employment Bureau, Mr. Grafton, telephoned to. Informant states that patient's "appearance and name queer him." Informant
has sent him out on at least a half dozen openings and though they did not
take on patient they did, however, take on some one else. He cited Hudson's as an example.

February 2.
   Y. M. C. A. secretary, Mr. Doyle, telephoned to, who knows of a temporary position for a man to do chiefly bookkeeping at Union Square,
Chelsea. He will telephone to get the present situation there and report
later to visitor. He volunteered that for some unknown reason it is harder
for a man out of a job to get a job than for a man who has a job to get
another one.

February 2.
   Y. M. C. A. secretary, Mr. Doyle, telephoned that he has just got in
touch with the Lambert Real Estate & Insurance Company, Chelsea, and
finds that the position is still vacant. About three weeks ago the firm
asked informant to find a man to hold the position for a few weeks.
Informant sent a man who filled the position very satisfactorily, but has
just left for a permanent position. Although this work is nominally temporary, the firm is a large and growing one, and if patient fits in well,
informant thinks there might be permanent work there. At all events, if
patient takes the position he could make it clear that he might have to
leave at any time for permanent work. Informant could reach neither
Mr. Lambert nor Mr. Hudson, but left word at the office about patient.
Visitor agreed to send patient in to the firm to-morrow to apply for the
position.

February 2.
   Patient telephoned to, telling him of the opening at the Lambert Real
Estate & Insurance Company. He agreed to apply first thing to-morrow.

February 3.
   Patient telephoned that he applied at Lambert's, but Mr. Lambert said
a young man was to apply in a day or so whom he would like to interview

1920
before deciding anything. It will take two or three days before Mr. Lambert decides.

February 3.
   Y. M. C. A., Mr. Doyle, telephoned to, who says that on the face of it it looks as if Mr. Lambert was not favorably impressed by patient. Informant will ask a man under whom patient would work directly at Lambert's details about the situation at Lambert's, as this man lives at the Y. M. C. A.

February 4.
   Patient telephoned that he will make the usual rounds to-day. He heard from Mr. Jackson that Mr. Fletcher does not need any men now.

February 4.
   Johnston-Abbott Mills, Chief Inspector, Mr. Fabian (visitor's brother-in-law) written to, asking him for advice as to possible openings in Lawrence for patient.

February 4.
   Boston University, Vocational Department, Mr. Warren seen by chance in the evening. He came over to visitor and asked whether patient had a job as yet. He suggested that it would be a good plan for patient to report to him so that informant could have him definitely on the waiting list for an opening.

February 5.
   International Optical Co., Lexington, heard from. Letter stated that at present the only clerical openings for patient would be in the Traffic Department at $20 and a probable one in the Shipping Department at $18, both of which informant thinks would not attract a man of patient's experience. If he is an Italian, that might bar him from office positions other than in workshops. An application blank was enclosed and informant states that possibly a better opening in the offices may later occur, of which visitor will be advised.

February 5.
   Patient written to, asking him to report to Boston University, Mr. Warren, and telling him of the reply from Lexington. Patient has sent the application blank and visitor stated that she was writing to the International Optical Company telling them that doubtless patient would consider an opening such as the one in the Traffic Department if promised definite advancement.

February 5.
   International Optical Company, Lexington, Miss Henderson written to, stating that patient would be glad to make the trip to Lexington if there should be a good opening or if the opening in the Traffic Department gave promise of advancement. The letter asked that patient be kept on the waiting list.

February 6.
   Patient telephoned. He has not received visitor's letter. He will go to Boston University to-day and to Wood & Berry, which he did not get around to as yet. His wife is feeling the strain of the children's illness. Emma is not yet up and around.

1920
February 6.

    Y. M. C. A. Secretary, Mr. Doyle, telephoned to, who forgot to inquire about the Chelsea opening but will telephone Mr. Lambert and report to visitor later.

February 7.

    Patient telephoned. He went to see Mr. Warren at Boston University yesterday and had a long talk with him. Mr. Warren advised him to apply at the Harvard Coal Company, Mr. Marsh, regarding an opening there as a bookkeeper. Patient applied, but Mr. Marsh was not there all day, but to-day patient found him in. Mr. Marsh was at first very enthusiastic and thought patient could do the work, but later on, finding patient could not do typewriting, said he would have to interview three or four others first.

February 7.

    Boston University, Mr. Warren, seen at Mr. Jenkins' class for employment managers, Boston University. He told visitor that there was a strong probability that one of the professors at the University would take patient on for temporary work and that informant would get in touch with patient about this on February 9.

February 9.

    Patient telephoned and was advised to get in touch with Mr. Warren, Boston University, at once regarding the possible temporary opening.

February 9.

    Y. M. C. A. secretary, Mr. Doyle, telephoned that he has got in touch with Mr. Lambert of the Lambert Real Estate Company, who says he has not interviewed patient and could not find out who has. The opening is still there and Mr. Lambert would be glad to consider patient if he can do the work.

February 9.

    Boston University, Mr. Warren, telephoned to, who states that the temporary opening at Boston University has been taken by a "young fellow just out of high school." Informant would be perfectly willing to have patient consider the opening in Chelsea.

February 9.

    Patient written to, asking him to apply at Lambert's and telling him that the opening at Boston University had been filled.

February 9.

    Patient telephoned to in the evening, asking him to get in touch with Mr. Lambert to-morrow morning.

February 10.

    Patient telephoned that he interviewed Mr. Lambert this morning and is to begin work there to-morrow morning. Mr. Lambert asked patient very few personal questions and told patient there would be a couple of weeks' work. He asked patient whether he was looking around for better opportunities and patient said he was. Patient was afraid if he put his salary too high he would not get the job so he gave $25.00 as his price and Mr. Lambert said "All right, if I have to pay that, I will." Patient seems pleased that he has a definite opening and agreed to get in touch with

1920
visitor soon to let her know how he likes it. He agreed to let the various agencies to which he applied for work know that he is temporarily employed, but that he is still looking about for better opportunities.

February 11.
Johnston-Abbott Mills, Chief Inspector, Mr. Fabian, writes that he saw his employment manager, Mr. John Durand, on February 9, who says he is taking on men right along and advises that patient call at his office so that he may talk with him and find out for what work he is adapted. Lawrence is not an unattractive city for a factory worker and but few of the workers need to pay carfare.

February 11.
Johnston-Abbott Mills, Chief Inspector, Mr. Fabian, written to, stating that visitor would let him know in about two weeks what patient's plans are and suggesting that possibly at that time patient would be glad to see Mr. Durand.

February 14.
Patient's wife telephoned that patient asked her to let visitor know that he liked his work very much and that he is "feeling good" and says the work is "pretty easy." His hours are 9 to 5 and Saturdays until one. Emma is well now and expects to return to school on February 16. Dr. Sullivan said Emma had had a bilious attack which she occasionally has about a week. He has advised about Emma's diet, and of a number of things Emma will not eat, such as cereals, and she has just begun to drink milk. The doctor says that her enlarged tonsils should be removed soon. Visitor urged her to take Emma to a hospital O. P. D. soon to make an appointment for tonsillectomy, as otherwise it might be difficult to make one before summer. Informant agreed to do this. Patient's wife is well now. Her back bothered her for a few days as she had strained it by some heavy lifting. Informant agreed to ask patient to telephone visitor on February 16 at noon.

February 14.
International Optical Company, Lexington, Employment and Service Department, Miss Henderson, writes that patient's application and visitor's letter have been received. Informant hopes to be able to find some work for patient and will keep him in mind, letting him know if she has an opening which she thinks patient would like.

February 16.
Patient telephoned at noon. He likes his present work which he says "is easy enough," there being "nothing complicated" about it. His boss is the head bookkeeper, Mrs. Judson. When asked how he gets along with her he replied, "I can get along with anybody," and that he pretends he doesn't know anything and does things her way. He is catching up with past bookkeeping as far back as last July which has been poorly done by his predecessors. There seems to be no question of permanent work and he says he sees about ten days more ahead. He asked visitor to get in touch with Boston University again, and to look into openings recently advertised, one at the Federal Furniture Company, 356 Benton St., and the other at Dunton-Berry's.
His wife begins work to-night, intending to keep at it until he has a permanent job. For the present, patient feels that she is better off there

1920
than not working as it distracts her mind from somewhat strained relations with the landlady.

February 16.
Federal Furniture Company, 356 Benton St., telephoned to. The man who does the hiring stated that the firm is a credit house needing a book-keeper, but a younger man than patient, as all the office force is young. He added, "They do all the work I want them to."

February 16.
Dunton-Berry's Department Store telephoned to. The employment manager was out, but the head bookkeeper, Mr. Hathaway, stated that he has an opening for an assistant auditor at $35.00. Considerable bookkeep-ing experience and a man of much common sense is required. There are about 40 applicants and informant will have to decide on them soon. Patient should send in a formal application.

February 17.
Patient telephoned to and agreed to write Dunton-Berry's to-day re-garding the opening in the bookkeeping department.

February 19.
Patient written to, suggesting that he take a half day off to apply for clerical opening at Allison's and enclosing a letter of introduction to the office manager there.

February 24.
Patient's wife telephoned that patient would telephone visitor at noon. Informant would like to live in North Beverly as she has friends of her girlhood living there. If patient should work in Beverly he would first commute from Boston before the family moved. They are all well.

February 24.
Patient telephoned stating that he will ask for a day off to look into openings at the Allison Manufacturing Company and the Johnston-Abbott Shops. Visitor agreed to mail patient a letter of introduction to the Johnston-Abbott shops.
Patient is sure his present work is temporary, lasting only a few days more, as the head bookkeeper practically said that this morning. Patient's job has been to catch up with her past bookkeeping. She has been careless, has let things slide, and does not fully understand her work. She has not made a trial balance for the last eight months. Patient has liked the work, however, and has felt well except that he has not slept very well. He is sure that when he has a permanent job he will be O. K.

February 24.
Johnston-Abbott Shops, Chief Inspector, Mr. Doyle, written to, stating that patient would apply soon to Mr. Durand.

February 26.
Patient telephoned that as he has to take off an hour to-morrow morn-ing to complete a piano deal, he will not visit Lawrence and Beverly until March 1. Yesterday he arranged for his landlady to purchase a piano at the Hotel Bellingham as a result of an advertisement he saw in the paper.

1920
This deal will give patient $20 commission. Patient is not yet sure when the work will terminate but says it may any time.

February 27.
Boston University, Mr. Warren, seen at Mr. Jenkin's class for employment managers. He knows of no opening for patient and admits that patient's age is much against him. Apparently no opening can be expected from this source.

March 1.
Patient telephoned early in the afternoon that he had spent the morning in Beverly at the Allison Manufacturing Co., but due to the present difficulties in transportation, could not reach Lawrence the same day. It is too late, however, to return to his work in Chelsea to-day.

This morning he waited one hour and a half for the office manager, Mr. Van Horn, who told patient he would look over various clerical positions to see whether patient would fit in. As most of the bookkeeping is done by girls, there would be no opportunity at bookkeeping. He was well impressed by patient's desire to live in Beverly and be permanent with the firm. He asked patient what salary he would require and patient said he would start at $25 if there was every opportunity for advancement; Mr. Van Horn assured patient that no employee was hired at Allison's without the idea of promotion in mind, and that the firm would not consider paying patient less than $25.

Patient suggested that visitor write a letter to Mr. Van Horn, who had asked patient to get in touch with him in about a week or ten days if patient had not heard from him.

When patient announced that he was not reporting to work this morning, the head bookkeeper was quite afraid that patient was leaving and felt much relieved that his absence was only temporary. Patient feels that he has given her a number of valuable suggestions for her bookkeeping, and that there is still a number of days' work there for patient. Patient seldom sees Mr. Lambert and apparently is responsible only to the head bookkeeper.

Patient plans to visit Lawrence soon, but would prefer to live in Beverly as his summer camp would be so near by.

March 2.
Allison Manufacturing Company, Manager, Mr. Van Horn, written to, asking him to let visitor know what he decides about patient, and assuring him that patient is ready for responsible work.

March 6.
Johnston-Abbott Shops, Chief Inspector, Mr. Doyle, writes that he spoke to Mr. Durand about patient and hopes patient gets a good job there. Some of the jobs are good and some seem hard to informant.

March 8.
Patient telephoned that he has not heard from the Allison Mfg. Co.

March 9.
Patient written to, reassuring him about Allison's and urging him to go to the Johnston-Abbott Shops at once.

March 11.
Patient telephoned that he sees several weeks ahead of work where he **is,** and suggested visitor's writing to Allison's to-day. He was very dis-

1920

appointed not hearing from Allison's. He thinks they may be waiting for his letter to decide on his merits. He plans to install new bookkeeping methods where he is. He will write Beverly to-day and visit Lawrence soon.

March 12.

Patient telephoned that he is very discouraged, having received a letter yesterday from Allison's, stating that there are no openings now suitable for patient, but if there are later, they will let patient know. Patient feels that other men with only half his ability are getting jobs without difficulty. (Patient apologizes for his conceit.) He wonders whether knowledge that he has been at the Psychopathic Hospital on the part of employers has anything to do with it, as he feels Allison's was so enthusiastic when he saw them ten days ago. Visitor reminded him that Allison's knew of his relations with the hospital at the time. His wife is not interested in Lawrence as she knew so many people in Beverly. Patient will, however, go to Lawrence this morning. He is already in the North Station and has forgotten to take visitor's letter with him.

March 11.

Allison Mfg. Co., Office Manager, Mr. Van Horn, written to, asking why patient was not taken on.

March 15.

Patient telephoned that he was much disappointed with his visit in Lawrence. He waited a long time for Mr. Durand who had only night work as a machinist to offer patient. This patient refused though wages were not discussed. Patient asked for Mr. Doyle as head office man, who was not so identified, but patient was referred to Mrs. Mahoney in charge of the clerks figuring the payroll. She told patient she had only young girls and boys at $15 and $16. Later patient talked with the head book-keeper, Mr. Hinton, who said most of the bookkeeping was done in Boston. Patient was not impressed favorably by the place, as even the office looked dirty and the young employees complained of the poor pay.

On returning to Boston patient applied to the Federal Employment Office and asked to be kept on the list. In his last letter to Boston University patient asked to be kept on their lists and visitor agreed to remind Boston University of this.

Patient feels it very much easier for visitor to advise than for him to carry out the advice, but says he tells himself he must keep up his courage. He will continue to look around for permanent positions as will visitor also.

March 17.

Allison Mfg. Co., Office Manager, Mr. Van Horn, writes that he could not now employ patient "in whom we are mutually interested" as there are no openings in the accounting division and the bookkeeping is done entirely by women. Informant wrote patient recently stating that there was no position now to "capitalize his previous experience" but that he would be kept on the waiting list until the situation became better defined.

March 18.

Johnston-Abbott Shops, Chief Inspector, Mr. Doyle, written to, explaining that patient's interview with Mr. Durand was not very satisfactory to patient and asking informant to keep patient in mind should any suitable openings appear soon.

1920
March 25.

Patient telephoned to ask visitor if there was any news regarding future openings. April 1 he plans to balance the books at Lambert's and says there may be more work there after that. When his work is finished there, he plans to go to the country a day or two, and will stop off via Allison's on his return home. "What's worth having is worth going after." He will tell Mr. Van Horn at Allison's that he will gladly start in anywhere in the firm. Patient inquired for Mr. Warren at Boston University. Patient has done nothing about membership in the Y. M. C. A. because unsettled as to location. He plans to drop his membership in the Elks which he never enjoyed and which costs him $12 annually. He feels it too expensive to play with the Elks. In two or three weeks he plans to go weekends to his camp.

March 26.

Boston University, Vocational Department, Mr. Warren, visited. Informant had an opening at the B. D. Cole Leather Company, 80 North Street, where Mr. Kelsey is looking for a bookkeeper at $25. Informant has sent over about six candidates, none of whom were accepted. One at $25 was too inexperienced and one at $30 was too expensive, but informant does not know what the drawback was with the others. If patient applies he can say he heard of the opening through Boston University.

March 26.

Patient written to, advising him to look into the opening at the B. D. Cole Leather Company at once and report back to visitor.

April 1.

Y. M. C. A., Mr. Doyle, telephoned to, who stated that he could quite easily find out from patient's employer how satisfactory his work is, and that he will make such inquiries soon.

April 1.

Boston University, Vocational Department, Mr. Warren, telephoned to, who stated that it was more to the point for visitor to telephone the B. D. Cole Leather Company than for informant as visitor knew patient so much better. Visitor agreed to do so.

April 1.

Patient writes that he has made several unsuccessful attempts to telephone visitor. On March 29 he called on Mr. Kelsey at the B. D. Cole Company who was very busy and talked with patient but a few minutes. Patient says "he was rather favorably impressed with me and gave me an application blank to fill out." Mr. Kelsey did not explain the position in detail. Patient thinks firm is "a very nice one" to work for. Patient thinks if Mr. Warren of B. U. would telephone Mr. Kelsey it might help to get him the position.

April 1.

B. D. Cole Leather Company, 80 North Street, Bookkeeping Dept., Mr. Kelsey, visited at 11 A. M.

Impression: Keen business man, human interest probably secondary to business.

Informant asked visitor her interest in patient. He is considering patient among two or three other candidates, but said patient did not im-

1920

press him very favorably. He would not explain this further than to say he felt patient might leave for the liquor business at any time prohibition took a turn and that informant preferred a younger candidate. In favor of patient he spoke of his neat handwriting. It is difficult now to get good material as bookkeepers though plenty of poor help is available. The position is for a man to work in as understudy to the head bookkeeper. His work would be to connect up between the factory and the office and the candidate would have to learn both the factory and office bookkeeping methods as well as have eight or nine men under him. Informant agreed to send for patient if he decided to consider him.

April 1.
Federal Employment Office, 4 Cherry St., visited. There is no opening for patient.

April 2.
Patient written to, explaining the result of the visit to the B. D. Cole Leather Company and advising patient not to expect the opening there though he can keep it in the back of his mind. Letter advised patient to visit Allison's soon with regard to future employment.

April 6.
Patient telephoned his wife is a little discouraged about his not having steady work but she does not say much. Patient will telephone Mr. Kelsey of the B. D. Cole Leather Company to-morrow to see if there are any chances there and will write Allison's that he plans to visit on April 12. Patient's wife has intended to make an appointment at the Children's Hospital for the removal of Emma's tonsils and patient will urge her to do so soon.

April 7.
Federal Employment Office, 4 Cherry Street, Mr. Brown, visited, who has no openings for patient as a bookkeeper. Prospects in this line have not improved.

April 8.
Allison Mfg. Co., Office Manager, Mr. Van Horn, written to, explaining that patient would visit on April 12 and that he would be willing to start in at any time in any line there, as he was especially interested in the firm because of its promise of advancement. Letter asked that informant put patient in touch with the employment department if informant had no openings himself.

April 8.
Patient written to, explaining that visitor was writing Allison's.

April 9.
Y. M. C. A., Mr. Doyle, telephoned, stating that patient has adapted himself very well to conditions, according to patient's employer, and has helped tide over the situation very well. Patient's work there will soon be finished and informant will keep patient in mind for a similar opening.

April 12.
Patient reported to visitor at 11:30, stating that his plans had been changed somewhat. In yesterday's *Globe* he saw an advertisement for

1920
various types of help at the Standard Drug Company, among them accountants and bookkeepers. He decided therefore to apply there the first thing in the morning, and waited with a "seething mob" from 8 A. M. until 10:30 before he was seen. The employment manager had him fill out an application blank and then told patient that undoubtedly they could fit him into the organization and that the man patient should see would not be in until to-morrow. The employment manager said he would look up patient's references in the' meantime. Patient put down as his minimum salary $27.50 per week. Patient seemed quite enthusiastic over the interview there. He plans to go at once to apply at Allison's this afternoon. He spent the week-end on his little farm and his farmer friend Henry told patient of an opening at $4 a day to clear the woods on the estate of the millionaire, Henderson, near Lexington, which would last until the summer. If no definite opening materializes in a week when patient expects the position at Lambert's to end, patient will take this job in the woods, as he does not want to be idle at all especially considering the high cost of living. Patient's wife cleaned up at the camp preparatory to living there for the summer. The family expect to go to camp again next week-end when patient will do his plowing. Patient says he feels pretty well but still sleeps only fairly well, waking up early and then only dozing for the rest of the morning.

Patient is sure his present employer will give him a good reference and when patient recently called up Mr. Stratton of the Stratton Piano Company relative to the sale of a piano, patient was reassured by Mr. Stratton that he would give patient a good reference at any time. Patient stated that it was difficult to reach visitor by telephone especially since there is no booth in his office. He will, however, let visitor know the results of his applications at Allison's and the Standard Drug Company. He telephoned the B. D. Cole Leather Company a few days ago and Mr. Kelsey said he had filled the position that morning. Patient then asked Mr. Kelsey why patient had not been selected, adding that perhaps patient was asking state secrets. Mr. Kelsey did say it was not because of patient's age but would give no further reply. Visitor agreed with patient that the position at clearing the woods would be good in case no further opening was at hand as patient said he would feel free to leave it at any time.

April 20.
  Patient's former employer, Lambert Real Estate Co., telephoned to. Patient left there on April 17. The clerk volunteered that patient had done very good work and that they thought he was going to work at Allison's and live at his camp.

April 20.
  Patient's wife telephoned to. Patient went out to Lexington to-day to look up Allison's and will be home to-night. Visitor left word for patient to write at once or telephone regarding his work plans. Further details could not be discussed over the telephone.

April 22.
  Patient's wife telephoned. A week ago patient was told at Allison's to report April 20 as the firm thought they could then place him in the stockroom. He planned to return home the evening of April 20 for his work clothes if put to work, but nothing has been heard from him. It is probably about a half hour's ride from his camp to Allison's, from which he planned to commute. Informant's plans will depend upon how well

1920

patient likes Allison's if he is working there. She will try to get news of patient for visitor as soon as possible.

April 26.

Patient reported to visitor, stating that he is well and busy, but that he still has vague fears at times, which he, however, has been able to control. His wife is still working, and his wife's sister is still helping somewhat financially. For example, she visited patient's camp last week-end, bringing out a good supply of food, and paying patient's son's transportation. Patient hopes to pay her back later.

Patient asked visitor's advice about his work. The last two times he applied at Allison's, word was sent to him from Mr. Van Horn that he was too busy to see patient, and that he should report back in a week. Patient wondered therefore if that was the real explanation or whether the firm has no interest in patient.

The Standard Drug Company, where he reported again to-day, said that patient's name is on the waiting list. They have selected no clerks or bookkeepers as yet, this being up to the department heads.

Mr. Lambert has sent for patient, asking patient what salary he would require to do the work he did temporarily as a permanent job. The present bookkeeper has already become nervous on the job since patient left, because she finds it beyond her ability to keep the books straight. Patient stated $35 as his salary and said to visitor if no other opening was available, he would take it, but he feels it is a "nerve-racking" job. The employer keeps one book where three are really necessary, hence making the bookkeeping complicated. Three books, though simpler, would entail extra work which the employer is unwilling to pay for. Complications come in through the fact that there are really three different funds to account for and the employer is constantly borrowing from one fund for another. If patient took the job, he fears he would need to start on overtime, but visitor firmly said he could not do this, and if overtime is necessary must have assistants. The present bookkeeper Mr. Lambert plans to shift into other work in the office. Patient wonders how she would feel toward patient's keeping her position. He suggested to Mr. Lambert that both Mr. Lambert and the insurance man spend too much time in the office, and that if patient took the position he thought he could undertake some of their office work, such as answering general questions about real estate, and making appointments for interested parties with his employer. Mr. Lambert will decide by noon of April 28 whether he can pay patient the salary of $35 or not.

Patient would prefer working for some large firm such as Allison's, as he feels a smaller firm can offer only a less secure job. After visitor's telephoning Allison's, patient agreed to get in touch with visitor late to-morrow morning.

April 26.

Allison Mfg. Company, Lexington, Office Manager, Mr. Van Horn, telephoned to, and stated that patient had reported the situation correctly to visitor, and that informant is very sorry he has been too busy to spend the hour required to see whether patient would fit into the stockroom. He is not willing to have patient take another position without informant's looking into the possibilities at Allison's, however. Informant agreed to telephone visitor to-morrow at 4 o'clock what the situation is.

April 27.

Patient telephoned late in the afternoon, and agreed to do so again to-morrow morning as Allison's had not been heard from.

1920
April 28.

Allison Mfg. Co., Lexington, Office Manager, Mr. Van Horn, telephoned to at 10:30 A. M. Informant apologized for not telephoning visitor yesterday. He had the memorandum on his desk and had done the preliminary work; namely, to see where patient would fit in.

At present there is no clerical opening for patient, but he can definitely be taken on in the stockroom giving out orders. This work is largely physical and is paid at an hourly rate, where patient would earn about $20 a week. Holidays and Sundays as well as vacations are not paid for. Informant would keep patient in mind while he worked in the stockroom for advancement to clerical work either in the stockroom or elsewhere. They are hard pressed now in the stockroom for clerical help but informant has not been able to "sell" patient to them for clerical work because of his age. Informant is confident, however, that clerical work will develop for patient later when his abilities are recognized in spite of his years.

Visitor stated that unless she notified informant to the contrary, patient would report to him on April 30. Informant said that at that time he would introduce patient to the employment department and arrange for patient to begin work on May 3. At first informant suggested that if patient had a good opening at Lambert's, he had better take it, but when visitor spoke of patient's fear of only temporary work there, informant admitted that at Allison's permanency could be expected.

April 28.

Patient telephoned and seemed somewhat depressed at the salary offered to start with at Allison's. Visitor reminded him that he could hardly have a better person than Mr. Van Horn interested in him, and pointed out the advantageous features of Allison's. Patient will telephone Lambert's about 12:30 to-day and will telephone visitor to-morrow morning. Patient himself will be allowed time by Lambert's to make a decision. Visitor told patient it was up to him to make the final decision.

April 29.

Patient telephoned, much discouraged. Mr. Lambert had telephoned to patient's brother-in-law in patient's absence yesterday that he could not meet patient's figure. Patient feels Allison's should offer him more as a starting figure (in fact, Mr. Van Horn told him he could expect a minimum of $25), and that the promise of advancement there is not definite enough. He is wondering whether he should telephone Mr. Lambert, but finally decided he would later. As Mr. Lambert had said he would be willing to pay $1,000 more a year, patient does not understand why he is "balking at $35 a week." He thinks all there is for him to do is to make the rounds of the employment offices. Visitor tried to assure him that the hardest part of his task was surely finished; namely, that he had gone the rounds of the employment offices and now had a good employer interested in him and that he could hardly hope to find a better firm than Allison's.

Visitor suggested that patient come out to talk with Dr. Jacobs. He first said he would gain nothing, and spoke in the tone of a spoiled child. When visitor reminded him that Dr. Jacobs was the doctor to sanction responsible work for him, he admitted he could lose nothing by coming out to see Dr. Jacobs and would do so.

April 29.

Patient reported at 3 P. M. to see Dr. Jacobs. Visitor first discussed the case with Dr. Jacobs, who felt that patient could rightly be discouraged

1920
with an offer of only $20 a week. After seeing patient, the doctor reported to visitor that patient is in very good condition, apparently now having full control of any fears. He is a typical psychasthenic, being introspective, overconscientious, hesitant about making decisions, and lacking self-confidence. Dr. Jacobs says patient's present problem to decide would be hard for a normal healthy person, and that if patient were not somewhat worried over prospects, considering his age, his judgment could be questioned. He told patient that he did not know the merits of the Allison opening, but that it likely was a good proposition for the summer at least.

Patient reported to visitor that he could get Dr. Jacobs' point of view; namely, that he must use "mental suggestions" to himself, but that it was harder to carry out than others realized. He will go to Allison's to-morrow morning and look into the situation for himself. If the promise of advancement is definite enough, he will take the position. He will write visitor to-morrow evening before going to camp for the week-end. He feels considerably worried about the support of his family as he hates to have his wife working, or his relatives assisting.

He telephoned Mr. Lambert this morning but found him out, but does not plan to telephone again as patient says "I have forgotten all about that place now," evidently considering the deal closed there.

May 3.
    Patient writes that he is to start in at the Allison Company on May 3, beginning in the stockroom, stating that "Mr. Van Horn promises to see that I get proper advancement if deserving of it."

May 3.
    Patient written to, stating that visitor feels he has made a wise choice, expressing the need of recreation, and asking him to report frequently regarding the progress of his work.

CASE 94

PSYCHOPATHIC HOSPITAL

SOCIAL SERVICE

NUMBERS 562

FILE NUMBER 5720   NAME   Harriet Nelson Farmer *

O. P. D. NUMBER 3838

RESIDENCE   44 Stevens St., Roxbury.

CORRESPONDENT   Mother, Frances Ordway Farmer, at above address.

SEX F	AGE 28 COLOR W
CIVIL CONDITION S	PLACE AND DATE OF BIRTH England,
RELIGION Protestant	1887
	OCCUPATION Compositor (typesetter)
TIME IN BOSTON 22 yrs.	IN MASS. 22 yrs. IN U. S. 22 yrs.

PREVIOUS ADDRESSES

    107 Downing Street, Boston

    63 Revere Street, Boston

WHEN KNOWN TO SOCIAL SERVICE   11/30/15; 3/12/18; 6/9/19

WHEN DISCHARGED FROM SOCIAL SERVICE   12/31/17; 4/24/18

REASON FOR BEING KNOWN TO SOCIAL SERVICE   Supervision

REPORT FROM CONFIDENTIAL EXCHANGE   No record

NAME OF FATHER   Henry (deceased)

ADDRESS

NAME OF MOTHER   Frances

ADDRESS   44 Stevens St., Roxbury

NAME OF SPOUSE

ADDRESS

NAMES AND AGES OF CHILDREN OR SIBLINGS

    Frederick (died in infancy)

    Florence, 34

    Benjamin, 32

    Bernard, 30

    Patient, 28

ADMITTED TO HOUSE 10/31/15	AUTHORITY CHAP. 174
DISCHARGED 12/8/15	ADMITTED TO O. P. D. 1/19/16
DIAGNOSIS	CONDITION Unchanged
Not insane—not feeble-minded	
(Psychopathic Personality)	
SOCIAL SYMPTOMS	DATE 3/1/16
Inebriety	
Fabrication	
Lying	
Suicidal attempt	
Non-support of mother	
Insufficient wage	
Friendlessness	
SOCIAL DIAGNOSIS	DATE 3/1/16

VITIA (Bad Habits) + Morbi (Disease)

    * All names used in this record are fictitious.

PSYCHOPATHIC HOSPITAL
SOCIAL SERVICE

NO. S-562   NAME   Harriet Nelson Farmer

ADDRESSES

Patient:
 Gordon Home,
 55 Dix Street.
Relatives:
 Mother, Mrs. Frances Ordway Farmer,
 44 Stevens St., Roxbury.

 Sister, Florence Farmer,
 44 Stevens St., Roxbury.

 Employer, Miss Nancy Stowell, Charles St.

 Brother, Benjamin Farmer,
 Newton St., Nashua, N. H.

 Brother, Bernard Farmer,
 Dover, Mass.

 Minister, Mr. Young, Channing Church,
 Day St., Roxbury.
 Residence, York St., Roxbury.

PSYCHOPATHIC HOSPITAL
SOCIAL SERVICE

NO. S-562   NAME   Harriet Nelson Farmer

EXPENSE SHEET

Expenditures

12/24/15	Tie for Christmas...$	.25
1/26/15	Material for sewing (for another patient)	1.29
2/19/16	Theater tickets	1.50
4/5/16	Theater tickets	1.00
4/6/16	Bath spray..........	.59
4/8/16	Out-of-work pay	.50

$5.13

PSYCHOPATHIC HOSPITAL
SOCIAL SERVICE

NO. S-562   NAME Harriet Nelson Farmer
SUMMARY

1916
January 30.
Social History:
   Patient is an English woman of 28, who has lived in the United States
22 years; in Boston 22 years. She has a sister, aged 34, and two brothers,
32 and 30 years of age. Patient was eight years old when her mother
separated from her father because he was found to be maintaining another
wife and family in the city. Children were boarded about a year by a
children's agency until the mother, who was and still is an invalid, gained
strength to reëstablish the home. Family were then supported by two
older children. Several years ago both brothers married and left patient
and sister to support the mother. In April, 1914, the mother was unable
to keep up her housework and the home was broken up. Patient lived in
lodging houses in the West End and sister and mother with a married
brother. A year later, April, 1915, patient was asked by mother and sister
to keep house with them, but she refused to go home to live until June,
1915, when she was unable to support herself on her low wages. Financial
struggle of the family has always been great. Patient did not contribute
after leaving home and only $2 a week when she returned.
   The mother is a frail woman, able to get about only on crutches. She
is religious, generous, and open-hearted. The sister has worked in the
same dressmaking establishment for many years. She is an earnest, upright, and matter-of-fact woman of excellent character. The older brother
who lives in Nashua has a wife and two young boys. The brother in
Dover has a wife and a daughter aged 1½. He is a machinist and irregularly employed. Several years ago he was discharged from one firm
for attempting to steal money from the safe. The family are all willing to
do whatever they can for patient and the mother especially is fond of her.
They are discouraged about her. They reprove her little and allow her to
have her own way because they are afraid of her tales of abuse.
   The mother and sister have two rooms, a bath and a kitchen in a
house on a pleasant, quiet residence street of Dorchester.
   Patient went to school in Boston through the grammar grades.
   Up to a year ago patient had been a typesetter in the same place for
eleven years and earned $12 a week. Since then she has worked in two
candy factories for $5 a week. Previously she worked in an office and a
laundry, a short time in each. Patient has about $50 savings.
   She is an ardent Episcopalian, though she was brought up a Unitarian.
   When the home was first broken up, a woman prominent in the Boston
school department was interested in the family and became guardian to

1916
the children. For the past two years St. James Church with the aid of York House has tried to supervise and guide patient.

Physical History:
Patient had normal birth and development, with exception of walking a little late. She had measles in childhood, diphtheria at five, and several attacks of appendicitis (no operation). Patient wears glasses. She has some headaches. Her teeth are in bad condition. She is subject to neuralgia. Examination here shows a poorly nourished condition. Question of anemia. Wassermann test, blood serum negative.

In appearance, she is short and slight, and is usually pale. She is the wiry type with normal endurance.

Father died in Westboro State Hospital of general paralysis. Mother is an invalid and has had spinal curvature from childhood. About twenty years ago she was treated for syphilis contracted from patient's father. Heredity otherwise negative or unknown.

Mental History:
Patient was an average scholar. She reads much good literature, *Les Miserables* and other classics. For the past two years patient has been excessively alcoholic, drinking alone in her own room and going several times to priest, or York House workers, under the influence of liquor. She has been untruthful and unreliable, telling many things about mistreatment by her family which have no basis in fact. She has told scandalous stories about the Episcopal priest to whom she confessed and about the other church members. She has fabricated stories of attentions of men. For a time, an unattractive young man paid her attention, but he soon let her alone. Patient talks constantly and is aggressive toward people with whom she comes in contact. Girls in church club would not come if she were to be there. She is lazy, slovenly, and thoughtless. At home, she leaves all the housework to her mother and sister, and expects them to sew and wash for her as well. She stays in bed late. Patient and sister are uncongenial, but patient is fond of mother. She is depressed at menstrual periods.

A short time before admission, she had put her name and address into a package of peanuts while working in a candy factory. As a result, she entered into correspondence with a man in Springfield whom she decided to marry. He turned out to be 65. Patient showed much disappointment at the outcome of this affair.

Patient was sent to this hospital after an attempt at suicide. On this day, nothing unusual had been noticed in patient's behavior. She had never threatened suicide, and had not shown great depression. After going to town that morning, she lunched with her mother, who then went to her room to rest. A few hours later the mother was notified that patient had taken Paris green, and had gone immediately to a doctor's office. She was taken to the City Hospital, and from there was sent here for observation. Patient said she had bought the Paris green for an insecticide and took it because she felt discouraged with her own life and her mother's physical condition.

In typesetting patient was fair, but was considered physically not fitted for the work. She was laid off from monotype with the introduction of more linotype machinery.

In other places of employment she was liked and considered good. Each place she left for a better place.

Examination here shows her to grade 15 years plus on the Point Scale and 12⅕ years on the Binet.

1916

Diagnosis: Not Insane—Not Feeble-minded (Psychopathic Personality).

November 30.

Recommendations in regard to:

Social Condition: Patient should be kept away from her own home except for visits. Her family should be made to understand and tolerate her peculiarities.

Keep her supplied with interesting handwork. Send to theater occasionally and try to have her be with girls her own age through living with them and through church clubs.

Next season try to arrange for night high school or some industrial class. Suggest books and keep patient supplied with list of free lectures.

Physical Condition: Regularity of meals and a proper diet should be arranged. Encourage daily bathing.

Further medical care at a general hospital (? of anemia) is recommended. Teeth should be filled.

Mental Condition: Encourage and commend patient in all her efforts. Congenial work should be found and signs of mental or physical fatigue watched for.

Patient should report to Out-Patient Department monthly in the beginning. Special attention should be given to any depression lest it lead to drinking. Patient's complaints and difficulties with family should be minimized and her friendly attitude maintained.

SUMMARY OF RESULTS IN SIX MONTHS

April 5.

Social:

Since leaving the hospital, patient has lived at the Gordon House in a double room. Every Saturday afternoon and Sunday she has spent at home and last two months she has been staying over night. Occasionally she has spent the day at her brother's in Dover. For two months she has been giving her mother 50 cents or $1 weekly. She takes her dainties often. She has put about $10 in the bank.

From December 28 to March 11 patient worked at piece work in a factory where the work was irregular and where she could earn a maximum of about $7.50 a week. On March 11 patient started time work in another factory where she pasted labels and packed bottles for $6 a week with advance in wage later. This work was uncongenial to her and on April 24 she found a position in her old trade of typesetting at $8.

Evenings patient stays in, usually either reading or sewing. She has been with her sister to a church entertainment, to the theater, and some public meetings. Occasionally she goes to the Settlement House forum meetings.

In the House the girls like her and come into her room evenings. They have spreads and very jolly times. In February her roommate, a blind girl to whom she was devoted, left, and she had a young Polish girl until May, when she has been alone. At work, she has made some girl friends.

1916
    In January patient joined her people's Unitarian Church, but she has attended only comparatively few times. She went to the Episcopal Church fairly regularly for four months without telling her family, but now goes less often.

Physical:
    On discharge, patient was referred to the Massachusetts General Hospital with a question of anemia. She was in the hospital from December 13 to 17 and was found to be not anemic. She has had her teeth cleaned and some fillings done at the Harvard Dental School at times when she has been out of work. She has reported monthly to the Out-Patient Department.
    Patient eats two meals at the House, and usually fruit and cocoa at night. Luncheon she takes with her to work.
    Patient walked to and from work a distance of about three miles in her first two places. Now she walks occasionally though it is about five miles. At present work she sits on a high stool, but stands from choice some of the time. She goes to bed early, particularly when work has been physically fatiguing. A bath spray has facilitated daily bathing.
    Patient had difficulty with menstruation and has been to consult Dr. Green, a woman physician at the hospital, about it.

Mental:
    There has been no evidence of patient's telling lies or elaborate fabrications. She exaggerates her own good efforts in everything she does and gives accounts of her excellent conduct. There has been no open conflict between her sister and herself. Patient has not been drinking, nor has she mentioned suicide.
    She has appeared to be happy and fairly contented except for her desire to stay at home over Saturday nights. This had not been allowed for several months because patient would stay in bed late and impose on the family. Her mother's invalidism worries her and often she gets discouraged or sad over it.
    Her last roommate was a rather stupid and ill-mannered girl and patient took much pleasure in training her manners and habits.
    Patient has shown herself to be very generous. She was glad to make two garments for another patient known to visitor and she has made several presents for visitor. She is good with handwork of all sorts and enjoys spending her time this way.
    When discouraged and blue she had two long talks with the Chief of Staff.
HA/C

PSYCHOPATHIC HOSPITAL

SOCIAL SERVICE

NO. S-562   NAME Harriet Nelson Farmer

HISTORY

1915
December 3.
    Patient's story: Patient gives following places of employment:
    1. T. S. Davis, 180 Young St., office work. Left for better wages.
    2. One year 1904-5—Charter Hill Laundry. Laundry work. (Place burned.) Left because work was too hard.

1915

3. Nine years to November, 1914—Sampson Press. Left with introduction of a new machine requiring fewer girls.

4. December, 1914—G. I. Eaves, candy work. Left because rush season was over.

5. February, 1914–October, 1915—Tyson Brand Co., Cross St., Cambridge, packing. Left because employees were rough and wages low. $5.50 a week.

Schools were as follows:

1. James B. Baker School (Grammar School), finished 1904.
2. East Boston High School (night), 1905.
3. Dixon's Commercial School (night), 1905, complete course.

Patient has always lived with her family until August, 1914, when they broke up because of mother's ill health. She has a married brother, Arthur, aged 32, living on Newton St., Nashua, N. H. Of his wife patient is fond and feels at home there. He has two boys. Another brother, Bernard, is married and has one girl and lives in Dover. Patient does not know his wife well nor feel at home with her. They have asked her to come and stay there when she leaves here, but she is anxious to go to work. "I think I might go insane if I stay out of work much longer." Patient and her sister Florence are not congenial. Sister is "older and more set in her ways" into which she tries to draw patient. Sister goes out and takes an interest in suffrage and such things while patient prefers to be at home and quiet.

Since family broke up housekeeping patient has lived in lodging houses, first at 107 Downing St. Room was $3 and when she took a $2.50 one in the same house it was ill-kept and had bugs and vermin. On September 18, 1914, she moved to 63 Revere St., where she stayed until June, 1915. At that time she returned to her family (mother and sister) who started to keep house.

Patient's family are Unitarians. She was confirmed in Christ Church, East Boston. The minister there, Rev. Y. K. Elden, has since left, but she keeps in close touch by correspondence with Mrs. Elden. Patient has been going to St. James Church, Cambridge St., for a little over a year. Confessions she has made to Father Cramer and had confidence in him until lately. When she confessed drinking he sent her to see Miss Kendall at York House, but patient did not feel she could enter there. She has seen Miss Kendall a good deal and trusted her. Has since heard that Miss Kendall said she was "mentally deranged" and this has hurt patient's feelings. Father Cramer told her she must do exactly as he said if he was to help her, but patient was unwilling to do this. At one time Father Cramer sent an immoral girl of 16 to her for advice. Patient thinks he must have had confidence in her to do such a thing. Lately, however, he has promised to see her, and has not done so, and said he went to Roxbury and found no one home, when in reality he saw her mother and upset her terribly. Her confession he used in his sermon. After the latter incident, she made up a lot of things to confess just to see whether he would tell them, and he did. Patient will discontinue connection with this church. She feels she ought to go to the Unitarian Church because Mr. Young, the pastor, is taking an interest in her and offering to help. She cannot believe their doctrines nor be satisfied with the service.

Patient goes out about two nights a week. The other nights she goes to bed 8 or earlier. She gets up about 6. Always she sleeps well and has a normal appetite. When she had a room, she cooked her own meals there, and on Sundays, when she went to see her mother at her brother's, they filled a travelling bag with home-cooked things for her. From August,

1915
1914, to May, 1915, patient took a glass of port wine ($1 a quart) a day to brace herself. She took raw eggs also. She found the wine made her nervous so she stopped it. Had one glass a few days before admission. She has no desire for it.

Patient averaged two books a week as well as all the books for which she set up type. She reads good books, naming as examples *Last Days of Pompeii* and Gilbert Parker's novels. She owns a number. Embroidery she likes to do and makes all her own clothes, mostly by hand, and trims her hats.

She likes to be alone and has never made any girl friends with the exception of Miss Kendall of York House. For six months in 1914 she knew Karl Cauldwell and was engaged to him, but he left town and wrote he would not see her again. Afterward, she found out he was not a good sort so has not cared that he went away. She had the friendship of Frank Illington, who in September, 1914, went away to study for Roman Catholic priesthood. He left his books to her. He was a fine, good young man. At one time patient belonged to the Girls' Friendly Society but dropped out because the meetings ceased to interest her. She never mixed with girls at St. James Church because she thought them two-faced. She would like industrial classes where work with the hands is done, but she does not care for dancing or exercise. Says she is a good girl.

Patient does not want to live away from home, but realizes it is better since she worries too much over her mother's suffering. She would want to go home every week.
HA/C

December 2.
Employer, Mr. D. I. Stern, Supt. of Sampson Press, seen at Cambridge St., Dorchester. No exact record kept of patient, but informant remembered her well. He had always taken an interest in her because he felt that she was delicate and that she was not suited to factory work. Exact dates of employment not kept. Informant thought she had been there for about five or six years. She was a compositor and set up and also corrected type. For the first few years she was in piece work and may have been paid from $7 to $17 per week, depending upon her speed. Later that system was abolished and for about a year she was a "weekly worker," and received $12 per week. The hours are from 7:20 to 5 with an hour for luncheon and every Saturday afternoon off. Patient was quite intermittent in her work. No record was kept of that either. Patient worked in a large, light, well-ventilated, clean room with about 75 other workers, men and women. The visitor saw this room and the processes used by the patient. There is no heavy lifting in the work. The patient selected type and arranged it in "sticks," these in turn being placed in a long pan. After the proof had been read it was returned to her. She then corrected any mistakes in setting up the type. Each worker sits on a high stool in front of a slanting desk arrangement on which the type is deposited. The only element of strain seemed to be that of remaining seated most of the time. A fair degree of skill is required in composition. The worker must have a good knowledge of the English language and be able to spell and punctuate fairly accurately. Patient was a fair worker, but "not distinguished" in speed or accuracy. She reached "about the middle mark" in efficiency. The informant thought her chief fault "lack of pep and steam." He said she did not seem to have physical energy. She was fairly attentive to her work and was not "a gad-about."

At the time when the piece-work system was abandoned a great many girls were dropped. In the natural course of events patient would also

1915
have been dropped because she was not particularly valuable, but when she told him that there was financial trouble at home and that "it was up to her" he let her stay on as a weekly worker. He felt that the work was too great a strain upon her and told her that she ought to get some kind of work in a private family and some place where she could be out of doors. She looked anemic. Informant heard that there was one member of the family who caused a lot of trouble and in addition there was illness. Patient was often out because of sickness.

She was always quiet and tractable, but if anything annoyed her she "got up and acted like a normal person." Informant thought that she was very proud and that she would take all trouble on her own shoulders and never give way under it. At one time she gave all the financial assistance that was given to her family. Her eyesight was poor and she had occasional treatment for it. Patient's work showed no deterioration. Patient resigned to take another kind of position. Informant would not care to take her back because she was not suited to the work, and was not particularly efficient.

Informant confirmed his own memory by talking with Mr. Quinn, patient's foreman, who gave a very similar report.

Impression: Unusually intelligent and understanding man, obviously interested in the welfare of his employees.
MBS/C

December 3.
Teacher, Miss Neide, seen at James B. Baker School, Roxbury. She did not have patient, but had had her brother, Benjamin, in her class. On her recommendation, Miss Neide's brothers, "The Three Neides," took Benjamin to work in their confectionery concern. He was there several years and it was finally discovered that he had been taking supplies for some time. He stole from the safe the last thing. The queer part was that he seemed to have no sense of the wrong of it. They all thought he might be "not responsible."
HA/C

York House Matron, Miss Kendall, who has known patient about two years, seen. Patient has been to her, to Miss Hunt, another matron, often. She has never had a sensible conversation with patient. She is most erratic, talks at great length about the men she intends to marry, or about injuries which various people have done her. Nothing that she says can be relied upon for she tells a different story to everyone. For example, she told Miss Kendall not to see her mother, because mother is a Unitarian. Mother was very cordial to Miss Kendall. She is very bold and boastful about her drinking. Has said she drank as much as two quarts of port wine in one night. She usually drinks alone. Has been seen under the influence of liquor though not actually drunk. She seldom takes anything without immediately going to one of the priests of St. James' about it.

Patient told the story of her father having contracted syphilis and having died in Westboro State Hospital. One maternal aunt was insane. Father disappeared at one time for several weeks. When he returned he gave mother syphilis. She soon found he had a wife and five children by the name of Farmers, living in the West End. Mother is now suffering from syphilis and tuberculosis. After death of father, patient and brothers and sisters were placed in home, patient going to Home for Orphan Children. Miss Kendall has not had the opportunity to verify these stories.

Patient has said a good deal about having men in her room and Miss Kendall has thought her to be immoral. Karl Cauldwell was a diseased-looking man; his face was covered with sores.

1915

In packing peanuts, patient put her name into a package. In September she had a letter from a man in Springfield who had bought the peanuts. She corresponded several weeks with him and then told Miss Kendall she wanted to marry him. Associated Charities in Springfield found he was about 60 and had a wife and children, and was somewhat "off" on the subject of women. Patient saw this letter from the Associated Charities a few days before she took poison. She had often said before that she would do so, but in an offhand way.

At home patient is troublesome. She stays out very late several nights a week and is quarrelsome.

HA/C

December 4.

Guardian, Miss George, of Public Schools, high school teacher, says she was made guardian of patient and other children when father died. She has known the family 25 years. When they first came to her attention through the children at school, they were underfed and it was found the family had been living on stale bread and water for several days.

Patient has never been a help to her family in a financial nor any other way. She should not go home now because she is too great a care and worry to her mother and sister. Mother has been sick all of 25 years Miss George has known her.

Patient graduated from grammar school at 17. Was a scholar below average.

HA/C

December 4.

Father Superior and Father Cramer of St. James' Church (Episcopal) seen. Patient has been known to them about two years, and was at that time drinking heavily. She has never been seen when she was unable to walk, but oftentimes was markedly under the influence of liquor and very unsteady on her feet. She has denied immoral sex conduct and they have no reason to believe she has been immoral. She has a "diabolical" and malicious way of starting and spreading scandal. She will tell one tale to one person and another to some one else. Among the parishioners, she is talkative and always ready to make friends. She is not bold. The girls of the church will have nothing to do with her because of her conduct, and have completely frozen her out. If she came to meetings, they would not.

The priests feel that sex is the basis of the whole matter. If she had married when younger she probably would have been comparatively normal. At one time last winter, Karl Cauldwell kept company with her and they were engaged. He was an uninteresting, somewhat slow young man, but not objectionable or bad. During the time patient kept company, she was a normal individual. He soon discovered what she was like and disappeared. Patient has been much worse since that, in February, 1915. Otherwise, her conduct has not shown any fluctuations.

Patient has taken her transfer letter from the church so is no longer a member of their parish.

Impressions: Father Cramer is a young man, probably looks younger than his years.

Father Superior did most of the talking and gave general statements chiefly. Interview was in the church, where the two fathers were on duty for hearing confessions.

HA/C

1915
December 6.
Landlady seen at 63 Revere St. Patient roomed there as stated and was recommended by Frank Illington. She had not known patient drank, until after patient had gone and Mr. Illington returned. He mentioned it and she then remembered smelling liquor on patient's breath once. In the beginning she was friendly with some church girls, but later had a falling out and asked landlady not to let them go to her room. Patient never made friends with other lodgers. "There are twelve rooms, two or three let to middle-aged men, and most rooms let for many years to same persons." Landlady never heard of her going out with men nor did she observe her coming home with any. She never had any in her room. Patient was out after twelve some nights when she went home and also she always went home on Saturday for Sunday. Other nights patient stayed home and sewed. She does this well.

Patient was a good lodger and always paid her rent ($2 a week) promptly and made no trouble. Landlady would not take her back now she knows she drinks. She had thought her queer because she talked so much, mostly about her disagreements with church people.

Landlady and her husband, old people, have lived in this place for years and have good old furniture and china and very homelike rooms of their own.

Impression: Unusually honest, frank, and dependable old lady. A well run, respectable house.

December 6.
Employer, Mr. Rawson, Mgr. T. S. Davis & Co., "Money to Loan," seen at his office, 180 Young St., Boston. Says he was there when patient was there for about six months in 1904. She did simple clerical work and some bookkeeping and informant can remember nothing except that patient was satisfactory and left for better wages in a laundry.

Impression: A middle-aged man of refined appearance and manner.

December 6.
Employer, Miss Ingham, in charge of packing room at G. I. Evans & Co., "Utopian Chocolates," seen at 98 Vernon St., Boston. She says patient worked under her several months, from September, 1914, through the Christmas rush season, and was entirely satisfactory, always on hand promptly. Informant knew patient was a church member and other women working there also lived near patient in South End and went to St. James. The women here are all Americans. Patient might be reëmployed after the rush season, but informant thinks it would not be wise for patient to work there during the rush. Patient wrote to informant several times since leaving, but informant has not answered or seen patient.

Impression: Young, but mature American woman, refined in appearance, manner, and speech, well dressed and of vigorous build.

Factory: Only the office seen. This was very neat and there were two other women of refined appearance.

December 6.
Employer, Mr. I. S. Henderson, Supt., Tyson Brand Co., salted nuts, etc., seen at the factory, Cross St., Cambridge. He says patient was one of the first to apply on opening of new factory last February. She was entirely satisfactory and was especially prompt at work. She did packing at a bench with Americans though there are some Italians. She earned $5.50 per week and might have had piece work if she had stayed and earned as much as $7.00 a week. He noticed particularly that she took no notice of the men about the factory as many women do. He would reemploy patient at any time.

1915
Impression: A young man of refined appearance and manners.

Factory: A new brick building, very well lighted, in neighborhood of other factories.
AEL/C

December 7.
Sister Florence seen in town after work by appointment. Patient's conduct has been the greatest trial to sister and mother. She talks so fast and so much it makes her mother nervous. She is superior and will never take any advice from them. Her connection with a different church is partly responsible because she has acted independently in this respect. She thinks she can in all others. She is stubborn.

Sister believes she drank a good deal with people whom she visited in South End.

Patient had a better chance than any of other children. She was the only one who graduated from grammar school. She was not petted and spoiled because she was the youngest. In money matters she is brighter than her sister, being quicker to add up her figures to get results.

Sister has worked years for Miss Nancy Stowell. Her physical health is not as good as patient's.

Impression: Open-minded, practical, and thoroughly sympathetic. She is a young woman of small stature and a somewhat nervous manner.
HA/C

December 8.
Family's minister, Mr. Young, Channing Church, seen. He says that the family feel that patient has gained nothing through her connection with St. James Church, and that it would be better if she discontinues going there any more. No matter what there was to be done at home, or how sick her mother was, patient always dropped everything to attend services. She was told that she must go every week.

The remainder of the Paris green was found in patient's trunk. She has very few clothes.

Sister Florence works for Nancy Stowell, dressmaker, on Charles St. Miss Stowell is very good about calling sister to the telephone.

Impression: Reliable, earnest man of about 35 years of age.
HA/C

December 17.
School report received.
HA/C

December 23.
Dixon's Commercial School reports no record of patient.
HA/C

1916
January 21.
State Board of Insanity telephoned to. They have no record of father, James Farmer.
MPC/C

January 21.
Patient's mother seen at home. Says that patient has always had her own way ever since she was a child; that she has had more opportunities and used them less than any other member of the family. Patient is only member of the family who went through the Grammar School. Patient was very ill during the voyage from England and has never been strong since, although she was a very healthy baby. Informant's husband, from whom she was separated, has been dead for 12 years. They have always

1916
had all they could do to get along. Patient always told people that she "slaved" at housework, but informant says that she never did any at all, not even to helping with the coal for the fire, etc. As informant has for many years been a cripple (six operations, one knee removed) she has not been able to do heavy work.

Five years ago they had to give up their home for a time during operation on informant's legs. The same thing has occurred a number of times since, the last time about a year ago. At one time when informant was "flat on her back" patient locked the door, went out saying that she would kill herself. Instead she went to her brother's, where she stayed for two weeks. At another time a year ago last October she and her sister went to look for a flat. Informant thought that she was able to have her own home again and that patient would live with them again. While they were out patient told her sister that she would never live with her family again. Patient and her sister never got along together. Informant blames patient who always expected her sister to do everything for her and who never did anything in return. Patient's brother never liked her.

While patient was living away from home she used to bring her washing home for her mother to do. She never did it herself. Informant says that her clothes were always in a disgracefully dirty condition; that it was too hard work for her to do again. Informant says that patient always talks a lot about being fond of her, but she does not show it much in her actions. Says that patient talks too much anyway. She used to make up stories about unkind things informant's friends said to her.

Informant thinks that Father Cramer allowed patient too much freedom; that if he had been more strict with her she would not have done so many foolish things. Informant says that patient got in with a poor lot of girls at St. James Church.

Informant says that when patient came home to live with them, as she did for a while, she spends all Sunday morning in bed, leaves the room where she sleeps (the "front" room) in an untidy state, and does not help with any of the work. Patient's sister gives $5 per week to informant who pays $3 for rent and makes the rest do. Patient's sister makes all her own clothes and in the past has made many of patient's. Patient thinks that she ought to make hers all the time.

Patient went out at all hours even when she lived at home and never told her family where she was going. They never knew where she spent her time unless she happened to mention it rather casually.

Impression: A very delicate old lady who cannot walk without crutches and then with great difficulty. She seems to be quite passive as though completely worn out with the whole situation with which she obviously feels unable to cope. She appeared convincing and aroused considerable sympathy.
HA/C

January 22.
    Vital Statistics Office gives following record of father: Died November 5, 1904, at Westboro State Hospital. Cause, General Paralysis. Resident of Boston, age 46. Inmate 1 year and 2 months at Westboro State Hospital.
FJC/C

January 27.
    Children's Home Society telephoned to. Patient and family are not known to them as was stated by sister in medical history in house record.

1916
March 27.

Mother seen. During the time that the patient lived at home, from June, 1915, until admission to the hospital, she paid in her $5 wages to her mother. Mother gave her $1 for spending money, used $3 and put aside $1 for patient's clothes. Patient later found out that her mother had saved $8 and was very disagreeable about it. She asked for it several times and said she saw no reason why she could not take care of her own money, so that mother gave it to her. She did not tell the family that she had any money saved. They all went to Nashua, N. H., to visit during patient's and her sister's two weeks' vacation and patient's sister-in-law found patient very difficult to deal with. She was disagreeable and lazy and impudent. While there she wrote often to the old man, Mr. Radnor, with whom she used to play cards about every week when she lived in the West End. She also wrote long letters to Father Cramer.

At one time patient was a member of the Girls' Friendly Society, but she had a quarrel with the leader (Christ Church, East Boston) and gave it up. Patient is apt to like people very well and talk about them all the time for a short time and later turn against them.
HA/C

Sister Edith seen by House Historian. See medical record for history.
HA/C

ACTION TAKEN

December 2.

Employer, Sampson Press, would not be willing to take patient back as he considers her unfit for factory work.
MBS/C

December 3.

Miss Kendall, York House, is willing to take patient into the Gales St. House to live until she can find work. She feels that St. James Church people should not let their responsibility end here. Though it seems best for patient to drop her connection with that church, they ought to stand expense of sending her away, if necessary.
HA/C

December 4.

Miss Kendall says there is room at the Roxbury House, if patient should decide to go there for six months. It would probably be the best plan.
HA/C

December 6.

Family's minister, Mr. Young of Channing Church (Unitarian), telephones. He has expected to take up the care of patient when she leaves. The family (mother and sister) are unwilling that patient should go to York House. They are anxious to have her sever connections with the Episcopal Church for reasons which Mr. Young cannot give by telephone. His plan is to place patient at the Gordon House of Working Girls. While she works in the day time, she should have some training business course at Y. W. C. A. at night as well as club or class work one or two evenings. He knows several workers at this house, whom he will interest in patient. He would like visitor to keep in touch with patient also.

Mr. Young feels that institutional restraint of such a girl who has been allowed so much freedom, will only make her rebellious and produce no results.
HA/C

1915
December 7.

Family's minister, Mr. Young, telephones that he will be able to arrange for patient to live at Gordon House, 44 Dix St.
HA/C

Mr. Young seen. He has been talking with Mrs. Dickinson, head of the House, and she will take an interest in patient. Miss Taylor of Canterbury Church will do what she can for her and take a friendly interest in her. Neither one of these people will be able to take definite and complete supervision of patient, and Mr. Young feels that he will not be able to do so himself.

He will, however, see the patient frequently and will naturally get the point of view of the family because he sees them often. He will be able to report to visitor anything which arises in patient's situation. He will pay for patient's board ten days or two weeks, but feels that she should have work by that time. He hopes that a definite schedule can be arranged for patient, so that she will have each evening planned for. He would suggest her taking some training, such as secretarial, at an evening school.

He would be glad to get some clothes for her so that she will not be ashamed when meeting the other girls at the House.

Patient taken to Gordon House and Mrs. Dickinson seen. Patient will go to-morrow morning to the Massachusetts General Hospital, Out-Patient Department, Female Medical Clinic, for a thorough examination. There is a question of anemia and tuberculosis.
HA/C

December 10.

Patient writes. She returns to Massachusetts General Hospital for examination to-day. Girls at Gordon House are not allowed out over night. See letter.
HA/C

December 11.

Massachusetts General Hospital, Social Service, Miss Davis, telephones that patient's lungs are negative, but that she has a severe anemia. Dr. Dawson advises patient going into the House for a few days. Patient is reluctant to do this as she says she is devoted to her roommate and does not want to leave her. Sister is at Out-Patient Department with patient and she says patient will stay.

Case will be transferred to House Social Service so that visitor may have reports directly.

Patient and sister telephoned. Patient did not want to enter hospital to-day and Dr. Young says he is not sure of a bed for Monday 12/13. Patient promises to go to Miss Davis on that date and enter hospital if possible. First asked to be treated by private physician.
HA/C

December 13.

Patient writes. See letter.
HA/C

December 14.

Massachusetts General Hospital, Miss Davis, telephoned to. Patient was admitted yesterday.

Minister, Mr. Young, and Mrs. Dickinson telephoned to. Arranged for patient to return to Gordon House on her discharge from Massachusetts General Hospital.
HA/C

1915
December 17.
Sister Florence seen in town by appointment. Patient is being discharged to-day and she will take her to Gordon House. Sister does not favor any domestic training for she thinks patient's place is at home if she can behave properly. For some time she has talked of stenography, but when aunt took a book to her she did not follow up the work by herself.

They like to have patient at home Sundays. She makes mother nervous because she talks so fast and so much, but they are both fond of patient and ready to do all they can to help her.
HA/C

December 18.
Massachusetts General Hospital, Social Service, telephones that patient is not anemic and can go to work. She needs no diet.

Patient seen at hospital. Is always able to find work for herself. Miss Taylor, Canterbury Church, saw her at Massachusetts General Hospital and said she might be able to get her into a private printing place. Patient wants to follow her printing trade, as she is used to it.

Patient intends to go home only a half day Sundays because the attitude at home wears on her. Her mother continually gives her good advice and harps on the past. They are "too strict." She cannot take off her dress and put on a kimono to rest until it is time to go to bed. She cannot have company because it wears on her mother. They are continually suspicious of her conduct.

Last night she stayed at home because she went out to get her things. They would not let her sleep on the cot in the parlor where she used to sleep, but had to share her mother's bed, so that all three were in the same room. Patient said nothing and does not know the reason for this except that they may not have trusted her to be alone.

At Gordon House, patient likes her roommate ever so much and her room too.

Sent patient to Harvard Dental School to have teeth examined. She will look for work Monday.
HA/C

December 23.
Patient writes. See letter and Christmas card.

Patient telephones. Hopes to get work in Newman's, 465 Denver St., at typesetting. Wages $12 a week. There is no vacancy now, but she is promised the next opportunity.

She will go to her own dentist, Dr. Day, Davis Square, Dorchester, who used to do work half price, since the Dental School is closed for vacation.
HA/C

December 27.
Patient telephones. She goes to work to-morrow at piece work in Dalton Fastener Co., 42 Belle Ave., Cambridge (near Kendall Square). Her first week's wages will have to go to the Mercantile Agency. Girls earn from $6–$12, according to their ability and skill. Hours are 7:30–5:30 and patient can have her breakfast at Gordon House and take her lunch.

Patient says she had a happier Christmas than for some time. "We never had happiness in the home before." She stayed all night there. Patient tells of going to Beacon Hill Christmas Eve to hear the carols. She went to Charles St. Jail and was much interested in that.
HA/C

1915
December 31.
Patient writes. See letter.
HA/C

1916
January 10 to January 17.
Patient writes. Asks to be allowed to go home Saturdays for over night. She writes she has joined the Unitarian Church. See letters.
HA/C

January 17.
Patient sends diet for past week by request.
HA/C

Monday:

BREAKFAST	LUNCH	DINNER	EVENING LUNCH
Wheatena	Thin egg sandwich	Cold sliced ham	Cocoa
Salt fish hash	Sponge cake	Boiled cabbage	Apples
Cup of coffee	Blueberry cake	Boiled carrots	Oat. cr.
	Apple	Mashed potatoes	Beef tea
			Uneedas

Tuesday:

BREAKFAST	LUNCH	DINNER	EVENING LUNCH
Oatmeal	Ham sandwich	Boiled cod and	Cocoa
Fried eggs	Doughnut	cream sauce	Oxtail soup
Mashed potatoes	Apple	Boiled onions	Uneedas
Coffee		Boiled potatoes	
		Apple tapioca	

Wednesday:

BREAKFAST	LUNCH	DINNER	EVENING LUNCH
Wheatena	Deviled ham sand-	Roast beef	Cocoa
Slice of salt	wich	Boiled lima beans	Oat. cr.
chipped beef	Half slice cake	Carrots	Uneedas
(tissue)	Apple	Boiled potatoes	Beef tea
Baked potatoes		Chocolate blanc	
Raised biscuit		mange	
Coffee			

Thursday:

BREAKFAST	LUNCH	DINNER	EVENING LUNCH
Corn meal	Roast beef sand-	Beef stew	Cocoa
Salt fish	wich	Cream pie	Oat. cr.
Fried potatoes	Half slice cake	Bread and butter	Uneedas
Raised biscuit	1 cookie		Beef tea
Coffee	Cocoa		Apples
	Apple		

Friday:

BREAKFAST	LUNCH	DINNER	EVENING LUNCH
Wheatena	Meat pie	Fried fish	Cocoa
3 slices bacon	Tea	Mashed potatoes	Oat. cr.
2 baked potatoes		Corn	Uneedas
Coffee		Bread pudding	Beef tea
			Apples
			Wash. pie

Saturday:

BREAKFAST	LUNCH	DINNER	EVENING LUNCH
Hash	Sliced ham	Baked beans	Cocoa
Muffin	Baked potatoes	Piccalilli	Oat. cr.
Coffee	Tea	Bread and butter	Uneedas
		Tea	Beef tea
			Macaroons

Sunday:

BREAKFAST	LUNCH	DINNER	EVENING LUNCH
Fish cakes	Tea	Canned cherries	Cocoa
Beans	Roast stuffed pork	Bread and butter	Beef tea
Brown bread	Pickles	Cake	Oat. cr.
Coffee	Bread and butter	Cocoa	Uneedas
	Potatoes		Frankfurters and
	Squash pie		bread
			Orange

$1.37 was spent extra for food.
HA/C

1916
January 18.

Mrs. Dickinson, Gordon House, telephoned to. She says patient is doing well. She takes an interest in the life at the House, enjoys the other girls, and has given no trouble in any way.

Mrs. Dickinson would be willing for her to go home Saturday if visitor arranges it.

HA/C

January 19.

Patient seen at hospital. Reported at evening clinic to Dr. Hatch. She is happy and says she is doing her best. Drinking she never thinks of. The life at the House is great fun. The girls always come into patient's room toward the end of the evening and leave things to eat, apples, cocoa. Patient spends her evenings sewing. She mends her roommate's clothes as well as her own and she has been doing some crocheting and embroidery for the nurse of the House, who is engaged. Mr. Young's church is to have a Fair, and she is making things for that as a surprise. She seldom goes out evenings though she went once to moving pictures. Sundays she goes home in the morning and returns in the afternoon. She washes her own shirtwaists at home, but her other clothes are done at the House and included in the board. Patient and her mother are devoted to one another and get on peaceably. Sister treats her better now, but patient has no fondness for her. Patient took her roommate, Fannie, home with her last Sunday and the family liked her.

Patient walks to and from work to Kendall Sq., Cambridge. She sleeps with windows open and eats heartily.

Work has been irregular. The largest wage made was some over $7, but it has been nearer $5 usually. There are many types of work and different machines and patient will make an effort to get on a machine with which she can earn most.

The foreman, Mr. James, is good to her, and when she complained he shifted her. This week, work has been slack because the firm is starting a new department next week. The old girls say one is seldom laid off, so patient will try it out another week. She can earn 80 cents for the other days this week. The board at Gordon House is $4. Patient owes Mr. Young $4 and the House $2 from a week she was not working (Mr. Young only paid the first two weeks). Patient has plenty of clothes. Mr. Young offered her more, but she did not need them. She still has some savings, but she does not wish to spend them for current expenses.

Patient is anxious to learn linotype because that was what put her out of work at the Sampson Press when she was setting type by hand. She thinks she cannot afford to go to a school for it this year.

Patient tells of a young man, whom she passes every morning going to work, asking her to meet him some night. She used to pass him when she worked at Tyson Brand and so she speaks to him. She does not intend to go out with him. Recently, she met Karl Cauldwell and he walked home with her. He offered to "keep company" with her again, but she "threw him over."

Patient seems happy, looks well, and is very friendly toward visitor.

HA/C

January 21.

Minister, Mr. Young, telephoned to. He thinks patient is doing well and has not been drinking. She is not really self-supporting yet. He was surprised and pleased to have her join the church.

HA/C

1916
January 21

Patient's mother seen at home. Informant thinks that patient gets along with sister somewhat better than previously, but notices no other change in her actions or attitude. Visitor asked informant about having patient return to her home to spend Saturday nights. Informant is willing to have her, but seems to feel that it may not be for patient's best good, as she thinks that patient is making the necessity of being at home in order to go to church an excuse to escape the early rising necessary at Gordon House. Informant says that patient can get to Church Sunday morning from where she is, that she did it last Sunday with her roommate whom she took to dinner at her home. Informant says that on day patient wrote to previous visitor (1/1) she spent the night at home and did not go to church the next morning, but read in bed. Informant thinks that patient will impose upon previous visitor unless she is most careful. Informant fears that patient will be most disagreeable to her if she finds out what informant has said. Informant is so tired of having fusses that she does not give a word of advice to patient now—whenever she does patient is ugly to her.

Informant suggests that if it is decided to be wise for patient to go home Saturday nights, it would be advisable to make it conditioned upon her attending church Sunday mornings, and in order not to make the patient angry at her family, to have the information obtained from Mr. Young, the minister. Informant says that patient cannot fool him. Patient joined the Unitarian Church the first Sunday of January, for which her mother is glad. Thinks it may do something toward keeping her with the family.

Informant says that patient should live as she is now with people and under rule; that otherwise she will become untidy again and will bring bad girls into her room. She thinks that if patient complains to visitor about conditions as she has at home that visitor should not pay too much attention to her, but should insist that she live with a roommate.

Informant says that patient was doing fairly well until last week when she made only $5 because the machine broke down and there was not enough work to do. Says that patient was discouraged Sunday. Informant thinks patient should try to get a position as monotype corrector as that is her trade.

Patient has never contributed to support of family, and does not consider the extra trouble it makes when she visits them, either in the matter of expense or work.

Informant is evidently rather afraid of patient and anxious not to displease her.
MBS

January 21.
Patient and mother written that she is not to go home Saturdays for the present.
HA/C

January 24.
Patient writes. See letter.

Patient telephones she is out of work for a day or so. Will go to Harvard Dental School this morning.

Linotype School sends literature. Evening course $50.

Patient seen at hospital. Is to go back to work 1/26 and to-morrow will have more work done on her teeth and will spend extra time mending.

1916

She made $4.40 last week and the foreman has promised to put her on a good machine when she goes back. She likes it so well there that she hates to leave and will give the place further trial. Mr. James urged her to stay on.

Patient wants to go home Saturday nights because it means such an early rising and such a hurry to get out to Roxbury in time for church Sundays. She stayed at home Friday night because she and sister went to an entertainment at Church.

Patient is very friendly indeed and assures visitor she wants to make as little trouble as possible.

Patient wants to go to Linotype School when she gets well established in work.

January 25.
Patient writes and asks to be allowed to help and do some sewing for visitor. See letter.

Patient written to, asking her to make two chemises for another patient.
HA/C

February 9.
Patient writes, 1/26 and 29, 2/5 and 9, and telephones 2/5. She is enthusiastic about her work, to which she went back 1/27. She made $1.75 and $1.80 for the first two days and over $7 for the past week. She expects to have all back board paid by 2/20. She has some neuralgia of the gums and if it is not improved in a few days, she will take time off to have her teeth seen to. Her roommate, Fannie, has been very sick and patient had to wait on her. Now she is away for a few weeks' rest.

February 9.
Patient writes, "It may seem strange to many people that my mother's illness should make such an impression on me, but it does. I am the youngest and think a whole lot of my mother, but instead of going out and seeing her enjoy life, I have to see her a cripple holding back her pain and trying to be happy. . . . I am sorry I was so bad, but I will be good always now to make up for it."
See letters.
HA/C

February 9.
Matron of Gordon House, Mrs. Dickinson, seen. She likes patient and thinks she is doing her very best. No indications that she has been drinking. The other girls like her, as she is always bright and jolly. Informant thinks she is happy there. She has a very lovely roommate, a blind girl, to whom she is devoted, and at present she is feeling pretty lonely, as the roommate has gone away to the country for two weeks. Informant chose this girl for patient's roommate, as she felt she would be a good influence.

Patient is orderly about picking up her things but the room is apt to be in need of dusting, but informant makes allowances for this as patient has to go off so early to work. Leaves the house at seven and does not come back till almost six.

The factory where she works is being enlarged and temporarily a good many people are working only part time. Last week patient worked only a few days and did not earn enough to pay her board. When she works full time she makes only about $8 at piece work. She is somewhat

1916
discouraged, and very restless when out of work. Talks of changing to Gillette Razor Factory, but Mrs. Dickinson is urging her to stick it out here in hopes that she will soon have regular full-time employment.

Informant feels she is devoted to her mother, but cannot get on well with her sister. Has told informant that she never could live with her. Informant thinks that probably patient teases sister, who retaliates.

There are no clubs or classes in Gordon House to which she can belong. There is a Friday Night Forum to discuss social questions, but patient has not attended. She does not go out evenings to movies, only occasionally for a few minutes to do an errand. Does not go with any former friends, but seems contented to be with her roommate, and sews a good deal.
EB/C

February 12.
Patient seen at hospital. Brought visitor a guest towel and face cloth which she had made as a present. Last week made $8 and was idle part of two half days. She would have made more, but was slow on account of a small injury to the tip of a finger.

Patient is lonely with roommate away.
HA/C

February 15.
Patient writes. Is going to a suffrage meeting with sister and a friend to-night. See letter.

February 21.
Patient and sister sent theater tickets to "It Pays to Advertise" to-night.
HA/C

March 9.
Patient writes often. See letters.
HA/C

March 10.
Patient seen at hospital. This week has been a bad one at work. They were laid off more than two hours one day, $1\frac{1}{2}$ the next, and patient made only 24 cents this morning. Patient is discouraged and would like to change to a firm that can give steady work.

Patient made two chemises by hand for another patient, made neatly and well.

Mr. Steadman, Delle Ink Co., telephoned to. He will see patient to-day and if she is good will start her there. She would make $6 a week for about two weeks and then go on to piece work at $33\frac{1}{3}$ per cent over regular piece work prices which would gradually be reduced until in about four or five weeks she would be at a regular rate. If she is good with her hands she might later work into piece work that gives $10 to $13 a week.
HA/C

March 13.
Patient's employer, Dalton Fastener Co., Mr. James, seen at factory, Belle Ave., Cambridge (near Central Sq.). Says patient returned to factory on 3/10/16 after employees had been dismissed early to tell him she had obtained other work, but he had gone, so she sent letter which he received next day. Patient was entirely satisfactory as a worker and got on well with other employees. She made about $9 a week on piece work, which is on ball and socket fasteners for automobile tops, tending machines, sorting and packing. Informant would reëmploy patient whenever they need help. She might make as high as $16 a week on piece work.

1916

Impression: A young man of intelligent appearance and kindly manner, apparently genuinely interested in the welfare of his employees.

Impression of Factory: Visitor was shown room where patient worked. A large, very bright room, not crowded with machinery or workers, but exceedingly noisy. Factory is a new one. Workers can eat lunch in room where they work, for which tables are cleared and machinery is stopped for an hour. Women employed are Americans.
AEL/C

March 21.

Patient writes about every other day. She says she likes her work and is receiving $6 a week for the first two weeks. Hours are 7:30–12; 12:45–5:30, or 9¼ hours a day, and 7:30–1, or 5½ hours, Saturdays; total, 51¾ hours a week. She is labelling and packing bottles. The work can be done faster standing. Stools are provided, but patient stands.

All patient's back board and two weeks' board advanced by Mr. Young was paid 3/6/16. Patient saved the money which would have gone to carfares and bought an attractive blue corduroy coat for about $5. Patient will keep an account book of all week's wages and expenditures. Board is now $4.

Patient now has a new roommate, Nancy Bornstein (also a patient, File No. 7246), who is under the care of Miss Stella Farrell, Massachusetts General Hospital Social Service. She is a great trial to patient who is trying to train her in manners, cleanliness, and industry. Nancy's diagnosis is Not Insane (Moron—Hysteria). Patient goes with her to see Miss Farrell.

Last week at visitor's suggestion patient offered her mother $1 which was refused. See letter of 3/20/16 from patient.
HA/C

March 27.

Massachusetts General Hospital Social Service, Miss Farrell, telephones about patient's roommate who is under her supervision. Nancy is under Dr. Fenmore's care at Massachusetts General Hospital nerve clinic. She is to stay on as long as possible at Gordon House.

Patient writes. See letters.

Mother seen at home. Patient has been in church very little in Roxbury, about three or four times, and mother suspects that she continues to go to St. James. When she used to go there she made friends with a girl who had an illegitimate child, and this child was boarded out with people who drank. Mother suspects that patient continues to see this girl, because she asked her sister about making a dress for a baby two years old. Patient was godmother to this child.

Patient wishes to stay at home Saturday nights and sometimes talks about going home to live. Mother is very unwilling to say that she does not want her at home, but it is evident that the patient is a trial to them. She stays in bed late and does not go to church and does a great deal of washing and odd jobs about the house which leaves a good deal of disorder. She once said she was staying at Gordon House as a punishment. Mother does not wish to take money from the patient, because in the past she has "thrown it up at them" for doing so. She does not want to be under any obligation to the patient. In regard to the incident about the tea mentioned in her letter of 3/20, mother says that she offered to pay for the tea from the beginning.

Mother thinks that the patient's present roommate is not good for her.

1916

She always has taken things hard and thinks too much about this girl. Thinks patient has improved somewhat, especially in her talk, which used to be profane and disagreeable. Mother thinks that the visitor has a good deal of influence over the patient, but that patient "puts on" a great deal of her own goodness.

HA/C

March 28.

Sister Florence met in town. She feels as mother does about the money, but is willing to have patient give $1 a week if it is necessary.

Patient told her employer at Dalton Fastener Co. that she could not support her invalid mother on what she earned. She is always misrepresenting family situations to sister's friends. Patient and her brother Bernard never got along together and sister is much amused at patient's pretending to take such an interest in him.

Sister will let visitor know the first time patient mentions the money she gives her mother.

Patient seen at Gordon House. Though 7 :30 she is ready for bed. She gets so tired standing at work that she usually goes to bed or reads after dinner. Patient bathes once a week at home and will not use the tub here because everyone uses it.

Patient does not go out evenings, both she and her roommate say. Nancy relates the fun which they have together evenings, eating oranges and joking. Nancy is apparently fond of patient and an admirer. She says "Harriet is smart." Patient is crocheting a large door mat out of heavy string. She is also making a complicated work bag. Patient has a library card and reads a good deal. The gas light is at one side and gives a poor light.

Patient goes to church every Sunday at some Episcopal church and has been to St. James several times. If she is allowed to go home Saturday nights, she will go to the Unitarian Church, but she does not take much interest in it. Patient begs to be allowed to go home Saturdays. She speaks of living at home later ; says one feels freer as to hours and all.

Patient continues on time work at $6 a week (third week) but the forelady praised her work. She has talked to Hilda Tibbets (also a patient here) and asks if she can do anything for her as she has noticed that no one talks to her.

HA/C

March 30.

Mother writes. See letter and copy of answer. Visitor suggests patient go home Saturdays for a trial.

HA/C

March 31.

Patient writes. See two letters.

Patient telephones to say she does not want to appear at a staff meeting of N. E. Hospital Social Workers' Association, but finally agrees. Patient will start staying at home Saturday nights.

Gordon House, Miss Dickinson, telephoned to about Saturday arrangement. Patient is in almost every evening or else comes in very early.

HA/C

April 3.

Employer, Mr. Steadman, Delle Ink Co., telephoned to. Patient is doing average work and though it is usually customary for new workers to stay six weeks on time work he will allow her to try piece work next week.

1916

Patient writes 3/30, 3/31, 4/3. See letters.. She gave her mother 50 cents this week.

Patient called at hospital this evening and left a present for visitor—crocheted slippers which she had made herself.
HA/C

April 4.
Patient's roommate writes. See letter.
HA/C

April 5.
Patient seen. She gave visitor her gold cross and chain because now she is a Unitarian she cannot wear it.

Patient presented at a clinic at the Massachusetts General Hospital meeting of N. E. Hospital Social Workers' Association. When asked to tell about her experiences she gave a very direct and clear account of how discouraged she had been before taking poison, of how much it meant to her to have someone take an interest and encourage her as the hospital people had, how the life and jolly times at Gordon House had made her happy.

Patient and her roommate given tickets to see "Grumpy."
HA/C

April 7.
Patient and her roommate write. See letters.
HA/C

Mother writes that patient gave her 50 cents last week. See letter.
HA/C

April 10.
Patient writes that she has lost her gold watch, the gift of her mother. She is much discouraged with everything.

Patient telephoned to.
HA/C

April 12.
Patient seen by Chief of Staff, Dr. Adler. He reports that she recognizes that her depression comes in six-month periods. She is now passing through the period—the previous one came in the fall when she took poison. She has no appetite, sleeps poorly, is disgusted with work and discouraged with everything. She is apt to go back to drink.

Patient seen. She wants to get back into printing trade. She cannot take much interest in ink work.

A shower spray was sent patient last week and she bathes twice a day now.
HA/C

April 17.
Patient writes to-day and 4/14. See letters.
HA/C

April 20.
Patient telephoned to every day. Her appetite is better. So far suggestions for work have been unsuccessful. She stayed out of Delle's this morning to go to two places for work. Patient's watch was found 4/16 at church.

1916

Mr. Norton of Sampson Press seen. They cannot take patient back because she was second or third rate worker, her attendance was very irregular, and they have no opening.

Mother seen at home. Visitor had already explained to sister by telephone last week that this is a critical time with patient. Mother seems to be a whiney individual. She repeats a good deal of past history in great detail.

Sister sat up until midnight last Saturday trimming a hat for patient to wear to church. She never came until after church.

Patient was at home over yesterday's holiday.
HA/C

April 22.

Patient seen at hospital. She feels encouraged about her work because she made $7 at piece work, even though there was a holiday. She will continue at least one week more. Then she may stop and try to find printing or some kind of work at which she can sit. The standing is difficult at Delle's. Patient has enough money in the bank to pay her own board while out of work. She cannot remember the exact amount.

Her roommate is more restless and queer of late so that patient has not had the proper amount of sleep. At midnight she got up and tried to go off so that patient had to call the matron.

Patient's appetite is good now and she has almost no desire for drink. She has made two tea aprons for another patient and done them well.
HA/C

April 26.

Patient has written and telephoned twice. She has secured work at Doherty's, 181 Norfolk Ave., hours 7:30–5:30. Thinks the pay will be $7 or $8 per week. She sets type for menus for hotels. She only worked until 3:30 to-day. Patient seems very happy over her new work, is much interested, and "the day simply flies."
MC/C

April 28.

Patient seen at Gordon House. She was tired and had a headache, and she went to bed early. She had had a tooth extracted. Nancy has refused to speak to her for several days.
MC/C

April 28.

Gordon House, Mrs. Dickinson seen. She has decided that Nancy cannot stay at the House any longer and she is waiting to hear from Miss Farrell. They all like patient very much. She does not think it is best for patient to have the care of Nancy.
MC/C

May 2.

Patient seen. At patient's invitation, visitor and patient attended recital at Jacob Sleeper Hall given by Curry School of Expression.
MC/C

May 5.

Patient seen at visitor's residence. She walks to her work every day now. She has to stay until 4:30 on Saturday afternoons, but will not have to do this in the summer.
MC/C

May 8.

Patient writes. See letter.
MC/C

1916
May 8.

Patient telephones. She is worrying for fear she will have to go home to live. Says she has been "thirsty all day and drinks a large quantity of water."
MC/C

May 12.

Patient writes. See letter.
MC/C

May 15.

Gordon House, Mrs. Dickinson, telephoned to. Nancy came back to the House for the night only. Miss Farrell said Nancy had no place to go so Mrs. Dickinson gave her the room for two days and a night. She did not see patient at dinner so she probably left immediately after she came home.
MC/C

May 15.

Patient telephones. She is at her mother's and wants to stay all night because she is angry because Nancy came back to room with her. She understood that she was to have a new roommate. Visitor advised patient to go back to the Settlement House.

Patient telephones later that she has decided to return and is on her way there now.
MC/C

May 28.

Patient telephones that she fainted at work yesterday because of menstruation. She is at home and resting to-day.
MC/C

Patient telephones and writes often. See letters. She likes her work and has made friends with girls at the shop.
HA/C

May 29.

Patient writes details of a medical nature. See letter. She has craving for drink and takes vinegar and water, lemon and limes, and anything she can think of.

She goes out to supper occasionally.
HA/C

May 31.

Patient writes and telephones. She tried to work Monday 5/29, but had to leave in early afternoon.
HA/C

June 2.

Patient seen at hospital. She is anxious to live at home now. She feels dissatisfied with the food at Gordon House because it is too salty and makes her thirsty. Visitor urged against going home, but left decision pending.

Patient gives her mother $1 a week; earns $8. She goes on the car now. She is able to save, out of the remaining $7, $2.40.

Patient says she is going out with a man older than herself. The affair is a serious one though patient has not yet decided to marry him. From everything she can hear, he is a good sort. She refuses further details on the ground that her previous affair with Karl Cauldwell was broken up by interference from other people.
HA/C

1916
June 5.
Patient writes that she has decided not to go home to live. This weekend she thought her mother and sister were very severe and strict with her. See letter.
HA/C

June 6.
Matron, Gordon House, Mrs. Dickinson, seen. Food is not salty. They always have fresh meat and fish and only occasionally ham. At dinner they have potatoes and two vegetables, or one vegetable and lettuce. Matron has found that patient exaggerates and cannot be depended upon to keep strictly to the truth. Illustrations given seemed to have discrepancy of detail rather than entire false basis.

There is no one to room with patient at present, but matron will have it in mind to put some one with her when she can. Patient is well liked by the girls, is friendly, agreeable to every one, and seems well behaved. She is in most of the time, but goes home to dinner occasionally on week nights.
HA/C

June 8.
Patient reported at hospital. Was seen by Dr. Green and given advice about menstrual period.

Dr. Wilson had a long talk with patient and says he thinks she is fairly contented; that there is nothing to the love affair. Patient is doing well.
HA/C

June 10.
Patient writes and telephones. She has a chance to work three evenings a week in a store in Kensington, but is advised not to do so, because of extra wear.

She has given up the young man by going off and leaving him looking in a store window. He wanted to give her a dog for which she had no place.
HA/C

June 13.
Patient writes.
HA/C

June 23.
Patient writes and telephones often. She went to Y. M. C. A. Entertainment one night with Henry Elkins, whom she knew at Sampson Press. He is a widower who is going to be married again next month.

Patient is writing short stories, a sample of which shows very wordy and flowery style with a romantic and imaginative background.
HA/C

June 23.
Minister, Mr. Young, telephones to inquire how patient is doing. He advises strongly that patient and family both be urged against patient's ever going home to live.
HA/C

June 23.
Patient seen at hospital. She wanted to explain to visitor about fellow employees who are not altogether agreeable with her. Patient and Martha Wilson, who soon leaves to be married, are the only Protestants. Since the other girls found this out, they have gone out of their way to be disagreeable and troublesome; for example, patient will just get her hand full of type and be seated on her stool, when they decide to get certain trays

1916
under her stool, so that she has to get down. They kick her standing box to the other side of the room whenever they get a chance. Patient will do her best to stand it and report to visitor before leaving.
HA/C

July 31.
Patient seen often in past month. She continues to write and telephone often. See letters. She has one friend, James V., who lives across the street from hospital. She "picked him up" through the window while she was on Ward V. Went out to suppers, several dances, and to ride with three or four different men, but would not tell visitor about them.

Patient once brought up question of going home to live, but after two days' consideration decided against it. Mother and sister have been in Dover part of month and patient went there for week-ends.

August 15.
Patient seen and writes often. James V. went to Bloomington, Ill., to work two days ago and patient has been quite blue ever since. She takes no interest in the other men and is going to give them up entirely. One made improper advances to her by saying something and patient will not have anything to do with him. Had a long talk with patient on this subject, but could get no definite account from her of her own affairs. She has never been "immoral"—her mother would put her out if she were, she says.
Patient is found to have pinworms. She reported to O. P. D., Dr. Samuels, who prescribed for her.

Employer, Mr. Simpson, a foreman at Doherty Printers, seen. He says patient's work is good. She has not shown any special discouragement (patient wrote she thought he saw her crying). He was not planning on giving her a vacation, but if visitor thinks she needs one he will arrange it. Employer is not given name of visitor or hospital, nor did he ask. Patient was not seen.
Impression: Intelligent young man who is kind and sympathetic.
HA/C

August 17.
Mother writes, saying that patient seems to be getting restless and talks of going home to live and she fears that as soon as visitor leaves patient will disarrange things.
Patient taken to dinner. A Mrs. Davis asked her to live with her. Patient would have the use of the kitchen and better meals. Room rent would be free. Mrs. Davis is an old friend as well as a fellow employee at Dalton Fastener Co. Patient also brings up the question of going home to live, but promised visitor to make no such change during her absence nor to talk about it to her mother.
Patient told of opportunity to go to Hampton Rest the first week in September and thinks that she would prefer to go to her brother's in Dover. She will write him and find out whether he can have her.
HA/C

August 26.
Matron, Mrs. Thompson, Gordon House, seen. She was surprised that patient complained of waiting on table because she has never seen her do it, although patient is supposed to do her share. She has not spoken of it because weather has been so warm and patient has seemed so tired. Patient

1916
seems worried and unhappy, probably because she would like to be at home,
but has decided to abide by the doctor's advice to stay away.
    Patient is to have a roommate, beginning to-night.
MW/C

August 26.
    Patient telephoned to at 1 :30. She has decided to go to her brother's
in Dover for her vacation. She sounded happy and seemed pleased at being
called up.

    Hampton Rest written to, saying patient will not take their place.
MW/C

August 31.
    Patient called at hospital in evening and asked advice about moving
from Gordon House. She is dissatisfied and says the new matron is too
strict. She has asked her repeatedly to wait on table, has not had a place
set for her when patient returned after a week-end at home, and told her
new roommate that patient has spells of depression. Patient thought of
taking her things home this week-end and living there after her vacation
until a new place can be found. Visitor advised leaving things as they are
and staying at the Gordon House until Miss Bemis returns and new arrangements can be made. Patient promised to abide by this and went away
happy.
MW/C

September 30.
    Patient seen two or three times and writes and telephones often. See
letters. At first she wished to move on return from her vacation at her
brother's in Dover; she had a new roommate and was content to stay on.
Roommate, Frances Caldwell, is a Church Home girl of 18, young, attractive, and not undesirable or bad. Patient is very superstitious and believed
what a fortune teller told her, interpreting that brother, Benjamin, was
working against her particularly with mother. She writes she intends to
make over her insurance to visitor.
    Patient had one crying spell at work before menstruation period. Has
been to Out-Patient Department and given treatment by Dr. Samuels for
pinworms.
    Patient has taken an account book and will keep track of her expenses.
Is interested in doing so.
    Room visited and patient keeps it cozy and pleasant.
HA/C

October 31.
    Mother visited 10/6. She does not want patient's financial assistance
of $1 because she is apt to throw it up to her that she gives money. Per-
suaded to continue taking it. Patient does not go to Unitarian Church.
When she comes home, she is as disagreeable and vulgar as ever.

    Patient seen three or four times. Moved 10/21 to the Inman House,
taking her roommate, Frances Caldwell, with her. Became dissatisfied with
new matron, Mrs. Thompson. Roommate was hot-tempered and saucy and
wanted to leave. Before going patient had a talk with matron who felt
more kindly disposed toward her. Patient has several young men with
whom she goes out to dinner and she claims she is not at the house many
times a week. 10/24 patient was disagreeable and sullen over telephone and
said she was going out on the streets. Wrote next day apologizing. Patient
telephones and writes often. See letters.

1916

Matron, Mrs. Thompson, seen. She has nothing to say against patient and thinks she is a nice girl. They had a good talk before patient left. Patient was not absent from meals that she noticed.
HA/C

November 30.

Patient seen twice, writes and telephones often. Has made several things for patients' Christmas tree, crochet baby sacks and slippers.

Patient is going to evening dental clinic at Boston Dispensary, referred by visitor. Was out of work a day at menses.

She complains of their third roommate, a nurse, who is not sociable and who they think tries to annoy them and be inconsiderate. Patient does not make friends with the others in the house and goes out evenings a good deal with men, coming in early. The boys' living club similar to this gave a party to the girls which patient seemed to enjoy.

Middle of month patient was determined to go home to live and would not promise visitor not to move. Three hours later telephoned she would stay where she was. Patient became angry at family and said she did not intend to go in to see them again, at least will not sleep there any more. See letters.

Former friend, Miss Simpson, governess of Mrs. M. C. Saunders' children, telephones to inquire for patient and says she expects to go to see her. She used to know her at St. James Church and had lost track of her until recently hearing of her coming to the hospital.

Mother writes patient brings her washing home and it is too much for her to do. (Laundry is not done at this house.) See letters.
HA/C

December 30.

Patient seen, telephones and writes. Has contributed 3 or 4 presents to the Christmas tree and takes much interest in doing so. The settlement club at Ferris Memorial, to which visitor referred patient, has not been active. Once patient went and it was a Jewish holiday and no others were there and last time only two or three, so that she is discouraged with it.

Patient was referred to Miss Harriet Martin (Boston Society for Care of Girls) for one of the new Girls' Protective Leagues. These are to be made from clubs already established, but Miss Martin will keep patient in mind. Patient has been to church with Miss Simpson. Is now going frequently to Episcopal Church.

December 31.

Patient seen three or four times. At end of month had a large and serious abscess in her tooth which gave her much pain and kept her from work a week. Spent a good deal of time at home.

Patient has a laundress and does not take washing home to mother. See letters.
HA/C

1917
January 31.

Patient seen a number of times. Patient became dissatisfied with Inman House because Matron, Mrs. Sawtelle, was not considerate of her when she was sick, because she did not like the third roommate, and because Frances Caldwell moved to her sister's. Effort was made to have patient return to Gordon House, but they refused to take her back but would give no reason. 1/11—After staying home three days patient moved to Warrenton St. Y. W. C. A. She has been very enthusiastic about it since.

1917

Patient knows several girls from Gordon House who room there. Patient introduced them to visitor and they seemed nice, wholesome working women, friendly toward patient.

Patient was out of work half a week with the abscess. 1/8 she went to Massachusetts General Hospital Out-Patient Department for advice in treatment of worms and was given medicine.

Mother wrote 1/8, fearing patient was planning to move home. See letter.

HA/C

February 28.

Patient seen. Writes often; see letters. 2/12 patient wrote "best of friends must part" and "I will not trouble you any more." Interview brought out fact that because patient was told over telephone that visitor was "out" she thought visitor did not wish to hear from her. Episode was smoothed over.

In past six weeks patient has not been going to church much. Is urged but does not wish to. Later writes she goes to Catholic Church at noons.

Patient made a chemise for a sick patient and called for another girl patient here to direct her to Y. W. C. A.

Friend, James V., who lives on Granville Road, is ill with mastoid and patient is quite upset over it. She has known him over a year, claiming to have picked him up while a patient in Ward V. They have been around together a good deal when he is in town. Patient tells of many invitations to go out with men.

HA/C

March 31.

Patient seen four times and writes. See letters. 3/4 patient wrote she was through with visitor and visitor did not go until 3/6 to see her. She continued to think she was abused in the telephone service, her chief grudge being that she could not reverse a business call because visitor was out. Thinks visitor could call her oftener. During month, patient has telephoned very little. Relationship continues strained through the month over telephone controversy, which patient insists is putting her down. She cites every instance when visitor said she was in a hurry or was out and enlarges on it.

Went with patient to see Mr. Mittelman, Vicar of St. Matthew's Church, and patient promises to go again and has already been to several services.

At work patient had $1 raise in pay with only two or three others in the shop, making $9 wage. She is saving money.

First of month Bertha Greenwood (also Social Service case) went to live across from patient. She had previously lived at Y. W. C. A. and old girls said horrid things about her so patient was snubbed for speaking to her. This lasted about ten days and is still a factor with patient's roommate, who now seldom speaks to her. Patient takes some pride in having befriended Bertha, who tells to patient untrue things about visitor and to visitor things which patient does not do.

April 30.

Patient seen three times. Early in month she talked of moving to a private family, but decided against it of her own accord. Reported that a girl in the house had offered her liquor last month.

After present of an Easter lily, patient was friendly and like herself until 4/24 she came unexpectedly in the evening and stayed 1½ hours. She was cross and sullen at first and would not look up. She criticized visitor

1917
and was very disagreeable. Later became jolly and chatty. Seemed to have come just to "let off steam" at some one and possibly to get a reaction from visitor, but visitor let her talk. She does not see brother, Bernard, now and plans not to visit there week-ends as she used to because she thinks he talks against her and dislikes her visits. Has not seen him since 3/25 at her mother's.

Patient says that last week she has taken a glass of porter every night (pays 5 cents for it). This week she has not taken it. She goes out and drinks it alone because it makes her sleep better. She has been restless and sleepless lately and has a loss of appetite. Patient promises not to drink at least to 4/30.

She is very discouraged and thinks visitor is only interested in order to find something on her to put her away. Has an idea which cannot be dispelled that visitor is a probation officer (view shared by Bertha Greenwood). Thinks she is followed by detectives because she has met the same man several successive mornings on the way to work. Another man was seen at Y. W. corner on several nights.

Patient was seen by Dr. Samuels, Out-Patient Department, 4/28, and had in the meanwhile written she would not drink again. 4/6 patient visits mother regularly on Sundays, but remains only 30 or 40 minutes and refuses to stay to meals. Patient was in a very disagreeable mood on last visit 4/1 and talked incessantly about quarrels with different girls at Y. W. C. A. Mother has not received any financial aid from patient since Christmas. For past two months patient has been cool and indifferent toward mother and sister. The sister usually met patient on way to business, but has not seen her during the past week. Both mother and sister are worried over the estrangement.
HA/C

May 31.
Patient seen 3 times. Was rather disagreeable 5/19 but the next day went to Marshfield Hills with visitor to see Fern Linnwood (also a Social Service case), a blind woman who was formerly her roommate. Patient is really devoted to her and suggests spending her vacation at the same house. Patient has been on excellent terms with visitor ever since. Does not put much trust in Bertha Greenwood, and sees as little of her as possible, but rooming across from her this is difficult to accomplish.

Patient would like to know if mother really needs her contribution. She would gladly give it, but has a feeling it is not wanted.
HA/C

June 15.
Patient seen twice. It is arranged that she will go 6/24 to Marshfield Hills with Fern Linnwood for her vacation at the rate of $7 a week. Patient has promised to room at the Y. W. C. A. during visitor's absence. The 1st of the month she insisted that she should live in a private family and while efforts were being made to find one patient changed her mind. She wrote that she realized if she came home tired she would make no effort to get proper food. See this and other letters.

Patient is friendly and responsive to visitor.
HA/C

July 5.
Patient seen at hospital. Patient says that she does not feel that her week's holiday rested her as much as it ought to have. Since coming back she has had a headache almost continually. She is quite sure this is from her eyes. She says she is going to see Dr. Nelson, an oculist on Irving

1917

Avenue, about them. Visitor urged her to go to the Bennett St. Dispensary and not spend so much money. She is skeptical of dispensaries. Patient says she may take three weeks' holiday soon, as work is slack and she feels the need of more rest. She would like to stay in her room and sleep and rest. She went to a dance Monday night at Nantasket with her young man friend. He is continually coming to see her and wanting her to go out with him. She finds him rather tiresome.
SPE/C

July 20.

Patient seen at work, 292 Nottingham Ave. Patient says the principal reason that she wanted to change her room was because her roommate was away and it was quite likely that a transient would be put with her. They are often brought in in the middle of the night and they are quite often girls that you cannot trust at all. Patient says that she has a nice room at the Y. W. C. A. and would hate to give it up as she feels as if it was quite like home. Says she will wait till Miss Bemis comes back and talks it over with her. Patient said she had spent a very happy Sunday with Fern Linnwood, a Social Service case. Patient seems to take a great interest in Bertha Greenwood and plans different things to keep her from getting into trouble. Patient did not seem as depressed as letter had indicated.
HA/C

Matron, Y. W. C. A., Mrs. Deneen, seen at 68 Warrenton St. Informant says as far as she knows patient has been going to her work and doing perfectly well in every way. A certain crowd of girls in the house were very noisy on Sunday, but there was no drinking. She knew patient was not in this crowd as she was away. Informant says she did not ask patient if she had been drinking as she does not know who it was. Informant thinks patient is very apt to exaggerate small incidents.

July 21.

Letter received from patient. See letter.
SPE/C

August 2.

Patient writes, asking advice in regard to medical examination. Family are anxious to have her see physician. Patient insists on woman physician.
MRW/C

August 6.

New England Hospital, O. P. D., telephoned to. Dr. Zearing reports no evening clinics.

August 7.

Dr. Margaret K. Deming telephoned to at 56 Chenoweth Road. Dr. Deming will see patient any Wednesday evening on her way home from work between 5–6:30 P. M. Will accept visitor's recommendation as to what fee should be.

Patient visited at Y. W. C. A. Patient very communicative and friendly. Talks much. Physical symptoms gone into. Nothing apparent save painful and too frequent menstruation with its accompanying depression. Patient thinks mother unnecessarily worried. Agrees to see Dr. Deming Wednesday evening, August 15, and give her frank history. Is rooming at present with Bertha Greenwood because she did not like transient who was put into her room. Hot weather created desire for drink, but claims she took nothing.
MRW/C

1917
August 8.
  Dr. Deming telephoned to.
MRW/C

August 13.
  Letter written to patient.

  Social summary sent to Dr. Margaret Deming.
MRW/C

August 14.
  Patient telephones in much disturbed condition because she has been told that Miss Bemis is not returning and feels that hospital has been trying to deceive her. Her point of view is that if the hospital lies to her in one thing it cannot be trusted in any. Situation finally explained after 10 or 15 minutes' conversation. Patient asks visitor to write Mrs. Deneen to see if it can be arranged for her to have a single room. Complains of being much upset by frequent arrival of transients.
MRW/C

August 15.
  Letter written to Mrs. Deneen, Y. W. C. A.
MRW/C

August 15.
  Telephoned to Dr. Margaret K. Deming, 56 Chenoweth Road. Dr. Deming reports that she gave a full physical examination to patient last evening and finds her lungs and heart negative. Patient eight pounds under weight. Dr. Deming considers that the pain experienced at the menstrual periods is due largely to her generally run-down physical condition. Has given her a tonic and is to see her again on September 5. If patient then continues to have much pain, Dr. Deming will give a local examination. Finds no evidence of any tubercular bone condition. Feels that patient is much relieved to learn this and also to know that her heart is normal. Patient paid Dr. Deming two dollars for the visit.
MRW/L

August 17.
  Letter received from patient. See letter.
MRW/L

August 17.
  Letter written to patient, urging her to follow Dr. Deming's directions conscientiously.
MRW/L

August 17.
  Letter written to Mrs. Deneen, Y. W. C. A., 68 Warrenton St., asking her, if possible, to arrange for patient to have a room by herself.
MRW/L

August 20.
  Letter from patient, stating that she is going to take a week off to rest. Liked Dr. Deming and is willing to do what she has advised. Is contented at the Y. W. C. A., although she still has occasionally longings to be with her own people. Dr. Deming has advised against this at present.
MRW/L

August 21.
  Patient seen at hospital. Mrs. Deneen has given patient a room by herself and she feels much better. Is resting this week, getting up late and going away for day trips. Agrees to see Dr. Dixon about her glasses soon.
MRW/L

1917
August 23.
   Letter from patient.
MRW/L

August 29.
   Letter from patient.   Seemed depressed.

   Letter to patient.
MRW/L

September 1.
   Letter from patient.
MRW/L

September 4.
   Letter from patient.
MRW/L

September 5.
   Letter to patient.
MRW/L

September 12.
   Patient seen at work during noon hour. Patient looked well and appeared in good spirits. Talked about several young men friends, especially about one named Young, whom she refused to say where she had met.
SPE/L

September 19.
   Patient seen at hospital. Patient appeared extremely "blue," played with her hands in a nervous way and cried. She said that she dreaded having the operation, but she supposed if it really would help her she would be willing to go through with it.
   Since she broke off with her friend, Young, she says a well-dressed man has been watching her on the street corner and making remarks to her. She has a feeling that this man may be a detective placed there by Young.
   Patient saw Dr. Harmon and after talking with him she appeared somewhat cheered.
SPE/L

September 25.
   Patient seen at hospital. Patient brought hat and shoes to be given away. She appeared in a much more cheerful mood since last seen in spite of the fact that a great family friend, whom she called uncle, had just died.
SPE/L

September 27.
   Dr. Simpson telephoned to. Informant said that the treatment that patient needed would only keep her in the hospital two or three days. After that she should have a week or two of convalescent care. Informant recommended patient going to the Massachusetts General Hospital, the Women's Free Hospital, or the New England Hospital.
SPE/L

   Patient seen at noon. Is willing to go to Massachusetts General Hospital for slight operation recommended by Dr. Simpson. She is very loath to go to a convalescent home for a week after, but finally consents to go to the country to board.
   She enjoys her single room at the Y. W. C. A. Her family are now treating her very well and she goes several times a week to see her mother. She has not been going out with the boys any during the summer. Has lost interest in such matters.

1917
　　Patient is entirely friendly and is in good spirits with the exception of believing that the matron, Mrs. Deneen, is not kindly disposed toward her.

　　Foreman, Mr. Simpson, seen at Doherty, Printers. It will be best for patient to be away the week of 10/15. He cannot readily spare her for this time, but is willing to do so in this case of sickness.
HA/L

October 13.
　　Patient writes several times, last two letters saying she has decided not to go to the Massachusetts General Hospital for the operation, as she has gotten the impression from a friend that this operation is a reflection upon her "character and her good name" and will "go against her" when she is married. Patient says that she intends to be married soon.

　　Patient seen at noon. Consents to go to the hospital when nature of operation is explained. Ingram Stone wishes her to be married soon. He is a man of 35, unmarried, and well able to support her. She has known him since her discharge from this hospital in 1915. Refused to introduce him to visitor.
HA/L

October 15.
　　Patient entered the Massachusetts General Hospital.
HA/L

October 16.
　　Mother seen at home. Patient has come in to see her every two weeks or month since last January. Last July she paid $1 for two or three weeks, but has not done so at any other time since January, 1917. She has taken no meals at the house with the exception of one breakfast. She has been fairly agreeable and not particularly troublesome. Mother seems to have a better conception of patient's needs and changeableness than previously, and to accept it as part of her character.
HA/L

　　Patient seen three or four times, and writes. October 15–21 patient was in the Massachusetts General Hospital for a slight gynecological operation. She paid $10 out of her own money for this. From Oct. 21–26 she was at home, going Oct. 26 to Marshfield Hills (Country Week paying fares), to spend the week-end with another patient, Fern Linnwood, a blind woman, formerly patient's roommate. She stayed only until the next day because of a disagreement with the boarding women. Fern later wrote a disagreeable letter, which has estranged patient from her. See letter.
　　Brother Bernard's wife had him arrested for abuse and non-support, and he was in jail a night in the end of October. Patient has been much upset over this. Agreement was made out of Court, and they are living together again.
　　Patient says that in the summer she went into Ukrane's Café, Pemberton Square, and ordered a drink. The waiter was a long time bringing it, and patient saw one speak to another, became suspicious that visitor had posted them not to serve her, but to get the police, and left hurriedly. She will not go back, and still thinks that visitor was in there to tell them.
　　Patient and Bertha Greenwood (another Social Service case) go several nights a week to a Soldiers' Mission on Isham Street.

November 15.
　　Patient's mother seen. She says that when patient was with them everything went well. Mother was given some army knitting to do, from which she is earning $2.30. They find it very hard to make both ends meet,

1917

especially as Florence's sewing season is dull, and living higher. Mother is not so well lately, and has pains in the side more often.

Patient seen four or five times, writes and telephones. Before Thanksgiving she drank something a couple of times, but did not tell visitor until two weeks later. She is most anxious to keep from it and will turn to some other visitor if she needs assistance in doing so.

She crocheted at the Mission, and was criticized by one of the men, so that she left. Patient has since been asked by the Matron, Mrs. Mentor, to return. She goes Saturday and Sunday evenings usually. Last Saturday she went with another girl to Underwood Chapel and stayed to Sunday School. Has not been to St. Matthew's church for several months, and no one has visited her from there, so that she thinks that she is not missed.

For the past two weeks, patient has been around evenings with Fannie Olson, who rooms across from her. She is a girl known to Miss Yonger, a social worker in the State House. Patient is afraid that she steals, so she will not go around the shops with her. They go to the Mission and Underwood Chapel.

HMA/A

November 15.

Patient's mother seen. She will write the Social Service if patient ever tries to move home, or makes any definite trouble. She is sometimes disagreeable to them, and on several occasions has spoken to Florence on the street. Her attitude is about as usual.

Brother Bernard now lives in Dover, Mass., to be nearer his employer, Introit Dillingham Electric Co.

See letters.

HA/S

December 31.

Case closed. Patient is doing well.

HA/S

1918

January 7.

Rev. Mr. Mittelman seen at St. Matthew's Church, Emmons St. Visitor tells informant that patient had not been going to St. Matthew's Church lately, but had been going to Underwood Chapel instead. Visitor asked informant if he would call on patient and get her interested in some organization. Informant did not remember patient's name, or know that she was a member of his church. He said he would be glad to do all he could for her. It was made known to informant that patient was a closed case to the hospital.

SPE/S

March 12.

Case reopened. Patient seen at hospital, said she was still living at Y. W. C. A., 68 Warrington St., but that she was very anxious to move. She is in debt to Y. W. C. A. for back room and board to the extent of $16 or $17, and would like to have arrangement made by which she could pay off this debt by paying $1 per week. Said she had between $40 and $50 in the bank, but did not want to take any money out as she was afraid she would never be able to save any more. Said she had become very intimate with a girl named Fannie Olson, who also lived at Y. W. C. A. Patient felt that this girl had bad influence over her. The girl steals, and spends a great deal of money for clothes. Patient tries to dress as well as Fannie Olson and consequently spends all her money for clothes. It was in this way that

1918
patient ran up bill at Y. W. C. A., as, instead of paying for board and room, she spent the money for clothes.

Patient seemed anxious to get a furnished room and take her meals out; thought it would be better for her to live alone, for when she lived with other girls she always got into difficulties. Said she had a married brother, Benjamin Farmer, living in North Dunning. She has always gotten along with him, although recently she has seen very little of him. Did not know whether they would consider giving her a home. Would like visitor to see them and will send visitor the exact address. Patient will stay at Y. W. C. A. until March 16. Is still working for Doherty Printers, 292 Nottingham Avenue, Boston, earning $10 a week.
MBH/H

Patient said she did not feel very well; had had a continuous cold all winter; said she was still subject to crying spells.
MBH/H

March 13.
Mrs. Dawson, Matron of Y. W. C. A., telephoned to. Said patient was a nice, quiet girl who gave no trouble in the house. Keeps to herself a great deal and has few friends in the house, although she is liked by everyone. To informant's knowledge, patient has not been drinking, and has been home a great deal, and has had several crying spells. Thought patient was in good condition physically, aside from a hard cold, which she had had all winter.

Informant said that patient and Fannie Olson had been very intimate, but quarreled about a month ago when a man who had been going with patient transferred his affections to Fannie. Patient and Fannie have not spoken since. Informant said Fannie was a very nice girl and did not believe patient's stories that Fannie stole could be true. Nothing had been taken from the house, and if Fannie was inclined to steal she would have excellent opportunity at the house.

Informant said that patient owed Y. W. C. A. a little over $16. Visitor asked if patient could pay this back in installments of $1 a week, to which informant readily agreed. Visitor told informant that patient was considering moving and informant was sorry to hear this, as she had enjoyed having patient in the house.
MBH/H

March 14.
See letter from patient.

March 14.
Inman House telephoned to. House is closing 3/30/18.

Gordon House telephoned to. Said they would not consider giving patient a room, as she had caused so much trouble when she was there formerly.
MBH/H

March 15.
Patient telephoned to. Said she had decided to stay at Y. W. C. A. Told her that arrangement had been made with Mrs. Dawson by which patient could pay $1 a week on her back board. Patient agrees to do this and said she would begin March 16. Said she liked living at Y. W. C. A. very much. The only reason she wished to move was because she thought Fannie Olson had bad influence on her. However, she has seen very little of Fannie lately, so did not feel it was necessary to move in order to get away from her.

1919
Mrs. Deneen, Matron Y. W. C. A., telephoned to. Told her that patient had decided not to move, and that she would begin paying back $1 a week on March 16. Informant said she was glad to have patient stay.
MBH/H

April 24.
Patient telephoned. Said she had been sick for a few days, but was now back at work. Said everything was going splendidly, both at work and at the Y. W. C. A. Said she was getting along well with the other girls, and seemed to be enjoying life very much. She is paying every week on her back board and now owes only about $10.
MBH/H

April 24.
Case closed.
MBH/H

June 9.
Case reopened. Patient interviewed at hospital. She came to talk over her job. She has been working steadily at the same job and living in the same place, but has recently become discouraged because she has had no advancement. She feels that the boss is hard on her and gives her a great deal more difficult and a greater amount of work than he gives to the other girls in the same department who have been there a shorter time and are earning more money. Seems quite depressed and discontented. Says that it is very difficult to get along on her present wage, which is still $10 a week.
Visitor advises patient to talk things over frankly with her Superintendent before giving up the job, asking him what he can do for her and calling to his attention the fact of how long she has been there. Patient promises to do this.
EW/MMM

June 11.
Patient telephones. States that she has talked with her Superintendent who could tell her nothing definite. Promises to see her again on June 14th and let her know the result.
EW/MMM

June 16.
Patient telephones. Says that the Superintendent was very nice to her and that he could not raise her wages until fall at any rate because the work was slack in the summer and he had to keep down expenses. States that he intended to raise all the girls' wages in the fall and will raise patient's. Meanwhile he gave her $6 surplus and promised to do what he could in this way during the summer, also to lighten her work somewhat.
EW/MMM

June 20.
Patient telephones. Things have been going fairly well as the Superintendent has lightened her work considerably and given the harder extra work to the other girls. She has not had overtime work since she spoke to him. She has not quite decided whether she will stay. Visitor advises her not to be precipitous in any case. Patient promises to let visitor know before she changes her job, or if she gets wind of any other position.
EW/MMM

APPENDIX B

SOCIAL SERVICE FORMS

Form I

PSYCHOPATHIC HOSPITAL
SOCIAL SERVICE
Memorandum Slip

Name   File number
Residence   O. P. D. number
Correspondent

Sex   Age   Color
Civil condition   Place and date of birth
Religion   Occupation
Time in Boston   In Mass.   In U. S.
Previous addresses

Name and address of father
Name and address of mother
Name and address of spouse
Names, addresses, and ages of children or siblings

Names and addresses of relatives or friends

Admitted to house   Authority
Discharged   Admitted to O. P. D.
Diagnosis   Examiner
Provisional diagnosis
Reason for referring to Social Service   Date
Report from the Confidential Exchange

Living conditions previous to admission

Remarks

                         Visitor's name

Form II

PSYCHOPATHIC HOSPITAL
SOCIAL SERVICE
Inquiry Slip

NAME OF PATIENT

DATE

CHECK WHEN DONE WITH INITIALS OF VISITOR	PERSONS TO BE SEEN (Give full name, address, and relationship to patient here and below)
	PERSONS TO BE TELEPHONED TO
	PERSONS TO BE WRITTEN TO

Form III

PSYCHOPATHIC HOSPITAL

SOCIAL SERVICE

Outline for History

I

Date
Name
Address
Age
Date and place of birth
Religion
Civil condition

Referred to hospital by
Brought by
Reason for coming
History obtained by

MEDICAL RECORD:
    Dates of admissions
    Dates of discharges
    Summary of physical examination
    Summary of mental examination
    Summary of intelligence tests
    Conduct on the wards
    Diagnosis
    Prognosis

SOCIAL HISTORY:

    Family:

Father		Address
Mother		Age and date of birth
		Nativity
Brothers and sisters	For each give	Religion
Spouse		Time in U. S., in state, in city
Children		Occupation
		Intelligence
		Character

    Date and place of marriage
    Other members of the household
    Attitude of the family toward patient
    Relatives

Social History:—Continued

Friends and References:
Friends, neighbors
Doctors, lawyers, clergymen
Institutions, courts, social agencies
Hospitals

Work:

Places of employment in chron-
ological order; and in each
{ Progress
Wages
Duration of the position
Character of associates

Recreation:
Opportunities
Companions

Schools (in order in which they were attended, with dates) :

Home and Neighborhood:
Character of locality (factory, business, tenement, suburban, etc.)
Character of street
Character of building
Character of the home } State as far as possible in specific term.
  (1) furnishings
  (2) neatness and cleanliness
Income and savings
Expenses — rent, insurance, benefit societies, etc.
Attitude of family toward their income

Habits of family in regard to eating and sleeping
Character of patient's bedroom (sleeps alone or with whom)
Character of patient's food

Physical History:
Developmental History:
Full term? Normal delivery?
Prenatal history:
  Work of mother during pregnancy
  Diseases of mother during pregnancy
  Injuries to mother during pregnancy
  Mental strain of mother during pregnancy
Birth weight
Feeding — breast or bottle
Age of sitting up
Age of first tooth
Age of creeping
Age of walking
Age of talking
Age of puberty
Illnesses:
  General
  Convulsions
  Injuries
  Hospital care

PHYSICAL HISTORY:—Continued

Personal Hygiene:
  Habits of sleeping (hours)
  Habits of eating
  Habits of bathing

Heredity:
  Relationship between parents
  Condition of health and cause of death of—
    Father
    Mother
    Sisters and brothers
    Maternal grandparents
    Paternal grandparents
    Uncles and aunts
  Tuberculosis, alcoholism, insanity, feeble-mindedness, epilepsy, or cancer
  Any mental or physical abnormalities in the family
  Any exceptional ability in the family

Physical Efficiency:
  Lazy or energetic?
  Frail or robust?
  How easily fatigued?
  Susceptibility to pain?

MENTAL HISTORY:

Education:
  Age of going to school
  School record
  Grade and age of leaving
  Special training (industrial, commercial, musical, etc.)
  Reading

Employment:
  Success or failure
  Reasons for resignations or discharges
  Patient's trade
  Work for which patient thinks he is best fitted

Disposition and Character:
  Likes and dislikes
  Habits
  Peculiarities
  Special abilities
  Attitude of patient toward his family
  Changes in character
  Onset of present trouble

SUMMARY:
  Social history
  Physical history
  Mental history

ANALYSIS OF SOCIAL SYMPTOMS

SOCIAL DIAGNOSIS

RECOMMENDATIONS IN REGARD TO —
  Social condition
  Physical condition
  Mental condition

II

HISTORY *(Interviews):*
  Patient's Story
  Statements of Others (with impression of informant at the end of each statement)

III

ACTION TAKEN *(Chronological record):*

SUMMARY OF RESULTS:

At the end of every three months $\begin{cases} \text{Social condition} \\ \text{Physical condition} \\ \text{Mental condition} \end{cases}$

APPENDIX C

LEGISLATION IN RELATION TO MENTAL DISEASE

FRANKWOOD E. WILLIAMS, M.D.

When hospitals for the insane were first opened in this country, admission to them was as informal and on the same basis as admission to any other hospital. Provision was made for the commitment by courts of those "so furiously mad as to be a danger to the community," but patients who desired admission or those whose friends desired admission for them were admitted freely.

During the early twenties of the nineteenth century, public interest in the care of the insane was aroused and states began to build public hospitals. This interest had come from England, where it had been shown that many of the insane if taken from the almshouses and jails, cages and pens, where many of the poorer were confined and neglected, and treated in proper hospitals, might be restored to reason. The object in building the state hospitals, therefore, was to provide this sort of care for those who could not otherwise afford it. The hospitals were regarded with great favor—the "state's greatest charity." It was believed that the earlier a patient could receive treatment the greater was the chance for his recovery and no obstacles, therefore, were put in the way of entrance to the hospital. On the contrary, the friends of patients, and patients themselves, were urged to come to the hospital as soon after the first signs of mental illness as possible; and when they came no question as to admission was raised except the possible one of an unoccupied bed.

This informality of admission continued, in Massachusetts, for example, for a period of forty-four years, or from the opening of the McLean Hospital in 1818 to 1862 when a law was passed requiring "in all cases the evidence and certificate of at least two reputable physicians . . . to establish the fact of insanity."

For some thirty years the hospitals had held the confidence of the community, but in the ten years previous to 1862 there had begun to develop a feeling first of disappointment and then of distrust. The disappointment was more or less warranted as the hospitals had not been able to bring about the happy results the community unfortunately had been led to expect; the distrust at this time was not warranted. Nevertheless, the fear became more or less general that patients were being wrongfully detained in hospitals and driven mad by their associates, that personal liberty was becoming of little consequence, and even that it might be possible to find two physicians who through interested motives might wrongfully certify to insanity, and that a superintendent might be bribed to keep the person in confinement. As a result, legal barriers were year by year built about the hospitals, until by 1874 the hospitals were almost completely isolated from the community; admission to them was a formal legal matter to be decided by court or jury. In consequence, admission was practically impossible for patients in the early stages of illness and the hospitals became asylums for the care of chronic patients about whose mental condition there could be no question, as it was obvious even to lay judges and juries.[1]

As the hospitals became more and more asylums for chronic patients, interest in them on the part of the medical profession lessened and the hospitals became the prey of the politician, positions in the hospitals from ward attendant and nurse to superintendent becoming the rightful spoils of successful candidates for public office. This situation obtained for many years and still obtains in certain states.

Legislatures that had been so aroused against the hospitals in 1874 had learned by 1882 that they had been badly advised; that it was to the interest neither of the community nor the patient to deny to the patient the only possible help there was for him until such time as his illness had become so chronic that any hope that there might have been in the first place was largely lost. A period of constructive legislation began about this time. Some states still have on their statute books the laws passed in this period of distrust, but in the past forty years many of the states have rewritten their "insanity laws" and in this rewriting two main objects have been kept in mind—to remove the hospitals from the field of political spoils and to place them in the hands of reputable physicians whose qualifications are their professional skill and knowledge of the special problems involved; and to make the hospitals as accessible as possible to those who may need them in order that the hospitals may serve their communities effectively. This desire to bring the hospitals back into the communities as dynamic forces in the interest of public health has been greatly increased in the past few years by the knowledge that has come from medical and social

[1] Legislation for the insane in Massachusetts with particular reference to the voluntary and temporary care laws. By Frankwood E. Williams, M.D. *Boston Medical and Surgical Journal*, vol. 173, no. 20, Nov. 11, 1915. Publication No. 5 of the Massachusetts Society for Mental Hygiene.

investigations showing the relationship that frequently exists between mental disease and defect and asocial conduct and likewise by medical research that has made possible a clearer conception of the nature of mental disease and indicated means by which such disease may be not only cured but avoided.' The barriers, therefore, that had unwisely been built about the hospitals until their usefulness had been largely destroyed are now being rapidly removed and the hospitals from being institutions of horror are becoming institutions of hope; professional skill of a very special kind instead of being locked inert within hospital walls is being brought through out-patient departments and social service departments out into the community where it can be of great service; and the community instead of drawing away in fear is seeking from the hospitals advice both in personal and community matters.

This development has been slow, although more rapid of recent years, and has developed differently and at a different pace in different states so that one may now find in this country an illustration of almost any stage from the more or less completely isolated and politically controlled asylum of the sixties and seventies to the most modern type of hospital scientifically equipped and staffed, with its social service and out-patient departments radiating to all points in its locality and its advice sought on many different matters.

In bringing about this accessibility of the hospitals three laws have been found particularly useful. These are known as the Voluntary Care, the Temporary Care, and the Observation Laws. In Massachusetts a fourth law, known as the Boston Police Law, has been found very useful.

Provision for the reception of voluntary patients in state and private hospitals has been made in the following twenty-nine states: California, Colorado, Connecticut, Georgia, Illinois, Indiana, Kansas, Maine, Maryland, Massachusetts, Michigan, Minnesota, Mississippi, Missouri, New Hampshire, New Jersey, New York, North Carolina, Ohio, Oklahoma, Oregon, Pennsylvania, Rhode Island, South Carolina, South Dakota, Vermont, Virginia, West Virginia, and Wisconsin.

The law ususally provides that the patient must sign an application for admission, that his mental condition must be such that he can understand the nature of this request as well as the need of treatment, and that he must be released on a demand in writing in from three to seven days after such application. In the case of six of these states his request for admission must be accompanied by the certificate of one or two physicians, and in some instances his application must be signed in the presence of a physician.

Fifteen states and the District of Columbia have laws authorizing commitment for temporary care and observation. They are Connecticut, Illinois, Maine, Massachusetts, Michigan, Minnesota, New Jersey, New York, North Carolina, Oklahoma, Pennsylvania, South Carolina, Tennessee, Washington, and Wisconsin.[1]

The best examples of Temporary Care Laws are probably those of Massachusetts, and they may well be used as illustrations here. Aside from the law permitting voluntary admission, Massachusetts has three laws that make it possible for a patient to obtain hospital care and treatment without formal court procedure and a fourth law under which the legal formalities are slight.

1. *Temporary Care Law* (Chapter 174, Acts 1915). This law provides that a superintendent may, when requested by a physician, by a member of the board of health or a police officer of a city or town, by an agent of the institutions-registration department of the city of Boston, or by a member of the district police, receive and care for in such hospital as a patient for a period not exceeding ten days, any person who needs immediate care and treatment because of mental derangement other than delirium tremens or drunkenness. Such patients are received on application in writing filed at the time of reception of the patient or within twenty-four hours thereafter and must be discharged or committed within ten days unless they make a request for voluntary care. This law is useful both as an emergency law and as an observation law as under it physicians may bring to the hospital for examination and advice patients about whose condition they have reason to be concerned, but whom they do not sufficiently understand to warrant a formal application for commitment as insane or those patients who, although clearly "insane" in a medical sense, are in such an early stage of their illness that a formal commitment would not be possible. Treatment is therefore provided at a time when it is likely to be of greatest help, but which could not be obtained except for the provisions of this law. The value of the law as an aid in restoring health and preventing chronic illness can scarcely be overestimated.

2. *Emergency Law* (Section 42, Chapter 504, Acts 1909). The superintendent of a hospital may receive and detain, for not more than five days without a court order, any person "certified to be one of violent and dangerous insanity or of other emergency" by two qualified medical examiners. Officers authorized to serve criminal processes, or police officers, must, on the request of the applicant or one of the examining physicians, bring such a person to the hospital. The applicant for this form of admission must within five days arrange for the commitment of the person so

---

[1] Laws controlling commitments to state hospitals for mental diseases, by James V. May, M.D., *Mental Hygiene*, vol. 5, no. 3, July, 1921.

received, or for his removal from the hospital. This law makes it unnecessary in an emergency to "arrest" a sick individual as a criminal and confine him in a local jail until such time as it may be possible to bring him before a court for commitment. Courts are frequently not in session at the time an individual becomes ill. When holidays fall at the end or the beginning of the week there may be several days without a session of the court. Through the provisions of this law, the patient may be brought at once to the hospital where he can be properly cared for until such time as the court may convene.

3. *Observation Law* (Chapter 145, Acts 1919). A person found by two qualified examiners to be in such mental condition that his commitment to a hospital is necessary for his proper care or observation may be committed to a state hospital for a period of thirty-five days pending the determination of his insanity. This law is particularly useful in legal and criminal proceedings in which the question of mental condition is raised. It is useful also in difficult cases in which more time is needed for a determination of the patient's mental condition than is provided in the Temporary Care Law.

4. *Boston Police Law* (Chapter 307, Acts 1910). Under the provisions of this law all persons suffering from "delirium, mania, mental confusion, delusions, or hallucinations under arrest or who come under the care or protection of the police of the city of Boston, shall be taken to the Boston Psychopathic Hospital in the same manner in which persons afflicted with other diseases are taken to a general hospital." Cases suffering from delirium tremens or drunkenness may be refused by the hospital authorities; otherwise all such persons are admitted, observed and cared for until they can be committed or admitted to the hospital or institution appropriate in each particular case unless the patient recovers or is discharged. Chapter 394 of the Acts of 1911 is complementary to the above in that it provides that no person suffering from insanity, mental derangement, delirium, or mental confusion, except delirium tremens or drunkenness, shall, except in an emergency, be placed or detained in a lockup, police station, city prison, house of detention, jail or other penal institution or place for the detention of criminals. If, in case of emergency, any such person is so placed or detained, he shall forthwith be examined by a physician and shall be furnished suitable medical care and nursing and shall not be detained for more than twelve hours. In Boston these patients are sent to the Psychopathic Hospital. In other parts of the state they are cared for by the board of health of the city or town in question until they can be admitted to a state hospital or cared for by relatives or friends.

A very considerable use of the voluntary and temporary care laws is made in Massachusetts. In fact, the temporary care laws have very largely determined the legal status of patients admitted to the Boston Psychopathic Hospital. During a period of six years, 6,499 patients, 57.5 per cent of all admissions, were admitted under the "ten-day" temporary care law. Nine thousand and seventy-four, or 80.3 per cent of the total number of admissions during the same period, were temporary-care patients of one kind or another. The voluntary patients represented 17.6 per cent of the 11,289 patients during the period.[1]

At the request of the Surgeon General of the United States Army, who during the war found embarrassing the lack of uniformity in the various state commitment laws, the National Committee for Mental Hygiene appointed in 1919 a special committee to make a study of the various state laws and to recommend such provisions as it seemed desirable to incorporate in a modern commitment law. The committee was composed of Dr. George M. Kline, Commissioner, Massachusetts State Department of Mental Disease; Dr. Charles W. Pilgrim, Chairman of the New York State Hospital Commission; Dr. Owen Copp, Superintendent, Pennsylvania Hospital, Department for Nervous and Mental Diseases; Dr. Frank P. Norbury of the Board of Public Welfare Commissioners of Illinois; and Major Frankwood E. Williams of the Office of the Surgeon General, Washington, D. C. The committee recommended in its report voluntary commitment, temporary care, emergency commitment, and commitment for observation.

[1] Laws controlling commitments to state hospitals for mental diseases, by James V. May, M.D., *Mental Hygiene*, vol. 5, no. 3, July, 1921.

BIBLIOGRAPHY

ABBOTT, EDITH and BRECKINRIDGE, SOPHONISBA. "The Delinquent Child and the Home." New York, Russell Sage Foundation, 1912.

ADDAMS, JANE. "The Spirit of Youth and the City Streets." New York, The Macmillan Company, 1914.

ADLER, HERMAN M. "Cook County and the Mentally Handicapped. A Study of the Provisions for Dealing with Mental Problems in Cook County, Ill." New York, National Committee for Mental Hygiene, 1918. Publication 13.

————. "A Psychiatric Contribution to the Study of Delinquency," *Journal of the American Institute of Criminal Law and Criminology*, May, 1917.

————. "Unemployment and Personality: A Study of Psychopathic Cases," *Mental Hygiene*, v. i, pp. 16–24, January, 1917.

————. "Medical Science and Criminal Justice." Section 5 of Report of the Cleveland Foundation's Survey of Criminal Justice. Cleveland, 1922.

————. "Organization of Psychopathic Work in the Criminal Courts," *Journal of the American Institute of Criminal Law and Criminology*, v. 8, pp. 362–374, 1917.

American Academy of Political and Social Science Annals, v. 72, whole no. 166, March, 1918. Social Work in Families. Edited by Frank D. Watson.

ANDERSON, V. V. "Mental Disease and Delinquency: A Report of a Special Committee of the New York State Commission on Prisons," *Mental Hygiene*, v. 3, pp. 177–198, April, 1919.

BACON, FRANCIS. "Novum Organum: or True Suggestions for the Interpretation of Nature." London, Routledge, 1893.

BALL, JAU DON. "Correlation of Neurology, Psychiatry, Psychology, and General Medicine as Scientific Aids to Industrial Efficiency," *American Journal of Insanity*, v. 75, pp. 521–55, April, 1919.

BARKER, LEWELLYS F. "The First Ten Years of the National Committee for Mental Hygiene, With Some Comments on its Future," *Mental Hygiene*, v. 2, No. 4, pp. 557–581, October, 1918.

BEISSER, PAUL T. "Social Work: An Outline of Its Professional Aspects." New York, American Association of Social Workers, 1922.

BERNHEIM, HIPPOLYTE. "Suggestive Therapeutics: A Treatise on the Nature and Uses of Hypnotism." Translated by Christian A. Herter. New York, G. P. Putnam's Sons, 1895.

BEVERIDGE, WILLIAM H. "Unemployment: A Problem of Industry." London, Longmans, Green & Company, 1912.

BINGHAM, ANNE T. "The Personal Problems of a Group of Workers," *Proceedings of the National Conference of Social Work*, 1920.

BOGARDUS, EMORY S. "History of Social Thought." Los Angeles, University of Southern California Press, 1922.

———. "Problems in Teaching Sociology," *Journal of Applied Sociology*, v. 6, No. 2, pp. 19–24, December, 1921.

BOSANQUET, HELEN. "The Family." London, The Macmillan Company, 1906.

BRECKINRIDGE, SOPHONISBA P. and ABBOTT, EDITH. "The Delinquent Child and the Home." New York, Russell Sage Foundation, 1912.

BRIGGS, L. VERNON. "The History of the Psychopathic Hospital of Boston, Massachusetts." (To be published.)

———. "The Manner of Man That Kills: Spencer—Czolgosz—Richeson." Boston, Badger, 1921.

BRILL, A. A. "Fundamental Conceptions of Psychoanalysis." New York, Harcourt, Brace & Company, 1921.

BRISTOL, LUCIUS MOODY. "Social Adaptation: A Study in the Development of the Doctrine of Adaptation as a Theory of Social Progress." Cambridge, Harvard University Press, 1915.

BRONNER, AUGUSTA F. "A Method of Case Presentation," *The Family*, v. 3, pp. 37–48, April, 1922.

———. "Psychology of Special Abilities and Disabilities." Boston, Little, Brown & Company, 1917.

BRONNER, AUGUSTA F. and HEALY, WILLIAM. "Case Studies." Series of twenty. Boston, Judge Baker Foundation, 1922.

BROWN, MABEL W. and WILLIAMS, FRANKWOOD E. "Neuropsychiatry and the War: A Bibliography with Abstracts." New York, National Committee for Mental Hygiene, 1918.

BURGESS, ERNEST W. and PARK, ROBERT E. "Introduction to the Science of Sociology." Chicago, University of Chicago Press, 1922.

BURNHAM, WILLIAM H. "Health Examination at School Entrance," *Journal of the American Medical Association*, v. 68, pp. 893–899, March 24, 1917. Massachusetts Society for Mental Hygiene, Publication 27.

———. "The Significance of the Conditioned Reflex in Mental Hygiene," *Mental Hygiene*, v. 5, pp. 673–706, October, 1921.

———. "Success and Failure as Conditions of Mental Health," *Mental Hygiene*, v. 3, pp. 387–397, July, 1919.

BYINGTON, MARGARET F. "The Confidential Exchange: A Form of Social Coöperation." New York, Russell Sage Foundation, 1912.
———. "What Social Workers Should Know About Their Own Communities," 3rd edition. New York, Russell Sage Foundation, 1916.
CABOT, RICHARD C. "Social Service and the Art of Healing." New York, Moffat, Yard & Company, 1909.
———. "Social Work: Essays on the Meeting-Ground of Doctor and Social Worker." New York, Houghton, Mifflin Company, 1919.
———. "Some Functions of Social Work in Hospitals," *Modern Hospital*, v. 4, pp. 188–191, March, 1915.
CAMPBELL, C. MACFIE. "Experiences of the Child: How They Affect Character and Behavior," *Mental Hygiene*, v. 4, pp. 312–319, April, 1920.
———. "Mental Health of the Community and the Work of the Psychiatric Dispensary,'' *Mental Hygiene*, v. 1, pp. 572–584, October, 1917.
———. "Nervous Children and Their Training," *Mental Hygiene*, v. 3, pp. 16–23, January, 1919.
———. "Psychiatric Contribution to Educational Problems," *Transactions of the Fourth International Congress on School Hygiene*, 1913.
CANNON, IDA M. "Social Work in Hospitals." New York, Russell Sage Foundation, 1913.
CANNON, M. ANTOINETTE. "Health Problems of the Foreign Born from the Point of View of the Hospital Social Worker," *Proceedings of the National Conference of Social Work*, 1920.
CANNON, WALTER B. "Bodily Changes in Pain, Hunger, Fear, and Rage: An Account of Recent Researches into the Function of Emotional Excitement." New York, D. Appleton and Company, 1920.
CARVER, THOMAS NIXON. "Essays in Social Justice." Cambridge, Harvard University Press, 1915.
———. "Sociology and Social Progress." Boston, Ginn & Company, 1905.
CHAPIN, F. STUART. "Field Work and Social Research." New York, The Century Co., 1920.
CLARK, L. PIERCE. "Treatment of the Epileptic Based on a Study of Fundamental Make-up," *Journal of American Medical Association*, v. 70, pp. 357–362, February 9, 1918.
Cleveland Foundation. Report of Survey of Criminal Justice directed by Roscoe Pound and Felix Frankfurter. Cleveland, 1922.
COBB, STANLEY. "Applications of Psychiatry to Industrial Hygiene," *Journal of Industrial Hygiene*, v. 1, pp. 343–347, November, 1919.

COLCORD, JOANNA C. "Broken Homes: A Study of Family Desertion and Its Social Treatment." New York, Russell Sage Foundation, 1919.

COPP, OWEN. "Community Organization for Mental Hygiene," Proceedings of National Conference of Social Work, 1917.

CURTIS, HANNAH. "Functions of Social Service in State Hospitals," Boston Medical and Surgical Journal, v. 175, pp. 271–275, August 24, 1916. Reprinted by Massachusetts Society for Mental Hygiene.

CUTLER, JAMES ELBERT. "Training for Social Work: The Correlation of the Profession of Social Work and the University in the Control of Training Schools." Published by School of Applied Social Sciences, Western Reserve University, Cleveland. Address at the meeting of the Association of Training Schools for Professional Social Work, Pittsburgh, December 30, 1921.

DAVIS, MICHAEL M. and WARNER, ANDREW R. "Dispensaries: Their Management and Development." New York, The Macmillan Company, 1918.

DERCUM, FRANCIS XAVIER. "A Clinical Manual of Mental Diseases," 2nd edition, revised. Philadelphia, W. B. Saunders Company, 1917.

———. "Rest, Mental Therapeutics, Suggestion." Philadelphia, Blakiston's Son & Company, 1903.

DEWEY, JOHN. "Human Nature and Conduct. An Introduction to Social Psychology." New York, Henry Holt & Company, 1922.

DEWEY, JOHN, and TUFTS, JAMES H. "Ethics." New York, Henry Holt & Company, 1908.

DONOHOE, MARIE L. "A Social Service Department in a State Hospital," Mental Hygiene, v. 6, No. 2, pp. 306–311, April, 1922.

EDER, M. D. "War Shock." Philadelphia, Blakiston's Son & Company, 1918

ELWOOD, CHARLES A. "Sociology in its Psychological Aspects," 2nd edition. New York, D. Appleton & Company, 1915.

EMERSON, CHARLES P. "Essentials of Medicine: A Textbook of Medicine for Students Beginning a Medical Course, for Nurses, and for Mothers Interested in the Care of the Sick," 3rd edition. Philadelphia, Lippincott Company, 1915.

EMERSON, HAVEN. "The Place of Mental Hygiene in the Public Health Movement," Mental Hygiene, v. 6, No. 2, pp. 225–233, April, 1922.

The Family (monthly). New York, American Association for Organizing Family Social Work, March, 1920—date.

FARMER, GERTRUDE. "A Form of Record for Hospital Social Work." Philadelphia, Lippincott Company, 1921.

FERNALD, WALTER E. "Burden of Feeble-mindedness." Boston, Massachusetts Society for Mental Hygiene, 1912. Publication 4.

———. "Growth of Provision for the Feeble-minded in the United States," *Mental Hygiene,* v. 1, pp. 34–57, January, 1917.

———. "An Out-patient Clinic in Connection with a State Institution for the Feeble-minded," *Mental Hygiene,* v. 4, pp. 848–856, April, 1917.

———. "Standardized Fields of Inquiry for Clinical Studies of Borderline Defectives," *Mental Hygiene,* v. 1, pp. 211–234, April, 1917.

———. "State Program for the Care of the Mentally Defective," *Mental Hygiene,* v. 3, pp. 566–574, October, 1919.

———. "What is Practicable in the Way of Prevention of Mental Defect," *Proceedings of National Conference of Social Work,* 1918.

FISHER, BOYD. "Has Mental Hygiene a Practical Use in Industry?" *Mental Hygiene,* v. 5, pp. 479–496, July, 1921.

FLEXNER, ABRAHAM. "Is Social Work a Profession?" *Proceedings of the National Conference of Social Work,* 1915.

———. "Medical Education in the United States and Canada: A Report to the Carnegie Foundation for the Advancement of Teaching." New York, 1910.

FOCH, FERDINAND. "The Principles of War." New York, H. K. Fly Company, 1918.

FRANKFURTER, FELIX. "Social Work and Professional Training." *Proceedings of the National Conference of Social Work,* 1915.

FRAZER, J. G. "The Golden Bough: A Study in Magic and Religion," 3rd edition. 7 pts. in 12 vols. London, Macmillan & Company, 1911–15.

FRINK, H. W. "Morbid Fears and Compulsions: Their Psychology and Psychoanalytic Treatment." New York, Moffat Yard & Company, 1918.

GAGE, HARRIET. "Place of Psychiatric Social Work in the Social Service Field," *Hospital Social Service,* v. 4, pp. 143–149, September, 1921.

GESELL, ARNOLD. "Mental Hygiene and the Public School," *Mental Hygiene,* v. 3, pp. 4–10, January, 1919.

GILLIN, JOHN LEWIS. "Poverty and Dependency: Their Relief and Prevention." New York, The Century Company, 1921.

GLUECK, BERNARD. "Concerning Prisoners," *Mental Hygiene,* v. 2, pp. 177–218, April, 1918.

———. "Recent Progress in Determining the Nature of Crime and the Character of Criminals," *National Conference of Social Work,* 1917.

GLUECK, BERNARD. "Special Preparation of the Psychiatric Social Worker," *Mental Hygiene*, v. 3, pp. 409–419, July, 1919.

――――. "Studies in Forensic Psychiatry." Boston, Little, Brown & Company, 1916. Criminal Science Monograph 2.

――――. "Types of Delinquent Careers," *Mental Hygiene*, v. 1, pp. 171–195, April, 1917.

GODDARD, HENRY H. "Feeble-mindedness: Its Causes and Consequences." New York, The Macmillan Company, 1914.

――――. "Human Efficiency and Levels of Intelligence." Princeton, Princeton University Press, 1920.

GOLDMARK, JOSEPHINE C. "Fatigue and Efficiency: A Study in Industry," 3rd edition. New York, Survey Associates, 1913.

GROSS, H. J. A. "Criminal Psychology: A Manual for Judges, Practitioners, and Students." Boston, Little, Brown & Company, 1911.

HALE, DOROTHY Q. "Inadequate Social Examinations in Psychopathic Clinics," *Mental Hygiene*, v. 5, pp. 794–806, October, 1921.

HALL, G. STANLEY. "Adolescence." New York, D. Appleton & Company, 1904.

HART, BERNARD. "Psychology of Insanity." New York, Putnam's Sons, 1914.

HAYES, ELIZABETH C. "Case Correspondence: A Method of Psychiatric Social Work," *Mental Hygiene*, v. 6, pp. 125–155, January, 1922.

HEALY, WILLIAM. "Honesty: A Study of the Causes and Treatment of Dishonesty Among Children." Indianapolis, Bobbs-Merrill Co., 1915.

――――. "The Individual Delinquent: A Test-book of Diagnosis and Prognosis for All Concerned in Understanding Offenders." Boston, Little, Brown & Company, 1915.

――――. "Mental Conflicts and Misconduct." Boston, Little, Brown & Company, 1917.

――――. "The Practical Value of Scientific Study of Juvenile Delinquents." Washington, U. S. Children's Bureau, 1922.

――――. "Psychiatry, Psychology, Psychologists, Psychiatrists," *Mental Hygiene*, v. 6, No. 2, pp. 248–256, April, 1922.

HEALY, WILLIAM and BRONNER, AUGUSTA F. "Case Studies." Series of twenty. Boston, Judge Baker Foundation, 1922.

HENRY, EDNA G. "The Sick," *Annals of the American Academy of Political and Social Science*, v. 77, pp. 45–59, May, 1918.

HOCH, AUGUST and AMSDEN, GEORGE S. "A Guide to the Descriptive Study of the Personality." New York State Hospital Bulletin, November, 1913.

HOCKING, WILLIAM ERNEST. "Human Nature and its Remaking." New Haven, Yale University Press, 1918.

HOLLINGWORTH, H. L. "Vocational Psychology: Its Problems and Methods." New York, D. Appleton & Company, 1916.

JAMES, WILLIAM. "Psychology." New York, Henry Holt & Company, 1892.

———. "The Varieties of Religious Experience: A Study in Human Nature." New York, Longmans, Green & Company, 1902.

JARRETT, MARY C. "Applications of Sociology in Psychiatry." Chap. 10 of "Manual of Psychiatry," edited by A. J. Rosanoff. New York, Wiley & Sons, 1920.

———. "Function of the Social Service of the Psychopathic Hospital, Boston," *Boston Medical and Surgical Journal*, v. 170, pp. 987–993, June 25, 1914.

———. "Further Notes on the Economic side of Psychopathic Social Service," *Boston Medical and Surgical Journal*, v. 171, pp. 852–854, December 3, 1914.

———. "Intensive Group of Social Service Cases," *Boston Medical and Surgical Journal*, v. 175, pp. 824–830, December 7, 1916.

———. "Mental Hygiene of Industry: Report of Progress on Work Undertaken under the Engineering Foundation of New York," *Mental Hygiene*, v. 14, No. 4, October, 1920.

———. "Possibilities in Social Service for Psychopathic Patients," *Boston Medical and Surgical Journal*, v. 176, pp. 201–204, February 8, 1917.

———. "Psychiatric Social Work," *Mental Hygiene*, v. 2, pp. 283–290, April, 1918.

———. "Psychiatric Thread Running Through All Social Case Work," *Mental Hygiene*, v. 3, pp. 210–219, April, 1919.

———. "The Psychopathic Employee: A Problem of Industry," *Medicine and Surgery*, v. 1, pp. 727–741, September, 1917.

———. "Shell-Shock Analogues: Neuroses in Civil Life Having a Sudden or Critical Origin," *Medicine and Surgery*, v. 2, pp. 266–280, March, 1918.

———. "The Significance of Psychiatric Social Work," *Mental Hygiene*, v. 5, pp. 509–518, July, 1921.

———. "War Neuroses After the War: Extra-Institutional Preparation," *Proceedings of National Conference of Social Work*, 1918.

JELLIFFE, S. E., and WHITE, W. A. "Diseases of the Nervous System: A Text-book of Neurology and Psychiatry," 2nd edition, revised and enlarged. Philadelphia, Lea and Febiger, 1917.

JUNG, C. G. "Psychology of the Unconscious." Authorized translation. New York, Moffat, Yard & Company, 1916.

KAMMERER, PERCY G. "The Unmarried Mother: A Study of Five Hundred Cases." Boston, Little, Brown & Company, 1918.

KELLOG, THEODORE H. "A Text-Book of Mental Diseases." New York, 1897.

KEMPF, E. J. "Autonomic Functions of the Personality." New York, Nervous and Mental Disease Publishing Company, 1918.

KIMBALL, EVERETT. "The National Government of the United States." Boston, Ginn & Company, 1920.

――――. "State and Municipal Government in the United States." Boston, Ginn & Company, 1922.

KING, W. L. MACKENZIE. "Industry and Humanity: A Study in the Principles Underlying Industrial Reconstruction." Boston, Houghton, Mifflin Company, 1918.

KLINE, GEORGE M. "Function of the Social Worker in Relation to a State Program," *Proceedings of National Conference of Social Work*, 1919; also in *Mental Hygiene*, October, 1919.

――――. "Social Service in the State Hospitals," *American Journal of Insanity*, v. 73, pp. 567–581, April, 1917.

KLINE, LILA. "Personal Psychiatric History," *Mental Hygiene*, v. 6, pp. 93–124, January, 1922.

KOBER, GEORGE MARTIN, and HANSON, WILLIAM CLINTON. "Diseases of Occupation and Vocational Hygiene." Philadelphia, Blackiston's Son & Company, 1916.

KRAEPELIN, EMIL. "Psychiatrie: Ein Lehrbuch fur Studirende und Aerzte," 5 Auflage. Leipzig, Barth, 1896.

KROPOTKIN, P. "Mutual Aid: A Factor in Evolution," revised edition. London, Heinemann, 1904.

LEE, JOSEPH. "Play in Education." New York, The Macmillan Company, 1916.

MACCURDY, J. T. "Psychiatric Clinics in the Schools," *American Journal of Public Health*, v. 6, pp. 1265–1271, December, 1916.

――――. "War Neuroses." Cambridge, Eng., University Press, 1918. Also, Psychiatric Bulletin, v. 2, pp. 243–354, July, 1917.

MACDONALD, J. B. "Community Value of the Out-Patient Department of the Hospital for the Insane," *Mental Hygiene*, v. 1, pp. 266–73, April, 1917. Massachusetts Society for Mental Hygiene, Publication No. 28.

McDOUGALL, WILLIAM. "An Introduction to Social Psychology." Boston, Luce, 1918.

――――. "The Group Mind: A Sketch of the Principles of Collective Psychology with Some Attempt to Apply Them to the Interpretation of National Life and Character." New York, G. P. Putnam's Sons, 1920.

MAGNAN, VALENTINE. "De l'alcoholisme, des diverses formes du délire alcoholique et de leur traitement." Paris, Delahaye, 1874.

MAROT, HELEN. "Creative Impulse in Industry: A Proposition for Educators." New York, E. P. Dutton & Company, 1918.

Mental Hygiene (quarterly). New York, National Committee for Mental Hygiene, January, 1917—date.

"A Mental Hygiene Primer": A Series of Brief Articles on the Symptoms and Especially the Prevention of the More Common Types of Mental Disorders. Boston, Massachusetts Society for Mental Hygiene, 1922.

MERZ, JOHN THEODORE. "A History of European Thought in the Nineteenth Century." Edinburgh and London, W. Blackwood & Sons, 1903–1914.

MEYER, ADOLF. "The Right to Marry: What Can a Democratic Civilization Do about Heredity and Child Welfare?" *Mental Hygiene*, v. 3, pp. 48–58, January, 1919. Originally printed in the *Survey*, v. 36, pp. 243–246, June 3, 1916.

MÜNSTERBERG, HUGO. "Psychology and Industrial Efficiency." Boston, Houghton Mifflin Company, 1913.

MYERSON, ABRAHAM. "The Foundations of Personality." Boston, Little, Brown & Company, 1921.

———. "The Nervous Housewife." Boston, Little, Brown, & Company, 1920.

———. "Psychiatric Family Studies," *American Journal of Insanity*, v. 73, pp. 355–486, January, 1917.

———. "Psychiatric Family Studies," Second Paper, *American Journal of Insanity*, v. 74, pp. 497–554, April, 1918.

———. "The Psychiatric Social Worker." Massachusetts Commission on Mental Diseases. Bulletin, v. 3, No. 2, pp. 113–217, April, 1919.

NEFF, IRWIN H. "Inebriety and How to Control It," *Boston Medical and Surgical Journal*, v. 176, pp. 337–341, March 8, 1917.

ORDWAY, MABEL D., and RYTHER, MARGHERITA. "Economic Efficiency of Epileptic Patients," *Journal of Nervous and Mental Diseases*, v. 47, No. 5, May, 1918.

OSLER, WILLIAM. "Principles and Practice of Medicine," 8th edition. New York, Appleton, 1918.

PARK, ROBERT E. and BURGESS, ERNEST W. "Introduction to the Science of Sociology." Chicago, University of Chicago Press, 1922.

PARKER, CARLTON H. "The Casual Laborer and Other Essays." New York, Harcourt, Brace & Howe, 1920.

PARKER, CORNELIA STRATTON. "An American Idyll: The Life of Carleton H. Parker." Boston, Atlantic Monthly Press, 1919.

PARMALEE, M. F. "Science of Human Behavior: Biological and Physiological Foundations." New York, The Macmillan Company. 1913.

PINEL, PH. "Nosographie philosophique ou la methode de l'analyse appliqué à la médecine." Paris, Brosson, 1818.

POUND, ROSCOE. "Criminal Justice in the American City." Section 8 of Report of the Cleveland Foundation's Survey of Criminal Justice. Cleveland, 1922.

————. "Individual Interests in the Domestic Relations," *Michigan Law Review*, v. 14, January, 1916.

————. "Interests of Personality," *Harvard Law Review*, February and March, 1915.

————. "The Future of the Criminal Law," *Columbia Law Review*, v. 21, January, 1921.

————. "Social Problems and the Courts," *American Journal of Sociology*, v. 18, November, 1912.

————. "A Theory of Social Interests," *Proceedings of the American Sociological Society*, v. 15, May, 1921.

POWERS, MARGARET J. "The Industrial Cost of the Psychopathic Employee," *Proceedings of the National Conference of Social Work*, 1920.

PUSEY, W. ALLEN. "Syphilis As a Modern Problem." Chicago, American Medical Association, 1915.

QUETELET, L. A. J. "Physique sociale, un essai sur le dévelopement des facultés de l'homme." Bruxelles, Muquardt, 1869.

RALPH, GEORGIA G. "Elements of Record Keeping for Child-Helping Organizations." New York, Russell Sage Foundation, 1915.

RAY, ISAAC. "Mental Hygiene." Boston, Ticknor & Fields, 1863.

READ, THOMAS T. "The Employment Manager and the Reduction of Labor Turnover," *Proceedings of the American Institute of Mining Engineers*, February, 1918.

REDLICH, JOSEF. "The Common Law and the Case Method: A Report to the Carnegie Foundation for the Advancement of Teaching." New York, 1914.

RICHMOND, MARY E. "Social Diagnosis." New York, Russell Sage Foundation, 1917.

————. "What is Social Case Work: An Introductory Description." New York, Russell Sage Foundation, 1922.

ROBESON, F. E. "A Progressive Course of Précis Writing." London, Oxford University Press, 1913.

ROBINSON, JAMES HARVEY. "The Mind in the Making: The Relation of Intelligence to Social Reform." New York, Harper & Brothers, 1921.

ROBINSON, VIRGINIA P. "Analysis of Processes in the Records of Family Case Working Agencies," *Proceedings of the National Conference of Social Work*, 1921; also *The Family*, July, 1921.

ROSANOFF, AARON J. "Manual of Psychiatry," 5th edition. New York, Wily & Sons, 1920.

Ross, E. A. "Foundations of Sociology." New York, The Macmillan Company, 1905.

———. "Principles of Sociology." New York, The Century Company, 1921.

———. "Social Control: A Survey of the Foundations of Order." New York, The Macmillan Company, 1904.

Rossy, C. S. "Feeble-mindedness and Industrial Relations," *Mental Hygiene*, January, 1918.

Royce, Josiah. "Fugitive Essays." Cambridge, Harvard University Press, 1920.

———. "Studies of Good and Evil: A Series of Essays upon Problems of Philosophy and Life." New York, D. Appleton & Company, 1915.

Ryther, Margherita. "Place and Scope of Psychiatric Social Work in Mental Hygiene," *Mental Hygiene*, v. 3, pp. 636–645, October, 1919.

Ryther, Margherita, and Ordway, Mabel D. "Economic Efficiency of Epileptic Patients," *Journal of Nervous and Mental Diseases*, v. 47, No. 5, May, 1918.

Salmon, Thomas W. "Care and Treatment of Mental Diseases and War Neuroses (Shell-Shock) in the British Army." New York, National Committee for Mental Hygiene, 1917.

———. "Importance of Social Service in Connection with the State Hospitals for the Insane," *New York State Hospital Quarterly*, v. 2, pp. 175–181, February, 1917.

———. "Some New Problems for Psychiatric Research in Delinquency," *Mental Hygiene*, v. 4, pp. 29–42, January, 1920; also in *Journal of Criminal Law and Criminology*, v. 10, pp. 375-384, November, 1919.

Sartorio, Enrico C. "Social and Religious Life of Italians in America." Boston, Christopher Publishing House, 1918.

Sears, Amelia. "The Charity Visitor: A Handbook for Beginners," 3rd edition. Chicago, School of Civics and Philanthropy, 1918.

Shand, A. F. "The Foundations of Character." London, The Macmillan Company, 1914.

Sheffield, Ada E. "Report on a Study of Applications for Illegitimacy Cases." Boston, Bureau on Illegitimacy, 1920.

———. "The Social Case History: Its Construction and Contents." New York, Russell Sage Foundation, 1920.

Singer, H. D. "Function of the Social Worker in Relation to the State Physician," *Mental Hygiene*, v. 3, pp. 609–617, October, 1919.

Small, Albion W. "General Sociology." Chicago, University of Chicago Press, 1905.

SMITH, G. E., and PEAR, T. H. "Shell Shock and its Lessons."
New York, Longmans, Green & Company, 1917.

SOLOMON, HARRY C. "Social Workers for Mental Hygiene," *Modern Medicine*, v. 2, No. 6, pp. 465–466.

——. "What Shall Be the Attitude of the Public toward the Recovered Insane Patient," *Boston Medical and Surgical Journal*, v. 174, No. 16, April 13, 1916.

SOLOMON, HARRY C. and MAIDA H. "The Effects of Syphilis on the Families of Syphilitics Seen in the Late Stages," *Social Hygiene*, v. 6, pp. 469–487, October, 1920.

——. "The Family of the Neurosyphilitic," *Mental Hygiene*, v. 2, January, 1918.

——. "A Study of the Economic Status of Forty-One Paretic Patients and Their Families," *Mental Hygiene*, v. 5, pp. 556–565, July, 1921.

SOLOMON, HARRY C., and SOUTHARD, E. E. "Neurosyphilis: Modern Systematic Diagnosis and Treatment." Boston, W. M. Leonard, 1917.

SOLOMON, MAIDA H. "Social Work and Neurosyphilis," *Social Hygiene*, v. 6, pp. 93–104, January, 1920.

——. "The Social Worker's Approach to the Family of the Syphilitic," *Hospital Social Service*, v. 3, p. 442, 1921.

SOUTHARD, E. E. "Alienists and Psychiatrists: Notes on Divisions and Nomenclature of Mental Hygiene," *Mental Hygiene*, v. 1, pp. 567–571, 1917.

——. "Cross-sections of Mental Hygiene, 1844, 1869, 1894. Presidential Address at Annual Meeting of American Medico-Psychological Association, 1919," *American Journal of Insanity*, v. 76, pp. 91–111, 1919.

——. "Diagnosis per Exclusionem in Ordine: General and Psychiatric Remarks." Bulletin of Massachusetts Commission on Mental Diseases, v. 2, No. 3, pp. 90–122, 1918.

——. "The Empathic Index in the Diagnosis of Mental Diseases," *Journal of Abnormal Psychology*, v. 13, pp. 199–214, 1918.

——. "Feeble-mindedness as a Leading Social Problem," *Boston Medical and Surgical Journal*, v. 170, pp. 781–784, May 21, 1914.

——. "Functions of a Psychopathic Hospital," *Canadian Journal of Mental Hygiene*, v. 1, pp. 4–19, 1919.

——. "Individual versus the Family as a Unit of Interest in Social Work," *Mental Hygiene*, v. 3, pp. 436–444, 1919.

——. "A Key to the Practical Grouping of Mental Diseases." Bulletin of Massachusetts Commission on Mental Diseases, v. 2, No. 1, pp. 5–24, 1918.

SOUTHARD, E. E. "The Kingdom of Evils: Advantages of an Orderly Approach in Social Case Analysis," *Proceedings of National Conference of Social Work,* 1918.

———. "Mental Hygiene and Social Work: Notes on a Course in Social Psychiatry for Social Workers," *Mental Hygiene,* v. 2, pp. 388–406, July, 1918; also in Massachusetts Commission on Mental Diseases, Bulletin, v. 3, No. 2, pp. 52–70, April, 1919.

———. "The Modern Specialist in Unrest: A Place for the Psychiatrist in Industry," *Journal of Industrial Hygiene,* v. 2, pp. 10–19, May, 1920; also *Industrial Management,* June, 1920. Reprinted by Engineering Foundation, New York.

———. "Movement for a Mental Hygiene of Industry," *Mental Hygiene,* v. 4, pp. 43–64, January, 1920; also *Industrial Management,* February, 1920. Reprinted by Engineering Foundation, New York.

———. "The Psychopathic Hospital Idea," *Journal of American Medical Association,* v. 61, pp. 1972–1974, 1913.

———. "Range of the General Practitioner in Psychiatric Diagnosis," *Journal of American Medical Association,* v. 73, pp. 1253–1256, 1919.

———. "Shell-Shock and Other Neuropsychiatric Problems, Presented in Five Hundred and Eighty-nine Case Histories from the War Literature, 1914–1918." Boston, W. M. Leonard, 1920.

———. "Sigmund Freud, Pessimist," *Journal of Abnormal Psychology,* v. 14, pp. 197–216, 1919.

———. "Trade Unionism and Temperament: Notes upon the Psychiatric Point of View in Industry," *Mental Hygiene,* v. 4, pp. 281–300, April, 1920; also *Industrial Management,* April, 1920. Reprinted by Engineering Foundation, New York.

SOUTHARD, E. E., and SOLOMON, H. C. "Neurosyphilis: Modern Systematic Diagnosis and Treatment." Boston, W. M. Leonard, 1917.

SPAULDING, EDITH R. "Training of the Psychiatric Social Worker," *Mental Hygiene,* v. 3, pp. 420–426, July, 1919.

"Statistical Manual for the Use of Institutions for the Insane." Prepared by the Committee on Statistics of the American Medico-Psychological Association in Collaboration with the Bureau of Statistics of the National Committee for Mental Hygiene, New York, 1918.

STEARNS, A. WARREN. "The Classification of Industrial Applicants," *American Journal of Insanity,* v. 76, pp. 409–417, April, 1920.

———. "Classification of Naval Recruits," *California State Journal of Medicine,* v. 17, p. 110, April, 1919.

STEARNS, A. WARREN. "The History as a Means of Detecting the Undesirable Candidate for Enlistment, with Special Reference to Military Delinquents." U. S. Naval Medical Bulletin, v. 12, pp. 413–418, July, 1918.

——. "Importance of a History as a Means of Detecting Psychopathic Recruits," Military Surgeon, v. 43, pp. 652–661, December, 1918.

——. "Psychiatric Examination of Recruits," Journal of the American Medical Association, v. 70, pp. 229–231, January 26, 1918.

——. "Social Work and Industrial Hygiene," Journal of Industrial Hygiene, v. 2, pp. 20–21, May, 1920.

——. "Suicide in Massachusetts," Mental Hygiene, v. 5, pp. 752–777, October, 1921.

——. "Value of Out-Patient Work among the Insane," American Journal of Insanity, v. 74, pp. 595–602, April, 1918; also in Massa-chusetts Commission on Mental Diseases. Bulletin, v. 3, No. 1, pp. 74–78, January, 1919.

STRECKER, E. A. "Bureau for Social Research," The Family, v. 2, pp. 177–179, December, 1921.

TAFT, JESSIE. "Mental Pitfalls in Industry and How to Avoid Them." Medicine and Surgery, v. 1, pp. 678–685, September, 1917.

——. "Problems of Social Case Work with Children," Mental Hygiene, v. 4, pp. 537–549, July, 1920.

——. "Qualifications of the Psychiatric Social Worker," Proceedings of the National Conference of Social Work, 1919; also Mental Hygiene, v. 3, pp. 427–435, July, 1919.

——. "What the Social Worker Learns from the Psychiatrist about her Problem Children," Modern Medicine, v. 1, pp. 240–245, July, 1919.

TARDE, GABRIEL. "Social Laws." Translated from the French by Howard C. Warren, with a preface by James Mark Baldwin. New York, The Macmillan Company, 1899.

TAUSSIG, F. W. "Inventors and Money-Makers: Lectures on Some Relations between Economics and Psychology." New York, The Macmillan Company, 1915.

TEAD, ORDWAY. "Development of the Guild Idea," Intercollegiate Socialist, April–May, 1918, pp. 16–19.

——. "Instincts in Industry: A Study of Working-Class Psychology." Boston, Houghton, Mifflin Company, 1918.

TERMAN, L. M. "The Hygiene of the School Child." Boston, Houghton, Mifflin Company, 1914.

TIMME, WALTER. "Indications for Internal Gland Therapy," New York Medical Journal, February 7, 1920.

TODD, Arthur J. "The Scientific Spirit and Social Work." New York, The Macmillan Company, 1919.

"Training School of Psychiatric Social Work at Smith College," by various authors, *Mental Hygiene*, v. 2, pp. 582–594, October, 1918.

TREDGOLD, A. F. "Mental Deficiency: Amentia," 2nd edition. New York, Wood & Company, 1914.

TROTTER, WILLIAM. "Instincts of the Herd in Peace and War." New York, The Macmillan Company, 1917.

TUFTS, JAMES H., and DEWEY, JOHN. "Ethics." New York, Henry Holt & Company, 1908.

VALENTINE, R. G. "Human Element in Production," *American Journal of Sociology*, v. 22, pp. 477–488, January, 1917.

VAN KLEECK, MARY. "Case Work and Social Reform," *Annals of the American Academy of Political and Social Science*, v. 77, pp. 9–12, May, 1918.

VAN KLEECK, MARY, and TAYLOR, G. R. "The Professional Organization of Social Work," *Annals of American Academy of Political and Social Science*, May, 1922.

VEBLEN, THORSTEIN. "Instinct of Workmanship, and the State of the Industrial Arts." New York, The Macmillan Company, 1914.

"The Visiting Teacher in the United States." A Survey by the National Association of Visiting Teachers. New York, Public Education Association, June, 1921.

WALLAS, GRAHAM. "The Great Society: A Psychological Analysis." New York, The Macmillan Company, 1914.

———. "Human Nature in Politics." Boston, Houghton, Mifflin Company, 1916.

WALLERSTEIN, HELEN C. "The Functional Relations of Fifteen Case Working Agencies as Shown by a Study of 421 Individual Families and The Report of the Philadelphia Intake Committee." Philadelphia, Bureau for Social Research, Seybert Institution, 1919.

WELLS, F. L. "Mental Adjustments." New York, D. Appleton & Company, 1917.

———. "The Status of Clinical Psychology," *Mental Hygiene*, v. 6, pp. 11–22, January, 1922.

WHITE, WILLIAM A. "Foundations of Psychiatry." New York and Washington, Nervous and Mental Disease Publishing Company, 1921.

———. "Mechanisms of Character Formation: An Introduction to Psychoanalysis." New York, The Macmillan Company, 1916.

———. "The Mental Hygiene of Childhood." Boston, Little, Brown & Company, 1919.

698   BIBLIOGRAPHY

WHITE, WILLIAM A. "Outlines of Psychiatry," 7th edition. Washington, Nervous and Mental Disease Publishing Company, 1919.

WHITE, WILLIAM A., and JELLIFFE, S. E. "Diseases of the Nervous System: A Text-book of Neurology and Psychiatry," 2nd edition. Philadelphia, Lea and Febiger, 1917.

WILLIAMS, FRANKWOOD E. "Legislation for the Insane in Massachusetts with Particular Reference to the Voluntary and Temporary Care Laws," *Boston Medical and Surgical Journal*, v. 173, pp. 723–734, November 11, 1915.

———. "Mental Hygiene and the College Student," *Mental Hygiene*, v. 5, pp. 283–301, April, 1921.

———. "The State Hospital in Relation to Public Health," *Mental Hygiene*, v. 4, pp. 885–896, October, 1920.

———. "Treatment of Mental Patients in the General Hospitals of the United States Army," *Proceedings of the American Medico-Psychological Association*, pp. 271–286, June, 1919.

WILLIAMS, FRANKWOOD E., and BROWN, M. W. "Neuropsychiatry and the War: A Bibliography with Abstracts." New York, National Committee for Mental Hygiene, 1918.

WOLF, ROBERT B. "Individuality: The Key to Conscious Life Purpose," *Survey*, v. 41, pp. 620–625, February 1, 1919.

———. "Making Men Like Their Jobs," System, v. 35, pp. 34–38, 222–226, January and February, 1919.

WORCH, MARGARET. "Psychiatric Social Work in a Red Cross Chapter," *Mental Hygiene*, v. 6, No. 2, April, 1922.

YERKES, ROBERT M. "How May We Discover Children Who Need Special Care?" *Mental Hygiene*, v. 1, pp. 252–259, April, 1917.

YERKES, ROBERT M., and others. "A Point Scale for Measuring Mental Ability." Baltimore, Warwick and York, Incorporated, 1915.

INDEX

MENTAL ILLNESS AND SOCIAL POLICY
THE AMERICAN EXPERIENCE

AN ARNO PRESS COLLECTION

Barr, Martin W. Mental Defectives: Their History, Treatment and Training. 1904.

The Beginnings of American Psychiatric Thought and Practice: Five Accounts, 1811-1830. 1973

The Beginnings of Mental Hygiene in America: Three Selected Essays, 1833-1850. 1973

Briggs, L. Vernon, et al. History of the Psychopathic Hospital, Boston, Massachusetts. 1922

Briggs, L. Vernon. Occupation as a Substitute for Restraint in the Treatment of the Mentally Ill. 1923

Brigham, Amariah. An Inquiry Concerning the Diseases and Functions of the Brain, the Spinal Cord, and the Nerves. 1840

Brigham, Amariah. Observations on the Influence of Religion upon the Health and Physical Welfare of Mankind. 1835

Brill, A. A. Fundamental Conceptions of Psychoanalysis. 1921

Bucknill, John Charles. Notes on Asylums for the Insane in America. 1876

Conolly, John. The Treatment of the Insane Without Mechanical Restraints. 1856

Coriat, Isador H. What is Psychoanalysis? 1917

Deutsch, Albert. The Shame of the States. 1948

Dewey, Richard. Recollections of Richard Dewey: Pioneer in American Psychiatry. 1936

Earle, Pliny. Memoirs of Pliny Earle, M. D. with Extracts from his Diary and Letters (1830-1892) and Selections from his Professional Writings (1839-1891). 1898

Galt, John M. The Treatment of Insanity. 1846

Goddard, Henry Herbert. Feeble-mindedness: Its Causes and Consequences. 1926

Hammond, William A. A Treatise on Insanity in Its Medical Relations. 1883

Hazard, Thomas R. Report on the Poor and Insane in Rhode-Island. 1851

Hurd, Henry M., editor. The Institutional Care of the Insane in the United States and Canada. 1916/1917. Four volumes.

Kirkbride, Thomas S. On the Construction, Organization, and General Arrangements of Hospitals for the Insane. 1880

Meyer, Adolf. The Commonsense Psychiatry of Dr. Adolf Meyer: Fifty-two Selected Papers. 1948

Mitchell, S. Weir. Wear and Tear, or Hints for the Overworked. 1887

Morton, Thomas G. The History of the Pennsylvania Hospital, 1751-1895. 1895

Ordronaux, John. Jurisprudence in Medicine in Relation to the Law. 1869

The Origins of the State Mental Hospital in America: Six Documentary Studies, 1837-1856. 1973

Packard, Mrs. E. P. W. Modern Persecution, or Insane Asylums Unveiled, As Demonstrated by the Report of the Investigating Committee of the Legislature of Illinois. 1875. Two volumes in one

Prichard, James C. A Treatise on Insanity and Other Disorders Affecting the Mind. 1837

Prince, Morton. The Unconscious: The Fundamentals of Human Personality Normal and Abnormal. 1921

Putnam, James Jackson. Human Motives. 1915

Russell, William Logie. The New York Hospital: A History of the Psychiatric Service, 1771-1936. 1945

Sidis, Boris. The Psychology of Suggestion: A Research into the Subconscious Nature of Man and Society. 1899

Southard, Elmer E. Shell-Shock and Other Neuropsychiatric Problems Presented in Five Hundred and Eighty-Nine Case Histories from the War Literature, 1914-1918. 1919

Southard, E[lmer] E. and Mary C. Jarrett. The Kingdom of Evils. 1922

Southard, E[lmer] E. and H[arry] C. Solomon. Neurosyphilis: Modern Systematic Diagnosis and Treatment Presented in One Hundred and Thirty-seven Case Histories. 1917

Spitzka, E[dward] C. Insanity: Its Classification, Diagnosis and Treatment. 1887

Supreme Court Holding a Criminal Term, No. 14056. The United States vs. Charles J. Guiteau. 1881/1882. Two volumes

Trezevant, Daniel H. Letters to his Excellency Governor Manning on the Lunatic Asylum. 1854

Tuke, D[aniel] Hack. The Insane in the United States and Canada. 1885

Upham, Thomas C. Outlines of Imperfect and Disordered Mental Action. 1868

White, William A[lanson]. Twentieth Century Psychiatry: Its Contribution to Man's Knowledge of Himself. 1936

Willard, Sylvester D. Report on the Condition of the Insane Poor in the County Poor Houses of New York. 1865